Cancer Drug Discovery and Development

Series editor:

Beverly A. Teicher

Bethesda, MD, USA

The Cancer Drug Discovery and Development series (Beverly A Teicher, series editor) is the definitive book series in cancer research and oncology, providing comprehensive coverage of specific topics and the field. Volumes cover the process of drug discovery, preclinical models in cancer research, specific drug target groups and experimental and approved therapeutic agents. The volumes are current and timely, anticipating areas where experimental agents are reaching FDA approval. Each volume is edited by an expert in the field covered and chapters are authored by renowned scientists and physicians in their fields of interest.

More information about this series at http://www.springer.com/series/7625

Xiaoting Zhang
Editor

Estrogen Receptor and Breast Cancer

Celebrating the 60th Anniversary
of the Discovery of ER

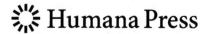 Humana Press

Editor
Xiaoting Zhang
Department of Cancer Biology
Vontz Center for Molecular Studies
University of Cincinnati College of Medicine
Cincinnati, OH, USA

ISSN 2196-9906   ISSN 2196-9914   (electronic)
Cancer Drug Discovery and Development
ISBN 978-3-030-07593-4   ISBN 978-3-319-99350-8   (eBook)
https://doi.org/10.1007/978-3-319-99350-8

This Humana Press imprint is published by the registered company Springer Nature Switzerland AG
The registered company address is: Gewerbestrasse 11, 6330 Cham, Switzerland

Preface

A lady with growth neoplastic
Thought castration was just a bit drastic.
She preferred that her ill could be cured with a pill.
Today it's no longer fantastic.

—Elwood V. Jensen, Ph.D. (1920–2012)

Breast cancer is one of the most frequent cancers and a leading cause of death for women with an estimated one in eight women in the USA diagnosed in their lifetime and more than 1.7 million new cases worldwide each year. Estrogen receptor (ER) is the key functional mediator of estrogen and plays prominent roles in breast cancer with about 75% of all breast cancer diagnosed as ER positive breast cancer. The discovery of ER by Dr. Elwood Jensen 60 years ago in 1958 through his "alternative thinking approach" mirrored his successful climbing of the mountain Matterhorn in the Swiss Alps. His enchantment of implementing unconventional approaches has not only led to the birth of a whole new nuclear receptor research field but also made a rapid, direct, and long-lasting impact on the diagnosis, treatment, and prevention of breast cancer. As appropriately illustrated in the limerick excerpt above by Dr. Jensen himself and further noted by the Lasker Foundation: "The work transformed the treatment of breast cancer patients and saves or prolongs more than a 100,000 lives annually." Since this landmark discovery, tremendous progress has been made in our understanding of the molecular functions of ER and in the development of targeted therapies against ER pathways for breast cancer treatment. However, there is currently no book available addressing these discoveries and the recent advancements in a historical and systematic fashion.

I appreciate the kind and timely invitation from Mr. William Helms, Associate Editor of Cancer Research, and Dr. Beverly Teicher for the task of spearheading this book. My goal for the book is to celebrate the 60th anniversary of the discovery of ER and the great achievements that have followed by providing comprehensive and most up-to-date information on the history and recent advancement of the field spanning from basic research to clinical practice. The chapters are contributed by world-renowned leaders in the field and include the history behind the discovery of

ER (Khan); physiological and pathological roles of ER (Korach); recent advancement of our understanding of ER-mediated gene transcription and cistrome (Zhang), Cryo-EM structural insights into ER coactivators (O'Malley), ER transcriptome (Kraus) and its regulation of newly classified noncoding RNAs in breast cancer (Nephew); personal account of the development of Tamoxifen as the first targeted cancer therapy and new generation of antiestrogens for breast cancer treatment (Jordan) and their current practice in clinics (Ellis); structural basis of ER and anti-estrogen actions (Burris); molecular insights into endocrine resistance (Schiff and Osborne); the role of ER-beta (Thomas and Gustafsson) and environmental estrogens, especially Bisphenol A (Ben-Jonathan), in breast cancer; and emerging state-of-the-art therapeutic regimens and approaches to overcome treatment resistance (Zhang).

I would like to sincerely thank all of the authors for their time, commitment, and highly enthusiastic devotion to this important book despite the short notice, their very busy schedules, and many administrative duties. With the outstanding work done by all of the contributors, I am happy to say that collectively we have fully accomplished our original goal of editing this book. We hope it will provide undergraduate and graduate students, basic scientists, clinical cancer researchers, residents, fellows, as well as clinicians, oncology educators, and the general public with a thorough and authoritative review of the key topics in this vital field of both basic and clinical significance. We would like to hear your feedback and look forward to incorporating those in our next edition of the book with an update of the new and most exciting developments in the field.

The past 60 years' work on estrogen receptor has been extraordinary in not only providing basic insights into estrogen receptor functions but also developing highly effective novel diagnostic and therapeutic approaches for the treatment of this devastating disease. With rapid technological advancement in emerging areas such as genomic, single cell and single molecule studies, we will be able to better understand estrogen receptor functions, breast cancer therapeutic resistance mechanisms, tumor heterogeneity, and interactions with the tumor microenvironment and immune system at both the individual and population levels. Combining the current development of creative targeted drug delivery systems and innovative therapeutic approaches, the knowledge gained will likely be translated into clinics more quickly and smoothly to further benefit patient care as well. We fully expect the next 60 years to be just as exciting and groundbreaking. Stay tuned!

Cincinnati, OH, USA   Xiaoting Zhang

Contents

Contributors

Balkees Abderrahman Department of Breast Medical Oncology, University of Texas, MD Anderson Cancer Center, Houston, TX, USA

Yukitomo Arao Receptor Biology Section, Reproductive and Developmental Biology Laboratory, National Institute Environmental Health Sciences, National Institutes of Health, Durham, NC, USA

Nira Ben-Jonathan Department of Cancer Biology, University of Cincinnati, Cincinnati, OH, USA

Gregory Bick Department of Cancer Biology, University of Cincinnati College of Medicine, Cincinnati, OH, USA

Thomas P. Burris Center for Clinical Pharmacology, Washington University School of Medicine and St. Louis College of Pharmacy, St. Louis, MO, USA

Mahmoud Charif Division of Hematology and Oncology, Department of Internal Medicine, University of Cincinnati College of Medicine, Cincinnati, OH, USA

Carmine De Angelis Lester and Sue Smith Breast Center, Baylor College of Medicine, Houston, TX, USA

Dan L. Duncan Comprehensive Cancer Center, Baylor College of Medicine, Houston, TX, USA

Ian Mitchelle S. de Vera Department of Pharmacology and Physiology, Saint Louis University School of Medicine, St. Louis, MO, USA

Matthew J. Ellis Lester and Sue Smith Breast Center, Baylor College of Medicine, Houston, TX, USA

Xiaoyong Fu Lester and Sue Smith Breast Center, Baylor College of Medicine, Houston, TX, USA

Dan L. Duncan Comprehensive Cancer Center, Baylor College of Medicine, Houston, TX, USA

Department of Molecular and Cellular Biology, Baylor College of Medicine, Houston, TX, USA

Marleny Garcia Receptor Biology Section, Reproductive and Developmental Biology Laboratory, National Institute Environmental Health Sciences, National Institutes of Health, Durham, NC, USA

Jan-Åke Gustafsson Department of Biology and Biochemistry, Center for Nuclear Receptors and Cell Signaling, University of Houston, Houston, TX, USA

Katherine J. Hamilton Receptor Biology Section, Reproductive and Developmental Biology Laboratory, National Institute Environmental Health Sciences, National Institutes of Health, Durham, NC, USA

Airi Han Lester and Sue Smith Breast Center, Baylor College of Medicine, Houston, TX, USA

Department of Surgery, Yonsei University Wonju College of Medicine, Wonju, South Korea

Sylvia C. Hewitt Receptor Biology Section, Reproductive and Developmental Biology Laboratory, National Institute Environmental Health Sciences, National Institutes of Health, Durham, NC, USA

V. Craig Jordan Department of Breast Medical Oncology, University of Texas, MD Anderson Cancer Center, Houston, TX, USA

Sohaib Khan Department of Cancer Biology, University of Cincinnati College of Medicine, Cincinnati, OH, USA

Kenneth S. Korach Receptor Biology Section, Reproductive and Developmental Biology Laboratory, National Institute Environmental Health Sciences, National Institutes of Health, Durham, NC, USA

W. Lee Kraus Laboratory of Signaling and Gene Regulation, Cecil H. and Ida Green Center for Reproductive Biology Sciences, University of Texas Southwestern Medical Center, Dallas, TX, USA

Division of Basic Research, Department of Obstetrics and Gynecology, University of Texas Southwestern Medical Center, Dallas, TX, USA

Marissa Leonard Department of Cancer Biology, University of Cincinnati College of Medicine, Cincinnati, OH, USA

Graduate Program in Cancer and Cell Biology, University of Cincinnati College of Medicine, Cincinnati, OH, USA

Yin Li Receptor Biology Section, Reproductive and Developmental Biology Laboratory, National Institute Environmental Health Sciences, National Institutes of Health, Durham, NC, USA

Elyse E. Lower Division of Hematology and Oncology, Department of Internal Medicine, University of Cincinnati College of Medicine, Cincinnati, OH, USA

Emilie Mathura Receptor Biology Section, Reproductive and Developmental Biology Laboratory, National Institute Environmental Health Sciences, National Institutes of Health, Durham, NC, USA

Ryoichi Matsunuma Lester and Sue Smith Breast Center, Baylor College of Medicine, Houston, TX, USA

First Department of Surgery, Hamamatsu University School of Medicine, Hamamatsu, Shizuoka, Japan

Hamamatsu Oncology Center, Hamamatsu, Shizuoka, Japan

Kenneth P. Nephew Molecular and Cellular Biochemistry Department, Indiana University, Bloomington, IN, USA

Medical Sciences Program, Indiana University School of Medicine, Bloomington, IN, USA

Department of Cellular and Integrative Physiology and Department of Obstetrics and Gynecology, Indiana University School of Medicine, Indianapolis, IN, USA

Bert W. O'Malley Department of Molecular and Cellular Biology, Baylor College of Medicine, Houston, TX, USA

C. Kent Osborne Lester and Sue Smith Breast Center, Baylor College of Medicine, Houston, TX, USA

Dan L. Duncan Comprehensive Cancer Center, Baylor College of Medicine, Houston, TX, USA

Department of Molecular and Cellular Biology, Baylor College of Medicine, Houston, TX, USA

Department of Medicine, Baylor College of Medicine, Houston, TX, USA

Nicholas Pulliam Molecular and Cellular Biochemistry Department, Indiana University, Bloomington, IN, USA

Medical Sciences Program, Indiana University School of Medicine, Bloomington, IN, USA

J. Tyler Ramsey Receptor Biology Section, Reproductive and Developmental Biology Laboratory, National Institute Environmental Health Sciences, National Institutes of Health, Durham, NC, USA

Tomas Reinert Programa de Pós-Graduação em Ciências Médicas, Universidade Federal do Rio Grande do Sul, Porto Alegre, Brazil

Rachel Schiff Lester and Sue Smith Breast Center, Baylor College of Medicine, Houston, TX, USA

Dan L. Duncan Comprehensive Cancer Center, Baylor College of Medicine, Houston, TX, USA

Department of Molecular and Cellular Biology, Baylor College of Medicine, Houston, TX, USA

Department of Medicine, Baylor College of Medicine, Houston, TX, USA

Jessica Tang Medical Sciences Program, Indiana University School of Medicine, Bloomington, IN, USA

Juan Tan Department of Cancer Biology, University of Cincinnati College of Medicine, Cincinnati, OH, USA

Christoforos Thomas Department of Biology and Biochemistry, Center for Nuclear Receptors and Cell Signaling, University of Houston, Houston, TX, USA

Yasmin M. Vasquez Laboratory of Signaling and Gene Regulation, Cecil H. and Ida Green Center for Reproductive Biology Sciences, University of Texas Southwestern Medical Center, Dallas, TX, USA

Division of Basic Research, Department of Obstetrics and Gynecology, University of Texas Southwestern Medical Center, Dallas, TX, USA

Jamunarani Veeraraghavan Lester and Sue Smith Breast Center, Baylor College of Medicine, Houston, TX, USA

Dan L. Duncan Comprehensive Cancer Center, Baylor College of Medicine, Houston, TX, USA

Zhao Wang Verna and Marrs McLean Department of Biochemistry and Molecular Biology, Baylor College of Medicine, Houston, TX, USA

Udayanga S. Wanninayake Department of Pharmacology and Physiology, Saint Louis University School of Medicine, St. Louis, MO, USA

Yongguang Yang Department of Cancer Biology, University of Cincinnati College of Medicine, Cincinnati, OH, USA

Ping Yi Department of Molecular and Cellular Biology, Baylor College of Medicine, Houston, TX, USA

Xiaoting Zhang Department of Cancer Biology, Vontz Center for Molecular Studies, University of Cincinnati College of Medicine, Cincinnati, OH, USA

Graduate Program in Cancer and Cell Biology, University of Cincinnati College of Medicine, Cincinnati, OH, USA

Dan Zhao Department of Cancer Biology, University of Cincinnati College of Medicine, Cincinnati, OH, USA

Estrogen Receptor and Breast Cancer: A Historical Perspective

Sohaib Khan

Abstract Sir George Beatson proposed a connection between breast cancer and ovary more than a century ago. It took several decades to the discovery of hormone estrogen and a few more decades when Elwood Jensen announced the discovery of estrogen receptor. His work led to our understanding of how hormones control target gene transcription via their receptors. Several laboratories made major contributions toward our understanding of hormone action. To date, 49 nuclear hormone receptors have been identified that form the nuclear receptor family and carry out a myriad of metabolic functions. Most notably, they are targets for therapy. Jensen and colleagues made ER antibodies that were used to develop ER assay kits in breast cancer specimens. ER contents in breast cancer patients proved to be useful in deciding mode of treatment. Soon after the discovery of ER, the antiestrogen, tamoxifen, which was originally developed as a female contraceptive, was repurposed for breast cancer management, and later it was used as a prophylactic in those women who were in high risk for breast cancer.

Keywords Hormones · Estrogen · Elwood Jensen · Estrogen receptor · Breast cancer · ER assay kits · Antiestrogen · Transcription factor and cofactors

Elwood Jensen's discovery of the estrogen receptor (ER) made a paradigm shift toward our understanding of steroid hormone action. It launched the field of nuclear receptors, which has profoundly impacted the discipline of molecular medicine. A perfect example of "Bench to Bedside" translational research, his work has saved thousands of lives of breast cancer patients. Moreover, his work has led to the understanding of how ligand-dependent transcription factors mediate the cell-type-specific gene expression in amplifying hormonal actions. It is fitting that many of his friends and colleagues, who are leaders in the field, have

S. Khan (✉)
Department of Cancer Biology, University of Cincinnati College of Medicine, Cincinnati, OH, USA
e-mail: Sohaib.Khan@UC.edu

© Springer Nature Switzerland AG 2019
X. Zhang (ed.), *Estrogen Receptor and Breast Cancer*, Cancer Drug Discovery and Development, https://doi.org/10.1007/978-3-319-99350-8_1

contributed chapters in this book. This is a testament that Elwood Jensen was regarded in high esteem among scientific contributions and their impact on the field with a historical perspective.

1   The Elusive Mechanism of Estrogen Action

Adolf Butenandt and Edward Doisy independently purified estrogen in 1929. Over the following decades, observations accumulated that tiny amount of the hormone could cause profound target tissue growth (e.g., uterus). However, the mechanism of its action remained elusive. In the 1950s, being the era of enzymology, research community assumed that enzymes mediate the hormone-dependent tissue growth. The popular belief was that the mechanism of estrogen action entailed trans-hydrogenation in which the 17-hydroxyl group of estradiol is oxidized by one coenzyme and the resulting estrone reduced by another, thus using NADH to produce NADPH [1]. However, there was one caveat with this thought process: such a mechanism would not explain the uterotropic actions of diethylstilbestrol (DES), a synthetic estrogen that lacks any aliphatic hydroxyl group and thus could not undergo that reversible oxidation/reduction [1].

2   Fellowship in Zurich and the Matterhorn Experience

While doing a steroid chemistry fellowship in Zurich with the Nobel Laureate, Professor Leopold Ruzicka, Elwood was fascinated by the natural beauty of the surrounding areas. He was particularly attracted toward the towering Matterhorn. Although never climbed a mountain, physically, he was in good condition from his collegiate sports activities (Boxing/Judo/Tennis) and decided to scale the Matterhorn. He teamed up with a lab colleague with mountaineering experience and a guide to climb the Matterhorn (Fig. 1) from an alternate route (Swiss side), rather than from the seemingly simple but more hazardous Italian side. The latter approach was used by Edward Whymper to scale the Matterhorn peak but at the cost of many unsuccessful attempts and a few human lives. Matterhorn was the last European mountain to be climbed. The successful Matterhorn experience by a novice like Elwood Jensen instilled a lifelong passion of applying "alternative strategy" approaches in his research pursuits [1].

3   Faculty Position at the University of Chicago: From Chemist to Endocrinologist

When Charles Huggins, who won the Nobel Prize for his work on prostate cancer, recruited Elwood at the University of Chicago, a vexing question in the endocrinology field was "how does tiny amount of estrogen induce massive uterine

Fig. 1 At the base of the Matterhorn with his first wife Mary Jensen

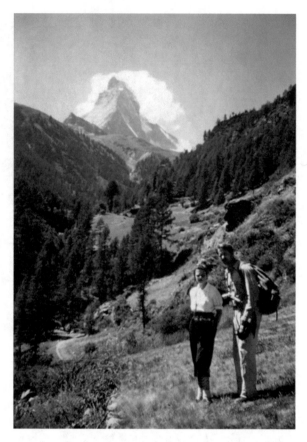

growth" [1]? Elwood Jensen, himself a chemist, and his postdoctoral fellow, Herbert Jacobson, who earned his PhD degree with the famous chemist Morris Kharasch at the University of Chicago, embarked upon solving an agelong endocrinology problem: what is the mechanism of estrogen action? Elwood invoked the "alternative approach" and decided to understand the fate of the hormone itself rather than what hormone does to the tissue—the prevailing approach in the field at the time. Because estrogens are active at such low doses (in nanomolar range), they planned to label the hormone with tritium and follow the radioactivity in various rat tissues. However, their experimental strategy entailed using the hormone radioactively labeled to prohibitively high specific activity, normally not permitted by the university regulatory authorities. But as luck would have it, the "Fermi Lab"—an epicenter of the Second World War "Atomic Bomb Project"—was located in the nearby Argonne National Laboratory and was made accessible to the Jensen team [1]. They built an apparatus, tritiumator (Fig. 2), to measure the uptake of tritium by a catalytic reduction of a double bond in the precursor. They reasoned that one could radiolabel the sixth and seventh position of the hormone with carrier-free tritium gas. Thus, using the Fermi Lab facilities to handle carrier-free tritium (60 Ci/mmole), they succeeded in labeling high specific activity estradiol. When they injected the tritiated estradiol to immature

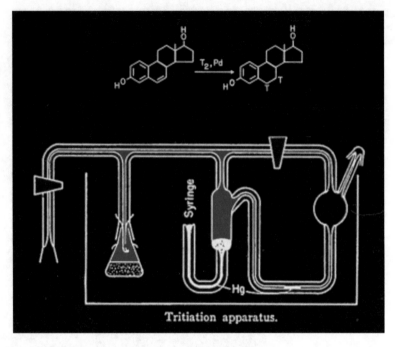

Fig. 2 Tritiation apparatus designed by Jensen and Jacobson

rats or to castrated rats, to their surprise, they found that the hormone remained biochemically unchanged and the uterus showed the usual massive growth. Moreover, when they examined various rat tissues for the uptake of radioactive estradiol (Fig. 3), they found uptake and retention was 100-fold higher in uterus and vagina than in nonreproductive tissue such as blood [1, 2]. Some skeptics raised the concern that estrogen might have undergone oxidoreduction of its 17-beta hydroxyl group such that the hydrogen atom lost during oxidation is not the same one that replaces it during reduction. Jensen and colleagues addressed this by injecting a mixture of 6,7 tritium-labeled estrogen plus 17-tritium-labeled estrogen in their rat model and clearly demonstrated that there was no loss of tritium from position 17 of estrogen during the hormone-induced uterotropic growth [1].

4   Birth of the Nuclear Receptor Family

When Elwood announced his groundbreaking findings at the International Congress in Vienna, five people came to listen to him—three of whom were speakers. Whereas, in a concurrent plenary session, hundreds went to hear the

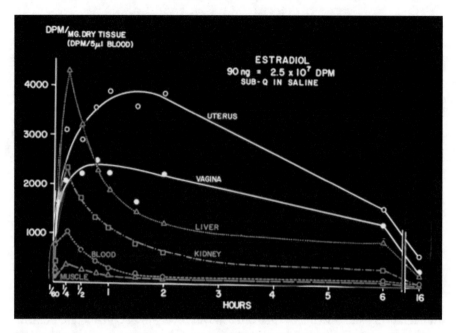

Fig. 3 Selective uptake and retention of tritiated estradiol by reproductive tissues (uterus and vagina)

now debunked enzymatic theories of estrogen action! The "factor" that Jensen initially termed "estrophilin" is now known as "estrogen receptor" (ER). This momentous discovery shifted attention away from the involvement of enzymes in the mechanism of hormone action. Subsequently, Elwood's contemporary, Jack Gorski at University of Illinois at Urbana/Champaign used state-of-the-art sedimentation gradient procedures to isolate and characterize a macromolecular component, which possessed the attributes of a specific receptor for estrogens [3]. The sedimentation density gradient would go on to play a critical role in the Jensen laboratory in research related to ER. These findings stimulated the search for other hormone receptors. The pioneering work by John Baxter, Pierre Chambon, Ron Evans, Jan-Ake Gustafsson, Bert O'Malley, and Keith Yamamoto led to the discoveries of the glucocorticoid receptor, progesterone receptor, retinoic acid receptor, and orphan receptors. In a remarkably short span of time, the 49 nuclear receptors described to date have become a family—"Nuclear Receptor Family" [4]. At the 2004 Lasker Award ceremony, Nobel Laureate, Joseph Goldstein, paid tribute to the discovery and called Elwood Jensen the patriarch and estrogen receptor the matriarch of the family [5]. The Lasker Foundation recognized these discoveries with Lasker Awards to Drs. Jensen, Chambon, and Evans; many in the field believe that it is deserving of recognition by the Nobel Committee as well because of its significant basic science and clinical impacts.

5 Estrogen Receptor and RNA Synthesis

After distinguishing two forms of the receptor [cytoplasmic and nuclear], Elwood Jensen, as well as Jack Gorski [3, 6], showed that the hormone-receptor complex becomes tightly bound in the nucleus and enhances RNA synthesis (transcription) in nuclei specifically isolated from hormone-dependent tissues [7]. Shortly thereafter, Bert O'Malley's group used estrogen-stimulated chicken oviduct system and published landmark papers not only describing the receptor for progesterone but also showing that it also stimulated transcription of specific mRNAs [8, 9]. This phenomenon of hormone-induced receptor activation has since proved to be a key step in the actions of various classes of steroid hormones, and it identified a definitive biochemical role for the steroid.

6 Estrogen Receptor Domain Structure and Ligand-Dependent Receptor Dimerization

In a relatively short period of time after the discovery of ER, many labs contributed toward identifying the domain structures of the receptor protein and establishing that indeed the family of steroid receptors shares several common features in their domain structures, enabling them to utilize a similar mode of action. Based on sequence homology and other criteria, the estrogen receptor protein can be divided into six functionally and physically independent domains (A–F). These domains are required for DNA binding (region C), nuclear localization (region D), and steroid binding (region E). The ER has two well-characterized transcriptional activation functions, which is located in the N-terminal A/B region and AF2 that is located in region E and whose activity is ligand dependent. The ER has been shown to form stable homodimers in solution [10], and several studies have provided evidence that a number of nuclear receptors including ER bind to their response elements as dimers [10–13]. However, Gorski et al. proposed a model where the ER protein bound to an ERE either as a monomer or with a heterodimeric partner [14, 15]. Most of the data for and against ER dimerization used in vitro experimental procedures such as gel mobility shift assays or complex assays requiring ER to bind DNA. It remained unclear whether estrogen was required [10] or not required [10–12] for high affinity ER/ERE interaction. More importantly, it remained unclear if the ER could form a dimer in vivo. Wang et al. approached this dilemma by using the yeast two-hybrid system, which is independent of the ER/ERE interaction, and showed that ER protein dimerization in vivo is ligand dependent [16].

7 Estrogen Receptor-Interacting Protein and Cloning of SRC-1

It was generally believed that accessory factors mediate hormone-dependent ER function in the nucleus, but their identity was elusive. Myles Brown used Southwestern blot analysis that indeed an ER coactivator protein, which he termed ER-associated protein (ERAP), exists in estrogen-sensitive cells [17] and acts as coactivator. A major advancement in the field occurred when O'Malley's group used the yeast two-hybrid system, using PR LBD as a bait, for the cloning of steroid receptor coactivator-1 (SRC-1). This discovery that has made a paradigm shift in our understanding of how ligand-induced activation of steroid receptors culminates into the assembly of multi-protein complexes on the target gene promoters and transcribe specific mRNAs. A majority of these proteins harbor enzymatic activities for chromatin modification. Several contributors in this book describe current status of their research that involves coactivators/corepressors. Such an intricate mechanism of steroid hormone action has broadened the scope of exploring new approaches to identify novel therapeutic approaches. One great example is that of AIB1/SRC3, which has been identified as an oncogene in breast cancer and is being explored for therapeutic values.

8 An Alternative Method to Detect Immune Complex Leads to the Production of Antibodies to Estrogen Receptor

Another major contribution of Elwood and his postdoctoral fellow, Geoffrey Greene, was the successful purification of the estrogen receptor, an achievement attributed to the first use of steroid affinity chromatography. Greene and Jensen then used the purified receptor to obtain monoclonal as well as polyclonal antibodies to ER. These were highly significant developments in the field, because, in collaboration with Pierre Chambon, they led to the cloning and structural determination of the cDNA for estrogen receptor and prompting an exponential increase in our understanding of how steroid receptors function as transcription factors [18]. Elwood credits the success in preparing the ER antibodies to the use of "alternative approach" to detect the immune complex of antigen and antibody. After many laboratories tried without success to prepare antibodies against estrogen or other steroid receptors, it had been considered that these proteins might be non-immunogenic "because they are so ubiquitous." Greene and Jensen suspected that antibodies to the estrogen receptor form soluble immune complexes, not detectable by the conventional immunoprecipitation techniques [19, 20].

They again invoked the "alternative approach" and used sucrose gradient sedimentation to identify ER antibodies by their ability to shift the sedimentation peak of the receptor with tritiated estradiol as a marker [21]. They succeeded in producing the first polyclonal as well as monoclonal antibodies to any steroid receptor.

9 Estrogen Signaling and Breast Cancer

More than 100 years ago, Sir George Beatson, a Scottish surgeon, noticed that severity of breast cancer strictly correlated with the menstrual cycle in his patients [1]. He reasoned that the culprit is in the ovary and decided to remove the ovary to manage his breast cancer patients. He successfully tried oophorectomy to manage advanced breast cancer, although not knowing the reason for his successful approach. Around late 1940s, the use of cortisol replacement had made it feasible to remove adrenal gland. Although known for his pioneering contributions with antiandrogenic treatment of prostate cancer for which he was awarded the Nobel Prize, Elwood's mentor, Dr. Charles Huggins at the University of Chicago, also revolutionized adrenalectomy to manage breast cancer in postmenopausal women [1]. However, there were no means to predict which breast cancer patients would respond. Jensen and colleagues exploited their success with the estrogen receptor research and described two types of breast cancers: ER-positive and ER-negative. His group later refined this finding, showing that estrogen receptor content of excised breast cancer tissue provides an indication of whether or not the tumor is hormone-dependent type, likely to be responsive to endocrine manipulation. Such predictive test had been the goal in the breast cancer field ever since the value of hormone therapy was recognized. Measurement of estrogen receptor in breast cancer specimens is now used routinely as a guide to prognosis and therapy selection. This development has been of immense value to breast cancer patients, not only to spare those with advanced disease from receiving unnecessary treatment that cannot help them but also in guiding the physician in the choice of adjuvant therapy following mastectomy. The following two immunoassays were developed for determining the estrogen receptor content of breast cancer specimens as a guide to therapy selection:

1. The enzyme immunoassay (EIA) measures the receptor in the cytosol fraction of a tumor homogenate by a "sandwich" technique. One monoclonal antibody (D547), bound to a Sepharose bead, absorbs the receptor from the diluted cytosol. The immobilized receptor is then treated with a second monoclonal antibody (H222), which binds to a different region of the receptor and is linked to the enzyme, horseradish peroxidase, which gives rise to a yellow color when exposed to a mixture of hydrogen peroxide and o-phenylenediamine. The color intensity is read in a colorimeter, and the receptor content of the cytosol calculated from a standard curve obtained with lyophilized cytosol from MCF-7 human breast cancer cells.

Fig. 4 Immunocyto-
chemical staining of breast
cancer tissue (right) and
control tissue (left). The
ER antibody H222 made in
Jensen Lab was used in
these assays

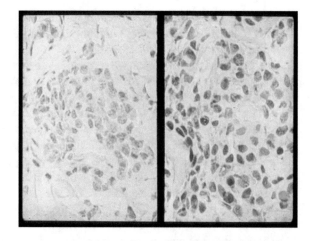

2. The immunocytochemical assay (ERICA) utilizes the peroxidase-antiperoxidase
   method in which frozen tumor sections, after gentle fixation, are treated first with
   an anti-receptor antibody (H222), then with a bridging antibody (goat anti-rat
   immuno-globulin), and finally with the peroxidase-antiperoxidase (PAP) reagent.
   Subsequent treatment with hydrogen peroxide and p-diaminobenzidine produces
   a brown stain in the cells where the receptor has retained the antibody and,
   thereby, the PAP reagent. Counterstaining is with hematoxylin to delineate cell
   nuclei (Fig. 4).

Because ER-positive tumors can be managed with antiestrogens, their studies
revealed that ER+ tumors had a better prognosis than ER-negative tumors. These
ER antibody-based assays were later developed as part of the diagnostic kit by
Abbott Laboratories and remained as a gold standard on the market until 2000,
when FDA put Abbott's diagnostic division under consent decree for some viola-
tion, not connected with ER assay kit. Abbott had to remove all its diagnostic kits
from the market, including the ER kits. When Elwood moved to University of
Cincinnati in 2002, he often felt sorry for the breast cancer patients that they were
deprived of the gold standard ER measurement kits. With a colleague of ours,
Elwood and I decided to reintroduce the kit in the market and set up a company—
Estrocept Diagnostics. Abbott cooperated with us and sublicensed the pair of cell
lines, producing ER antibodies to Estrocept for developing the ER assay kits.

10 Antiestrogens as a "Selective Estrogen Receptor Modulator (SERM)": *A Novel Concept to Treat Breast Cancer*

Elwood Jensen also left his marks in the development of antiestrogens as a therapeutic agent for breast cancer. For the first time, he "demonstrated that the antiutero-
tropic activity of MER-25, a non-steroidal antiestrogen, partly depends on its ability

to prevent the incorporation and retention of administered estradiol in the rat uterus. Thus, a foundation for the molecular mechanism of action of antiestrogen was established."

Due to its toxicity, MER-25 never qualified as a therapeutic agent. During the 1960s, antiestrogens were the focus of attention to develop them as female contraceptives, and the best-known antiestrogen for this purpose at the time was tamoxifen. When tamoxifen failed as contraceptive, Craig Jordan, a pioneer in the science of antiestrogens, repurposed tamoxifen as a therapeutic agent to treat breast cancer. In his initial career, Craig Jordan established a highly productive collaboration with Elwood Jensen, whose own discovery of estrogen receptor would play a pivotal role in advancing the concept of developing tamoxifen as a SERM and targeted therapeutic agent for managing breast cancer. The success of tamoxifen led to one of the largest clinical trials led by NIH (NASBP) to evaluate if tamoxifen could also be used as a prophylactic agent in women with high risk for breast cancer. Craig Jordan was among the first ones to raise concerns of developing endometrial cancer in those women taking tamoxifen as a prevention measure. Our own experiments using the rat model indicated that tamoxifen induced the expression of protooncogene c-fos and fosb [22]. However, Jordan showed that the second-generation antiestrogen raloxifene did not show uterotropic activity [23]. Jensen and Jordan have exemplified the concept of Bench to Bedside research and in recognition received several coveted awards: they shared the AACR's inaugural Dorothy Landen Award in 2003.

An avid Limerick composer, Elwood wrote:

A lady with growth neoplastic
thought castration was just a bit drastic
She preferred that her ill
could be cured with a pill
Today it's no longer fantastic.

11 Estrogen Receptor Harbors Two Antiestrogen Binding Sites

For many years, type I antiestrogens were noted to display unusual pharmacological behavior compared with type II "pure" antiestrogens [24]. Furthermore, ER was shown to bind nearly twice as much antiestrogen when compared with estradiol [25]. This provocative model relates to the agonist activity of type I antiestrogens to the occupancy of the cognate ligand-binding site, whereas antagonist activity results from an additional interaction with a secondary location. Depending on the particular species and tissue studied, tamoxifen exhibits properties of a pure agonist, a partial agonist/antagonist, or a pure antagonist [26]. For example, tamoxifen displays mixed agonist/antagonist behavior in human and rat tissues but under certain circumstances is a pure agonist in mouse and guinea pig [26, 27]. Tamoxifen also displays differential effects in human tissues, where it is an antagonist in breast and an agonist in uterine and bone tissues [28, 29]. By contrast, type II antiestrogens, including U11110A, LY 117018, and ICI 164384, display exclusively antagonist behavior. Type I and type II antiestrogens were shown to expose an ER epitope specific for the monoclonal ER antibody H222 [25, 30, 31]. These studies, which were carried out in the presence of a saturating amount of E2, led to the hypothesis that exposure of the H222-specific epitope results from the interaction of the antiestrogens at a distinct site from the cognate ligand-binding site. This alleged second ligand-binding site appeared to have a lower affinity for ligand, when compared with the cognate ligand-binding site for E2. In support, sucrose sedimentation and tritiated ligand experiments revealed that ER from MCF-7 cytosol binds approximately twice the amount of type I (HT) or type II (RU 58668) antiestrogens when compared with E2 and studied in the low nM range [25]. Interestingly, the concentration at which the second site-binding event occurs correlates to approximately the same concentration where agonism changes to antagonism [32] thus suggesting a two-site model for antiestrogen action [24].

12 Structural Validation of a Second ER Ligand-Binding Site

This second 4OHT ligand-binding site was recently corroborated in a report of the structure of human ERβ LBD bound to two molecules of 4OHT [33]. The overall fold of ERβ LBD structure (Fig. 5a) is similar to previously published NR LBD structures, namely, a three-layered α-helical sandwich. One 4OHT molecule is located in the cognate ligand-binding pocket, whereas the second 4OHT molecule

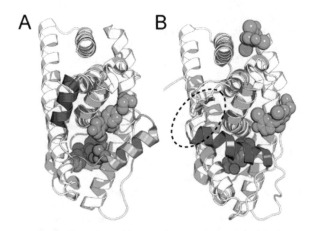

Fig. 5 Structures of human ERα and ERβ, depicting the positioning of helix 12 and ligand-binding site locations in various NR protein structures. (**a**) 4OHT-ERβ (second 4OHT-binding site; PDB 2FSZ) (**b**) DHT/4HY-AR (PDB 2PIU). Display is similar to Fig. 2. Helix 12 from a neighboring molecule of 4OHT-ERβ is orange, and the AR C-terminal extension of helix 12 is circled

is located in the hydrophobic groove of the AF-2 coactivator-binding surface, comprising helices 3, 4, 5, and 12—the surface that provides a binding site for coactivator proteins containing the LXXLL recognition motif. Thus, this structure suggests a direct means of antagonism: a ligand blocking the coactivator-binding surface of ERβ. The binding of the second 4OHT molecule in the AF-2 surface primarily involves hydrophobic and van der Waals interactions. The unsubstituted phenyl group of the second 4OHT molecule is buried deep into the hydrophobic cavity of the coactivator surface, which was noted to likely provide the main contribution to binding in the AF-2 surface. Consistent with the aforementioned biological data suggesting a second lower-affinity binding site, the second 4OHT molecule has higher crystallographic B-factors and is not fully buried when compared with the 4OHT molecule in the cognate ligand-binding site. Charge clamp residues K314 and E493, important for recognition of the LXXLL motif, do not interact with the second 4OHT. Similar second-site ligand interactions were reported for androgen receptor (AR) [34] (Fig. 5b) and thyroid receptor (TR) [35].

References

1. Jensen EV, Jacobson HI, Walf AA, Frye CA (2010) Estrogen action: a historic perspective on the implications of considering alternative approaches. Physiol Behav 99(2):151–162. https://doi.org/10.1016/j.physbeh.2009.08.013
2. Jensen EV, Jacobsonk HI (1962) Basic guides to the mechanism of estrogen action. Recent Prog Horm Res 18:387–414
3. Toft D, Gorski J (1966) A receptor molecule for estrogens: isolation from the rat uterus and preliminary characterization. Proc Natl Acad Sci U S A 55(6):1574–1581
4. Khan S, Lingrel JB (2010) Thematic minireview series on nuclear receptors in biology and diseases. J Biol Chem 285(50):38741–38742. https://doi.org/10.1074/jbc.R110.196014
5. Goldstein JL (2004) Towering science: an ounce of creativity is worth a ton of impact. Nat Med 10(10):1015–1017. https://doi.org/10.1038/nm1004-1015
6. Jensen EV, Suzuki T, Kawashima T, Stumpf WE, Jungblut PW, DeSombre ER (1968) A two-step mechanism for the interaction of estradiol with rat uterus. Proc Natl Acad Sci U S A 59(2):632–638
7. Jensen EV, DeSombre ER (1973) Estrogen-receptor interaction. Science 182(4108):126–134
8. O'Malley BW, Sherman MR, Toft DO (1970) Progesterone "receptors" in the cytoplasm and nucleus of chick oviduct target tissue. Proc Natl Acad Sci U S A 67(2):501–508
9. O'Malley BW, McGuire WL, Middleton PA (1968) Altered gene expression during differentiation: population changes in hybridizable RNA after stimulation of the chick oviduct with oestrogen. Nature 218(5148):1249–1251
10. Kumar V, Chambon P (1988) The estrogen receptor binds tightly to its responsive element as a ligand-induced homodimer. Cell 55(1):145–156
11. Wrange O, Eriksson P, Perlmann T (1989) The purified activated glucocorticoid receptor is a homodimer. J Biol Chem 264(9):5253–5259
12. Fawell SE, Lees JA, White R, Parker MG (1990) Characterization and colocalization of steroid binding and dimerization activities in the mouse estrogen receptor. Cell 60(6):953–962
13. Forman BM, Samuels HH (1990) Dimerization among nuclear hormone receptors. New Biol 2(7):587–594
14. Gronemeyer H (1991) Transcription activation by estrogen and progesterone receptors. Annu Rev Genet 25:89–123. https://doi.org/10.1146/annurev.ge.25.120191.000513

15. Gorski J, Furlow JD, Murdoch FE, Fritsch M, Kaneko K, Ying C, Malayer JR (1993) Perturbations in the model of estrogen receptor regulation of gene expression. Biol Reprod 48(1):8–14
16. Wang H, Peters GA, Zeng X, Tang M, Ip W, Khan SA (1995) Yeast two-hybrid system demonstrates that estrogen receptor dimerization is ligand-dependent in vivo. J Biol Chem 270(40):23322–23329
17. Halachmi S, Marden E, Martin G, MacKay H, Abbondanza C, Brown M (1994) Estrogen receptor-associated proteins: possible mediators of hormone-induced transcription. Science 264(5164):1455–1458
18. Walter P, Green S, Greene G, Krust A, Bornert JM, Jeltsch JM, Staub A, Jensen E, Scrace G, Waterfield M et al (1985) Cloning of the human estrogen receptor cDNA. Proc Natl Acad Sci U S A 82(23):7889–7893
19. Greene GL, Closs LE, Fleming H, DeSombre ER, Jensen EV (1977) Antibodies to estrogen receptor: immunochemical similarity of estrophilin from various mammalian species. Proc Natl Acad Sci U S A 74(9):3681–3685
20. Greene GL, Nolan C, Engler JP, Jensen EV (1980) Monoclonal antibodies to human estrogen receptor. Proc Natl Acad Sci U S A 77(9):5115–5119
21. Jensen EV (2004) From chemical warfare to breast cancer management. Nat Med 10(10): 1018–1021. https://doi.org/10.1038/nm1004-1018
22. Nephew KP, Polek TC, Akcali KC, Khan SA (1993) The antiestrogen tamoxifen induces c-fos and jun-B, but not c-jun or jun-D, protooncogenes in the rat uterus. Endocrinology 133(1):419–422. https://doi.org/10.1210/endo.133.1.8319588
23. O'Regan RM, Gajdos C, Dardes RC, De Los Reyes A, Park W, Rademaker AW, Jordan VC (2002) Effects of raloxifene after tamoxifen on breast and endometrial tumor growth in athymic mice. J Natl Cancer Inst 94(4):274–283
24. Jensen EV, Khan SA (2004) A two-site model for antiestrogen action. Mech Ageing Dev 125(10–11):679–682. https://doi.org/10.1016/j.mad.2004.08.006
25. Hedden A, Muller V, Jensen EV (1995) A new interpretation of antiestrogen action. Ann N Y Acad Sci 761:109–120
26. Jordan VC (1984) Biochemical pharmacology of antiestrogen action. Pharmacol Rev 36(4):245–276
27. Furr BJ, Jordan VC (1984) The pharmacology and clinical uses of tamoxifen. Pharmacol Ther 25(2):127–205
28. Gottardis MM, Robinson SP, Jordan VC (1988) Estradiol-stimulated growth of MCF-7 tumors implanted in athymic mice: a model to study the tumoristatic action of tamoxifen. J Steroid Biochem 30(1–6):311–314
29. Wijayaratne AL, Nagel SC, Paige LA, Christensen DJ, Norris JD, Fowlkes DM, McDonnell DP (1999) Comparative analyses of mechanistic differences among antiestrogens. Endocrinology 140(12):5828–5840. https://doi.org/10.1210/endo.140.12.7164
30. Berthois Y, Pons M, Dussert C, Crastes de Paulet A, Martin PM (1994) Agonist-antagonist activity of anti-estrogens in the human breast cancer cell line MCF-7: an hypothesis for the interaction with a site distinct from the estrogen binding site. Mol Cell Endocrinol 99(2):259–268
31. Martin PM, Berthois Y, Jensen EV (1988) Binding of antiestrogens exposes an occult antigenic determinant in the human estrogen receptor. Proc Natl Acad Sci U S A 85(8):2533–2537
32. Katzenellenbogen BS, Kendra KL, Norman MJ, Berthois Y (1987) Proliferation, hormonal responsiveness, and estrogen receptor content of MCF-7 human breast cancer cells grown in the short-term and long-term absence of estrogens. Cancer Res 47(16):4355–4360
33. Wang Y, Chirgadze NY, Briggs SL, Khan S, Jensen EV, Burris TP (2006) A second binding site for hydroxytamoxifen within the coactivator-binding groove of estrogen receptor beta. Proc Natl Acad Sci U S A 103(26):9908–9911. https://doi.org/10.1073/pnas.0510596103
34. Estebanez-Perpina E, Arnold LA, Nguyen P, Rodrigues ED, Mar E, Bateman R, Pallai P, Shokat KM, Baxter JD, Guy RK, Webb P, Fletterick RJ (2007) A surface on the androgen receptor that

allosterically regulates coactivator binding. Proc Natl Acad Sci U S A 104(41):16074–16079. https://doi.org/10.1073/pnas.0708036104

35. Estebanez-Perpina E, Arnold LA, Jouravel N, Togashi M, Blethrow J, Mar E, Nguyen P, Phillips KJ, Baxter JD, Webb P, Guy RK, Fletterick RJ (2007) Structural insight into the mode of action of a direct inhibitor of coregulator binding to the thyroid hormone receptor. Mol Endocrinol 21(12):2919–2928. https://doi.org/10.1210/me.2007-0174

Physiological and Pathological Roles of Estrogen Receptor

Kenneth S. Korach, Sylvia C. Hewitt, Katherine J. Hamilton, Yin Li, J. Tyler Ramsey, Marleny Garcia, Emilie Mathura, and Yukitomo Arao

Abstract Estrogen produces a variety of physiological functions in numerous tissues in both females and males. The actions can occur through cytoplasmic and nuclear activities of two receptor protein isoforms, ERα and ERβ, and multiple cell signaling mechanisms, including non-genomic and genomic actions. Genomic actions involve either direct DNA binding or tethered gene regulation. We describe herein some of the physiological responses of estrogen occurring through a particular receptor by way of gene targeting experimental models. We describe additional experimental models that isolate specific estrogen receptor activities to determine and evaluate the physiological responses, in reproductive/gonadal tissues, neuroendocrine actions, and obesity related to adipose tissue and bone as some examples, linked to that receptors' functional domains and tissue specificity.

Keywords Reproduction · Metabolic syndrome · Clinical estrogen insensitivity · Pulmonary · Cardiovascular

1 Introduction

Elwood Jensen's original observations made a seminal, profound, and highly significant contribution to science in general. Discovering receptor proteins for steroid/thyroid hormones with the plausible explanation for their potential mode of action answered a long-standing question of these secreted substances from their initial discovery, some 70 years earlier [1]. Jensen's proposal was that the specific uptake and tissue retention of his radiolabeled reagent might be due to receptor interactions. Ultimately, this observation did essentially create the field of "nuclear receptors" and spawned many successful research careers for investigators. Significantly, it answered many biomedical questions, and uncovered a variety of unknown effects

K. S. Korach (✉) · S. C. Hewitt · K. J. Hamilton · Y. Li · J. T. Ramsey · M. Garcia
E. Mathura · Y. Arao
Receptor Biology Section, Reproductive and Developmental Biology Laboratory, National Institute Environmental Health Sciences, National Institutes of Health, Durham, NC, USA
e-mail: korach@niehs.nih.gov

© Springer Nature Switzerland AG 2019
X. Zhang (ed.), *Estrogen Receptor and Breast Cancer*, Cancer Drug Discovery and Development, https://doi.org/10.1007/978-3-319-99350-8_2

of hormones, with application to solving clinical problems, thereby explaining the spectrum of both specific and differential actions of different steroid hormones in different tissues. Although estrogen was the first steroid hormone analyzed, his initial synthesis of high specific activity radiolabeled estradiol was the key to determining the detection of receptors for a natural steroid hormone. Subsequent use of columns, sucrose gradients, and unlabeled competitor analysis provided evidence of a molecular form and hormone specificity for the entire family of nuclear receptor proteins. Parallel studies and confirmation of his findings by Jack Gorski's group were only possible because of Elwood Jensen's extreme generosity to share with Gorski the only source of his radiolabeled estradiol that allowed studies to move forward. Jensen's discovery of nuclear receptors also led to his development of a major diagnostic advance for breast cancer in the form of diagnostic estrogen receptor analysis. Elwood Jensen was quite a lyricist and at times gave statements and answers in rhyme. So, not in any respect as good as Elwood, I just might want to add this phrase.

> Many actions occur in a cell
> But how do we know how well
> Is ER part of the game?
> If so, is alpha or beta to blame?
> Through research we keep on yearning
> In tissues with hopes of learning
> How estrogen does it so well

Our group's interest for a number of years has been in determining and understanding the physiological actions of estrogens. Molecular mechanisms and structural analysis of estrogen and its receptors are described in other chapters of this book. Herein, we describe some of the biological actions associated with estrogen receptor activity gleaned from characterization of phenotypes from estrogen receptor knockout and mutant experimental mouse models. Since these experimental model systems have been developed, hundreds of studies from a multitude of investigators have bene published utilizing these various models. We can only give a description of general conclusions and examples of effects. For more details on specific topics and studies, we provide additional review references [2, 3].

2   Molecular Mechanisms of Estrogen Receptor-Mediated Signaling

Estrogen (E2) is the primary phenolic steroid hormone synthesized by mammalian ovaries and secreted into the blood [4] and is also synthesized peripherally in cells expressing the enzyme aromatase. Its lipophilic nature allows it to freely pass through cell membranes, accessing cells within many tissues. How E2 is able to specifically target certain cells in a variety of tissues (Fig. 1) occurs with its ability to act through the estrogen receptor (ER) as a transducer of its hormonal activity.

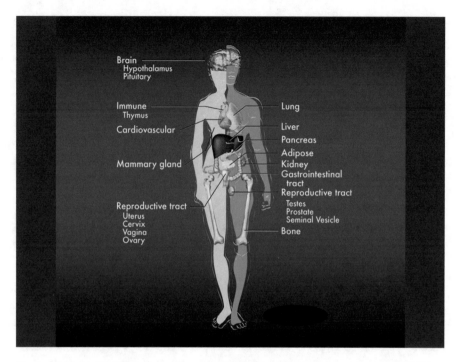

Fig. 1 Diagrammatic illustration of the various known target and organ systems where estrogens have been linked to biological actions. Some of the tissues have been linked to estrogens influence on cancer

In mammals there are two ERs, ERα and ERβ, both members of the nuclear receptor superfamily of hormone-inducible transcription factors [5–7]. As the name indicates, nuclear receptors work in the cell by multiple mechanisms illustrated schematically in Fig. 2. Nuclear receptors are primarily within the nucleus of cells and are receptors for various specific hormones. A clear manner to illustrate how ERs function is to describe their protein domain structure (Fig. 3). All nuclear receptor family members share a general multi-domain structure, with each domain directing the mechanistic interactions and functions necessary for hormone response. The ERs have six domains, A–F [6–8]. The two key functions of high affinity and high specificity binding to (1) its hormonal activator E2 and (2) its target gene DNA motif, the estrogen-responsive element (ERE), are located in the ligand-binding domain (LBD) and the DNA-binding domain (DBD), respectively. Each of these domains, along with the four other domains, encodes structural features critical to their activity, which will be described in more detail in other chapters.

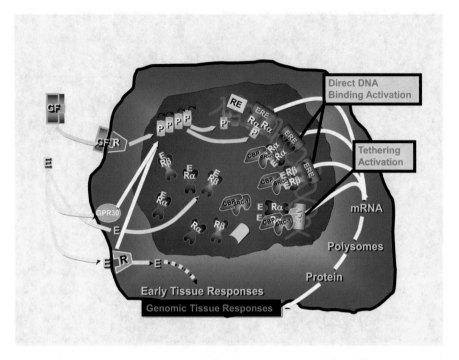

Fig. 2 Illustration of the two forms of the nuclear estrogen receptors ERα and ERβ and the various modes of estrogen action occurring in a target cell. Membrane forms of the estrogen receptor and the G-protein-coupled estrogen-binding receptor producing non-genomic activities. Ligand-dependent activation involving either direct DNA binding of the receptor or the tethering activation. Example of a possible general mode of ligand-independent activation of the ER

3   Mouse Models to Study Physiological Roles of Estrogen Receptors

In order to study the physiological roles of estrogen receptors, multiple genetic models have been developed and characterized. These models include global knock-out strains lacking functional ERα (αERKO) [9], ERβ (βERKO) [10], or both estrogen receptors (αβERKO) [11, 12]. All three global knockouts are viable to adulthood and harbor distinct phenotypes. As such, they have allowed researchers an opportunity to discern many physiological roles of each receptor. Due to the technology used at the time, the original global knockouts expressed trace amounts of splice variants which complicated data interpretation; however, new global knockout models were created with the cre-loxP system which provided complete global knockouts: Ex3αERKO, Ex3βERKO, and αβERKO [13]. The introduction of the cre-loxP system further allowed generation of multiple tissue- or cell-type-specific

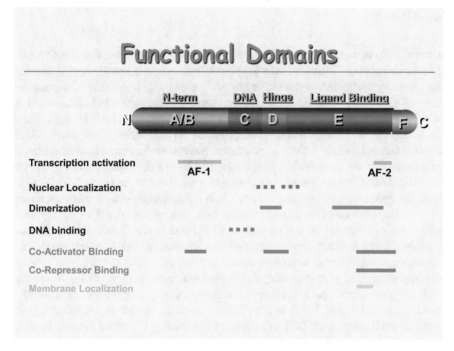

Fig. 3 Diagrammatic illustration depicting the positions of the six functional domains of the estrogen receptor and their proposed cellular and biochemical activities

knockouts which have given us a wealth of information on the tissue-specific functionality of the ERs, which was not possible with the global knockout alone. Specific examples of tissue-specific models will be discussed in later sections of this chapter. Furthermore, many estrogen receptor mutants have been developed which alter a specific domain functionality of ERα, thereby allowing for evaluating the physiological relevance to a domain function. These include models which disrupt binding to the estrogen-responsive DNA element due to alterations in the DNA-binding domains (NERKI and EAAE), as well as a model which disrupts estradiol-mediated transcription activation by inhibiting estradiol binding due to a point mutation in the ligand-binding domain (ENERKI) [14–16]. Additional models have included the deletion of AF-1 or AF-2 (AF-1^0 and AF-2^0) and point mutations in helix 12 of AF-2 (AF2ERKI) [16–18]. Most recently, models have been created to evaluate non-genomic ERα signaling (NOER, MOER, C451-ERα, H2NES) [19]. Due to the breadth and spectrum of estrogen action, use of these mouse models has been an extremely valuable tool in evaluating the physiological roles of the estrogen receptors.

4   Uterus

Uterine cells contain abundant ERα, so it is not surprising, then, that the endometrium responds rapidly and robustly to cyclical fluctuations in circulating E2 released by the ovary during the menstrual or estrous cycle [20, 21]. Because of the expression of ERα and robust E2 response, the uterus has become a valuable model in which to study mechanisms underlying uterine responses, at both biological and molecular levels. Uterine tissue is comprised of several different cell types, which confer essential functions during growth and the establishment and maintenance of pregnancy and for parturition. Embryos implant by invading through a layer of epithelial cells that line the lumen, an opening in the interior of the uterus [22]. In addition, the epithelial cell structures extend into the endometrium, forming secretory glands. The exterior of the uterus consists of a muscular level, called the myometrium, which contracts during parturition to allow delivery. Between the epithelial and myometrial structures are stromal cells, which undergo an E2- and progesterone-dependent decidual transformation during pregnancy, which is critical to support the implanting and growing embryo [21]. Endothelial cells lining blood vessels, as well as general and specialized immune cells, are key components of a healthy endometrium. ERα is found in myometrial, stromal, epithelial, endothelial, and some of the immune cells [23]. In response to increasing E2 during the proliferative phase of the menstrual cycle, or during the proestrous phase of the estrous cycle, epithelial cells proliferate and secrete important factors, and fluid and immune cells are brought into the uterine tissue by increased vascular permeability, all of which serve to substantially increase the size of the uterus and the thickness of the epithelial layer.

This response was the basis for the development of the ovariectomized rodent uterus as a model to study E2 response in a controlled manner and separate from effects caused by progesterone, the other major ovarian hormone impacting uterine cells. Early studies using ovariectomized rats and mice began by surgically removing the ovaries and then treating the animals with E2 which was used as a classical bioassay for characterizing the biological activity of estrogens [24]. Several hours after injection of E2, production of ERα-mediated changes in RNA transcription and protein synthesis are observed, as well as a uterine weight increase because of increased vascular permeability and uptake of fluid into the tissue. Later, 18–24 h after the E2 treatment, proliferation of epithelial cells and a further increase in uterine weight are observed. Some experiments extend the response by injecting E2 daily for 3 days, which results in substantial tissue weight increase and a thickened epithelial layer. Although this experimental scheme is not completely physiological, as it introduces an environment of ovarian hormone depletion followed by E2 alone, it has been an important tool in understanding ERα mechanisms in an intact tissue.

Development of techniques to disrupt or replace mouse and rat genes, first using homologous recombination, and later with Cre-driven recombination of "floxed" alleles, or with gene editing techniques, facilitates study of the roles of the whole ERα as well as specific functional features of the ERα. Initial studies looked at the impact of deleting, or "knocking out," the ERα, resulting in a mouse, the αERKO (ERα knockout), with a hypoplastic uterus that lacked both growth and gene transcription responses following E2 treatments [25, 26]. The tissue has a normal cellular composition, indicating that ERα is not needed for embryonic uterine development but is critical for postpubertal development and function. αERKO females are sterile, in part due to impaired ovulation; however, exogenous E2 and progesterone were used to experimentally mimic pregnancy to study decidualization and implantation. αERKO uteri failed to implant embryos and decidual response could not be induced [7].

Interesting studies using separation and reconstitution of neonatal uterine epithelial and stromal cells from αERKO and WT mice showed that for the E2-induced growth of uterine epithelial cells, ERα need not be present in the epithelial cells, but is needed in the stromal cells [27]. This was shown because mixing αERKO epithelial cells with WT stromal cells and treating with E2 caused epithelial growth, whereas the converse combination (WT epithelial cells with αERKO stromal cells) did not have epithelial growth after E2 treatment. This affirms a hypothesized paracrine mechanism, in which E2 induces stromal cell secretion of growth factors, such as EGF and IGF1, which then interact with growth factor receptors on epithelial cells, leading to the growth responses. To affirm if paracrine mechanisms occurred in adult intact tissues and to extend these studies in un-disrupted uterine tissue, ERα was deleted using a uterine epithelial-selective promoter (Wnt7aCre), with floxed ERα creating Wnt7aCre;Esr1$^{f/f}$ mice. Uterine transcriptional and growth responses of ovariectomized Wnt7aCre;Esr1$^{f/f}$ mice are initially like those of WT mice, with epithelial growth [28]. This observation confirmed that epithelial cell ERα is not needed for stimulating uterine growth response to E2. However, after multiple days of E2 treatment, the uterine weight increase of mice lacking uterine epithelial cell ERα is blunted compared to WT mice, and the tissue exhibits indications of epithelial cell apoptosis, showing a requirement for epithelial cell ERα activity for maintaining epithelial cell stature for optimal uterine response [28]. Wnt7aCre;Esr1$^{f/f}$ mice are sterile, and are unable to implant embryos, showing the importance of uterine epithelial cell ERα for uterine function [28]. Mice in which stromal ERα was deleted were created by crossing with a uterine stromal-selective promoter (Amhr2Cre) to Esr1$^{f/f}$ mice, creating Amhr2Cre;Esr1$^{f/f}$ mice. Uterine ERα deletion in the Amhr2Cre; Esr1$^{f/f}$ mice was predominant in stromal cells in the antimesometrial region of the uterus, where embryos implant. Consequently, epithelial cell proliferation did not occur when ovariectomized mice are treated with E2, except in epithelial cells that were adjacent to mesometrial stromal cells that still contain ERα [29]. This mouse model provided essentially an internal tissue control for evaluating the role of stromal ERα in uterine growth. The observation clearly indicates that paracrine factors secreted by uterine stromal cells mainly act on adjacent epithelial cells for stimulating proliferation.

Several other "knock-in" mouse models have been generated by replacing the WT ERα with mutation-bearing substitutes. This allows examination of different activities of the ERα in the uterine environment. Mutations in the zinc finger region of the DBD that disrupt the ability of the ERα to bind ERE DNA motifs (EAAE) result in a uterine phenotype that mirrors that of the αERKO [15, 30]. The uterus is hypoplastic and does not respond to E2 treatment, lacking both transcriptional and growth responses. This indicates that although tethering has been described using in vitro cell reporter assay-based systems, in an intact uterine environment, direct ERE binding is essential for E2 responses. Mutations that disrupt AF-1 of the ERα do not appear to impact uterine development, but do result in a blunted response to E2 [31, 32]. Mutations in the AF-2 region of the ERα cause a hypoplastic uterine phenotype, are insensitive to E2, but show a blunted response to ERα antagonists [17, 33]. These findings indicate that AF-1 and AF-2 together contribute to a full uterine response to E2. Two different research groups introduced ERα mutations that removed the palmitoylation site involved in membrane localization of the ERα, thus restricting the ERα to its nuclear activities. One of the groups reported that uterine development and response to E2 were unaltered [34], whereas the second group reported and found hypoplastic uterine development and lack of E2 response [35], but subsequently in later work, they reported a uterine growth response [36]. The differences in observations between these two mouse models are not understood and make it impossible to draw conclusions regarding the importance of extranuclear ERα signaling in uterine development and E2 responsiveness. Two complementary models, which both exclude the ERα from the nucleus, via mutations in the NLS in one case [19] or through fusion of multiple palmitoylation sites to the ERα LBD [37], exhibit hypoplastic uteri that lack both the early and late phases of E2 responses. Thus, extranuclear ERα signaling alone is not sufficient for uterine development and E2 response.

5   Uterine Cancer

Two major types of uterine cancer are adenocarcinoma and sarcoma. A retrospective study showed an increased relative risk of endometrial carcinoma in women who received exogenous estrogen treatment during menopause and/or postmenopause. This risk was highest in women who were not already predisposed to endometrial cancer due to other health factors [38, 39]. Estrogen receptors and/or progesterone receptors are reportedly expressed in 40–80% of cases of uterine leiomyosarcoma [40–43]. Moreover, enhanced survival has been associated with uterine expression of estrogen receptors and/or progesterone receptors compared to their lack of expression in high-grade uterine leiomyosarcoma [42]. Another retrospective study showed that endometrial carcinomas lacking ERα are correlated with epithelial-mesenchymal transition and worse prognosis [44]. The E2 antagonist and partial agonist molecule, tamoxifen, is used in hormone therapy in ERα-positive breast cancer to decrease tumor cell growth [45]. However, in postmenopausal women, tamoxifen can cause malignant changes in the endometrium [46]. A study used ChiP-Seq analysis and found differences in the ERα-binding sites and ERα gene expression regulation between tamoxifen-associated endometrial tumors and endometrial tumors not associated with tamoxifen use [47]. Hence, ERα expression regulation in uterine tissue is critical for uterine tissue health and can be altered by hormonal environment.

6 Endometriosis

Endometriosis is a common estrogen-dependent gynecological condition described by endometrial tissue invasion into extrauterine sites creating painful, inflammatory lesions [48–51]. It is known that ERα and ERβ are aberrantly expressed in women with endometriosis [52–54]. To investigate the role of ER signaling in endometriosis lesions, an immunocompetent mouse model of endometriosis was used [55]. To create this mouse model, uterine tissue was taken from a donor mouse, crushed, and dispersed into the peritoneal cavity of a recipient mouse. Mice used as donors or recipients were WT, αERKO, and βERKO. The mouse models were treated with vehicle or E2. Subsequently, endometriosis-like lesion quantity, localization, and size were taken into account. The results of this study suggest that endometriosis-like estrogen-dependent signaling is predominately mediated through ERα [56].

On a positive note, the ER ligands chloroindazole (CLI) and oxabicycloheptene sulfonate (OBHW) reportedly suppress endometriotic lesion development and stimulate a size reduction of established lesions without altering the estrous cycle or fertility in preclinical models of endometriosis [57]. CLI predominantly acts through ERβ while OBHS mainly exhibits its effects through ERα [58–61]. Hence, both ligands are involved in suppressing the estrogen-dependent phenomena that come with endometriosis, such as cell proliferation, cyst formation, vascularization, and lesion growth [57].

7 Ovary

Since the ovary is the primary source of estrogen in the female, the classical experimental paradigm to evaluate a role, if any, for ER in the ovary was impossible to test. The ERKO mouse models helped to solve this conundrum. Immunohistochemical studies concluded that rodents have distinct localization of the estrogen receptors within the ovary: theca cells primarily express ERα while ERβ is primarily localized to the granulosa cells, which have undetectable levels of ERα expression [62]. Individual estrogen receptor knockout (αERKO and βERKO) mice have grossly normal ovaries at birth; however, the mice have unique ovarian and ovulatory phenotypes that become apparent as they mature [2].

Adult αERKO mice are anovulatory and ovarian histology is characterized by multiple large hemorrhagic cysts that likely arise from antral follicles that fail to ovulate [63] ERα-null mice have severe disruptions to their hormonal milieu as a result of loss of ERα in the hypothalamic-pituitary axis (elevations in estradiol, testosterone, and LH) and therefore are acyclic, with the lack of an LH surge. FSH levels are normal, but ovariectomy results in increased levels, likely a result of the loss of ovarian inhibin which is elevated in αERKO mice [64]. Taken together this represents both the cause and effect of the ovarian phenotypes. As expected with such disruptions in the hormonal environment, the ovaries exhibit thecal hypertrophy and elevated steroidogenic enzyme expression [65, 66]. Notably, ovaries of ERα-null mice have elevated Cyp17, Cyp19, and aberrant Hsd17b3 expression [66]. The aberrant expression of Hsd17b3 is quite surprising because this enzyme is unique to the testes, so it represents a form of endocrine sex reversal and is also an explanation for the elevated testosterone levels in the mice. When treated with a GnRH-antagonist, the cystic follicles and elevated steroidogenesis in ERα-null mice are prevented, which indicates that the phenotypes are indirectly caused by a lack of ERα as a mediator of estradiol actions in the HPG axis. Of note, there is evidence that intraovarian actions of estradiol on theca cells change Cyp17 expression which is involved in androgen synthesis [63, 67]. There are several different reports of superovulation studies where mice lacking ERα were treated with exogenous PMSG and hCG to induce ovulation. While the conclusions of the reports differ, it seems likely that ovulation was only observed in strains with the presence of an ERα splice variant, and complete loss of ERα greatly reduces the number of oocytes recovered after superovulation [12, 65, 68, 69]. To look more specifically at loss of ERα from the theca cells in the ovary, Bridges et al. generated a theca cell-specific ERα knockout using a Cyp17-cre mouse [70]. Two-month-old mice lacking ERα in the theca cells (thEsr1KO) did not have an altered estrus cycle and were fertile, but by 6 months, these measures were reduced and the mice have a significantly diminished response to exogenous gonadotropins [70]. Furthermore, thEsr1KO mice have a reduction of LH which confirms that LH excess in the global ERα KO is due to loss of the receptor in the pituitary and suggests that ERα in the ovary may play a role in LH secretion [70]. Mice with altered DNA-binding activity (EAAE, NERKI) are infertile, have elevated LH, and have hemorrhagic and cystic ovaries suggesting that DNA binding is essential for ERα activities in the ovary and HPG axis [15, 71]. ENERKI mice, with a point mutation preventing ligand binding, do not ovulate, also have cystic follicles, and have an increased number of atretic antral follicles [16]. To examine the importance of the AF2 domain in the ovary, mice with a point mutation in helix 12 were analyzed [33]. AF2ER mice have an ovarian phenotype and hormonal profile very similar to the global ERα KO. Historically, the focus of estrogen's role in the ovary has focused on ERβ due to the high expression in granulosa cells and the resulting phenotypes discussed below. Taken together these data from many different mutant ERα models show that ERα is critical to fertility, regulation of steroidogenesis, and ovulation, although more work needs to be done to determine the precise role of ERα in ovulation.

Several aspects of ovarian physiology, which are thought to be dependent on paracrine actions of estradiol, are maintained in ERα-null mice suggesting a dependence on ERβ in the ovary [65, 66]. Ovaries from ERβ-null mice develop normally as neonates and display no gross abnormalities [2]. Adult ERβ-null mice have all stages of follicles, but corpora lutea are scarce and there is a slight increase in atretic follicles [10, 67, 72]. Female ERβ mice are severely subfertile, but there is variability in this finding where some females are completely infertile and some have one or more litters during a continuous mating scheme [10, 73]. Despite variability in both fertility and response to superovulation studies, the ERβ-null mice are consistently impaired in ovulation, suggesting the importance of ERβ in normal ovarian function. The fertility defect appears to be due to disrupted ovulation function that results in inefficient ovulation despite a normal hormonal environment [2]. In granulosa cells isolated from mice lacking ERβ, the response to FSH and LH is impaired, with reduced levels of cAMP accumulation in response to FSH stimulation [74, 75]. This coincides with a reduction of LH-receptor mRNA accumulation and suggests that granulosa cells from ERβ-null mice are unable to properly stimulate an increase in LH receptor which could be the cause of the ovulation defect seen in these mice [75]. In fact, ERβ-null mice have a severely blunted LH surge, and when ovaries are transplanted from WT to ERβ-null mice, the surge and fertility are rescued which demonstrates the essential role for ERβ in the ovary [76]. Lack of gonadotropin stimulation affecting poor ovulation in ERβ-null mice can be overcome with forskolin treatment, thereby circumventing the cAMP stimulation [77].

Mice null for both estrogen receptors, αβERKO, are infertile, do not ovulate spontaneously, and have a similar disrupted hormonal profile to the ERα-null mice [11, 12]. Adult ovaries from the "double" knockout have a unique phenotype not seen in any of the other ERKO lines. They show follicles of various stages and also can have some cystic follicles similar to those seen in the ERα-null mice; however, they are not as large or hemorrhagic suggesting an intraovarian role for ERβ in this pathology. Unique to the αβERKO ovary when compared to the single receptor knockouts is a sex-reversal phenotype characterized by the postpubertal development of structures that are seminiferous tubule-like structures that have cells that resemble Sertoli cells of the testis [11, 12]. The Sertoli-like cells express *Sox9*, which is critical to normal Sertoli cell development in the testis of humans and rodents [11]. This novel phenotype does indicate that the proper differentiation state of the granulosa cells requires functionality of both ERα and ERβ signaling pathways. The link between loss of ER function and postnatal sex reversal in the ovary is still unclear [11].

8 Hypothalamic-Pituitary-Gonadal Axis

The hypothalamic-pituitary-gonadal axis, commonly known as the HPG axis, consists of three organs which are crucial to the homeostatic endocrine feedback of steroid hormones. Hypothalamic secretion of GnRH stimulates responses from the anterior pituitary to secrete FSH and LH, which then act on the ovary. Presence of FSH and LH promote folliculogenesis and the synthesis of estradiol (E2). Serum E2 then completes the negative feedback loop by acting on both the hypothalamus and the pituitary gland to inhibit production of gonadotropins, FSH, and LH [66]. Both ERα and ERβ are expressed throughout the neuroendocrine tissues. In the pituitary gland and hypothalamus, there is expression primarily of ERα, while GnRH neurons are reported to solely express ERβ.

The phenotypes characterized with these mice reveal proposed functions of each receptor form. When comparing αERKO mice to βERKO mice, αERKO have a distinctly more severe phenotype indicating that ERα appears to be the predominant receptor form in maintaining homeostasis of negative feedback in the female HPG axis. Prior studies had used pharmacological agents in attempts to investigate the neurological identity of the neuroendocrine sites but have yielded inconclusive results. In general, based on the ensuing phenotypes, it appears that ERα not ERβ is involved in maintaining homeostasis between the negative feedback loops of the HPG axis since only mutations in the *Esr1* gene exhibit loss of negative feedback, elevated LH, and hyper-stimulated cystic ovaries. A novel finding from the characterization of αERKO ovaries was the discovery of the aberrant expression of Hsd17b3 in both the αERKO and αβERKO ovaries. Ovaries customarily express 17β-Hsd1 while the testes express Hsd17b3. The aberrant expression is reflective of an endocrine sex reversal resulting from the loss of ERα [9].

9   Mammary Gland

In mammals, development of the mammary gland could be divided into five distinct stages, embryonic and fetal/neonatal, prepubertal, pubertal, sexually mature adult, and pregnancy/lactation [2]. The mammary gland is essentially undeveloped at birth and does not undergo full ductal development until puberty and then lactation during pregnancy. Fetal/neonatal mammary glands of rodents are responsive to gonadal steroids [78]. In males, the fetal glandular structures are destroyed via the "masculinization" effects of testicular androgens, an effect that can be reproduced in males by prenatal exposure to testosterone [78]. In female mice, aberrant neonatal exposure to estradiol, testosterone, or PRL has been reported to result in an apparent increased sensitivity of the gland to mammographic hormones during adulthood, leading to varied degrees of excessive ductal growth and differentiation [78, 79]. The later four stages of mammary gland development occur after birth and terminate in a gland composed of ductal glands and alveoli capable of milk production. The endogenous ovarian hormones regulate the five stages of mammary gland development. Upon pregnancy and the onset of lactation, the gland becomes dramatically differentiated, producing milk-secreting structures throughout the ductal network [2]. Therefore, the mammary gland provides a unique system in which to study ER-mediated hormone signaling.

In adult WT female mice, the mammary glands consist of a network of epithelial ducts originating from the nipple and forming a treelike structure. The growth of the epithelial ducts begins during prepuberty and continues during puberty until the branches of the gland have reached the limits of the fat pad [2]. The mammary glands of adult αERKO female mice are undeveloped and exhibit a phenotype like the glands of a newborn WT female [2]. However, the αERKO gland does possess the component structures necessary for mammary gland development [80] and does not undergo ductal morphogenesis or alveolar development [81], confirming that ERα plays an important role for ductal growth during mammary gland development. Studies have shown that the estradiol-ERα complex increases progesterone receptor (PR) expression in various tissues, including the mammary gland [82]. Combined loss of PR-mediated progesterone functions results in lack of alveolar development consistent with the PRKO mammary gland phenotype [83]. Our study indicates that prolonged progesterone treatment of the mammary glands in adult αERKO female mice results in the formation of terminal end buds and differentiation in the mammary gland, suggesting that the lack of progesterone action caused by disruption of the ERα gene could be partially overcome with treatment of superphysiological levels of exogenous progesterone [2]. However, unlike αERKO mammary gland development, there is no such phenotype observed in adult βERKO female mice who have normal ductal glandular development. Furthermore, βERKO females appear to have undergone normal differentiation and exhibit the lobuloalveolar structures for lactation [2]. The findings from the ERKO models indicate that ERα is the predominant receptor for mediating the estrogen action in the mouse mammary glands.

10 ER Status and Breast Cancer

Both ERα and ERβ are normally expressed and present in the mammary gland. Normal human mammary gland tissue from premenopausal women shows that ERα, PR-A, PR-B, and AR localize mostly to the inner layer of epithelial cells lining acini and intralobular ducts and to myoepithelial cells in the external layer of interlobular ducts [84]. However, ERβ expression is more widespread, showing staining of stromal, epithelial, and myoepithelial cells in acini and ducts [84]. Estrogen signaling is reported to be mediated by ERα and ERβ in hormone dependent breast cancer. ERα is a prognostic marker in breast cancer, but the role of ERβ is less clear [85]. Jensen and colleagues were some of the first to determine ER expression in breast cancer correlated with ERα-positive status of the tumor for treatment responses and survival outcomes, but no overall prognostic significance was demonstrated for ERβ. A detailed study of ERβ expression examining localizations of ERβ1, ERβ2, and ERβ5 isoforms suggests that the cellular localization of these isoforms differentially affects some patient's outcome [86, 87]. The relationship of ERα phosphorylation to clinical outcome after tamoxifen therapy suggest that high phosphorylation status of the ERα protein is associated with increased mortality [85]. In breast cancer, ER, PR, HER2, and Ki67 are biological makers for predicting prognosis and treatment decisions, but other nuclear receptors and transcription factors also play a role in breast cancer progression. In HER2-positive tumors, ERα and PR are associated with androgen receptor (AR) co-expression and lower proliferative activity, while AR/ERα-negative tumors are associated with the highest proliferation, suggesting that co-expression of AR and ERα provides a protective effect [85]. Male breast cancer is a rare disease, accounting for around 1% of all breast cancers [88]. In contrast to female breast cancer, the majority of all male cases are ERα-positive (91–95%) and/or PR-positive (80–81%) [89, 90]. Consequently, adjuvant treatment of male breast cancer revolves around inhibition of ERα. A recent review has summarized that mutational and epigenetic similarities and differences between male and female breast cancer do exist, further suggesting that some features are strongly conserved between the two diseases [91].

11 Male Reproductive Tract

Estrogens have always been historically associated with female reproduction. However, recent studies have established that estrogens and the primary receptors, ESR1, ESR2, and G-protein-coupled estrogen receptor (GPER), are also important for male reproductive tract and nonreproductive tissues [92]. E2 has been found in circulating male blood and tests seminal fluids at levels comparable to E2 levels in females. The testis produces approximately 20% of circulating estrogen in males; other organs (adipose, brain, skin, and bone) are responsible for aromatase activity and conversion of testosterone into estrogen [92]. Before KO mice were available, estrogen was known to affect male behavior as well as alter development and function of the testis, prostate, and seminal vesicles. It was also documented that estrogen played a role in altering circulating testosterone and luteinizing hormone (LH) levels. At that time, however, little was known about the mechanisms regulating these hormone levels [92].

In humans, the aromatase pathway is essential for estrogen production in males. The pathway can be detected in reproductive tissues such as immature germ cells, spermatozoa, epithelium of efferent ductules, and the epithelium of the proximal epididymis. According to Cooke et al., ESR1 was found in the following organs: the testis, Leydig cells, Sertoli cells, germ cells, myoid cells, rete testis, efferent ducts, and vas deferens. Additionally, immunohistochemistry showed that ESR2 was found in Leydig, peritubular, germ, and Sertoli cells [92].

To observe the physiological changes that occur as a result of the absence of ERα, Esr1KO mice were characterized. The most surprising and interesting observation of Esr1KO mice was that they were completely infertile. From the phenotype characterization, the two predominant physiological roles of ESR1 appear to be (1) fluid resorption by efferent ductule epithelium and (2) maintenance of sperm morphology, activation, and motility. Both of these processes are dependent upon various ion and water transporter proteins, which establish luminal environments that maintain proper pH, osmolality, and sperm concentration. One of the major morphological changes observed was diminished fluid resorption due to impaired efferent ductile epithelial differentiation, which resulted in decreased epithelial height and loss of cellular structures associated with fluid reabsorption. These increased fluid changes cause an enlarged luminal seminiferous tubule dilation compared to WT mice. This fluid accumulation was seen in the rete testes and seminiferous tubules. Thus, ESR1 plays a significant role in the efferent ducts [92]. Additionally, with age, the initial testicular dysmorphogenesis swelling results in significant decreases in testis weight, atrophy, and epididymis/vas deferens size. However, seminal vesicle/coagulating glands and all the prostate lobes appeared normal in size [2], which was surprising since the prostate has measurable amounts of both ER forms, but no phenotype. Studies using the αERKO and AF2ERKI mouse models have shown that the regulation of the fluid absorption was mediated by the sodium/proton exchanger (NHE3), whose regulation is under control by the AF-1 function of ERα [93, 94]. When observing Esr2KO mice, there were no dramatic differences when compared to WT mice and they were completely fertile. Double-Esr1/Esr2KO mice showed similar physiological changes to the Esr1KO mice, indicating that Esr1 is the dominant and most important ER isoform in male reproductive tissues [2, 92].

Since estrogen seems to have a role in male reproductive physiology, ArKO mice with no endogenous estrogen were also analyzed. Surprisingly, these male mice were completely fertile, and testicular weight was normal when compared to WT mice. Thus, this data suggests that ESR1 needs to be present, but its activity does not appear to require estrogen hormone and may be a physiological example of ligand-independent regulation [2, 92]. More recent studies have shown in other nonreproductive tissues that unliganded ER can contribute to regulation and function and is therefore likely performing similar roles in the reproductive tract of males. The precise reason for such action is unclear, but one speculation is to maintain the functionality of the male system by ER. The only requirement is for the receptor protein itself and the hormone is just a possible supplementation to the activities. But if hormone is not present, then male fertility is able to be sustained.

12 Bone/Skeletal System

Estrogen (E2) has been known to play a key role in the growth, regulation, and maintenance of nonreproductive organs, such as the bone, in both women and men [2, 95]. Multiple studies have confirmed that postmenopausal women and ovariectomized women and female rodents experience significant decreases in bone mass due to the absence of estrogen [2, 96]. Recently, more research has become available involving estrogen and its role in maintaining bone mass in males. Previously, it was thought that androgens were the essential regulator for bone tissue in males. However, it has become known that declining estrogen levels in elderly men have been associated with a decrease in bone mass and are a large predictor for fracture risks [95, 97]. These findings indicate that estrogen plays a major role in maintaining healthy bone in both sexes [95, 98, 99].

Bone is a dynamic tissue that constantly fluctuates as it is turned over, with micro areas of bone loss and formation, for maintenance of skeletal strength in order to sustain mineral supplies. Osteoporosis and the pathology associated with this disease are thought to be a result of an imbalance between bone formation and loss as a dynamic process to preserve a normal amount of bone tissue. Estrogens, vitamin D, calcitonin, and bisphosphates have been used as a therapy to establish and maintain a healthy balance of bone tissue [2].

In male mice, cortical and trabecular peak bone mass was found to be dependent on the activity of both AR and ERα. ERβ, however, appears to have no substantial role in this process [95]. These results were confirmed using ERKO, BERKO, and ERαβERKO ("double" ERKO or DERKO) mice [95, 100]. To further confirm ERα's major role in bone tissue of males, ArKO mice were tested. This mouse phenotype displayed decreased bone mineral density (BMD), even with high circulating androgen levels, and symptoms were reversed upon treatment with estrogen, thus indicating that the synthesis of estrogen hormone through the aromatase pathway is mostly dependent on ERα functionality [100]. Estrogen plays a major role in preventing the increase in bone reabsorption, and both estrogen and testosterone are equally important in maintaining bone formation [96]. When observing distinct regions of ERα using ERαAF-1 and ERαAF-2 mice, it was found that the AF-1 region was crucial for cortical bone growth, but no effect was observed in trabecular bone [95, 97].

In female mice, ERα was found to be essential for cortical and trabecular bone development. The AR can maintain trabecular, but not cortical bone mass. In contrast to males, in females ERβ is reported to have some inhibitory effects on ERα, which was linked to activities in osteoblast cells. ERα is also important for osteoblast lineage and is necessary for cortical bone in female mice. Additionally, ERα regulates mature osteoblasts in female mice. When comparing critical regions for the function of ERα to males, AF-1 was also crucial for cortical bone development but not trabecular bone [2, 96].

13 Brain

From the earliest stages of life, the estrogen receptor affects the brain and its development. The dose and timing of exposure to steroid hormones that a fetus experiences have a major effect on the developing brain. As mentioned earlier in this chapter, the HPG axis and its function are hugely influenced by the types of estrogen receptors present in its respective tissues. In the brain, but outside of the HPG axis, estrogen receptors can be found in many brain regions including the hypothalamus, intralaminar thalamic nuclei, and deep layers of the cerebral cortex. The presence of ER throughout the brain could indicate that it modulates many neural behaviors outside of reproduction [101]. This concept is exemplified in the presence of ER in the hippocampus and how that affects memory. In the study, WT mice, αERKO mice, and βERKO mice were compared at middle age after either hormone deprivation or E2 treatment. After hormone deprivation, αERKO mice exhibited a decrease in the expression of genes associated with the blood-brain barrier. The expression of these genes increased with cyclic E2 treatment, and learning was improved when tested with a water maze. βERKO mice when treated with E2 had a profile comparable to WT mice. However, during hormone deprivation, their learning was preserved when given the water maze challenge. These findings would indicate that ERα and ERβ may be influencing the transcriptional regulation, depending on hormone levels, to maintain memory and function of the hippocampus during aging [102]. A selective effect in the hippocampus from the loss of ERβ has been reported related to anxiety. βERKO females show an age-related increase in anxiety, which has not been reported for αERKO mice [103, 104].

14   Behavior

Changes in behavior due to ER activity have been documented in mice for several decades. In 1979 it was found that castration of male mice at birth results in a feminized adult male that exhibits female behavioral patterns when treated with E2 and progesterone [105]. It is also well known that neonatal testosterone exposure to females can result in a masculinized adult female that exhibits male reproductive behaviors [10]. The characterization of αERKO phenotypic behavior reveals a receptor-mediated role that affects physiological behavior. Gonadotropin-induced progesterone surge following ovulation is imperative for activating the display of lordosis for successful mating. The exhibition of lordosis is unique to female mice and relies on feminization of the brain during development [106]. αERKO female mice do not exhibit lordosis and are not recognized as a potential mate by a stud male. Instead, αERKO females are sometimes attacked as an intruder, most likely due to a result of their abnormally high testosterone levels and to the pheromone effect from stimulation of the clitoral glands. Lordosis can be induced in WT females by treating with E2. However, αERKO females require both a dose of E2 and progesterone to achieve lordosis. Probably, again, due to high serum testosterone levels, αERKO females are often more aggressive and prone to infanticide. Male αERKO mice still exhibited mounting behavior but had reduced levels of intromissions and ejaculations in comparison to the βERKO males which exhibited sexual behavior consistent with WT [107]. By comparison αβERKO males have no sexual mounting response indicating some compensatory activity of the two ER isoforms in maintaining male mounting responses [107]. This is another of the few examples of a unique physiological effect from the loss of both ER signaling systems.

15   Cardiovascular System

Cardiovascular disease (CVD) is the leading cause of death in the United States for both men and women [108, 109]. Estrogen has been identified to have protective effects in the development of CVD, such as atherosclerosis and restenosis [2, 108]. The risk for premenopausal women to develop CVD is significantly lower than for males, even though women have higher risk factors overall such as obesity, diabetes, elevated blood pressure, and plasma cholesterol [2]. Many studies have been performed to confirm the protective effects of estrogen in the cardiovascular system.

Estrogen has been known to decrease proliferation of vascular smooth muscle cells (VSMCs). Over proliferation of VSMCs has been linked to the development of vascular occlusive disease. Additionally, estrogen also regulates vascular endothelial cell growth and in return also attenuates vascular occlusive disease [110]. When observing the specific roles of the estrogen receptors (ERα and ERβ) in protection against CVD, these receptors play different roles. It was found that ERα has a much more significant role in the CVS and is required for protection against CVD. ERα inhibited smooth muscle cell proliferation and vascular thickening when vascular injury occurred. Additionally, ERα promoted reendothelialization, prevented atherosclerosis [111, 112] by inhibiting plaque formation, and was found to contribute in the reduction of circulating cholesterol. ERβ was only found to contribute to regulating peripheral vascular tone and blood pressure [2, 110], while being linked to effects in the heart associated with myocardial hypertrophy [112, 113]. The compilation of CVS studies and effects involving ERα and ERβ suggest that the protective effects of estrogen and ER signaling on the CVS are selectively segregated to ERβ in the heart and ERα to the peripheral vasculature.

In a recent study, unliganded ERα was found to inhibit proliferation and migration of endothelial cells (ECs), promote VSMCs, promote inflammatory effects in ECs and VSMCs in vitro, and regulate expression of many genes involved in vascular cell proliferation, thus indicating that the cardiovascular protective effects of estrogen may be connected to its ability to counteract these effects of unliganded ERα [110]. New reports have shown that nonnuclear estrogen receptor signaling has been a major contributor to the cardiovascular system. Mentioned previously, VSMCs are inhibited upon estrogen treatment. Phosphorylation levels of Akt and extracellular kinase induced by platelet-derived growth factor were significantly inhibited when treated with estrogen in wild-type mice [114]. Estrogen increased complex formation between ERα and phosphatase 2A (PP2), which enhanced PP2A activity. These findings would indicate that rapid nonnuclear ER signaling is involved in estrogen-induced inhibition of VSMC proliferation and PP2A activation by which estrogen mediates antiproliferative effects [108].

In previous studies, estrogen was shown to effectively clear cholesterol from serum blood and consequently reduce the risk of CVD [2]. After menopause, serum low-density lipoprotein (LDL) cholesterol and triglyceride levels rise, and high-density lipoprotein (HDL) cholesterol levels fall [109]. Studies have shown that patients with hypercholesterolemia have a reduction in the protective effects of estrogen on the CVS [115]. According to Umetani et al., 27-hydroxycholesterol (27HC) is the most abundant oxysterol and is used as a measure of cholesterol levels in humans. Interestingly, 27HC displayed competitive antagonistic effects on estrogen receptor action in vascular cells, decreased the estrogen-dependent production of nitrogen oxide synthase (NOS), and repressed reendothelialization in the carotid artery [115]. Endothelial NOS (eNOS) is the primary isoform involved in estrogen-mediated vasodilation. Hence, nitrogen oxide (NO) is critically important for CVS health, as it is produced to increase vasodilation [109, 114]. Liver X receptors (LXR) are stimulated by cholesterol-derived oxysterols and serve as transcription factors to regulate gene expression in response to alterations in cholesterol levels. It has been discovered that LXRβ has nonnuclear functions and stimulates EC migration by activating eNOS. When LXR becomes activated, LXRβ was promoted to the ligand-binding domain of ERα and initiated an extranuclear signaling cascade that required ERα phosphorylation by PI3/AKT. Thus, LXRβ and ERα were found to be dependent with each other for *successful reendothelialization* of the carotid artery [114].

16 Lung

The estrogen receptor and its target tissues are not limited to tissues in primary and secondary reproductive organs or classical endocrine target tissues. Outside of the reproductive tissues and HPG axis, ER is also detectable in bone, cardiovascular system, and regions of the brain. In this section, we evaluate how the ER affects lung tissue. It is known that female sex hormones have some function in modulating lung development [116]. Epidemiological evidence suggests that gender plays a role in the incidence and severity of certain lung diseases. The expression of both forms of ER in the lungs allows for regulatory effects on human lung development in response to neonatal exposure to hormones. Neonatal female mice produce surfactant before their male counterparts. ERα and ERβ are critical for proper respiratory alveolar development. Based on the respiratory phenotype of αERKO, it seems that ERα may play a crucial role in modulating lung function and airway hyperresponsiveness which is the major symptom of asthma and the leading risk factor for chronic obstructive pulmonary disease (COPD) [117]. When compared to their wild-type littermates, αERKO mice have multiple lung abnormalities, increased airway responsiveness, and significant reduction in breathing frequency. This finding may help explain the increased incidence of sleep apnea in postmenopausal women and the positive corrective effect of hormone replacement therapy. Hyperresponsive airways in αERKO mice are attributed to defects in the airway smooth muscle. The publication of studies linking hormone signaling and lung cancer began to uncover a relationship between ER and cancer prognosis. It was shown by Kawai et al. [118] that ERα expression in a tumor and the absence of ERβ expression were negative prognostic factors in non-small-cell lung cancer. Although still controversial, evidence suggests that circulating female hormones may play a role in decreasing hormone receptor-positive lung tumor growth [119].

17 Immune System

A connection between reproduction and immunology was not reported until 1898 [120]. Today the hypothesis that reproductive and immune system interactions are regulated by gonadal steroids estrogen, androgen, and progesterone is well supported [121]. Clinical and experimental studies have concluded the following observations in support of this hypothesis: there is a sexual dimorphism in immunity, the change in immune response after a gonadectomy and sex steroid hormone replacement, the change in immune response during pregnancy due to altered sex steroid production, and the specific receptors for gonadal steroid hormones are found in organs of the immune system [121].

Estrogens specifically contribute a significant role in immunity. For example, estradiol-induced antibody production appears to be due to estradiol's ability to inhibit suppressor T-cell activity, hence allowing B-cells to mature and produce antibodies [122]. Furthermore, estrogenic compounds such as diethylstilbestrol (DES) can compromise immune status. Neonatal exposure to DES results in decreased antibody production in adult female mice due to a DES-induced developmental halt of T-helper cell production [123]. Immunomodulatory actions are also observed with E2 and xenoestrogens due to an inhibitory capacity of chemoattractant cytokine production in MCF-7 cells [124]. In relation to gender and age, comparable amounts of ER expression are found in thymocytes of young, middle-aged, and old female and male mice [125]. However, in vivo analysis of ER in thymocytes has demonstrated male mice lack the E2-induced creatine kinase activity that is observed in females [125]. Although ER expression in thymocytes did not decline with age, the same study showed that E2 activity only contributes to thymocytopoiesis of young donor-derived thymocytes, suggesting a difference of ER functionality in immunity throughout aging.

18 Gastrointestinal Tract (GI)

Conditions associated with reduced estrogen in women, such as late puberty onset [126], older menopause, and nulliparity, are associated with cystic bowel disease [127], colon carcinoma [128], and an increased risk of gastric carcinoma [129]. A retrospective study found a lower incidence of gastric cancer in men who received exogenous estrogen treatment for prostate cancer compared to non-estrogen-treated men of the same age and population [130]. Thus, although controversial, estrogen appears to have some protective role against gastric cancer. In addition, intracellular

E2 presence was confirmed in cancerous gastric cells, and an absence was confirmed in non-cancerous gastric cells [131]. Although a malignant function of ER in gastric adenocarcinoma is contentious, cathepsin D, an E2-regulated lysosomal protease, has been associated with a tumor-progressive role in diffuse-type gastric carcinoma [132]. Compared to ERα, only ERβ is detected in gastric adenocarcinomas and non-cancerous gastric mucosa Hence, E2 is suggested to mediate its effects through ERβ in the gastric mucosa [133].

As seen with gastric and esophageal cancer, colorectal cancer appears to be more prevalent in men compared to women [88]. Compared to ERα, ERβ is reportedly more abundant in colonic epithelium and thought to be responsible for inhibiting estrogen-induced proliferation and inhibiting malignant transformation of the colonic mucosa [134]. Another cancer-inhibitory function of ERβ in the colon is induction of apoptosis, which has been proposed through mechanisms including increased DNA fragmentation, p53 signaling initiation, involving caspase-dependent pro-apoptotic cascade initiation [135]. Experimental studies with ERKO mice have indicated a role of ERα in colon cancer models [136].

Compared to women, men with Barrett's esophagus are twice as likely to progress to invasive carcinoma [137]. Furthermore, while ERβ is expressed in esophageal adenocarcinoma and Barrett's esophagus cells, it is significantly overexpressed in esophageal adenocarcinoma compared to its precursor, Barret's metaplasia [138]. Still, an epidemiological study showed no relationship between hormonal treatment (increased E2 and decreased testosterone) and a reduced risk to developing esophageal adenocarcinoma in males [126]. Hence, a protective estrogen effect on esophageal cancer was not confirmed. In regard to gallbladder cancer, this rare condition, like other sexually dimorphic conditions, is more prevalent in women compared to men [139]. Malignant properties such as metastatic potential, tumor progression, and poor prognosis of gallbladder cancer have been correlated with a lack of ERβ expression [39]. Therapeutic implications for a role for ERβ in gallbladder cancers, however, remain understudied and inconclusive at the present time.

19   Estrogen Effects on Metabolic Regulation

The consequences from the loss of either estrogen or ERα activity can be seen from the phenotypes of the *Cyp19* (aromatase) knockout (KO) mice unable to synthesize E2 from androgen precursors or the αERKO mice. Treatment of *Cyp19*KO mice with exogenous E2 restores the E2 protective effect in both male and female mice against the development of metabolic syndrome [140]. Studies using the estrogen receptor (ERα and ERβ) knockout mice have demonstrated that ERα plays a more essential role in estrogen-mediated metabolic regulation than ERβ [141]. Metabolic phenotypes of αERKO females have been shown as obese, with impaired glucose tolerance (IGT) and insulin resistance [142]. They have significant fat deposition of gonadal and inguinal white adipose tissues compared to wild-type (WT) littermates, but such differences are not observed in perirenal white fat and brown adipose tissue. Increases are also detected in both adipocyte volume and adipocyte number in gonadal and inguinal fat [142]. βERKO mice of both sexes are not obese or insulin resistant compared to wild type [143]. These observations suggested that ERα is involved in the adipogenesis; however, the precise mechanisms responsible for ERα-dependent regulation remain unclear. Energy intake was equal and appears not to be a cause, but in contrast, energy expenditure was reduced in αERKO compared with WT, thereby suggesting that loss of ERα and the obesity may be occurring through altered energy expenditure [142].

Other forms of ERα mutants have been used to identify functional signaling activity to metabolic regulation. ERα DNA-binding domain mutant mice (KIKO) were analyzed to characterize the non-genomic and indirect DNA-binding transcription-mediated metabolic regulations [144, 145]. KIKO mice had a restoration of metabolic parameters dysregulated in αERKO mice to normal values when put on high fat diet, suggesting that the nonclassical ERα signaling rescues body weight and metabolic function. Normalization of energy expenditure, including voluntary locomotor activity, would indicate nonclassical ERα signaling can normalize metabolic regulation [144]. However, when on a higher fat diet, the metabolic phenotypes of KIKO females were identical with αERKO females [145]. The phenotypes of KIKO mice suggest that the nonclassical ERα signaling could be a potential target for selective modulation of ERα-mediated metabolic regulation.

The two transactivation functions of ERα have also been evaluated using the deleted ERα AF-1 (ERaAF-1°) or ERα AF-2 (ERaAF-2°) [146]. ERaAF-2° females presented with obesity, IGT, and insulin resistance, similar to αERKO females. In contrast, ERaAF-1° mice had metabolic phenotypes identical to WT. Estrogen administration protected ERaAF-1° and WT mice, whereas the estrogen treatment was totally abrogated in ERaAF-2° and αERKO mice. Thus, use of these models indicates that the protective effect of estrogen against obesity and insulin resistance is selectively ERα AF-2 dependent but not AF-1 [146]. As described, various functional domains of ERα contribute to differential estrogen-mediated metabolic regulations. Further studies with tissue-specific analyses have implicated ERα activity in muscle is regulating energy metabolism through mitochondrial actions [147]. Future development of ERα functional domain selective regulators may be a therapeutic approach to reduce the risks of obesity and metabolic disturbances in postmenopausal women without appreciable side effects.

20 Clinical Cases of Disrupted Estrogen Receptor Signaling

ER gene mutations were thought to be lethal until a 28-year-old male patient with estrogen resistance was identified and described and underwent studies revealing he carried a homozygous nonsense C157T mutation in exon 2 of the ERα gene (*ESR1*) resulting in a premature stop codon and the lack of synthesis of ERα protein [148]. This patient experienced typical pubertal development, was normally masculinized, and had normal serum testosterone concentrations, but low sperm viability. His main phenotypes were osteopenia, incomplete epiphyseal closure, a tall stature (204 cm), and abnormal gonadotropin secretion [148]. He had impaired glucose tolerance and hyperinsulinemia and compromised endothelial vasodilatory responsiveness [149]. He showed no signs of estrogen response after receiving high-dose transdermal estrogen for 6 months. These main phenotypes are all in accordance with the *Esr1* knockout mouse model described earlier in this chapter.

Male patients with androgen insensitivity syndrome (AIS) with corresponding mutations in the androgen receptor gene have helped characterize androgen resistance in humans [150]. Up until 2013, sex steroid insensitivity had been studied more heavily in men than women due to its clinical prevalence. The male patient with a mutation in the estrogen receptor gene (ESR1) was the only clue of non-lethality, but how the disruption of this receptor protein may affect women was unknown. Not until the discovery of an 18-year-old female with delayed puberty and a different homozygous missense mutation in the ligand-binding domain of *ESR1* that estrogen insensitivity in a woman could be properly clinically characterized. The mutation (Q375H) changed a neutral polar glutamine to a basic polar histidine leading to the apparent inability of the hormone to be bound by the receptor [151].

The presentation of multiple severe symptoms following delayed puberty since the age of 15 was the cause for medical consultation leading to the discovery of the Q mutation. At the time of detection, the patient was 18 years of age and reported experiencing intermittent lower abdominal pain, primary amenorrhea, Tanner stage 1 breast development, Tanner stage 4 pubic hair development, severe facial acne, and astronomically high serum E2 levels (3500 pg/mL). Upon further examination, it was discovered that she had a small uterus with no endometrial stripe as well as enlarged multicystic ovaries. Her growth chart revealed lack of an estrogen-induced growth spurt at the time of puberty and radial and ulnar epiphyseal plates that remained unfused. These signs were all consistent with estrogen insensitivity.

In attempt to induce breast development, exogenous estrogen in the form of conjugated equine estrogen and micronized estradiol were then administered orally to the patient. After 3 months of a standard dose and 2 months of an increased dose, her breasts remained at Tanner stage 1 so she was then treated with norethindrone only for 5 months. This resulted in a drop in her serum estradiol level from 3500 pg/mL at the time of detection to 114 pg/mL. Her ovaries and ovarian cysts reduced in size indicating that her progesterone receptor was likely functional. When treatment was discontinued, her ovaries returned to their enlarged and cystic state. She also took 25 µg of levothyroxine for mild hypothyroidism. The levothyroxine treatment did not influence the presence or size of her ovarian cysts or high estrogen and estrone levels but did indicate that thyroid function was normal via thyroid function testing.

This case was instrumental to the characterization of ERα mutations in women and how subsequent estrogen insensitivity can affect female patients. The study identified a highly conserved glutamine residue in the ligand-binding domain. It also demonstrated that negative feedback in the hypothalamus and pituitary is consistent with the αERKO mouse and regulation principally by ERα and not ERβ due to the fact that the patient's ERβ was unaffected by the mutation. An in vitro cell-based analysis of the mutant receptor showed no effect on nuclear localization but did show markedly impaired estrogen gene transcriptional signaling [151].

The final example is quite unusual and involves a familial case of two sisters and one brother with estrogen insensitivity which has been reported, revealing they each carried a homozygous missense R394H mutation which occurred through an autosomal recessive mode of transmission in the ligand-binding domain of *ESR1*. The mutation resulted in significantly reduced ERα transcriptional activity and a proposed effect of this mutant receptors' inability to anchor estradiol in the ligand-binding pocket, its main activating hormone. When tested for a possible therapeutic treatment, other ERα activating ligands, such as ethinyl estradiol, DES, and raloxifene, did not overcome the estrogen insensitivity in R394H ERα in vitro. An alternative therapeutic approach the authors proposed to activate R394H ERα is the use of transcriptional coactivator small molecules that could potentially stabilize the defective ligand-receptor complex [152].

The eldest sister of the affected siblings, 25 years old at the time of the study, was of normal stature; experienced primary amenorrhea, Tanner stage 1 breast development, mild adipomastia, chest acne, enlarged multicystic ovaries, and a small uterus with a thin endometrium; and had a history of intrauterine growth restriction. The younger affected sister, 21 years old at the time of the study, also experienced similar clinical effects such as primary amenorrhea, enlarged multicystic ovaries, and Tanner stage 1 breast development. As opposed to her older affected sister, she was tall (175 cm) and had a normal birth weight. The affected brother, 18 years old, had normal stature, Tanner stage 1 gonadal development, a cryptorchid right testis, and an underdeveloped left testis. All affected siblings had elevated levels of 17β estradiol, luteinizing hormone (LH), and follicle-stimulating hormone (FSH). The affected brother had low levels of dehydroepiandrosterone sulfate and testosterone. Both affected sisters had normal levels of dehydroepiandrosterone sulfate and high levels of testosterone [152].

The parents of this family of patients were both heterozygous carriers of the respective estrogen receptor mutation. Abnormalities shown by these patients further demonstrate estrogen's essential role in skeletal development and mineralization during puberty in both females and males. They also further illustrate the critical role of negative estrogen feedback on gonadotropin levels and regulation in both sexes and ovarian cyst formation in females. Most clearly, all cases so far reported of estrogen receptor insensitivity or resistance, the patients all arose from consanguineous pairings. Such a relationship may be one explanation for the clinical rarity of this condition. As heterozygous carriers, the parents are fertile and have no apparent dysfunctions, similar to the experimental models, although it raises the possibility that more clinical examples of ER mutations may be present in the population. Combinatorial studies will need to be done in order to assess the clinical and physiological consequences of multiple different mutations of the estrogen receptors.

References

1. Jensen EV, Jacobson HI (1962) Basic guides to the mechanism of estrogen action. Recent Prog Horm Res 18:387–414
2. Couse JF, Korach KS (1999) Estrogen receptor null mice: what have we learned and where will they lead us? Endocr Rev 20(3):358–417
3. Hewitt SC, Korach KS (2018) Estrogen receptors: new directions in the new millennium. Endocr Rev. https://doi.org/10.1210/er.2018-00087
4. Cui J, Shen Y, Li R (2013) Estrogen synthesis and signaling pathways during aging: from periphery to brain. Trends Mol Med 19(3):197–209. https://doi.org/10.1016/j.molmed.2012.12.007
5. Aranda A, Pascual A (2001) Nuclear hormone receptors and gene expression. Physiol Rev 81(3):1269–1304
6. Gibson DA, Saunders PT (2012) Estrogen dependent signaling in reproductive tissues - a role for estrogen receptors and estrogen related receptors. Mol Cell Endocrinol 348(2):361–372
7. Hewitt SC, Winuthayanon W, Korach KS (2016) What's new in estrogen receptor action in the female reproductive tract. J Mol Endocrinol 56(2):R55–R71. https://doi.org/10.1530/JME-15-0254
8. McEwan IJ (2016) The nuclear receptor superfamily at thirty. Methods Mol Biol 1443:3–9. https://doi.org/10.1007/978-1-4939-3724-0_1
9. Lubahn DB, Moyer JS, Golding TS, Couse JF, Korach KS, Smithies O (1993) Alteration of reproductive function but not prenatal sexual development after insertional disruption of the mouse estrogen receptor gene. Proc Natl Acad Sci U S A 90(23):11162–11166
10. Krege JH, Hodgin JB, Couse JF, Enmark E, Warner M, Mahler JF, Sar M, Korach KS, Gustafsson JA, Smithies O (1998) Generation and reproductive phenotypes of mice lacking estrogen receptor beta. Proc Natl Acad Sci U S A 95(26):15677–15682
11. Couse JF, Hewitt SC, Bunch DO, Sar M, Walker VR, Davis BJ, Korach KS (1999) Postnatal sex reversal of the ovaries in mice lacking estrogen receptors alpha and beta. Science 286(5448):2328–2331
12. Dupont S, Krust A, Gansmuller A, Dierich A, Chambon P, Mark M (2000) Effect of single and compound knockouts of estrogen receptors alpha (ERalpha) and beta (ERbeta) on mouse reproductive phenotypes. Development 127(19):4277–4291
13. Hamilton KJ, Arao Y, Korach KS (2014) Estrogen hormone physiology: reproductive findings from estrogen receptor mutant mice. Reprod Biol 14(1):3–8. https://doi.org/10.1016/j.repbio.2013.12.002
14. Jakacka M, Ito M, Martinson F, Ishikawa T, Lee EJ, Jameson JL (2002) An estrogen receptor (ER)alpha deoxyribonucleic acid-binding domain knock-in mutation provides evidence for nonclassical ER pathway signaling in vivo. Mol Endocrinol (Baltimore, MD) 16(10):2188–2201
15. Ahlbory-Dieker DL, Stride BD, Leder G, Schkoldow J, Trolenberg S, Seidel H, Otto C, Sommer A, Parker MG, Schutz G, Wintermantel TM (2009) DNA binding by estrogen receptor-alpha is essential for the transcriptional response to estrogen in the liver and the uterus. Mol Endocrinol 23(10):1544–1555. https://doi.org/10.1210/me.2009-0045
16. Sinkevicius KW, Burdette JE, Woloszyn K, Hewitt SC, Hamilton K, Sugg SL, Temple KA, Wondisford FE, Korach KS, Woodruff TK, Greene GL (2008) An estrogen receptor-alpha knock-in mutation provides evidence of ligand-independent signaling and allows modulation of ligand-induced pathways in vivo. Endocrinology 149(6):2970–2979. https://doi.org/10.1210/en.2007-1526
17. Billon-Gales A, Krust A, Fontaine C, Abot A, Flouriot G, Toutain C, Berges H, Gadeau AP, Lenfant F, Gourdy P, Chambon P, Arnal JF (2011) Activation function 2 (AF2) of estrogen receptor-alpha is required for the atheroprotective action of estradiol but not to accelerate endothelial healing. Proc Natl Acad Sci U S A 108(32):13311–13316. https://doi.org/10.1073/pnas.1105632108

18. Billon-Gales A, Fontaine C, Filipe C, Douin-Echinard V, Fouque MJ, Flouriot G, Gourdy P, Lenfant F, Laurell H, Krust A, Chambon P, Arnal JF (2009) The transactivating function 1 of estrogen receptor alpha is dispensable for the vasculoprotective actions of 17beta-estradiol. Proc Natl Acad Sci U S A 106(6):2053–2058. https://doi.org/10.1073/pnas.0808742106

19. Stefkovich ML, Arao Y, Hamilton KJ, Korach KS (2017) Experimental models for evaluating non-genomic estrogen signaling. Steroids. https://doi.org/10.1016/j.steroids.2017.11.001

20. Jabbour HN, Kelly RW, Fraser HM, Critchley HO (2006) Endocrine regulation of menstruation. Endocr Rev 27(1):17–46. https://doi.org/10.1210/er.2004-0021

21. Wang H, Dey SK (2006) Roadmap to embryo implantation: clues from mouse models. Nat Rev 7(3):185–199. https://doi.org/10.1038/nrg1808

22. Teixeira J, Rueda BR, Pru JK (2008) Uterine stem cells. In: StemBook. Harvard Stem Cell Institute, Cambridge. https://doi.org/10.3824/stembook.1.16.1

23. Blesson CS, Masironi B, Sahlin L (2012) Effects of selective estrogen receptor agonists on estrogen receptor expression in the uterus of ovariectomized rats. Open J Mol Integrative Physiol 2(2):9. https://doi.org/10.4236/ojmip.2012.22006

24. Diel P, Schmidt S, Vollmer G (2002) In vivo test systems for the quantitative and qualitative analysis of the biological activity of phytoestrogens. J Chromatogr B Analyt Technol Biomed Life Sci 777(1–2):191–202

25. Couse JF, Curtis SW, Washburn TF, Lindzey J, Golding TS, Lubahn DB, Smithies O, Korach KS (1995) Analysis of transcription and estrogen insensitivity in the female mouse after targeted disruption of the estrogen receptor gene. Mol Endocrinol 9:1441–1454

26. Hewitt SC, Kissling GE, Fieselman KE, Jayes FL, Gerrish KE, Korach KS (2010) Biological and biochemical consequences of global deletion of exon 3 from the ER alpha gene. FASEB J 24(12):4660–4667. https://doi.org/10.1096/fj.10-163428

27. Cooke PS, Buchanan DL, Young P, Setiawan T, Brody J, Korach KS, Taylor J, Lubahn DB, Cunha GR (1997) Stromal estrogen receptors mediate mitogenic effects of estradiol on uterine epithelium. Proc Natl Acad Sci U S A 94(12):6535–6540

28. Winuthayanon W, Hewitt SC, Orvis GD, Behringer RR, Korach KS (2010) Uterine epithelial estrogen receptor alpha is dispensable for proliferation but essential for complete biological and biochemical responses. Proc Natl Acad Sci U S A 107(45):19272–19277. https://doi.org/10.1073/pnas.1013226107

29. Winuthayanon W, Lierz SL, Delarosa KC, Sampels SR, Donoghue LJ, Hewitt SC, Korach KS (2017) Juxtacrine activity of estrogen receptor alpha in uterine stromal cells is necessary for estrogen-induced epithelial cell proliferation. Sci Rep 7(1):8377. https://doi.org/10.1038/s41598-017-07728-1

30. Hewitt SC, Li L, Grimm SA, Winuthayanon W, Hamilton KJ, Pockette B, Rubel CA, Pedersen LC, Fargo D, Lanz RB, DeMayo FJ, Schutz G, Korach KS (2014) Novel DNA motif binding activity observed in vivo with an estrogen receptor alpha mutant mouse. Mol Endocrinol 28(6):899–911. https://doi.org/10.1210/me.2014-1051

31. Billon-Gales A, Fontaine C, Filipe C, Douin-Echinard V, Fouque MJ, Flouriot G, Gourdy P, Lenfant F, Laurell H, Krust A, Chambon P, Arnal JF (2009) The transactivating function 1 of estrogen receptor alpha is dispensable for the vasculoprotective actions of 17 beta-estradiol. Proc Natl Acad Sci U S A 106(6):2053–2058. https://doi.org/10.1073/pnas.0808742106

32. Abot A, Fontaine C, Raymond-Letron I, Flouriot G, Adlanmerini M, Buscato M, Otto C, Berges H, Laurell H, Gourdy P, Lenfant F, Arnal JF (2013) The AF-1 activation function of estrogen receptor alpha is necessary and sufficient for uterine epithelial cell proliferation in vivo. Endocrinology 154(6):2222–2233. https://doi.org/10.1210/en.2012-2059

33. Arao Y, Hamilton KJ, Ray MK, Scott G, Mishina Y, Korach KS (2011) Estrogen receptor alpha AF-2 mutation results in antagonist reversal and reveals tissue selective function of estrogen receptor modulators. Proc Natl Acad Sci U S A 108(36):14986–14991. https://doi.org/10.1073/pnas.1109180108

34. Adlanmerini M, Solinhac R, Abot A, Fabre A, Raymond-Letron I, Guihot AL, Boudou F, Sautier L, Vessieres E, Kim SH, Liere P, Fontaine C, Krust A, Chambon P, Katzenellenbogen

JA, Gourdy P, Shaul PW, Henrion D, Arnal JF, Lenfant F (2014) Mutation of the palmitoylation site of estrogen receptor alpha in vivo reveals tissue-specific roles for membrane versus nuclear actions. Proc Natl Acad Sci U S A 111(2):E283–E290. https://doi.org/10.1073/pnas.1322057111

35. Pedram A, Razandi M, Lewis M, Hammes S, Levin ER (2014) Membrane-localized estrogen receptor alpha is required for normal organ development and function. Dev Cell 29(4):482–490. https://doi.org/10.1016/j.devcel.2014.04.016

36. Gustafsson KL, Farman H, Henning P, Lionikaite V, Moverare-Skrtic S, Wu J, Ryberg H, Koskela A, Gustafsson JA, Tuukkanen J, Levin ER, Ohlsson C, Lagerquist MK (2016) The role of membrane ERalpha signaling in bone and other major estrogen responsive tissues. Sci Rep 6:29473. https://doi.org/10.1038/srep29473

37. Pedram A, Razandi M, Kim JK, O'Mahony F, Lee EYHP, Luderer U, Levin ER (2009) Developmental phenotype of a membrane only estrogen receptor alpha(MOER) mouse. J Biol Chem 284(6):3488–3495

38. Smith DC, Prentice R, Thompson DJ, Herrmann WL (1975) Association of exogenous estrogen and endometrial carcinoma. N Engl J Med 293(23):1164–1167. https://doi.org/10.1056/NEJM197512042932302

39. Sumi K, Matsuyama S, Kitajima Y, Miyazaki K (2004) Loss of estrogen receptor beta expression at cancer front correlates with tumor progression and poor prognosis of gallbladder cancer. Oncol Rep 12(5):979–984

40. Bodner K, Bodner-Adler B, Kimberger O, Czerwenka K, Leodolter S, Mayerhofer K (2003) Estrogen and progesterone receptor expression in patients with uterine leiomyosarcoma and correlation with different clinicopathological parameters. Anticancer Res 23(1B):729–732

41. Kelley TW, Borden EC, Goldblum JR (2004) Estrogen and progesterone receptor expression in uterine and extrauterine leiomyosarcomas: an immunohistochemical study. Appl Immunohistochem Mol Morphol 12(4):338–341

42. Leitao MM Jr, Hensley ML, Barakat RR, Aghajanian C, Gardner GJ, Jewell EL, O'Cearbhaill R, Soslow RA (2012) Immunohistochemical expression of estrogen and progesterone receptors and outcomes in patients with newly diagnosed uterine leiomyosarcoma. Gynecol Oncol 124(3):558–562. https://doi.org/10.1016/j.ygyno.2011.11.009

43. Leitao MM, Soslow RA, Nonaka D, Olshen AB, Aghajanian C, Sabbatini P, Dupont J, Hensley M, Sonoda Y, Barakat RR, Anderson S (2004) Tissue microarray immunohistochemical expression of estrogen, progesterone, and androgen receptors in uterine leiomyomata and leiomyosarcoma. Cancer 101(6):1455–1462. https://doi.org/10.1002/cncr.20521

44. Wik E, Raeder MB, Krakstad C, Trovik J, Birkeland E, Hoivik EA, Mjos S, Werner HM, Mannelqvist M, Stefansson IM, Oyan AM, Kalland KH, Akslen LA, Salvesen HB (2013) Lack of estrogen receptor-alpha is associated with epithelial-mesenchymal transition and PI3K alterations in endometrial carcinoma. Clin Cancer Res 19(5):1094–1105. https://doi.org/10.1158/1078-0432.CCR-12-3039

45. Osborne CK, Hobbs K, Clark GM (1985) Effect of estrogens and antiestrogens on growth of human breast cancer cells in athymic nude mice. Cancer Res 45(2):584–590

46. Kedar RP, Bourne TH, Powles TJ, Collins WP, Ashley SE, Cosgrove DO, Campbell S (1994) Effects of tamoxifen on uterus and ovaries of postmenopausal women in a randomised breast cancer prevention trial. Lancet 343(8909):1318–1321

47. Droog M, Nevedomskaya E, Dackus GM, Fles R, Kim Y, Hollema H, Mourits MJ, Nederlof PM, van Boven HH, Linn SC, van Leeuwen FE, Wessels LF, Zwart W (2017) Estrogen receptor alpha wields treatment-specific enhancers between morphologically similar endometrial tumors. Proc Natl Acad Sci U S A 114(8):E1316–E1325. https://doi.org/10.1073/pnas.1615233114

48. Asante A, Taylor RN (2011) Endometriosis: the role of neuroangiogenesis. Annu Rev Physiol 73:163–182. https://doi.org/10.1146/annurev-physiol-012110-142158

49. Bulun SE (2009) Endometriosis. N Engl J Med 360(3):268–279

50. Giudice LC (2010) Clinical practice. Endometriosis. N Engl J Med 362(25):2389–2398. https://doi.org/10.1056/NEJMcp1000274
51. Han SJ, Hawkins SM, Begum K, Jung SY, Kovanci E, Qin J, Lydon JP, DeMayo FJ, O'Malley BW (2012) A new isoform of steroid receptor coactivator-1 is crucial for pathogenic progression of endometriosis. Nat Med 18(7):1102–1111. https://doi.org/10.1038/nm.2826
52. Bulun SE, Monsavais D, Pavone ME, Dyson M, Xue Q, Attar E, Tokunaga H, Su EJ (2012) Role of estrogen receptor-beta in endometriosis. Semin Reprod Med 30(1):39–45. https://doi.org/10.1055/s-0031-1299596
53. Trukhacheva E, Lin Z, Reierstad S, Cheng YH, Milad M, Bulun SE (2009) Estrogen receptor (ER) beta regulates ERalpha expression in stromal cells derived from ovarian endometriosis. J Clin Endocrinol Metab 94(2):615–622. https://doi.org/10.1210/jc.2008-1466
54. Xue Q, Lin Z, Cheng YH, Huang CC, Marsh E, Yin P, Milad MP, Confino E, Reierstad S, Innes J, Bulun SE (2007) Promoter methylation regulates estrogen receptor 2 in human endometrium and endometriosis. Biol Reprod 77(4):681–687. https://doi.org/10.1095/biolreprod.107.061804
55. Hirata T, Osuga Y, Yoshino O, Hirota Y, Harada M, Takemura Y, Morimoto C, Koga K, Yano T, Tsutsumi O, Taketani Y (2005) Development of an experimental model of endometriosis using mice that ubiquitously express green fluorescent protein. Hum Reprod 20(8):2092–2096. https://doi.org/10.1093/humrep/dei012
56. Burns KA, Rodriguez KF, Hewitt SC, Janardhan KS, Young SL, Korach KS (2012) Role of estrogen receptor signaling required for endometriosis-like lesion establishment in a mouse model. Endocrinology 153(8):3960–3971. https://doi.org/10.1210/en.2012-1294
57. Zhao Y, Gong P, Chen Y, Nwachukwu JC, Srinivasan S, Ko C, Bagchi MK, Taylor RN, Korach KS, Nettles KW, Katzenellenbogen JA, Katzenellenbogen BS (2015) Dual suppression of estrogenic and inflammatory activities for targeting of endometriosis. Sci Transl Med 7(271):271ra279. https://doi.org/10.1126/scitranslmed.3010626
58. De Angelis M, Stossi F, Carlson KA, Katzenellenbogen BS, Katzenellenbogen JA (2005) Indazole estrogens: highly selective ligands for the estrogen receptor beta. J Med Chem 48(4):1132–1144. https://doi.org/10.1021/jm049223g
59. Nettles KW, Bruning JB, Gil G, Nowak J, Sharma SK, Hahm JB, Kulp K, Hochberg RB, Zhou H, Katzenellenbogen JA, Katzenellenbogen BS, Kim Y, Joachmiak A, Greene GL (2008) NFkappaB selectivity of estrogen receptor ligands revealed by comparative crystallographic analyses. Nat Chem Biol 4(4):241–247. https://doi.org/10.1038/nchembio.76
60. Saijo K, Collier JG, Li AC, Katzenellenbogen JA, Glass CK (2011) An ADIOL-ERbeta-CtBP transrepression pathway negatively regulates microglia-mediated inflammation. Cell 145(4):584–595. https://doi.org/10.1016/j.cell.2011.03.050
61. Zhou HB, Comninos JS, Stossi F, Katzenellenbogen BS, Katzenellenbogen JA (2005) Synthesis and evaluation of estrogen receptor ligands with bridged oxabicyclic cores containing a diarylethylene motif: estrogen antagonists of unusual structure. J Med Chem 48(23):7261–7274. https://doi.org/10.1021/jm0506773
62. Sar M, Welsch F (1999) Differential expression of estrogen receptor-beta and estrogen receptor-alpha in the rat ovary. Endocrinology 140(2):963–971
63. Couse JF, Yates MM, Sanford R, Nyska A, Nilson JH, Korach KS (2004) Formation of cystic ovarian follicles associated with elevated luteinizing hormone requires estrogen receptor-beta. Endocrinology 145(10):4693–4702
64. Lindzey J, Jayes FL, Yates MM, Couse JF, Korach KS (2006) The bi-modal effects of estradiol on gonadotropin synthesis and secretion in female mice are dependent on estrogen receptor-alpha. J Endocrinol 191(1):309–317
65. Schomberg DW, Couse JF, Mukherjee A, Lubahn DB, Sar M, Mayo KE, Korach KS (1999) Targeted disruption of the estrogen receptor-alpha gene in female mice: characterization of ovarian responses and phenotype in the adult. Endocrinology 140(6):2733–2744
66. Couse JF, Yates MM, Walker VR, Korach KS (2003) Characterization of the hypothalamic-pituitary-gonadal axis in estrogen receptor (ER) Null mice reveals hypergonadism and

endocrine sex reversal in females lacking ERalpha but not ERbeta. Mol Endocrinol 17(6):1039–1053. https://doi.org/10.1210/me.2002-0398

67. Emmen JM, Couse JF, Elmore SA, Yates MM, Kissling GE, Korach KS (2005) In vitro growth and ovulation of follicles from ovaries of estrogen receptor (ER){alpha} and ER{beta} null mice indicate a role for ER{beta} in follicular maturation. Endocrinology 146(6):2817–2826

68. Couse JF, Bunch DO, Lindzey J, Schomberg DW, Korach KS (1999) Prevention of the polycystic ovarian phenotype and characterization of ovulatory capacity in the estrogen receptor-alpha knockout mouse. Endocrinology 140(12):5855–5865

69. Rosenfeld CS, Murray AA, Simmer G, Hufford MG, Smith MF, Spears N, Lubahn DB (2000) Gonadotropin induction of ovulation and corpus luteum formation in young estrogen receptor-alpha knockout mice. Biol Reprod 62(3):599–605

70. Bridges PJ, Koo Y, Kang D-W, Hudgins-Spivey S, Lan Z-J, Xu X, DeMayo F, Cooney A, Ko C (2008) Generation of Cyp17iCre transgenic mice and their application to conditionally delete estrogen receptor alpha (Esr1) from the ovary and testis. Genesis 46(9):499–505. https://doi.org/10.1002/dvg.20428

71. O'Brien JE, Peterson TJ, Tong MH, Lee EJ, Pfaff LE, Hewitt SC, Korach KS, Weiss J, Jameson JL (2006) Estrogen-induced proliferation of uterine epithelial cells is independent of estrogen receptor alpha binding to classical estrogen response elements. J Biol Chem 281(36):26683–26692. https://doi.org/10.1074/jbc.M601522200

72. Cheng G, Weihua Z, Makinen S, Makela S, Saji S, Warner M, Gustafsson JA, Hovatta O (2002) A role for the androgen receptor in follicular atresia of estrogen receptor beta knockout mouse ovary. Biol Reprod 66(1):77–84

73. Antal MC, Krust A, Chambon P, Mark M (2008) Sterility and absence of histopathological defects in nonreproductive organs of a mouse ERbeta-null mutant. Proc Natl Acad Sci U S A 105(7):2433–2438. https://doi.org/10.1073/pnas.0712029105

74. Couse JF, Yates MM, Deroo BJ, Korach KS (2005) Estrogen receptor-beta is critical to granulosa cell differentiation and the ovulatory response to gonadotropins. Endocrinology 146(8):3247–3262

75. Deroo BJ, Rodriguez KF, Couse JF, Hamilton KJ, Collins JB, Grissom SF, Korach KS (2009) Estrogen receptor beta is required for optimal cAMP production in mouse granulosa cells. Mol Endocrinol 23(7):955–965. https://doi.org/10.1210/me.2008-0213

76. Jayes FL, Burns KA, Rodriguez KF, Kissling GE, Korach KS (2014) The naturally occurring luteinizing hormone surge is diminished in mice lacking estrogen receptor beta in the ovary. Biol Reprod 90(2):24. https://doi.org/10.1095/biolreprod.113.113316

77. Rodriguez KF, Couse JF, Jayes FL, Hamilton KJ, Burns KA, Taniguchi F, Korach KS (2010) Insufficient luteinizing hormone-induced intracellular signaling disrupts ovulation in preovulatory follicles lacking estrogen receptor-{beta}. Endocrinology 151(6):2826–2834. https://doi.org/10.1210/en.2009-1446

78. Mori T, Nagasawa H, Bern HA (1979) Long-term effects of perinatal exposure to hormones on normal and neoplastic mammary growth in rodents: a review. J Environ Pathol Toxicol 3(1–2):191–205

79. Bocchinfuso WP, Korach KS (1997) Mammary gland development and tumorigenesis in estrogen receptor knockout mice. J Mammary Gland Biol Neoplasia 2(4):323–334

80. Arendt LM, Kuperwasser C (2015) Form and function: how estrogen and progesterone regulate the mammary epithelial hierarchy. J Mammary Gland Biol Neoplasia 20(1–2):9–25. https://doi.org/10.1007/s10911-015-9337-0

81. Bocchinfuso WP, Lindzey JK, Hewitt SC, Clark JA, Myers PH, Cooper R, Korach KS (2000) Induction of mammary gland development in estrogen receptor-alpha knockout mice. Endocrinology 141(8):2982–2994

82. Chauchereau A, Savouret JF, Milgrom E (1992) Control of biosynthesis and posttranscriptional modification of the progesterone receptor. Biol Reprod 46(2):174–177

83. Conneely OM, Lydon JP (2000) Progesterone receptors in reproduction: functional impact of the A and B isoforms. Steroids 65(10–11):571–577

84. Li S, Han B, Liu G, Li S, Ouellet J, Labrie F, Pelletier G (2010) Immunocytochemical localization of sex steroid hormone receptors in normal human mammary gland. J Histochem Cytochem 58(6):509–515. https://doi.org/10.1369/jhc.2009.954644
85. Burns KA, Korach KS (2012) Estrogen receptors and human disease: an update. Arch Toxicol 86(10):1491–1504. https://doi.org/10.1007/s00204-012-0868-5
86. Chen JQ, Russo PA, Cooke C, Russo IH, Russo J (2007) ERbeta shifts from mitochondria to nucleus during estrogen-induced neoplastic transformation of human breast epithelial cells and is involved in estrogen-induced synthesis of mitochondrial respiratory chain proteins. Biochim Biophys Acta 1773(12):1732–1746. https://doi.org/10.1016/j.bbamcr.2007.05.008
87. Mandusic V, Nikolic-Vukosavljevic D, Tanic N, Kanjer K, Neskovic-Konstantinovic Z, Celeketic D, Dimitrijevic B (2007) Expression of estrogen receptor beta wt isoform (ERbeta1) and ERbetaDelta5 splice variant mRNAs in sporadic breast cancer. J Cancer Res Clin Oncol 133(8):571–579. https://doi.org/10.1007/s00432-007-0209-x
88. Siegel RL, Miller KD, Jemal A (2016) Cancer statistics, 2016. CA Cancer J Clin 66(1):7–30. https://doi.org/10.3322/caac.21332
89. Giordano SH, Buzdar AU, Smith TL, Kau SW, Yang Y, Hortobagyi GN (2004) Is breast cancer survival improving? Cancer 100(1):44–52. https://doi.org/10.1002/cncr.11859
90. Anderson WF, Jatoi I, Tse J, Rosenberg PS (2010) Male breast cancer: a population-based comparison with female breast cancer. J Clin Oncol 28(2):232–239. https://doi.org/10.1200/JCO.2009.23.8162
91. Severson TM, Zwart W (2017) A review of estrogen receptor/androgen receptor genomics in male breast cancer. Endocr Relat Cancer 24(3):R27–R34. https://doi.org/10.1530/ERC-16-0225
92. Cooke PS, Nanjappa MK, Ko C, Prins GS, Hess RA (2017) Estrogens in Male Physiology. Physiol Rev 97(3):995–1043. https://doi.org/10.1152/physrev.00018.2016
93. Arao Y, Hamilton KJ, Goulding EH, Janardhan KS, Eddy EM, Korach KS (2012) Transactivating function (AF) 2-mediated AF-1 activity of estrogen receptor alpha is crucial to maintain male reproductive tract function. Proc Natl Acad Sci U S A 109(51):21140–21145. https://doi.org/10.1073/pnas.1216189110
94. Hess RA, Bunick D, Lubahn DB, Zhou Q, Bouma J (2000) Morphologic changes in efferent ductules and epididymis in estrogen receptor-alpha knockout mice. J Androl 21(1):107–121
95. Vanderschueren D, Laurent MR, Claessens F, Gielen E, Lagerquist MK, Vandenput L, Borjesson AE, Ohlsson C (2014) Sex steroid actions in male bone. Endocr Rev 35(6):906–960. https://doi.org/10.1210/er.2014-1024
96. Khosla S (2013) Pathogenesis of age-related bone loss in humans. J Gerontol A Biol Sci Med Sci 68(10):1226–1235. https://doi.org/10.1093/gerona/gls163
97. Farman HH, Wu J, Gustafsson KL, Windahl SH, Kim SH, Katzenellenbogen JA, Ohlsson C, Lagerquist MK (2017) Extra-nuclear effects of estrogen on cortical bone in males require ERalphaAF-1. J Mol Endocrinol 58(2):105–111. https://doi.org/10.1530/JME-16-0209
98. Smith EP, Specker B, Bachrach BE, Kimbro KS, Li XJ, Young MF, Fedarko NS, Abuzzahab MJ, Frank GR, Cohen RM, Lubahn DB, Korach KS (2008) Impact on bone of an estrogen receptor-alpha gene loss of function mutation. J Clin Endocrinol Metab 93(8):3088–3096. https://doi.org/10.1210/jc.2007-2397
99. Vanderschueren D, Vandenput L, Boonen S, Lindberg MK, Bouillon R, Ohlsson C (2004) Androgens and bone. Endocr Rev 25(3):389–425
100. Lindberg MK, Moverare S, Skrtic S, Alatalo S, Halleen J, Mohan S, Gustafsson JA, Ohlsson C (2002) Two different pathways for the maintenance of trabecular bone in adult male mice. J Bone Miner Res 17(4):555–562. https://doi.org/10.1359/jbmr.2002.17.4.555
101. Simerly RB, Chang C, Muramatsu M, Swanson LW (1990) Distribution of androgen and estrogen receptor mRNA-containing cells in the rat brain: an in situ hybridization study. J Comp Neurol 294(1):76–95. https://doi.org/10.1002/cne.902940107
102. Han X, Aenlle KK, Bean LA, Rani A, Semple-Rowland SL, Kumar A, Foster TC (2013) Role of estrogen receptor alpha and beta in preserving hippocampal function during aging. J Neurosci 33(6):2671–2683. https://doi.org/10.1523/JNEUROSCI.4937-12.2013

103. Tomihara K, Soga T, Nomura M, Korach KS, Gustafsson J-A, Pfaff DW, Ogawa S (2009) Effect of ER-beta gene disruption on estrogenic regulation of anxiety in female mice. Physiol Behav 96(2):300–306. https://doi.org/10.1016/j.physbeh.2008.10.014
104. Krezel W, Dupont S, Krust A, Chambon P, Chapman PF (2001) Increased anxiety and synaptic plasticity in estrogen receptor beta-deficient mice. Proc Natl Acad Sci U S A 98(21):12278–12282
105. Baum MJ (1979) Differentiation of coital behavior in mammals: a comparative analysis. Neurosci Biobehav Rev 3(4):265–284
106. Ogawa S, Eng V, Taylor J, Lubahn DB, Korach KS, Pfaff DW (1998) Roles of estrogen receptor-alpha gene expression in reproduction-related behaviors in female mice. Endocrinology 139(12):5070–5081. https://doi.org/10.1210/endo.139.12.6357
107. Ogawa S, Chester AE, Hewitt SC, Walker VR, Gustafsson JA, Smithies O, Korach KS, Pfaff DW (2000) Abolition of male sexual behaviors in mice lacking estrogen receptors alpha and beta (alpha beta ERKO). Proc Natl Acad Sci U S A 97(26):14737–14741. https://doi.org/10.1073/pnas.250473597
108. Ueda K, Lu Q, Baur W, Aronovitz MJ, Karas RH (2013) Rapid estrogen receptor signaling mediates estrogen-induced inhibition of vascular smooth muscle cell proliferation. Arterioscler Thromb Vasc Biol 33(8):1837–1843. https://doi.org/10.1161/ATVBAHA.112.300752
109. Ueda K, Karas RH (2013) Emerging evidence of the importance of rapid, non-nuclear estrogen receptor signaling in the cardiovascular system. Steroids 78(6):589–596. https://doi.org/10.1016/j.steroids.2012.12.006
110. Lu Q, Schnitzler GR, Vallaster CS, Ueda K, Erdkamp S, Briggs CE, Iyer LK, Jaffe IZ, Karas RH (2017) Unliganded estrogen receptor alpha regulates vascular cell function and gene expression. Mol Cell Endocrinol 442:12–23. https://doi.org/10.1016/j.mce.2016.11.019
111. Hodgin JB, Krege JH, Reddick RL, Korach KS, Smithies O, Maeda N (2001) Estrogen receptor alpha is a major mediator of 17 beta-estradiol's atheroprotective effects on lesion size in Apoe(−/−) mice. J Clin Investig 107(3):333–340
112. Wang M, Crisostomo PR, Markel T, Wang Y, Lillemoe KD, Meldrum DR (2008) Estrogen receptor beta mediates acute myocardial protection following ischemia. Surgery 144(2):233–238. https://doi.org/10.1016/j.surg.2008.03.009
113. Gabel SA, Walker VR, London RE, Steenbergen C, Korach KS, Murphy E (2005) Estrogen receptor beta mediates gender differences in ischemia/reperfusion injury. J Mol Cell Cardiol 38(2):289–297. https://doi.org/10.1016/j.yjmcc.2004.11.013
114. Ishikawa T, Yuhanna IS, Umetani J, Lee WR, Korach KS, Shaul PW, Umetani M (2013) LXRbeta/estrogen receptor-alpha signaling in lipid rafts preserves endothelial integrity. J Clin Invest 123(8):3488–3497. https://doi.org/10.1172/JCI66533
115. Umetani M, Domoto H, Gormley AK, Yuhanna IS, Cummins CL, Javitt NB, Korach KS, Shaul PW, Mangelsdorf DJ (2007) 27-Hydroxycholesterol is an endogenous SERM that inhibits the cardiovascular effects of estrogen. Nat Med 13(10):1185–1192. https://doi.org/10.1038/nm1641
116. Carey MA, Card JW, Voltz JW, Arbes SJ Jr, Germolec DR, Korach KS, Zeldin DC (2007) It's all about sex: gender, lung development and lung disease. Trends Endocrinol Metab 18(8):308–313. https://doi.org/10.1016/j.tem.2007.08.003
117. Thun MJ, Henley SJ, Burns D, Jemal A, Shanks TG, Calle EE (2006) Lung cancer death rates in lifelong nonsmokers. J Natl Cancer Inst 98(10):691–699. https://doi.org/10.1093/jnci/djj187
118. Kawai H, Ishii A, Washiya K, Konno T, Kon H, Yamaya C, Ono I, Minamiya Y, Ogawa J (2005) Estrogen receptor alpha and beta are prognostic factors in non-small cell lung cancer. Clin Cancer Res 11(14):5084–5089. https://doi.org/10.1158/1078-0432.CCR-05-0200
119. Alexiou C, Onyeaka CV, Beggs D, Akar R, Beggs L, Salama FD, Duffy JP, Morgan WE (2002) Do women live longer following lung resection for carcinoma? Eur J Cardiothorac Surg 21(2):319–325
120. Calzolari A (1898) Recherches experimentales sur un rapport probable entre la function du thymus et celle des testicules. Arch Ital Biol 30:71–77

121. Grossman CJ (1985) Interactions between the gonadal steroids and the immune system. Science 227(4684):257–261
122. Paavonen T, Andersson LC, Adlercreutz H (1981) Sex hormone regulation of in vitro immune response. Estradiol enhances human B cell maturation via inhibition of suppressor T cells in pokeweed mitogen-stimulated cultures. J Exp Med 154(6):1935–1945
123. Kalland T (1980) Alterations of antibody response in female mice after neonatal exposure to diethylstilbestrol. J Immunol 124(1):194–198
124. Inadera H, Sekiya T, Yoshimura T, Matsushima K (2000) Molecular analysis of the inhibition of monocyte chemoattractant protein-1 gene expression by estrogens and xenoestrogens in MCF-7 cells. Endocrinology 141(1):50–59. https://doi.org/10.1210/endo.141.1.7233
125. Kohen F, Abel L, Sharp A, Amir-Zaltsman Y, Somjen D, Luria S, Mor G, Knyszynski A, Thole H, Globerson A (1998) Estrogen-receptor expression and function in thymocytes in relation to gender and age. Dev Immunol 5(4):277–285
126. Lagergren J, Nyren O (1998) Do sex hormones play a role in the etiology of esophageal adenocarcinoma? A new hypothesis tested in a population-based cohort of prostate cancer patients. Cancer Epidemiol Biomark Prev 7(10):913–915
127. Jin H, Wen G, Deng S, Wan S, Xu J, Liu X, Xie R, Dong H, Tuo B (2016) Oestrogen upregulates the expression levels and functional activities of duodenal mucosal CFTR and SLC26A6. Exp Physiol 101(11):1371–1382. https://doi.org/10.1113/EP085803
128. Topi G, Ehrnstrom R, Jirstrom K, Palmquist I, Lydrup ML, Sjolander A (2017) Association of the oestrogen receptor beta with hormone status and prognosis in a cohort of female patients with colorectal cancer. Eur J Cancer 83:279–289. https://doi.org/10.1016/j.ejca.2017.06.013
129. Freedman ND, Chow WH, Gao YT, Shu XO, Ji BT, Yang G, Lubin JH, Li HL, Rothman N, Zheng W, Abnet CC (2007) Menstrual and reproductive factors and gastric cancer risk in a large prospective study of women. Gut 56(12):1671–1677. https://doi.org/10.1136/gut.2007.129411
130. Lindblad M, Ye W, Rubio C, Lagergren J (2004) Estrogen and risk of gastric cancer: a protective effect in a nationwide cohort study of patients with prostate cancer in Sweden. Cancer Epidemiol Biomark Prev 13(12):2203–2207
131. Nishi K, Tokunaga A, Shimizu Y, Yoshiyuki T, Wada M, Matsukura N, Tanaka N, Onda M, Asano G (1987) Immunohistochemical study of intracellular estradiol in human gastric cancer. Cancer 59(7):1328–1332
132. Ikeguchi M, Fukuda K, Oka S, Yamaguchi K, Hisamitsu K, Tsujitani S, Sakatani T, Ueda T, Kaibara N (2001) Clinicopathological significance of cathepsin D expression in gastric adenocarcinoma. Oncology 61(1):71–78. https://doi.org/10.1159/000055356
133. Matsuyama S, Ohkura Y, Eguchi H, Kobayashi Y, Akagi K, Uchida K, Nakachi K, Gustafsson JA, Hayashi S (2002) Estrogen receptor beta is expressed in human stomach adenocarcinoma. J Cancer Res Clin Oncol 128(6):319–324. https://doi.org/10.1007/s00432-002-0336-3
134. Foley EF, Jazaeri AA, Shupnik MA, Jazaeri O, Rice LW (2000) Selective loss of estrogen receptor beta in malignant human colon. Cancer Res 60(2):245–248
135. Hogan AM, Collins D, Baird AW, Winter DC (2009) Estrogen and gastrointestinal malignancy. Mol Cell Endocrinol 307(1–2):19–24. https://doi.org/10.1016/j.mce.2009.03.016
136. Cleveland AG, Oikarinen SI, Bynote KK, Marttinen M, Rafter JJ, Gustafsson JA, Roy SK, Pitot HC, Korach KS, Lubahn DB, Mutanen M, Gould KA (2009) Disruption of estrogen receptor signaling enhances intestinal neoplasia in Apc(Min/+) mice. Carcinogenesis 30(9):1581–1590. https://doi.org/10.1093/carcin/bgp132
137. Yousef F, Cardwell C, Cantwell MM, Galway K, Johnston BT, Murray L (2008) The incidence of esophageal cancer and high-grade dysplasia in Barrett's esophagus: a systematic review and meta-analysis. Am J Epidemiol 168(3):237–249. https://doi.org/10.1093/aje/kwn121
138. Akgun H, Lechago J, Younes M (2002) Estrogen receptor-beta is expressed in Barrett's metaplasia and associated adenocarcinoma of the esophagus. Anticancer Res 22(3):1459–1461

139. Lazcano-Ponce EC, Miquel JF, Munoz N, Herrero R, Ferrecio C, Wistuba II, Alonso de Ruiz P, Aristi Urista G, Nervi F (2001) Epidemiology and molecular pathology of gallbladder cancer. CA Cancer J Clin 51(6):349–364

140. Jones ME, Thorburn AW, Britt KL, Hewitt KN, Wreford NG, Proietto J, Oz OK, Leury BJ, Robertson KM, Yao S, Simpson ER (2000) Aromatase-deficient (ArKO) mice have a phenotype of increased adiposity. Proc Natl Acad Sci U S A 97(23):12735–12740. https://doi.org/10.1073/pnas.97.23.12735

141. Naaz A (2003) Effect of ovariectomy on adipose tissue of mice in the absence of estrogen receptor alpha (ER alpha): a potential role for estrogen receptor beta (ER beta) (vol 34, pg 758, 2002). Horm Metab Res 35(4):271–271

142. Heine PA, Taylor JA, Iwamoto GA, Lubahn DB, Cooke PS (2000) Increased adipose tissue in male and female estrogen receptor-alpha knockout mice. Proc Natl Acad Sci U S A 97(23):12729–12734

143. Ohlsson C, Hellberg N, Parini P, Vidal O, Bohlooly M, Rudling M, Lindberg MK, Warner M, Angelin B, Gustafsson JA (2000) Obesity and disturbed lipoprotein profile in estrogen receptor-alpha-deficient male mice. Biochem Biophys Res Commun 278(3):640–645

144. Park CJ, Zhao Z, Glidewell-Kenney C, Lazic M, Chambon P, Krust A, Weiss J, Clegg DJ, Dunaif A, Jameson JL, Levine JE (2011) Genetic rescue of nonclassical ERalpha signaling normalizes energy balance in obese Eralpha-null mutant mice. J Clin Invest. https://doi.org/10.1172/JCI41702

145. Hart-Unger S, Arao Y, Hamilton KJ, Lierz SL, Malarkey DE, Hewitt SC, Freemark M, Korach KS (2017) Hormone signaling and fatty liver in females: analysis of estrogen receptor alpha mutant mice. Int J Obes 41(6):945–954. https://doi.org/10.1038/ijo.2017.50

146. Handgraaf S, Riant E, Fabre A, Waget A, Burcelin R, Liere P, Krust A, Chambon P, Arnal JF, Gourdy P (2013) Prevention of obesity and insulin resistance by estrogens requires ERalpha activation function-2 (ERalphaAF-2), whereas ERalphaAF-1 is dispensable. Diabetes 62(12):4098–4108. https://doi.org/10.2337/db13-0282

147. Ribas V, Drew BG, Zhou Z, Phun J, Kalajian NY, Soleymani T, Daraei P, Widjaja K, Wanagat J, de Aguiar Vallim TQ, Fluitt AH, Bensinger S, Le T, Radu C, Whitelegge JP, Beaven SW, Tontonoz P, Lusis AJ, Parks BW, Vergnes L, Reue K, Singh H, Bopassa JC, Toro L, Stefani E, Watt MJ, Schenk S, Akerstrom T, Kelly M, Pedersen BK, Hewitt SC, Korach KS, Hevener AL (2016) Skeletal muscle action of estrogen receptor alpha is critical for the maintenance of mitochondrial function and metabolic homeostasis in females. Sci Transl Med 8(334):334ra354. https://doi.org/10.1126/scitranslmed.aad3815

148. Smith EP, Boyd J, Frank GR, Takahashi H, Cohen RM, Specker B, Williams TC, Lubahn DB, Korach KS (1994) Estrogen resistance caused by a mutation in the estrogen-receptor gene in a man. N Engl J Med 331(16):1056–1061. https://doi.org/10.1056/NEJM199410203311604

149. Sudhir K, Chou TM, Messina LM, Hutchison SJ, Korach KS, Chatterjee K, Rubanyi GM (1997) Endothelial dysfunction in a man with disruptive mutation in oestrogen-receptor gene [letter]. Lancet 349(9059):1146–1147

150. Quigley CA, De Bellis A, Marschke KB, el-Awady MK, Wilson EM, French FS (1995) Androgen receptor defects: historical, clinical, and molecular perspectives. Endocr Rev 16(3):271–321. https://doi.org/10.1210/edrv-16-3-271

151. Quaynor SD, Stradtman EW Jr, Kim HG, Shen Y, Chorich LP, Schreihofer DA, Layman LC (2013) Delayed puberty and estrogen resistance in a woman with estrogen receptor alpha variant. N Engl J Med 369(2):164–171. https://doi.org/10.1056/NEJMoa1303611

152. Bernard V, Kherra S, Francou B, Fagart J, Viengchareun S, Guéchot J, Ladjouze A, Guiochon-Mantel A, Korach KS, Binart N (2016) Familial multiplicity of estrogen insensitivity associated with a loss-of-function ESR1 mutation. J Clin Endocrinol Metabol 102(1):93–99

Estrogen Receptor-Mediated Gene Transcription and Cistrome

Gregory Bick, Dan Zhao, and Xiaoting Zhang

Abstract The discovery of the estrogen receptor 60 years ago radically transformed the field of hormonal signaling and led to the recognition of ER as a prototype nuclear receptor that primarily functions as a transcription factor. In this chapter, we will first describe the conserved domain architecture of ER and its regulation through various modifications by diverse intracellular pathways. We will then discuss the history and most recent advancement in the understanding of ER regulation of target genes at both individual gene and whole genome levels. A number of new concepts emanated from these studies, including ER cistrome, pioneer factors, chromosome looping and enhancer RNA, etc. and their potential impact on the fight against breast cancer therapeutic resistance all will be discussed in detail in this chapter.

Keywords ER domain structure · Posttranslational modification (PTM) · Cistrome · Pioneer factors · Chromosome looping · Enhancer RNA

1 Introduction

The paradigm shifting discovery of estrogen receptor (ER) by Dr. Elwood Jensen in 1958 revolutionized the popular view that estrogen functions through affecting enzymatic activities [1, 2]. Instead, the steroid hormone estrogen can directly diffuse through the plasma membrane to interact with its intracellular receptor to elicit its biological functions in the nucleus [3, 4]. Not until 10 years later, Dr. Bert O'Malley further discovered that the primary function of ERα is to regulate the expression of a subset of mRNAs [5, 6]. The cloning of ERα further established its

G. Bick · D. Zhao
Department of Cancer Biology, University of Cincinnati College of Medicine,
Cincinnati, OH, USA

X. Zhang (✉)
Department of Cancer Biology, Vontz Center for Molecular Studies,
University of Cincinnati College of Medicine, Cincinnati, OH, USA
e-mail: zhangxt@ucmail.uc.edu

© Springer Nature Switzerland AG 2019

X. Zhang (ed.), *Estrogen Receptor and Breast Cancer*, Cancer Drug Discovery and Development, https://doi.org/10.1007/978-3-319-99350-8_3

role as a ligand-dependent transcription factor and continued to open up a whole nuclear receptor field [7–9]. Since its discovery, the estrogen receptor has been extensively studied both for its own function and as a model for our understanding of other nuclear receptor family members. We will focus on ERα in this chapter as ERβ will be discussed in chapter "Estrogen Receptor β and Breast Cancer." We will first briefly discuss the basic ERα domain structure and its regulation by posttranslational modifications such as phosphorylation, ubiquitination, acetylation, and methylation. We are then putting our main emphasis on the current understanding of how ERα binds to specific estrogen regulatory element (EREs) to regulate its target gene expression and the recent advancement in utilizing state-of-the-art approaches to map its genome-wide binding sites (cistrome). New concepts and insights emerging from these genome-wide studies that included the roles for pioneer factors, chromosome looping, and enhancer RNAs (eRNAs) in ERα-mediated transcription will be discussed in detail. Finally, we will discuss how cellular signaling pathways affect the ERα cistrome and how these studies could provide not only new insights into molecular mechanisms underlying ERα-mediated transcription and antiestrogen resistance but may also provide potential new avenues for the development of innovative strategies for overcoming therapeutic resistance.

2   Estrogen Receptor α Domain Structure

Estrogen receptor α is 595 amino acids long and contains six functional domains including two transactivation domains (Fig. 1). The activation function 1 (AF1 domain, aa 51–149) is responsible for ligand-independent interaction with many cofactors to drive gene transcription [10, 11]. AF-1 is a common target for growth factor-driven phosphorylation cascades, allowing diverse inputs to affect the activity of estrogen receptor α. The DNA-binding domain (DBD, aa 183–246),

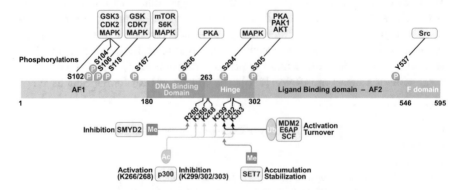

Fig. 1 Domain structure and modification landscape of estrogen receptor α. Layout of the domains of ERα with selected phosphorylation (activation/green, repression/red), methylation, acetylation, and ubiquitination sites. The responsible enzymatic pathways and effects on estrogen receptor functions are also shown

which follows AF1, is highly conserved between ERα and other nuclear receptors and contains two zinc fingers which specify DNA-binding sequences [12]. DNA binding is further stabilized by amino acids through 282, indicating that the following domain also plays a role in DNA binding [13]. Amino acids 263–302 constitute the hinge domain which also contains the nuclear localization sequence (NLS) of ERα [14]. The hinge domain has been shown to be important for optimal synergy between the AF1 and AF2, possibly by allowing them to interact with shared cofactors [15]. The C-terminus of ERα is made up of the ligand-binding domain (LBD) that can also act as a transactivation domain (AF2) and the c-terminal F domain. The ligand-binding domain of ERα is bound by protein folding chaperones such as HSP90 and is released after ligand binding [16]. Crystal structures of the ERα ligand-binding domain show that it is made of 12 helixes [11]. Helix 10 is primarily responsible for the dimer interface, while the 12th helix acts as an activation gatekeeper. When bound to estrogen, helix 12 adopts an open conformation allowing for the binding of coactivator proteins. Interestingly when bound to inhibitors such as tamoxifen, helix 12 prevents this opening to cover the sites where coactivators typically bind and allows for the binding of corepressors [17, 18]. Finally, the extreme c-terminal F domain of ERα appears to play a role in dimerization and cofactor binding as well, but its role is not very well defined [17, 19, 20].

3 Regulation of ERα Activity by Posttranslational Modifications

3.1 Phosphorylation

The activity of ERα has been found to be regulated by a number of posttranslational modifications such as phosphorylation, ubiquitination, acetylation, and methylation (Fig. 1). To date, more than 15 phosphorylation sites on ERα have been characterized, with many of them located in the AF-1 domain. Phosphorylation of Serine 118 is among the best-studied posttranslational modification of the AF-1 domain. The initial characterization of pS118 found that estrodiol (E2) treatment can increase the levels of pS118, while later studies found it is also induced by growth factors (such as EGF or IGF-1) even in the absence of hormone [21, 22]. S118 has also been found to be targeted by several additional pro-growth pathways including the MAP kinase, CDK7, and glycogen synthase kinase (GSK) to promote ERα-mediated transactivation [23]. To understand how pS118 affects ERα function mechanistically, many groups examined its role in affecting protein-protein interactions. By using yeast as a model, it was found that mutation of 118 in human ERα led to a dramatic reduction in ERα homodimerization [24]. In human cell lines, phospho-Serine 118 has been found to mediate interactions with important ERα coactivators such as p300 [23, 25]. Additionally, ERα S118A mutant shows reduced recruitment to nonclassical sites that require protein-protein interactions with other transcription factors such as AP-1 as described later in this chapter.

Most ERα-AF-1 phospho-target sites are similar to S118 in that they are targeted by pro-growth pathways and serve to increase the activation potential of ERα. A cluster of serines, S102, 104, and 106, are also targeted by pathways including MAPK, GSK3, and Cdk2, and mutation of these sites to alanine reduces transactivation activity of ERα [23]. S167 is a target of the MAPK, mTOR, and S6K pathways, and phosphorylation of this residue increases transactivation from the AF-1 domain of ERα [23]. Outside of the AF-1 domain, serine 236, in the second zinc finger of the DNA-binding domain, is targeted by the PKA (protein kinase A) pathway. This phosphorylation appears to inhibit activation, as mutating this residue to glutamic acid (a phosphoserine mimic) prevented homodimer formation, DNA binding, and the ability to activate reporter gene expression [26, 27]. PKA and PAK1 and AKT phosphorylate ERα at serine 305, which has been found to promote cofactor binding and transactivation [23, 28]. In addition, serine 305 phosphorylation has also been shown to moderate modifications on other residues of ERα such as S118 phosphorylation and K303 acetylation [29]. Importantly, high PAK1 protein expression and S305 phosphorylation in breast cancers have been found to correlate with sensitivity to tamoxifen [23, 28]. Interestingly, S294 can be phosphorylated by MAPK, which activates ERα through increased ubiquitination at nearby lysines as will also be discussed below. In addition to all these serine phosphorylations, a tyrosine residue in the F domain (Tyr537) has been found to be phosphorylated by Src kinase to regulate the dimerization ability and transcription [23]. Phosphorylation mapping by mass spectrometry has uncovered additional phosphorylation sites, but their functions and the pathways responsible for their phosphorylation remain to be explored [30].

3.2   Ubiquitination

Interestingly, the half-life of ERα is significantly decreased after the administration of E2 (3–5 days versus 3–5 h), suggesting that ERα turnover is an important step in the cellular response to estrogens [31]. ERα is degraded by the ubiquitin proteasome system after treatment by E2, linking its degradation to its transcriptional function [31, 32]. This relationship was supported by the discovery that treating cells with MG132, a proteasome inhibitor, reduced expression of E2-responsive reporter genes, despite stabilization of ERα at protein levels [33]. Further studies indicated that E2 induction results in a cyclical recruitment of ERα and its cofactors on the TFF1 promoter [34, 35], a pattern that was abrogated by MG132 treatment [36]. The lysines responsible for ubiquitin-dependent degradation, 302 and 303, were found to be essential for E2-induced degradation, while mutation of these lysines to alanines led to both stabilization of ERα and a reduction in its transcriptional activities [37]. Knockdown experiments have found that several E3-ubiquitin ligases, including MDM2, E6AP, and SCF, are responsible for ubiquitination of ERα [38–40]. As discussed previously, phosphorylation of ERα on S294 allows

ERα to be recognized by SKP2, a member of the SCF ubiquitin ligase complex. SKP2 recognizes the phosphorylation site, bridging the E2 ubiquitin ligase SCF complex and ERα [41]. This has been found to be particularly important in late response genes such as E2F-1 [40]. Inhibition of MAPK or mutation of S294 to alanine reduced ubiquitination of ERα and transcription of its target genes. In addition, ERα coactivators, including AIB1 and SRC-1, have also been shown to be able to enhance ubiquitination of ERα and recruit the proteasomal subunit LMP2, respectively [42, 43]. Conversely, ERα function can be inhibited by the deubiquitinating enzyme OTUB1. As might be expected, OTUB1 overexpression drastically reduces ubiquitination and activation of ERα, while knockdown of OTUB1 led to higher rates of ubiquitination and transcription [44]. Together, these studies indicate that ERα turnover is a highly regulated step required for its transactivation activities.

3.3   Acetylation and Methylation

Estrogen receptor α activity can also be regulated by acetylation and methylation on these ubiquitination sites (K302, K303) as well as other lysines. Protein acetyltransferases such as p300 and P/CAF are well-characterized ERα cofactors that acetylate histones and activate transcription. Wang and colleagues found that p300 but not P/CAF can also directly acetylate ERα preferentially at lysines 302 and 303 with additional sites such as lysine 299 [45]. Interestingly, mutation of these lysines to arginine, glutamic acid, or threonine did not alter the expression of ERα but affected both ERα-mediated transactivation and the sensitivity to E2 stimulation [45]. In addition, p300 has also been found to acetylate K266 and 268 to increase ERα DNA binding and transactivation [46]. Furthermore, ERα is also known to recruit a number of histone methyltransferases and demethylases. It is therefore not surprising that ERα itself is also subjected to regulation by methylation and demethylation. Through a functional screening of different methyltransferase catalytic domains, SMYD2 was found to be able to methylate ERα at lysine 266. Knockdown of SMYD2 increased E2-induced transcription of target genes and recruitment of ERα to enhancer elements, while also leading to marked increases in acetyl-K266 and 268. Meanwhile, the lysine demethylase LSD1 acts as the demethylase of K266/268. Knockdown of LSD1 was shown to increase levels of methyl-K266 and a subsequent decrease in the acetyl-K266 [47]. ERα K302 has been shown to be a target of the SET7 methyltransferase, and methylation of K302 has been found to prevent ERα polyubiquitination and degradation and enhance the accumulation of ERα at target genes [48]. Together, these studies indicate that additional modifications such as acetylation and methylation could provide further mechanisms to regulate ERα functions through diverse signaling inputs, which is important given that ERα can directly feed from hormone and signaling stimulation and quickly translate into transcriptional regulations.

4   Estrogen Receptor α Binding Modes

Once activated, ERα recognizes and binds to specific sequences on DNA to regulate its target gene transcription. ERα can either directly bind to DNA at specific sequences in enhancer elements in a "classical" mode or by tethering with other transcription factors such as AP-1 that themselves are recruited in a sequence-specific manner in a "nonclassical" mode. In the classical mode, ERα binds to specific DNA motifs called estrogen response elements (ERE) to regulate its target gene expression. EREs are palindromic or near-palindromic sequences and can function as typical enhancer elements in both directions and in a distance-independent manner. The ERE was first discovered on the *Xenopus* vitellogenin genes A1, A2, B1, and B2 as the estrogen-responsive and estrogen receptor-binding regulatory elements [49]. Subsequently, human EREs have been identified in other estrogen-induced target genes such as TFF-1/pS2, GREB1, Cathepsin D, TGFα, etc. The consensus ERE core sequence has been deduced to be composed of GGTCAnnnTGACC in which n can be any nucleotide (Fig. 2a, b) [49]. These sites are bound by mirrored homodimers, in which the two zinc fingers in the DNA-binding domain are essential for ERα recognition of the proper ERE. The first zinc finger contains a helix structure that is inserted into the major groove to identify the proper sequence. Three amino acids (Glu203, Gly204, and Ala207) with the proximal box (P-box) have been shown to be particularly important for sequence

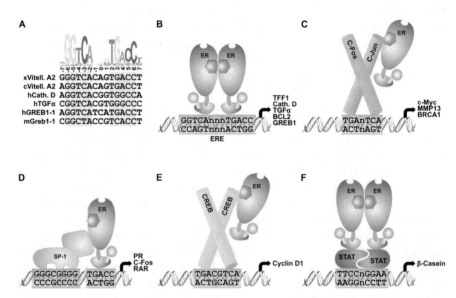

Fig. 2 Schematics of classical and nonclassical ERα binding modes. (**a**) Estrogen receptor consensus binding sequence with representative ERE sites. (**b**) Classical binding of an estrogen receptor dimer to the canonical estrogen response element, (**c–f**) nonclassical tethering of ERα binding with AP-1 (**c**), SP-1 (**d**), CREB (**e**), and STAT (**f**) to their respective response elements. Genes known to be regulated by enhancer elements are shown for each element

determination. The second zinc finger promotes ERα dimerization as a mechanism for recognition of the spacing between the half sites [11, 12, 50, 51].

While many E2-responsive genes are activated from EREs, the nonclassical recruitment ERα onto target gene promoters represents an additional layer of complexity [52]. In this nonclassical mode, ERα may or may not bind DNA directly but instead is recruited through interacting with a variety of other DNA-binding transcription factors, such as AP-1, SP-1, cAMP-like elements, and STAT dimers (Fig. 2c–f). For example, ERα is able to transactivate through the AP-1 site through interacting with AP-1 dimer (Fos and Jun proteins), regulating genes including matrix metalloproteinase 13 and BRCA1 (Fig. 2c) [53, 54]. The in vitro interaction studies have mapped the interaction site with Jun to the central hinge region of ERα, while interaction between ERα and Fos was undetected [55]. C-Myc is another well-known ERα target regulated by a combined AP-1 site with a half-ERE, indicating a possible ERα monomer interaction with the DNA in this configuration. Deletion of either enhancer element reduced estrogen inducibility of a reporter gene from this enhancer [56, 57]. Other nonclassical activation sites function in similar ways to AP-1 sites. Well-known SP-1-recruited ERα target genes include progesterone receptor, c-Fos, and the retinoic acid receptor [58, 59]. Similar to the c-Myc enhancer, these enhancer elements also include half-EREs and require binding of both SP-1 and ERα for full expression of the target genes. Other response elements can also function by similar mechanisms through proteins such as the cAMP-response element binding protein (CREB) and STATs to regulate the target genes such as cyclin D1 or β-casein, respectively [52]. Overall, this nonclassical mode of action of ERα in mediating gene transcription greatly expands the repertoire and complexity of estrogen receptor α-regulated target genes and transcriptional programs.

5   Dynamic and Cyclic Recruitment of ERα Cofactors in ERα-Mediated Gene Transcription

Once estrogen-bound and activated, ERα recognizes and binds to these specific EREs to recruit diverse transcriptional cofactors to regulate its target gene expression. These cofactors play essential roles in regulating the expression of ERα target genes by facilitating the recruitment and/or the function of the RNA polymerase II and general transcription machinery [60, 61]. The better-characterized class of nuclear receptor-interacting coactivators includes ATP-dependent chromatin-remodeling SWI/SNF complexes and histone-modifying enzymes including p160/SRC family members (SRC1, 2, and 3), p300/CBP, PGC-1, PRMT1, CARM1, HDACs, and LSD1, among many others [62, 63]. These coactivators have intrinsic enzymatic activities (e.g., ATP-dependent remodeling functions, histone acetyltransferase, methyltransferase, deacetylases, demethylase, etc.) and are thought to act, at least in part, through chromatin remodeling or histone modifications to open up the chromatin structure that in turn facilitate the recruitment and function of the general transcription machinery [64, 65]. Furthermore, ERα-dependent transcription also requires another class of coactivators to send the signal directly to the general transcription machinery to activate transcription [66–68]. Among these coactivators, Mediator has recently emerged as the main bridge for direct communication between ERα and RNA polymerase II through direct interaction between ERα and MED1 subunit of the Mediator complex [69–74]. Moreover, a number of other ERα cofactors have also recently been reported to play roles in transcription elongation, splicing, etc., further linking ERα to not only transcription initiation but also these other processes in regulating target gene expression [62, 64]. Interestingly, studies found that the recruitment of these diverse cofactors by ERα is a rather dynamic process, occurring in a sequential and cyclical fashion. It was first reported by Shang et al. that ERα promoter occupancy peaked first followed by p160, p300, MED1, and then RNA pol II upon estrogen stimulation and released in a cyclic mode by using a kinetic chromatin IP method [35]. This phenomenon was further confirmed by a number of other studies using the similar and additional approaches [34, 75–77]. Although the exact functional significance of this cyclic recruitment has just started to be deciphered and will be extensively discussed in the next chapter (Chapter "Structural Studies with Coactivators for the Estrogen Receptor"), it is consistent with the findings that the degradation of ERα and its cofactor is required for their optimal activation of target genes. It further reflects the precise and tightly controlled nature of the ERα-mediated target gene transcription at multiple levels.

6 Genome-Wide Analyses of Estrogen Receptor α Binding Cistrome

With the completion of the Human Genome Project and development of computational tools, scientists began to search for EREs near promoter regions to identify potential ERα target genes [78–80]. One such genome-wide analysis of consensus or near consensus EREs found over 70K potential EREs in the human and mouse genomes [81]. By eliminating the EREs that are not conserved among species, they identified 660 genes with one or more conserved ERE in their proximal promoter regions (708 conserved EREs in total) [81]. Most of these conserved EREs were located in the 0 to +2-kb region; but there are also a significant number of conserved EREs (24.6%) mapped to between −5 and −10 kb of the transcriptional start sites. Further, gel shift and chromatin IP experiments were able to confirm the binding of ERα to most of these ERE sites both in vitro and in vivo. Interestingly, another study also combining computational prediction and experimental validation estimated the total ERα direct binding EREs to be between 5000 to 10,000 [82].

The combination of chromatin IP with high-throughput sequencing methodologies like DNA microarray (ChIP-on-chip) and next-generation sequencing (ChIP-seq) has further accelerated the identification of genome-wide ERα-binding cistrome. By using the ChIP-on-chip method, Carroll et al. examined the ERα binding sites, initially on chromosomes 21 and 22, and later expanded on the whole genome [83, 84]. Overall, they identified 3665 ERα binding sites using a stringent threshold with a false discovery rate of ~1%. Interestingly while a majority of RNA pol II (67%) bound at proximal promoter regions (−800 bp to +200 bp), only 4% of ERα binding sites could be mapped to these 1-kb regions. Instead, the majority of ERα binding sites were found in intronic or distal upstream locations within 100 kb of the transcription start site. These studies also revealed enrichment of binding sites for ERα cofactors like FOXA1, C/EBP, and OCT adjoining ERE sequences in the ERα binding regions. Interestingly, although there is a strong negative correlation of ERE and AP-1 elements, C/EBP, Oct, and Forkhead transcription factors showed equal likelihood of occurrence with both motifs, suggesting that these factors are important for both classical and nonclassical ERα activation.

Since then, a number of additional genome-wide characterizations of the ERα cistrome have been carried out using varying approaches and cell lines [85–92]. For example, Lin et al. performed ChIP-PET (paired-end tags) experiments and identified 1234 high-confidence ERα binding sites, approximately 95% of which were farther than 5 kb from a TSS [86]. Of these regions, most (~71%) contained at least one ERE-like sequence, and a large minority (~25%) contained putative half-EREs with the rest containing no discernible ERE sequences [86]. In addition to FOXA1 sites, they also found several more enriched motifs like Sp1 and PAX3 motifs in the ERα binding sites. However, they found that only 22–24% of ERα binding sites were conserved among vertebrates [86, 93]. Joseph et al. [92] mapped the ERα cistrome using ChIP-seq and found the majority of ERα binding sites were located in the intragenic regions (39.5%) and 5′-distal (17.4%) and 3′-distal regions (14.3%), with only 9.3% found in promoter regions. While not all of the ERα binding sites identified were consistent among these experiments, a common theme that emerged is that ERα binds preferentially not to the promoter regions but to distal enhancer regions to regulate its target gene expression in response to estrogen stimulation [94].

7   ERα Genome-Wide Binding and Pioneer Factors

These genome-wide analyses of ERα binding sites have also revealed another previously unexpected mode of action for ERα-mediated gene transcription in terms of the pioneer factors. As discussed above, in one of the first chromosome-wide mappings of ERα binding studies, ChIP analysis was combined with the use of tiled oligonucleotide microarrays that cover the entire non-repetitive chromosomes 21 and 22 at a 35-bp resolution [83]. This analysis revealed 57 ERα binding sites within 32 clusters in chr 21 and 22, far less than the 5500 predicted elements, suggesting that ERE sequences alone are insufficient to predict ERα binding sites. Further in-depth analysis of the surrounding sequences of these ERα binding sites for enriched motifs revealed that Forkhead factor binding sites were present in over half of the 57 ERα binding regions. Subsequent ChIP experiments have verified the FOXA1 binding to these sites, and siRNA-mediated knockdown of FOXA1 has confirmed the requirement for FOXA1 in both ERα recruitment and target gene expression [83]. FOXA1 is known to be a pioneer factor that can interact with and open compact chromatin due to its structural similarity to linker histones [95]. Subsequent studies confirmed the requirement of FOXA1 for ERα-chromatin interactions and transcription in multiple breast cancer cell lines [96]. Together, these studies have therefore established a new model for ERα-mediated transcription in which pioneer factor FOXA1 binds to the chromatin prior to estrogen treatment and functions to guide and provide accessibility for the binding of ERα to regulate the expression these target genes upon estrogen stimulation (Fig. 3).

Since the discovery of FOXA1, additional proteins such as TLE, Ap2γ, and PBX1 have also been reported to be able to act as pioneer factors. Like FOXA1, the Groucho/transducin-like enhancer of split (TLE) proteins are known to interact with chromatin independent of other factors. Holmes et al. explored the role of TLE proteins in ERα-mediated transcriptional activation and functions [97]. Similar to FOXA1, they found that TLE1 is associated with ERα binding sites with or without estrogen treatment. Additionally, knockdown of TLE1 affected 45% of all ERα

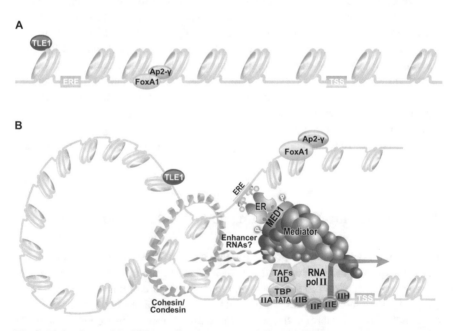

Fig. 3 Molecular model of ERα-mediated gene transcription. (**a**) Prior to estrogen treatment, pioneer factors such as FoxA1, AP2-γ, and TLE1 are present near estrogen response elements to facilitate ERα binding. (**b**) After estrogen treatment, ERα binds to enhancer elements and recruits cofactors (e.g., MED1/Mediator and SRC-1), as well as condensin/cohesin and enhancer RNAs to form chromosome loop to activate transcription by RNA Pol II and the general transcription factors (GTFs)

binding events and significantly impaired both ERα-mediated gene transcription and cell proliferation. Interestingly, TLE1 knockdown does not affect the binding of FOXA1, and most of the ERα binding events affected by TLE1 knockdown are on those target sites not cobound by FOXA1. In another study, Tan et al. observed that AP-2 motifs are enriched in the ERα binding sites [98]. They demonstrated that AP-2γ binds to ERα binding sites in a ligand-independent manner, while perturbation of AP-2γ expression significantly impaired ERα binding, long-range chromatin interactions, and target gene transcription. Unlike TLE1, AP-2γ colocalizes with FoxA1 on ERα binding sites that are associated with long-range chromatin interactions, and their functions are mutually dependent. More recently, PBX1 (pre-B-cell leukemia homeobox 1) has also been implicated to function as a pioneer factor promoting an ERα-dependent transcriptional program favorable to drive breast cancer progression and metastasis [99, 100].

8 ERα-Driven Chromosome Looping

Given that ERα predominantly binds to distal enhancers upon estrogen stimulation, an important question is raised as to how ERα regulates target gene expression from tens to hundreds of kilobases away. One proposed model hypothesized that PolII might be recruited to enhancers and then translocate along the DNA until it hits the promoter and transcriptional start site to initiate transcription. A second model hypothesized that transcription factors and cofactors could curve the DNA to bring enhancers and promoters close to one another in a three-dimensional space through a process called "chromosome looping." Recently developed methods and technologies such as chromosome conformation capture (3C) [101, 102] have provided crucial evidence supporting the latter model. Basic 3C methods and their derivatives such as ChIP-3C, 4C, 5C, and 6C approaches usually involve chemically cross-linked chromatin treated with restriction enzymes or sonication similar to ChIP [103]. Unlike ChIP, the DNA fragments are religated allowing sequences connected by protein bridges to be ligated together. These novel combined fragments can then be identified through PCR or sequenced and mapped to the genome. By using such technologies, chromosome looping has been detected and confirmed between the promoter and enhancer of ERα target genes such as TFF1 and GREB1 [83, 84, 104].

Using a 3C-based technique called ChIA-PET, Fullwood and colleagues generated a genome-wide map of the ERα-bound chromatin interactome [105]. The ChIA-PET approach enriches cross-linked DNA-protein complexes through ChIP after sonication to shear the chromatin. The immunoprecipitated DNA fragments are then ligated to paired-end tags (PET) which can be ligated more easily and also bypasses the use of restriction enzymes to reduce the inherent bias caused by only allowing digestion at specific sites. Through this approach, they identified a total of 1451 intrachromosomal interactions and a small set of 15 interchromosomal interactions. They also found many nearby duplex interactions (1036) in which two anchor loci are interconnected to form a complex interaction. Interestingly, they found that most (86%) of the duplex interactions span a genomic region of less than 100 kb, while 13% span 100 kb to 1 Mb; however, the complex interactions have genomic spans in the range of 100 kb to 1 Mb. They were able to verify these results by additional ChIA-PET using a different antibody against ERα and further experimental confirmation by ChIP-qPCR, 3C, ChIP-3C, 4C, FISH, etc. Overall, the study found that most high-confidence remote ERα binding sites are indeed anchored through long-range chromosome interactions, supporting chromosome looping as a primary mechanism for ERα-mediated transcription.

ER-driven loop formation has been found to involve a number of additional proteins including cohesin, condensin, as well as some ERα cofactors (e.g., Mediator, LSD1) [106]. Cohesin and condensin are evolutionarily conserved protein complexes which form ring-like structures to keep DNA strands organized in close proximity during replication in preparation for mitosis [107]. Interestingly, it was found that they also play important roles in mediating the chromosomal looping between distal enhancers and promoters. Cohesin has been found to be involved in repressing gene expression through promoting CTCF-mediated insulator function, but it has also been found to work independently of CTCF to promote gene looping. Schmidt et al. [108] found that in MCF7 cells, cohesin can be recruited to distal EREs in an estrogen-dependent manner. Further, ERα and cohesin co-recruitment was more successful at predicting estrogen-responsive genes than ERα binding alone. Importantly, knocking down the cohesin subunit, Rad21, in MCF7 cells leads to a decrease in looping and expression of ERα target genes [109]. Similarly, the condensin 1 and 2 subunits NCAPG and NCAPH2 have been shown to be required for optimal activation of ERα target genes such as GREB1 and FOXC1. These subunits are localized to ERα-bound EREs in an estrogen-dependent manner and are required for looping of ERE enhancers and TSSs [104]. Several lines of evidence also support the involvement of the ERα coactivator Mediator complex in chromosome looping. The Mediator complex was shown to interact with the cohesin-loading protein Nipbl on the ERα target gene enhancers and promoters. In addition, RNAi-mediated knockdown of condensin subunits in MCF7 cells can also reduce the recruitment of ERα cofactor and Mediator subunit MED1 [104, 110, 111]. Moreover, it has been shown that in castration-sensitive prostate cancer cells, MED1 phosphorylation and activation are required for androgen receptor-dependent chromosome looping [112]. Although direct evidence for MED1 in ERα-mediated chromosome looping still remains to be seen, a similar mechanism is likely to exist. In addition, another recent study has also supported the involvement of another ERα cofactor LSD1 in ERα-mediated long-range chromatin interactions and looping [113]. Together these studies support chromosome looping as a key step involved in ERα-mediated transactivation from ERα-bound distal enhancers.

9 Enhancer RNA and ERα-Mediated Transcription

While chromosome looping provides an elegant model for how distal enhancers can feed into PolII activity at promoters to regulate ERα-mediated transcription, interestingly global ChIP experiments also found that these distal enhancer regions are highly enriched in active transcription marks and have high levels of RNA polymerase II recruitment [114]. Using the global run-on sequencing (GRO-seq) method to examine nascent transcripts, it has been found that noncoding RNAs are actively transcribed from the enhancer region in a regulated manner. These noncoding RNAs have been termed enhancer RNAs (eRNAs), although it has been debated as whether these are functional or merely indicative of active enhancers [115]. Comparing enhancer RNA (eRNA) expression data with data gathered from ChIP and chromosome conformation capture (3C) experiments across multiple tissue types, several patterns emerged. First, eRNAs are usually long and transcribed in both directions from the enhancer elements. These eRNAs tend to be expressed from enhancers with high levels of H3K4mono- and di-methylation, but not trimethylation, and high H3K27 acetylation. In addition, eRNA levels are highly correlated with the transcription levels of the cognate gene [116], and highly expressed enhancers participate in more chromosomal looping and have higher POLII occupancy levels. Functionally, knocking down eRNAs has been found not to reduce POLII recruitment to the enhancer elements, but does reduce RNA Pol II recruitment to the gene body and subsequent gene transcription [117]. Together, these data support that eRNAs could play important roles in gene expression and regulation.

Interestingly, estrogen-responsive enhancers are not only enriched with RNA Pol II and the activating histone mark H3K27ac but also express higher levels of enhancer RNAs (Fig. 3) [104, 118, 119]. The expression of these eRNAs, like the genes they regulate, also depends on estrogen stimulation. Li et al. [118] found that knockdown of ERα-driven enhancer RNAs causes a sharp decrease in the level of cognate mRNA expression, while tethering enhancer RNAs to an engineered enhancer region was sufficient to increase expression from that enhancer. The mechanism by which eRNAs impact expression of their cognate mRNAs is unclear but may involve chromosome looping. In vitro binding assays showed that E2-responsive eRNAs, but not a control RNA, could pull down cohesin subunits RAD21 and SMC3. Further, knockdown of enhancer RNAs caused a significant reduction in estrogen-induced localization of these cohesin subunits to the respective enhancer elements and caused a reduction in enhancer-promoter looping at ERα target genes such as NRIP1 and GREB1 [118]. These studies support the hypothesis that eRNAs may enhance transcription by stabilizing cohesins at promoter-enhancer looping sites. However, in another study, it was found that treatment of a global transcription inhibitor flavopiridol did not inhibit ERα-mediated chromosome looping or recruitment of coactivators in MCF7 cells [120]. Different conclusions from these studies could be due to different methods used (RNAi-mediated knockdown or transcription inhibition, respectively), but it is clear that further understanding of molecular mechanisms of eRNA functions and their binding partners could provide deeper understanding into ERα-mediated transcription and functions.

10 Growth Factor Signaling Regulation of ERα Cistrome

Interestingly, studies have found that the ERα genome-wide binding cistrome can also undergo reprogramming in response to other signaling pathways such as EGF, PKA, and AKT. As we have discussed earlier in this chapter, the transcriptional activity of ERα can be regulated by distinct posttranslational modifications such as phosphorylation. However, how such changes impacted the ERα cistrome was not known. In one early study, Bhat-Nakshatri et al. investigated this by focusing on the phosphorylation of ERα by the serine/threonine kinase AKT/PKB [121], which is aberrantly activated in ~50% of human malignancies and plays key roles in antiestrogen resistance. Using ChIP-on-chip, they compared ERα binding sites in MCF7s transduced with a retroviral control vector (MCF-7p) or constitutively active AKT (MCF-7AKT). They found that while the control MCF7 cells and the AKT-overexpressing cells displayed a similar number of ERα binding sites (4349 and 4359, respectively), about 40% of ERα binding sites were unique to either cell line. This suggested that AKT activation has a significant effect on ERα cistrome. Importantly, they found a similar percentage of differentially expressed genes between these two cell types. These AKT-induced estrogen-regulated genes were linked to transforming growth factor β (TGF-β), NF-κB, and E2F pathways, which are known to be involved in tumor progression and antiestrogen resistance. These results highlight a unique role of AKT in modulating estrogen signaling that changes the landscape of ERα binding to the genome and the expression pattern of its downstream target genes.

Another such example is the regulation of the ERα cistrome by protein kinase A. PKA can phosphorylate ERα at two target sites Ser236 and Ser305. Importantly, the predominant phosphorylation of ERα is at position S305 and is known to induce a conformational arrest of ERα upon tamoxifen treatment, causing tamoxifen to act as an agonist and inducing breast cancer cell growth [122]. In fact, immunodetection of pS305 in tumor sections has been successfully used to identify tamoxifen-resistant breast cancer patients. To determine the effects of pS305 on ERα genome-wide binding, De Leeuw et al. [123] activated PKA by treating cells with forskolin and then performed ChIP-seq using anti-ERα-pS305 antibody. They found that ERα-pS305 shows 3327 binding events, of which only about 912 overlap with previously reported ERα binding sites. In addition, there was a striking enrichment for ERα-pS305 for promoter regions, 3'-UTRs and 5'-UTRs, in contrast to the total ERα that generally prefers distal enhancers. Further, only a subset of these PKA-induced pS305 binding sites overlap with above EGF-induced ERα binding sites, suggesting distinct ERα cistrome patterns can form through activation of different kinase pathways. By integrating ERα-pS305 chromatin binding and gene expression analyses, De Leeuw and colleagues have identified a 26-gene signature of ERα-pS305 targets that significantly correlate with poor disease outcome in breast cancer patients [123].

ERα is also known to be stimulated by a variety of growth factors such as epidermal growth factor (EGF) in breast cancer cells. To assess the impact of EGF on the ERα cistrome, Lupien et al. compared EGF and estrogen-induced ERα cistromes in MCF7 breast cancer cells [124]. They found that both estrogen and EGF can induce ERα recruitment to many of the same sites as expected but EGF activation can also induce ERα recruitment to a significant number of unique sites. For the shared estrogen and EGF-induced ERα cistromes, there is an enrichment in Forkhead (FKH) motif binding sites, which is consistent with the central role of FoxA1 as a pioneer factor for ERα recruitment. However, the EGF-unique sites were instead enriched for AP-1 binding sites, suggesting a nonclassical tethering binding mode through AP-1 family members. Interestingly, the EGF-induced ERα cistrome is enriched in genes that are overexpressed in ERBB2-positive human breast cancers, and these EGF-specific ERα target genes are significantly associated with poor patient outcomes such as metastasis, recurrence, death, and high grade. These data are significant since hormone-refractory tumors are often dependent on the overexpression of the EGFR or ERBB2 and this study supported a new strategy to overcome such resistance through blocking both estrogen- and growth factor-stimulated activities. Together, the above studies not only highlight the dynamic regulation of the ERα cistrome by diverse signaling pathways but also reveal novel molecular mechanisms underlying antiestrogen resistance and potential new avenues for the development of innovative strategies to overcome such resistance.

Acknowledgments We thank Zhang lab members for helpful discussion and Mr. Glenn Doerman for figure illustrations. This study was supported by NCI R01 CA197865, University of Cincinnati Cancer Center Startup and College of Medicine Innovation Seed Grant (to X.Z). G.B was supported by NCI training grant T32CA117846.

References

1. Jensen EV (1958) Studies of growth phenomena using tritium-labeled steroids. In: Proc. 4th Int. Congress of Biochem, vol 15. Pergamon Press, Vienna, p 119
2. Jensen EV, Jacobson H (1962) Basic guides to the mechanism of estrogen action. Recent Prog Horm Res 18:318–414
3. Jensen EV (2005) The contribution of "alternative approaches" to understanding steroid hormone action. Mol Endocrinol 19:1439–1442. https://doi.org/10.1210/me.2005-0154
4. Jensen EV (2004) From chemical warfare to breast cancer management. Nat Med 10:1018–1021
5. O'Malley BW, McGuire WL (1968) Studies on the mechanism of estrogen-mediated tissue differentiation: regulation of nuclear transcription and induction of new RNA species. Proc Natl Acad Sci U S A 60:1527–1534. https://doi.org/10.1073/pnas.60.4.1527
6. O'Malley BW, McGuire W, Middleton P (1968) Altered gene expression during differentiation: population changes in hybridizable RNA after stimulation of the chick oviduct with oestrogen. Nature 218:1249–1251

7. Greene GL, Gilna P, Waterfield M, Baker A, Hort Y, Shine J (1986) Sequence and expression of human estrogen receptor complementary DNA. Science 231:1150–1154
8. Green S, Walter P, Kumar V, Krust A, Bornert J-M, Argos P, Chambon P (1986) Human oestrogen receptor cDNA: sequence, expression and homology to v-erb-A. Nature 320:134–139
9. O'Malley BW, Khan S (2013) Elwood V. Jensen (1920-2012): father of the nuclear receptors. Proc Natl Acad Sci 110:3707–3708. https://doi.org/10.1073/pnas.1301566110
10. Lavery DN, Mcewan IJ (2005) Structure and function of steroid receptor AF1 transactivation domains: induction of active conformations. Biochem J 391:449–464. https://doi.org/10.1042/BJ20050872
11. Yaşar P, Ayaz G, User SD, Güpür G, Muyan M (2017) Molecular mechanism of estrogen–estrogen receptor signaling. Reprod Med Biol 16:4–20. https://doi.org/10.1002/rmb2.12006
12. Schwabe JW, Chapman L, Finch JT, Rhodes D (1993) The crystal structure of the estrogen-receptor DNA-binding domain bound to DNA - how receptors discriminate between their response elements. Cell 75:567–576. https://doi.org/10.1016/0092-8674(93)90390-C
13. Mader S, Chambon P, White JH (1993) Defining a minimal estrogen receptor DNA binding domain. Nucleic Acids Res 21:1125–1132. https://doi.org/10.1093/nar/21.5.1125
14. Leclercq G, Lacroix M, Laïos I, Laurent G (2006) Estrogen receptor alpha: impact of ligands on intracellular shuttling and turnover rate in breast cancer cells. Curr Cancer Drug Targets 6:39–64. https://doi.org/10.2174/156800906775471716
15. Zwart W, de Leeuw R, Rondaij M, Neefjes J, Mancini MA, Michalides R (2010) The hinge region of the human estrogen receptor determines functional synergy between AF-1 and AF-2 in the quantitative response to estradiol and tamoxifen. J Cell Sci 123:1253–1261. https://doi.org/10.1242/jcs.061135
16. Echeverria PC, Picard Didier D (2010) Molecular chaperones, essential partners of steroid hormone receptors for activity and mobility. Biochim Biophys Acta, Mol Cell Res 1803:641–649. https://doi.org/10.1016/j.bbamcr.2009.11.012
17. Kumar R, Zakharov MN, Khan SH, Miki R, Jang H, Toraldo G, Singh R, Bhasin S, Jasuja R (2011) The dynamic structure of the estrogen receptor. J Amino Acids 2011:1. https://doi.org/10.4061/2011/812540
18. Shiau AK, Barstad D, Loria PM, Cheng L, Kushner PJ, Agard DA, Greene GL (1998) The structural basis of estrogen receptor/coactivator recognition and the antagonism of this interaction by tamoxifen. Cell 95:927–937. https://doi.org/10.1016/S0092-8674(00)81717-1
19. Montano MM, Müller V, Trobaugh A, Katzenellenbogen BS (1995) The carboxy-terminal F domain of the human estrogen receptor: role in the transcriptional activity of the receptor and the effectiveness of antiestrogens as estrogen antagonists. Mol Endocrinol 9:814–825
20. Patel SR, Skafar DF (2015) Modulation of nuclear receptor activity by the F domain. Mol Cell Endocrinol 418:298–305. https://doi.org/10.1016/j.mce.2015.07.009
21. Ali S, Metzger D, Bornert J, Chambon P (1993) Modulation of transcriptional activation by ligand-dependent phosphorylation of the human oestrogen receptor A/B region. EMBO J 12:1153–1160. https://doi.org/10.1002/j.1460-2075.1993.tb05756.x
22. Bunone G, Briand PA, Miksicek RJ, Picard D (1996) Activation of the unliganded estrogen receptor by EGF involves the MAP kinase pathway and direct phosphorylation. EMBO J 15:2174–2183. https://doi.org/10.1016/j.jsbmb.2015.07.018
23. Le Romancer M, Poulard C, Cohen P, Sentis SP, Renoir JM, Corbo L (2011) Cracking the estrogen receptor's posttranslational code in breast tumors. Endocr Rev 32:597–622. https://doi.org/10.1210/er.2010-0016
24. Sheeler C, Singleton DW, Khan SA (2003) Mutation of serines 104, 106, and 118 inhibits dimerization of the human estrogen receptor in yeast. Endocr Res 29:237–255
25. Ward RD, Weigel NL (2009) Steroid receptor phosphorylation: assigning function to site-specific phosphorylation. Biofactors 35:528–536. https://doi.org/10.1002/biof.66
26. Chen D, Pace PE, Coombes RC, Ali S (1999) Phosphorylation of human estrogen receptor alpha by protein kinase A regulates dimerization. Mol Cell Biol 19:1002–1015

27. Shindo S, Sakuma T, Negishi M, Squires J (2012) Phosphorylation of serine 212 confers novel activity to human estrogen receptor α. Steroids 77:448–453. https://doi.org/10.1016/j.steroids.2012.01.001

28. Anbalagan M, Rowan BG (2015) Estrogen receptor alpha phosphorylation and its functional impact in human breast cancer. Mol Cell Endocrinol 418:264–272. https://doi.org/10.1016/j.mce.2015.01.016

29. Cui Y, Zhang M, Pestell R, Curran EM, Welshons WV, Fuqua SAW (2004) Phosphorylation of estrogen receptor α blocks its acetylation and regulates estrogen sensitivity. Cancer Res 64:9199–9208. https://doi.org/10.1158/0008-5472.CAN-04-2126

30. Atsriku C, Britton DJ, Held JM, Schilling B, Scott GK, Gibson BW, Benz CC, Baldwin MA (2009) Systematic mapping of posttranslational modifications in human estrogen receptor-alpha with emphasis on novel phosphorylation sites. Mol Cell Proteomics 8:467–480. https://doi.org/10.1074/mcp.M800282-MCP200

31. Tecalco-Cruz AC, Ramírez-Jarquín JO (2017) Mechanisms that increase stability of estrogen receptor alpha in breast cancer. Clin Breast Cancer 17:1–10. https://doi.org/10.1016/j.clbc.2016.07.015

32. Nawaz Z, Lonard DM, Dennis AP, Smith CL, O'Malley BW (1999) Proteasome-dependent degradation of the human estrogen receptor. Proc Natl Acad Sci U S A 96:1858–1862. https://doi.org/10.1073/pnas.96.5.1858

33. Lonard DM, Nawaz Z, Smith CL, O'Malley BW (2000) The 26S proteasome is required for estrogen receptor-alpha and coactivator turnover and for efficient estrogen receptor-alpha transactivation. Mol Cell 5:939–948. https://doi.org/10.1016/S1097-2765(00)80259-2

34. Métivier R, Penot G, Hübner MR, Reid G, Brand H, Koš M, Gannon F (2003) Estrogen receptor-α directs ordered, cyclical, and combinatorial recruitment of cofactors on a natural target promoter. Cell 115:751–763. https://doi.org/10.1016/S0092-8674(03)00934-6

35. Shang Y, Hu X, DiRenzo J, Lazar MA, Brown M (2000) Cofactor dynamics and sufficiency in estrogen receptor–regulated transcription. Cell 103:843–852. https://doi.org/10.1016/S0092-8674(00)00188-4

36. Reid G, Hübner MR, Métivier R, Brand H, Denger S, Manu D, Beaudouin J, Ellenberg J, Gannon F (2003) Cyclic, proteasome-mediated turnover of unliganded and liganded ERα on responsive promoters is an integral feature of estrogen signaling. Mol Cell 11:695–707. https://doi.org/10.1016/S1097-2765(03)00090-X

37. Berry NB, Fan M, Nephew KP (2008) Estrogen receptor-α hinge-region lysines 302 and 303 regulate receptor degradation by the proteasome. Mol Endocrinol 22:1535–1551. https://doi.org/10.1210/me.2007-0449

38. Duong V, Boulle N, Daujat S, Chauvet J, Bonnet S, Neel H, Cavaillès V (2007) Differential regulation of estrogen receptor α turnover and transactivation by Mdm2 and stress-inducing agents. Cancer Res 67:5513–5521. https://doi.org/10.1158/0008-5472.CAN-07-0967

39. Li L, Li Z, Howley PM, Sacks DB (2006) E6AP and calmodulin reciprocally regulate estrogen receptor stability. J Biol Chem 281:1978–1985. https://doi.org/10.1074/jbc.M508545200

40. Zhou W, Srinivasan S, Nawaz Z, Slingerland JM (2014) ERα, SKP2 and E2F-1 form a feed forward loop driving late ERα targets and G1 cell cycle progression. Oncogene 33:2341–2353. https://doi.org/10.1038/onc.2013.197

41. Bhatt S, Xiao Z, Meng Z, Katzenellenbogen BS (2012) Phosphorylation by p38 mitogen-activated protein kinase promotes estrogen receptor α turnover and functional activity via the SCF(Skp2) proteasomal complex. Mol Cell Biol 32:1928–1943. https://doi.org/10.1128/MCB.06561-11

42. Shao W, Keeton EK, McDonnell DP, Brown M (2004) Coactivator AIB1 links estrogen receptor transcriptional activity and stability. Proc Natl Acad Sci U S A 101:11599–11604. https://doi.org/10.1073/pnas.0402997101

43. Zhang H, Sun L, Liang J, Yu W, Zhang Y, Wang Y, Chen Y, Li R, Sun X, Shang Y (2006) The catalytic subunit of the proteasome is engaged in the entire process of estrogen receptor-regulated transcription. EMBO J 25:4223–4233. https://doi.org/10.1038/sj.emboj.7601306

44. Stanišić V, Malovannaya A, Qin J, Lonard DM, O'Malley BW (2009) OTU domain-containing ubiquitin aldehyde-binding protein 1 (OTUB1) deubiquitinates estrogen receptor (ER)α and affects ERα transcriptional activity. J Biol Chem 284:16135–16145. https://doi.org/10.1074/jbc.M109.007484

45. Wang C, Fu M, Angeletti RH, Siconolfi-Baez L, Reutens AT, Albanese C, Lisanti MP, Katzenellenbogen BS, Kato S, Hopp T, Fuqua SAW, Lopez GN, Kushner PJ, Pestell RG (2001) Direct acetylation of the estrogen receptor α hinge region by p300 regulates transactivation and hormone sensitivity. J Biol Chem 276:18375–18383. https://doi.org/10.1074/jbc.M100800200

46. Kim MY, Woo EM, Chong YTE, Homenko DR, Kraus WL (2006) Acetylation of estrogen receptor α by p300 at lysines 266 and 268 enhances the deoxyribonucleic acid binding and transactivation activities of the receptor. Mol Endocrinol 20:1479–1493. https://doi.org/10.1210/me.2005-0531

47. Zhang X, Tanaka K, Yan J, Li J, Peng D, Jiang Y, Yang Z, Barton MC, Wen H, Shi X (2013) Regulation of estrogen receptor α by histone methyltransferase SMYD2-mediated protein methylation. Proc Natl Acad Sci 110:17284–17289. https://doi.org/10.1073/pnas.1307959110

48. Subramanian K, Jia D, Kapoor-Vazirani P, Powell DR, Collins RE, Sharma D, Peng J, Cheng X, Vertino PM (2008) Regulation of estrogen receptor α by the SET7 lysine methyltransferase. Mol Cell 30:336–347. https://doi.org/10.1016/j.molcel.2008.03.022

49. O'Lone R, Frith MC, Karlsson EK, Hansen U (2004) Genomic targets of nuclear estrogen receptors. Mol Endocrinol 18:1859–1875. https://doi.org/10.1210/me.2003-0044

50. Klinge CM (2001) Estrogen receptor interaction with estrogen response elements. Nucleic Acids Res 29:2905–2919. https://doi.org/10.1093/nar/29.14.2905

51. Gruber CJ, Gruber DM, Gruber IML, Wieser F, Huber JC (2004) Anatomy of the estrogen response element. Trends Endocrinol Metab 15:73–78. https://doi.org/10.1016/j.tem.2004.01.008

52. Björnström L, Sjöberg M (2005) Mechanisms of estrogen receptor signaling: convergence of genomic and nongenomic actions on target genes. Mol Endocrinol 19:833–842. https://doi.org/10.1210/me.2004-0486

53. Lu T, Achari Y, Sciore P, Hart DA (2006) Estrogen receptor alpha regulates matrix metalloproteinase-13 promoter activity primarily through the AP-1 transcriptional regulatory site. Biochim Biophys Acta Mol basis Dis 1762:719–731. https://doi.org/10.1016/j.bbadis.2006.06.007

54. Jeffy BD, Hockings JK, Kemp MQ, Morgan SS, Hager JA, Beliakoff J, Whitesell LJ, Bowden GT, Romagnolo DF (2005) An estrogen receptor-α/p300 complex activates the BRCA-1 promoter at an AP-1 site that binds Jun/Fos transcription factors: repressive effects of p53 on BRCA-1 transcription. Neoplasia 7:873–882. https://doi.org/10.1593/neo.05256

55. Teyssier C, Belguise K, Galtier F, Chalbos D (2001) Characterization of the physical interaction between estrogen receptor α and JUN proteins. J Biol Chem 276:36361–36369. https://doi.org/10.1074/jbc.M101806200

56. Kushner PJ, Agard DA, Greene GL, Scanlan TS, Shiau AK, Uht RM, Webb P (2000) Estrogen receptor pathways to AP-1. J Steroid Biochem Mol Biol 74:311–317. https://doi.org/10.1016/S0960-0760(00)00108-4

57. Wang C, Mayer JA, Mazumdar A, Fertuck K, Kim H, Brown M, Brown PH (2011) Estrogen induces c-myc gene expression via an upstream enhancer activated by the estrogen receptor and the AP-1 transcription factor. Mol Endocrinol 25:1527–1538. https://doi.org/10.1210/me.2011-1037

58. Petz LN, Nardulli AM (2000) Sp1 binding sites and an estrogen response element half-site are involved in regulation of the human progesterone receptor A promoter. Mol Endocrinol 14:972–985. https://doi.org/10.1210/mend.14.7.0493

59. Rishi AK, Shao ZM, Baumann RG, Li XS, Sheikh MS, Kimura S, Bashirelahi N, Fontana JA (1995) Estradiol regulation of the human retinoic acid receptor α gene in human breast carcinoma cells is mediated via an imperfect half-palindromic estrogen response element and sp1 motifs. Cancer Res 55:4999–5006

60. Roeder RG (1996) The role of general initiation factors in transcription by RNA polymerase II. Trends Biochem Sci 21:327–335. https://doi.org/10.1016/0968-0004(96)10050-5
61. Roeder RG (1998) Role of general and gene-specific cofactors in the regulation of eukaryotic transcription. Cold Spring Harb Symp Quant Biol 63:201–218
62. Glass CK, Rosenfeld MG (2000) The coregulator exchange in transcriptional functions of nuclear receptors. Genes Dev 14:121–141. https://doi.org/10.1101/gad.14.2.121
63. McKenna NJ, O'Malley BW (2002) Combinatorial control of gene expression by nuclear receptors and coregulators. Cell 108:465–474. https://doi.org/10.1016/S0092-8674(02)00641-4
64. Lonard DM, O'Malley BW (2007) Nuclear receptor coregulators: judges, juries, and executioners of cellular regulation. Mol Cell 27:691–700. https://doi.org/10.1016/j.molcel.2007.08.012
65. Nilsson S, Mäkelä S, Treuter E, Tujague M, Thomsen J, Andersson G, Enmark E, Pettersson K, Warner M, Gustafsson J-Å (2001) Mechanisms of estrogen action. Physiol Rev 81:1535–1565. https://doi.org/10.1152/physrev.2001.81.4.1535
66. Malik S, Baek HJ, Wu W, Roeder RG (2005) Structural and functional characterization of PC2 and RNA polymerase II-associated subpopulations of metazoan mediator. Mol Cell Biol 25:2117–2129. https://doi.org/10.1128/MCB.25.6.2117
67. Conaway RC, Sato S, Tomomori-Sato C, Yao T, Conaway JW (2005) The mammalian mediator complex and its role in transcriptional regulation. Trends Biochem Sci 30:250–255. https://doi.org/10.1016/j.tibs.2005.03.002
68. Kornberg RD (2005) Mediator and the mechanism of transcriptional activation. Trends Biochem Sci 30:235–239. https://doi.org/10.1016/j.tibs.2005.03.011
69. Zhang X, Krutchinsky A, Fukuda A, Chen W, Yamamura S, Chait BT, Roeder RG (2005) MED1/TRAP220 exists predominantly in a TRAP/mediator subpopulation enriched in RNA polymerase II and is required for ER-mediated transcription. Mol Cell 19:89–100. https://doi.org/10.1016/j.molcel.2005.05.015
70. Jiang P, Hu Q, Ito M, Meyer S, Waltz S, Khan S, Roeder RG, Zhang X (2010) Key roles for MED1 LxxLL motifs in pubertal mammary gland development and luminal-cell differentiation. Proc Natl Acad Sci U S A 107:6765–6770. https://doi.org/10.1073/pnas.1001814107
71. Yang Y, Leonard M, Zhang Y, Zhao D, Charif M, Khan S, Wang J, Lower E, Zhang X (2018) HER2-driven breast tumorigenesis relies upon interactions of the estrogen receptor with coactivator MED1. 78:422–435
72. Wärnmark A, Almlöf T, Leers J, Gustafsson JÅ, Treuter E (2001) Differential recruitment of the mammalian mediator subunit TRAP220 by estrogen receptors ERalpha and ERbeta. J Biol Chem 276:23397–23404. https://doi.org/10.1074/jbc.M011651200
73. Kang YK, Guermah M, Yuan C-X, Roeder RG (2002) The TRAP/mediator coactivator complex interacts directly with estrogen receptors and through the TRAP220 subunit and directly enhances estrogen receptor function in vitro. Proc Natl Acad Sci 99:2642–2647. https://doi.org/10.1073/pnas.261715899
74. Fondell JD, Ge H, Roeder RG (1996) Ligand induction of a transcriptionally active thyroid hormone receptor coactivator complex. Proc Natl Acad Sci U S A 93:8329–8333. https://doi.org/10.1073/pnas.93.16.8329
75. Mcnally JG, Walker D, Wolford R, Hager GL (2000) The glucocorticoid receptor: rapid exchange with regulatory sites in living cells. Science 287:1262–1266. https://doi.org/10.1126/science.287.5456.1262
76. Yi P, Wang Z, Feng Q, Chou CK, Pintilie GD, Shen H, Foulds CE, Fan G, Serysheva I, Ludtke SJ, Schmid MF, Hung MC, Chiu W, O'Malley BW (2017) Structural and functional impacts of ER coactivator sequential recruitment. Mol Cell 67:733–743.e4. https://doi.org/10.1016/j.molcel.2017.07.026
77. Voss TC, Schiltz RL, Sung MH, Yen PM, Stamatoyannopoulos JA, Biddie SC, Johnson TA, Miranda TB, John S, Hager GL (2011) Dynamic exchange at regulatory elements during chromatin remodeling underlies assisted loading mechanism. Cell 146:544–554. https://doi.org/10.1016/j.cell.2011.07.006

78. Watanabe T, Inoue S, Hiroi H, Orimo A, Kawashima H, Muramatsu M (1998) Isolation of estrogen-responsive genes with a CpG island library. Mol Cell Biol 18:442–449. https://doi.org/10.1128/MCB.18.1.442

79. Dubik D, Dembinski TC, Shiu RP (1987) Stimulation of c-myc oncogene expression associated with estrogen-induced proliferation of human breast cancer cells. Cancer Res 47:6517–6521

80. Sabbah M, Courilleau D, Mester J, Redeuilh G (1999) Estrogen induction of the cyclin D1 promoter: involvement of a cAMP response-like element. Proc Natl Acad Sci 96:11217–11222. https://doi.org/10.1073/pnas.96.20.11217

81. Bourdeau V, Deschênes J, Métivier R, Nagai Y, Nguyen D, Bretschneider N, Gannon F, White JH, Mader S (2004) Genome-wide identification of high-affinity estrogen response elements in human and mouse. Mol Endocrinol 18:1411–1427. https://doi.org/10.1210/me.2003-0441

82. Vega VB, Lin C-Y, Lai KS, Kong SL, Xie M, Su X, Teh HF, Thomsen JS, Yeo AL, Sung WK, Bourque G, Liu ET (2006) Multiplatform genome-wide identification and modeling of functional human estrogen receptor binding sites. Genome Biol 7:R82. https://doi.org/10.1186/gb-2006-7-9-r82

83. Carroll JS, Liu XS, Brodsky AS, Li W, Meyer CA, Szary AJ, Eeckhoute J, Shao W, Hestermann EV, Geistlinger TR, Fox EA, Silver PA, Brown M (2005) Chromosome-wide mapping of estrogen receptor binding reveals long-range regulation requiring the forkhead protein FoxA1. Cell 122:33–43. https://doi.org/10.1016/j.cell.2005.05.008

84. Carroll JS, Meyer CA, Song J, Li W, Geistlinger TR, Eeckhoute J, Brodsky AS, Keeton EK, Fertuck KC, Hall GF, Wang Q, Bekiranov S, Sementchenko V, Fox EA, Silver PA, Gingeras TR, Liu XS, Brown M (2006) Genome-wide analysis of estrogen receptor binding sites. Nat Genet 38:1289–1297. https://doi.org/10.1038/ng1901

85. Kwon Y-S, Garcia-Bassets I, Hutt KR, Cheng CS, Jin M, Liu D, Benner C, Wang D, Ye Z, Bibikova M, Fan J-B, Duan L, Glass CK, Rosenfeld MG, Fu X-D (2007) Sensitive ChIP-DSL technology reveals an extensive estrogen receptor alpha-binding program on human gene promoters. Proc Natl Acad Sci U S A 104:4852–4857. https://doi.org/10.1073/pnas.0700715104

86. Lin CY, Vega VB, Thomsen JS, Zhang T, Kong SL, Xie M, Chiu KP, Lipovich L, Barnett DH, Stossi F, Yeo A, George J, Kuznetsov VA, Lee YK, Charn TH, Palanisamy N, Miller LD, Cheung E, Katzenellenbogen BS, Ruan Y, Bourque G, Wei CL, Liu ET (2007) Whole-genome cartography of estrogen receptor alpha binding sites. PLoS Genet 3:e87. https://doi.org/10.1371/journal.pgen.0030087

87. Hua S, Kallen CB, Dhar R, Baquero MT, Mason CE, Russell BA, Shah PK, Liu J, Khramtsov A, Tretiakova MS, Krausz TN, Olopade OI, Rimm DL, White KP (2008) Genomic analysis of estrogen cascade reveals histone variant H2A.Z associated with breast cancer progression. Mol Syst Biol 4. https://doi.org/10.1038/msb.2008.25

88. Hurtado A, Holmes KA, Geistlinger TR, Hutcheson IR, Nicholson RI, Brown M, Jiang J, Howat WJ, Ali S, Carroll JS (2008) Regulation of ERBB2 by oestrogen receptor-PAX2 determines response to tamoxifen. Nature 456:663–666. https://doi.org/10.1038/nature07483

89. Kininis M, Chen BS, Diehl AG, Isaacs GD, Zhang T, Siepel AC, Clark AG, Kraus WL (2007) Genomic analyses of transcription factor binding, histone acetylation, and gene expression reveal mechanistically distinct classes of estrogen-regulated promoters. Mol Cell Biol 27:5090–5104. https://doi.org/10.1128/MCB.00083-07

90. Welboren W-J, van Driel MA, Janssen-Megens EM, van Heeringen SJ, Sweep FC, Span PN, Stunnenberg HG (2009) ChIP-Seq of ERα and RNA polymerase II defines genes differentially responding to ligands. EMBO J 28:1418–1428. https://doi.org/10.1038/emboj.2009.88

91. Hah N, Danko CG, Core L, Waterfall JJ, Siepel A, Lis JT, Kraus WL (2011) A rapid, extensive, and transient transcriptional response to estrogen signaling in breast cancer cells. Cell 145:622–634. https://doi.org/10.1016/j.cell.2011.03.042

92. Joseph R, Orlov YL, Huss M, Sun W, Li Kong S, Ukil L, Pan YF, Li G, Lim M, Thomsen JS, Ruan Y, Clarke ND, Prabhakar S, Cheung E, Liu ET (2010) Integrative model of genomic factors for determining binding site selection by estrogen receptor-α. Mol Syst Biol 6. https://doi.org/10.1038/msb.2010.109

93. Lin C-Y, Ström A, Vega VB, Kong SL, Yeo AL, Thomsen JS, Chan WC, Doray B, Bangarusamy DK, Ramasamy A, Vergara LA, Tang S, Chong A, Bajic VB, Miller LD, Gustafsson J-Å, Liu ET (2004) Discovery of estrogen receptor alpha target genes and response elements in breast tumor cells. Genome Biol 5:R66. https://doi.org/10.1186/gb-2004-5-9-r66

94. Cheung E, Kraus WL (2010) Genomic analyses of hormone signaling and gene regulation. Annu Rev Physiol 72:191–218. https://doi.org/10.1146/annurev-physiol-021909-135840

95. Cirillo LA, Lin FR, Cuesta I, Friedman D, Jarnik M, Zaret KS (2002) Opening of compacted chromatin by early developmental transcription factors HNF3 (FoxA) and GATA-4. Mol Cell 9:279–289. https://doi.org/10.1016/S1097-2765(02)00459-8

96. Hurtado A, Holmes KA, Ross-Innes CS, Schmidt D, Carroll JS (2011) FOXA1 is a key determinant of estrogen receptor function and endocrine response. Nat Genet 43:27–33. https://doi.org/10.1038/ng.730

97. Holmes KA, Hurtado A, Brown GD, Launchbury R, Ross-Innes CS, Hadfield J, Odom DT, Carroll JS (2012) Transducin-like enhancer protein 1 mediates estrogen receptor binding and transcriptional activity in breast cancer cells. Proc Natl Acad Sci U S A 109:2748–2753. https://doi.org/10.1073/pnas.1018863108

98. Tan SK, Lin ZH, Chang CW, Varang V, Chng KR, Pan YF, Yong EL, Sung WK, Sung WK, Cheung E (2011) AP-2γ regulates oestrogen receptor-mediated long-range chromatin interaction and gene transcription. EMBO J 30:2569–2581. https://doi.org/10.1038/emboj.2011.151

99. Magnani L, Ballantyne EB, Zhang X, Lupien M (2011) PBX1 genomic pioneer function drives ERα signaling underlying progression in breast cancer. PLoS Genet 7:1–15. https://doi.org/10.1371/journal.pgen.1002368

100. Magnani L, Patten DK, Nguyen VTM, Hong S-P, Steel JH, Patel N, Lombardo Y, Faronato M, Gomes AR, Woodley L, Page K, Guttery D, Primrose L, Fernandez Garcia D, Shaw J, Viola P, Green A, Nolan C, Ellis IO, Rakha EA, Shousha S, Lam EW-F, Gyorffy B, Lupien M, Coombes RC (2015) The pioneer factor PBX1 is a novel driver of metastatic progression in ERalpha-positive breast cancer. Oncotarget 6:21878–21891. https://doi.org/10.18632/oncotarget.4243

101. Hagège H, Klous P, Braem C, Splinter E, Dekker J, Cathala G, de Laat W, Forné T (2007) Quantitative analysis of chromosome conformation capture assays (3C-qPCR). Nat Protoc 2:1722–1733. https://doi.org/10.1038/nprot.2007.243

102. Simonis M, Kooren J, de Laat W (2007) An evaluation of 3C-based methods to capture DNA interactions. Nat Methods 4:895–901

103. Davies JOJ, Oudelaar AM, Higgs DR, Hughes JR (2017) How best to identify chromosomal interactions: a comparison of approaches. Nat Methods 14:125–134. https://doi.org/10.1038/nmeth.4146

104. Li W, Hu Y, Oh S, Ma Q, Merkurjev D, Song X, Zhou X, Liu Z, Tanasa B, He X, Chen A, Ohgi K, Zhang J, Liu W, Rosenfeld MG (2015) Condensin I and II complexes license full estrogen receptor α-dependent enhancer activation. Mol Cell 59:188–202. https://doi.org/10.1016/j.molcel.2015.06.002

105. Fullwood MJ, Liu MH, Pan YF, Liu J, Xu H, Mohamed YB, Orlov YL, Velkov S, Ho A, Mei PH, Chew EGY, Huang PYH, Welboren W-J, Han Y, Ooi HS, Ariyaratne PN, Vega VB, Luo Y, Tan PY, Choy PY, Wansa KDSA, Zhao B, Lim KS, Leow SC, Yow JS, Joseph R, Li H, Desai KV, Thomsen JS, Lee YK, Karuturi RKM, Herve T, Bourque G, Stunnenberg HG, Ruan X, Cacheux-Rataboul V, Sung W-K, Liu ET, Wei C-L, Cheung E, Ruan Y (2009) An oestrogen-receptor-α-bound human chromatin interactome. Nature 462:58–64. https://doi.org/10.1038/nature08497

106. Wood AJ, Severson AF, Meyer BJ (2010) Condensin and cohesin complexity: the expanding repertoire of functions. Nat Rev Genet 11:391–404. https://doi.org/10.1038/nrg2794

107. Yuen KC, Gerton JL (2018) Taking cohesin and condensin in context. PLoS Genet 14:1–14. https://doi.org/10.1371/journal.pgen.1007118

108. Schmidt D, Schwalie PC, Ross-Innes CS, Hurtado A, Brown GD, Carroll JS, Flicek P, Odom DT (2010) A CTCF-independent role for cohesin in tissue-specific transcription. Genome Res 20:578–588. https://doi.org/10.1101/gr.100479.109

109. Antony J, Dasgupta T, Rhodes JM, McEwan MV, Print CG, O'Sullivan JM, Horsfield JA (2015) Cohesin modulates transcription of estrogen-responsive genes. Biochim Biophys Acta 1849:257–269. https://doi.org/10.1016/j.bbagrm.2014.12.011

110. Kagey MH, Newman JJ, Bilodeau S, Zhan Y, Orlando DA, van Berkum NL, Ebmeier CC, Goossens J, Rahl PB, Levine SS, Taatjes DJ, Dekker J, Young RA (2010) Mediator and cohesin connect gene expression and chromatin architecture. Nature 467:430–435. https://doi.org/10.1038/nature09380

111. Ebmeier CC, Taatjes DJ (2010) Activator-mediator binding regulates mediator-cofactor interactions. Proc Natl Acad Sci 107:11283–11288. https://doi.org/10.1073/pnas.0914215107

112. Chen Z, Zhang C, Wu D, Chen H, Rorick A, Zhang X, Wang Q (2011) Phospho-MED1-enhanced UBE2C locus looping drives castration-resistant prostate cancer growth. EMBO J 30:2405–2419. https://doi.org/10.1038/emboj.2011.154

113. Saramäki A, Diermeler S, Kellner R, Laitinen H, Väisänen S, Cariberg C (2009) Cyclical chromatin looping and transcription factor association on the regulatory regions of the p21 (CDKN1A) gene in response to 1α,25-dihydroxyvitamin D3. J Biol Chem 284:8073–8082. https://doi.org/10.1074/jbc.M808090200

114. Plank JL, Dean A (2014) Enhancer function: mechanistic and genome-wide insights come together. Mol Cell 55:5–14. https://doi.org/10.1016/j.molcel.2014.06.015

115. Kim TK, Hemberg M, Gray JM (2015) Enhancer RNAs: a class of long noncoding RNAs synthesized at enhancers. Cold Spring Harb Perspect Biol 7:2015–2018. https://doi.org/10.1101/cshperspect.a018622

116. Shiekhattar R (2013) Opening the chromatin by eRNAs. Mol Cell 51:557–558. https://doi.org/10.1016/j.molcel.2013.08.033

117. Li W, Notani D, Rosenfeld MG (2016) Enhancers as non-coding RNA transcription units: recent insights and future perspectives. Nat Rev Genet 17:207–223. https://doi.org/10.1038/nrg.2016.4

118. Li W, Notani D, Ma Q, Tanasa B, Nunez E, Chen AY, Merkurjev D, Zhang J, Ohgi K, Song X, Oh S, Kim H-S, Glass CK, Rosenfeld MG (2013) Functional roles of enhancer RNAs for oestrogen-dependent transcriptional activation. Nature 498:516–520. https://doi.org/10.1038/nature12210

119. Liu Z, Merkurjev D, Yang F, Li W, Oh S, Friedman MJ, Song X, Zhang F, Ma Q, Ohgi KA, Krones A, Rosenfeld MG (2014) Enhancer activation requires trans-recruitment of a mega transcription factor complex. Cell 159:356–373. https://doi.org/10.1016/j.cell.2014.08.027

120. Hah N, Murakami S, Nagari A, Danko CG, Kraus WL (2013) Enhancer transcripts mark active estrogen receptor binding sites. Genome Res 23:1210–1223. https://doi.org/10.1101/gr.152306.112

121. Bhat-Nakshatri P, Wang G, Appaiah H, Luktuke N, Carroll JS, Geistlinger TR, Brown M, Badve S, Liu Y, Nakshatri H (2008) AKT alters genome-wide estrogen receptor binding and impacts estrogen signaling in breast cancer. Mol Cell Biol 28:7487–7503. https://doi.org/10.1128/MCB.00799-08

122. Michalides R, Griekspoor A, Balkenende A, Verwoerd D, Janssen L, Jalink K, Floore A, Velds A, Van't Veer L, Neefjes J (2004) Tamoxifen resistance by a conformational arrest of the estrogen receptor after PKA activation in breast cancer. Cancer Cell 5:597–605. https://doi.org/10.1016/j.ccr.2004.05.016

123. De Leeuw R, Flach K, Toaldo CB, Alexi X, Canisius S, Neefjes J, Michalides R, Zwart W (2013) PKA phosphorylation redirects ERα to promoters of a unique gene set to induce tamoxifen resistance. Oncogene 32:3543–3551. https://doi.org/10.1038/onc.2012.361

124. Lupien M, Meyer CA, Bailey ST, Eeckhoute J, Cook J, Westerling T, Zhang X, Carroll JS, Rhodes DR, Liu XS, Brown M (2010) Growth factor stimulation induces a distinct ER(alpha) cistrome underlying breast cancer endocrine resistance. Genes Dev 24:2219–2227. https://doi.org/10.1101/gad.1944810

Structural Studies with Coactivators for the Estrogen Receptor

Ping Yi, Zhao Wang, and Bert W. O'Malley

Abstract Coactivators play essential roles in nuclear receptor-mediated gene transcription. To date, a variety of coactivators have been identified. They can be scaffolding proteins, chromatin remodelers, posttranslational modification enzymes, or RNA splicing factors. Different coactivators are recruited to a nuclear receptor to form large protein complexes at different stages of transcription, and they often act synergistically. Structural analyses on these coactivators and their complex formation with nuclear receptors provide valuable information on understanding nuclear receptor-mediated gene regulation. Here we review recent structural studies on three well-documented nuclear receptor coactivators: steroid receptor coactivators (SRCs), CBP/p300, and CARM1, and their assembly into active DNA-bound estrogen receptor/coactivator complexes for initiation and for the subsequent step of elongation. This review specifically emphasizes the structural interaction within the estrogen receptor (ER) coactivator complex.

Keywords Estrogen receptor · Coactivators · Structure · Complex · Protein-protein interaction

1 Introduction

Transcription is a fundamental cellular process that controls gene expression. Precise regulation of transcription is essential for normal cell growth, differentiation, and function. Central players in this process are the general transcription machinery including RNA polymerase and its associated factors, DNA sequence-specific

P. Yi · B. W. O'Malley (✉)
Department of Molecular and Cellular Biology, Baylor College of Medicine, Houston, TX, USA
e-mail: berto@bcm.edu

Z. Wang
Verna and Marrs McLean Department of Biochemistry and Molecular Biology, Baylor College of Medicine, Houston, TX, USA

© Springer Nature Switzerland AG 2019   71
X. Zhang (ed.), *Estrogen Receptor and Breast Cancer*, Cancer Drug Discovery and Development, https://doi.org/10.1007/978-3-319-99350-8_4

transcription factors, and a plethora of coregulators, which include coactivators that assist transcription activation and corepressors that repress transcription. Nuclear receptors are ligand-dependent transcription factors that are activated upon ligand binding. They interact with a variety of coactivators and recruit them to target gene promoter/enhancer regions to form large protein complexes and activate transcription. More than 300 coregulators have been identified so far (Nuclear Receptor Signaling Atlas, www.Nursa.org). They have diverse functions and are involved in different steps of transcription on different genes. These proteins can be chromatin remodeling enzymes, posttranslational modification enzymes, RNA splicing factors, or scaffolding proteins/bridging factors to bring other enzymatic coregulators to nuclear receptor complexes and stabilize general transcription machinery [1]. Understanding the structural basis of nuclear receptor/coactivator complexes provides valuable information on how different types of coactivators precisely contribute to nuclear receptor-mediated transcriptional activation.

Most nuclear receptor family members have generally similar domain structures. They have a conserved DNA-binding domain (DBD) at the central region that recognizes specific DNA-responsive elements, a C-terminal ligand-binding domain (LBD) that binds ligands and recruits ligand-dependent coactivators (AF-2), and a N-terminal variable region that often contains constitutive activation functions (e.g., AF-1) that the specific receptor also can bind coactivators. Crystal structures of certain regions of nuclear receptors especially the LBD have attracted much attention. Such studies provide valuable insights for understanding ligand-activated receptor function and therapeutic design of nuclear receptor antagonists. The X-ray structural studies of nuclear receptor domains have been reviewed recently [2–4] and will not be discussed here. Crystal structural studies of coactivators, however, are very limited due to the presence of intrinsically disordered regions, artifacts caused by a large amount of reduction from their large sizes, and conformational modification due to packing during the process of various chemical conditions in crystallization. Here we will focus on current understanding of several coactivator structures in context with our recent progress on structural organization of nuclear receptor/coactivator complexes.

2 Structural Studies of Individual Coactivators

2.1 Steroid Receptor Coactivator (SRC)

The existence of common limiting intermediary factors shared by different steroid receptors was long speculated following the observation of a squelching effect between different receptors or different activation function domains [5, 6]. Steroid receptor coactivator-1 (SRC-1/NCOA1) was the first coactivator identified through a yeast two-hybrid screen using the progesterone receptor LBD as a bait. Its overexpression enhances the receptor activity without altering basal activity of the promoter and inhibits the squelching effect [7]. Two other steroid receptor coactivator family members were later identified as SRC-2 (TIF2/GRIP1/NCOA2) [8, 9] and SRC-3 (ACTR/AIB1/RAC3/pCIP/TRAM1/NCOA3) [10–14]. They have similar domain structures and are approximately 160KDa size proteins and thus often are referred to as the p160 family. These three coactivators interact and activate many different nuclear receptors. They serve as primary coactivators and scaffolding proteins to recruit other secondary coactivators to nuclear receptor-targeted DNA-binding sites. The SRCs play important roles in regulating reproduction, metabolism, circadian biology, and cancer development [15–18].

The structure of SRCs can be divided into five domains (Fig. 1a). The N-terminus is a highly conserved bHLH-PAS (basic helix-loop-helix-Per Arnt Sim) domain. This domain is involved in the interaction between SRC and several secondary coactivators [19–22], as well as regulating SRC nuclear localization and protein turnover [23]. A Ser/Thr-rich region is targeted by many different posttranslational modifications (e.g., phosphorylation, monoubiquitination, and polyubiquitination) to control a SRC transcriptional time clock (activation and degradation) [24]. The central region is a RID domain (receptor-interacting domain); it interacts with a nuclear receptor LBD upon ligand activation. The C-terminal region of SRCs contains two activation domains: the CID domain (CBP/p300 interaction domain)

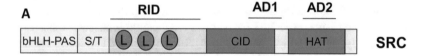

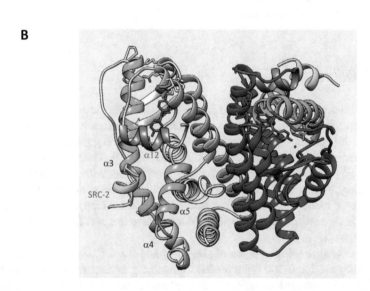

Fig. 1 SRC domain organization. (**a**) Schematic representation of SRCs. L represents LXXLL motif. (**b**) Crystal structure of SRC-2 LXXLL motif (NR box II, yellow) interacting with diethylstilbestrol (magenta)-bound ER LBD dimer (PDB 3ERD). The LXXLL motif binds to a hydrophobic groove in ER LBD formed by helices 3, 4, 5 (light blue) and helix 12 (green)

that interacts with the histone acetyltransferase CBP/p300 to promote histone acetylation (AD1) and the HAT domain (AD2) that contains a weak acetyltransferase activity [13, 25] and later recruits histone methyltransferases CARM1 (coactivator-associated arginine methyltransferase) and PRMT1.

Most of the prior SRC structural studies have been focused on the RID domain. There are three conserved LXXLL motifs (L represents leucine and X represents any amino acid) present in the RID domain. These motifs also are named NR boxes for their specific interactions with ligand-bound nuclear receptors [26]. Crystallographic studies of the binding NR box peptides to various nuclear receptors demonstrate that these peptides form amphipathic α-helices with leucine residues lined up on one side to contact a hydrophobic groove formed at the surface of agonist-bound receptor LBD [27] (Fig. 1b). The NR LBD is usually a three-layer sandwich-shaped structure consisting of 12 α-helices. Helix 12 is highly mobile in the absence of ligand binding (see review [4]). Agonist binding induces its transition from disordered to ordered structure [4], which then forms the SRC NR box-interacting hydrophobic groove together with helices 3, 4, and 5 [27–29]. Two highly conserved glutamate and lysine residues outside the hydrophobic groove also form a "charge clamp" with the LXXLL motifs to orient and pack the motifs into the coactivator-binding site [29].

The structures of other regions of SRCs remain undetermined. A NMR study on SRC-3 and CBP interaction domains indicates that both domains are intrinsically disordered when isolated [30]. However, they cooperate with each other to fold "synergistically" into a helical heterodimer [30]. This induced structure upon contact is not unique to SRC-CBP interaction domains. Many transcription factors interacting with CBP/p300 also have this structural feature to allow specific protein-protein interactions [31] (see below).

2.2   CBP/p300

CBP (CREB-binding protein [32]) and its paralog E1A-associated p300 proteins [33, 34] are essential coactivators for many transcription factors including nuclear receptors [35–38]. They play important roles in regulating cell growth, transformation, differentiation, apoptosis, and development [37, 39, 40]. The two proteins can function as bridging factors to connect transcription factors with basal transcriptional machinery, as protein scaffolds to build up multicomponent transcription factor complexes or mainly as protein and histone acetyltransferases to transfer an acetyl group from acetyl CoA to lysine residues in histones and their component substrates [39, 41] (Fig. 2a).

CBP and p300 have a high degree of similarity and share 63% identical amino acids [39]. They are large 300 KDa proteins containing several folded functional domains (Fig. 2b) connected through regions predicted to be intrinsically disordered [31, 42]. The bromodomain, CH2 region (cysteine-histidine-rich region 2), and HAT domain constitute the catalytic core of CBP/p300. The CH1/TAZ1 (transcriptional adaptor zinc finger 1), KIX (CREB-binding domain), CH3/TAZ2, and NCBD (nuclear coactivator-binding domain) domains mainly mediate the interaction of

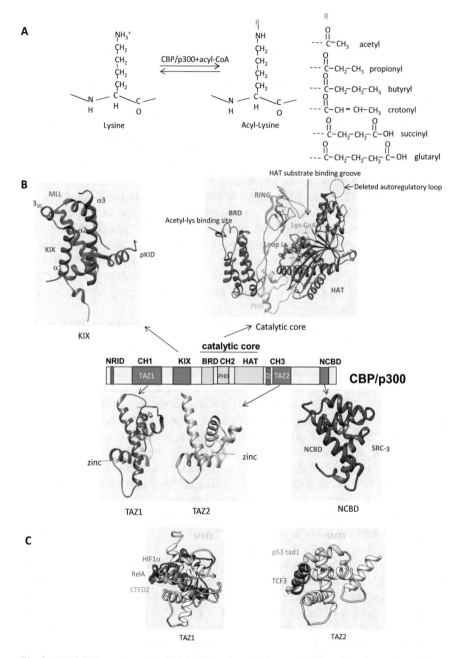

Fig. 2 CBP/p300 structures. (**a**) CBP/p300 catalyzes lysine acylation. R represents different acyl groups. (**b**) Schematic representation of CBP/p300 domains and folded domain structures. TAZ1 (PDB 1U2N); KIX (PDB 2LXT, KIX (blue) binds to MLL activation domain peptide (red) and CREB pKID peptide (purple)); catalytic core (PDB 4BHW); TAZ2 (PDB 1F81); NCBD (PDB 1KBH, NCBD (blue) binds to SRC-3 peptide (purple)). (**c**) Comparison of TAZ1 (left panel, white,

Fig. 2 (continued) PDB 2KA4) and TAZ2 (right panel, white, PDB 3T92) binding to TADs from different transcription factors. STAT2 (yellow, PDB 2KA4); HIF1α (purple, PDB 1L8C); RelA (blue, PDB 2LWW); CTED2 (green, PDB 1R8U); STAT1 (yellow, 2KA6); p53 (green, PDB 2K8F); TCF3 (blue, PDB 2MH0)

CBP/p300 with a variety of transcription factors, viral oncoproteins, basal transcription machinery, and coactivators.

CBP and p300 are KAT3 (lysine acetyltransferase 3 family) enzymes, which are different from other KATs (HATs) in that they use a "hit-and-run" (Theorell-Chance) catalytic mechanism [43]. They do not form a stable ternary complex with substrates and acetyl CoA cofactors. After acetyl CoA binding, substrates associate with the CBP/p300 surface transiently to allow acetyl group transfer to lysine residues. This mechanism is proposed to contribute to a broad CBP/p300 substrate specificity unlike other KATs which require a more specific substrate-binding pocket [43, 44]. CBP and p300 acetylate both histones and nonhistone proteins. Histone tail acetylation neutralizes lysine-positive charges and decondenses chromatin; it is generally associated with transcriptional activation [45, 46]. CBP and p300 are able to acetylate all core histones [47]. Their HAT activity is essential for ligand-induced nuclear receptor-target gene transcription [48]. CBP and p300 also acetylate a number of transcription factors and coactivators, such as p53 [49], CREB [50], E2F [51, 52], GATA-1 [53], TFIIE, TFIIF [54], SRC-3 [55], and regulate their transcriptional activities.

In addition to catalyzing acetylation on a broad set of substrates, CBP and p300 also utilize a variety of acyl-CoAs as cofactors to mediate histone propionylation, butyrylation, crotonylation, succinylation, glutarylation, and β-hydroxybutyrylation [56] (Fig. 2a). These non-acetyl acylations are believed to be functionally different from acetylation and exert unique regulations on gene transcription and chromatin structure [56]. P300-mediated histone butyrylation and crotonylation also were shown to strongly stimulate gene transcription in vitro [57, 58]. The relative concentrations of different acyl-CoAs regulated by cellular metabolism can determine the preference for p300 over different cofactors [56]. For example, under low glucose condition, non-acetyl histone acylations are more common [59, 60]. Crystal structures of the p300 HAT domain in a complex with different acyl-CoA cofactors demonstrate that p300 has a deep aliphatic pocket present in its active site to accommodate short-chain acyl groups that is not present in other HATs such as GCN5. This unique feature also explains the broad acyltransferase activity of p300 [61]. The preferred HAT for ER complex and SRC-3 is p300.

The HAT domain contains 380 residues. The X-ray structure of the HAT domain and Lys-CoA inhibitor complex demonstrates that it consists of seven central β-strands surrounded by nine α-helices and several loops (Fig. 2b) [43]. The Lys moiety of Lys-CoA mimics the substrate Lys residue. An unusual long substrate-binding loop L1 in the HAT domain, which is only found in CBP/p300 but not in other HATs, covers the Lys-CoA and appears to influence substrate binding [43]. CBP/p300 HAT activity is regulated by its autoacetylation. Hyperacetylated CBP/p300 is much more active than the hypoacetylated form [62]. Hyperacetylation occurs in an autoregulatory loop, which is a lysine-rich intrinsically disordered region in the HAT domain [62, 63]. When hypoacetylated, the autoregulatory loop competes with substrate binding to the HAT active site. Its autoacetylation releases its binding and thus enhances the HAT activity [62].

In addition to the loop L1 and the autoregulatory loop, domains flanking the HAT domain also play an important role in regulating the HAT activity. X-ray structures of CBP/p300 HAT and flanking domains, bromodomain, and the CH2 region [63, 64] show that they form a compact module with intimate association between flanking domains and the HAT domain (Fig. 2b). The bromodomain recognizes acetylated substrates. It is a left-handed four-helix bundle linked by two interspersed loops, which form an active acetyl-lysine binding pocket [65, 66] (Fig. 2b). This domain is required for CBP/p300 binding to its substrate, chromatin binding, and its full HAT activity [63, 67–70]. The CH2 region contains a PHD (plant homeodomain) finger interrupted by a RING (Really Interesting New Gene) domain [64]. The PHD finger is connected to the HAT domain and also makes multiple contacts with the bromodomain through hydrogen bonds and hydrophobic interactions [63, 64]. It also plays a role in recruiting p300 to chromatin [70, 71]. RING domains are often found in E3 ubiquitin ligases to mediate substrate ubiquitination. The RING domain in p300, however, does not have ubiquitination activity [64]. Instead, it has an inhibitory role on the HAT activity. It contacts the loop L1 and is positioned over the HAT active site, partially blocking access to the HAT substrate-binding groove [64]. Deletion of the RING domain significantly increases p300 autoacetylation and substrate acetylation [64].

CBP/p300 serves as a docking platform for numerous other transcription factors, components of the general transcription machinery, and coactivators, through its transactivation domains engaging in protein-protein interaction. Many of their interaction partners contain intrinsically disordered transactivation domains and adopt folded structures upon binding to CBP/p300 [31, 42]. The KIX domain was originally identified based on its interaction with the KID (kinase-inducible domain) domain of CREB [72]. It is a 90-residue long bundle of three α-helices and two additional 3_{10} helices [73]. In addition to CREB, it also interacts with p53 [74], c-Myb [75], MLL [76], c-Jun [77], FOXO3a [78], BRCA-1 [79], SREBP [80], and STAT-1 [81] transcription factors. This domain has two binding surfaces for interacting with different transcription factors or with different transactivation domains in one protein simultaneously. Unstructured phosphorylated KID of CREB and the c-Myb activation domain fold into helical structures upon binding to a common binding site, a shallow hydrophobic groove formed by helices 1 and 3, at the KIX surface (Fig. 2b) [73, 75]. A second binding site at the opposite surface of KIX formed by helices 2, 3, and 3_{10} is also a hydrophobic groove allowing the binding of the MLL or Jun activation domain [76, 77]. It was reported that MLL and c-Myb or MLL and p-KID form a stable ternary complex with KIX and the two binding events act cooperatively to enhance the protein-protein affinity [76, 82]. This interaction mechanism provides a structural basis for synergistic activation of transcription when CBP/p300 interacts with different transcription factors simultaneously. Some proteins, such as p53 and FOXO3a, have two disordered activation domains that each can interact with one of the KIX binding surfaces to enhance their binding affinities with the KIX domain [78, 83].

The TAZ1 at the CH1 region and TAZ2 at the CH3 region are also major domains interacting with transcription factors. They are zinc finger motifs having similar folding structures with four amphipathic α-helices stabilized by binding of three zinc atoms. TAZ1 and TAZ2 differ in that their fourth helix adopts opposite orientations resulting in different binding surfaces (Fig. 2b) [84]. They have different binding specificities to different subsets of intrinsically disordered transcription factor activation domains [42]. Comparison of structures of TAZ1 in a complex with trans-activation domains from HIF1α, CITED2, STAT2, and NFκB reveals that these unstructured TADs usually have multiple amphipathic regions and fold into helical structures when interacting with TAZ1, but they do not have a fixed binding site. Instead, they wrap around the entire TAZ1 molecule along a hydrophobic groove depending on the amino sequences of amphipathic regions [31] (Fig. 2c). TAZ2 is located close to the HAT domain. It interacts with numerous transcription factors [37]. Unlike TAZ1, TAZ2 has a hydrophobic docking site at the interface of helices 1, 2, and 3 for interacting with various disordered TADs and inducing helical structure folding [31] (Fig. 2c).

The NCBD domain at the C-terminus of CBP/p300 interacts with SRCs [30, 85], p53 [86] and IRF-3 [87]. Unlike other well-structured protein-protein interaction domains mentioned above, it has characteristics of a molten globule when not contacting its binding partners [30, 88]. NMR studies suggest that the free NCBD undergoes rapid reversible conformational exchange [89] and adopts different conformations upon binding to different proteins. It folds into a three-α-helix bundle when in contact with a SRC-3 CID region, which also transits from a disordered state into a three-helix structure. The two regions pack together to create an extensive leucine-rich hydrophobic core to stabilize the complex structure (Fig. 2b) [30]. When interacting with IRF-3, the NCBD folds into a three-helix structure, but contacts between these helices are different resulting in a different tertiary structure compared to SRC-bound NCBD [87, 89]. This feature of conformational flexibility could allow the NCBD to interact with different partners with optimized structural fit.

Since CBP/p300 interacts with numerous transcription factors and has a limited concentration in cells, it is important for a mechanism to exist that regulates its binding specificity with different proteins in response to external signals. The binding affinities of CBP/p300 with different partners can be positively or negatively regulated by partner protein phosphorylation, hydroxylation, and S-nitrosylation [42] as well as by PTMs on CBP/p300. For example, CARM1-mediated CBP/p300 methylation switches off its interaction with CREB and turns on a NR-activated gene transcription function [90, 91]. Similarly, phosphorylation of CBP S436 inhibits the interaction with CREB while enhancing its association with AP-1 and Pit-1 [92, 93]. Posttranslational modifications thus provide an important layer of regulation to control CBP/p300 specificity.

2.3   CARM1

CARM1 was originally identified in a yeast two-hybrid screen for proteins interacting with the AD2 domain of SRC-2/GRIP1 [94]. It synergizes with SRCs and CBP/p300 to activate NR-mediated target gene transcription [95, 96]. Loss of CARM1 in a mouse embryo significantly reduced estrogen-regulated gene transcription [97],

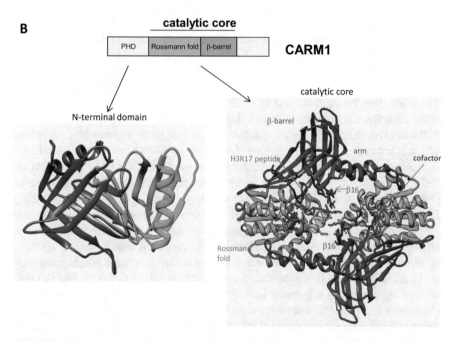

Fig. 3 CARM1 structures. (**a**) CARM1 catalyzes arginine mono- and dimethylation. (**b**) Schematic representation of CARM1 domains and structures. N-terminal domain dimer (PDB 2OQB); catalytic core dimer (PDB 5DX0)

indicating its important role in ER-mediated function. CARM1 belongs to a protein arginine methyltransferase (PRMT) family. It is a type I PRMT (PRMT4) that asymmetrically dimethylates arginines. It transfers methyl groups from S-adenosylmethionine (AdoMet) to a guanidino nitrogen of arginine leading to the formation of methylated arginine and S-adenosylhomocysteine (AdoHcy) (Fig. 3a). CARM1 methylates histones H3R17, H3R26 [98], and H3R42 [99], as well as non-histone proteins including SRC [100], CBP/p300 [90, 91, 101], Sox2 transcription factor [102], Notch1 [103], several RNA-binding proteins [104, 105], and splicing and transcription elongation factors [106]. CARM1 knockout mice are smaller than wild-type littermates and die shortly after birth [97]. It plays an important role in T cell development [107], neural development [108], and proliferation and differentiation of adipocyte [109], chondrocyte [110], and pulmonary epithelial cells [111].

CARM1 has three individual domains (Fig. 3b). The central region is a catalytic core that forms a head-to-tail dimer that is conserved in PRMTs. The catalytic PRMT core is folded into two domains that are connected by a conserved proline residue [112, 113]. The N-terminal part of the catalytic core is involved in cofactor binding. It contains a Rossmann fold structure [114], a sandwich-structure consisting of four α-helices and five β-strands, and two terminal α-helices (αX and αY) (Fig. 3b) [112, 113]. This structure is conserved for AdoMet binding in SAM-dependent methyltransferases [115]. Cofactor binding induces a structural change of the αX region from disordered structure to an α-helix, which then forms a deep binding pocket with other terminal helices and three β-strands in the Rossmann fold to bury the cofactor, restricting its accessibility only to the substrate arginine [113]. The C-terminal part of the catalytic core is a β-barrel (11 β-strands and 6 α-helices) and an arm (2 α-helices and 2 short 3_{10} helices) involved in CARM1 dimerization. The interaction between the arm in one monomer and the Rossmann fold structure in the other monomer is important for the dimer formation. Both N- and C-domains of the catalytic core participate in the formation of an active arginine binding pocket which is located close to the cofactor-binding site. CARM1 has unique sets of substrates including histone H3R17. Structural comparison of CARM1 with PRMT1, PRMT3, and yeast Hmt1 catalytic cores demonstrates that CARM1 has a unique C-terminal extension (β_{16}) that affects substrate-binding specificity [113]. Unlike PRMT1/PRMT3/Hmt1, CARM1 does not recognize a conserved substrate sequence motif. It does not have an acidic rich area at the surface to provide initial binding affinity for basic rich substrates. Rather, it is proposed that a narrow opening between the potential substrate-binding groove and the cofactor-binding site only accommodates a tight β-turn substrate conformation, which could explain the lack of flanking consensus sequences among CARM1 substrates [113]. Recent crystal structures of CARM1 in a complex with five different peptide substrates, including unmethylated and monomethylated H3R17 and nonhistone protein PABP1, indicate that all the substrates display a conserved core binding mode despite their different primary sequences [116]. The enzyme-substrate interactions are made primary through hydrogen bonds between an Arg residue, the backbone of substrate flanking residues with a variety of sequences, and active site residues in CARM1. This unique backbone recognition may explain CARM1 substrate sequence diversity [116]. In addition to methyltransferase activity and dimerization, the catalytic core is also required for interacting with SRCs and its coactivator function [117].

Compared to other PRMTs, CARM1 has a unique N- and C-terminal domain flanking the conserved catalytic core [118]. The N-terminal domain (28–140 aa) adopts a PH (pleckstrin homology) domain fold (two nearly perpendicular β-sheets capped by an amphipathic α-helix) and behaves as a dimer (Fig. 3b) [112]. The PH domain structure is found in a large family of proteins often involved in transient protein-protein interactions in response to upstream signals [119]. Interestingly, the density of this PH domain is not observed in a larger CARM1 protein structure (28–507 aa), suggesting that the PH domain is wobbly [112]. We recently demonstrated that the N-terminal domain of CARM1 is mobilized upon formation of an estrogen receptor/coactivator complex and it is involved in the interaction with p300 in the complex [120]. The C-terminal domain of CARM1 is intrinsically disordered [112]. It has strong autonomous activation function [117]. Deletion of either of the N- or C-terminal domains abolishes CARM1 coactivator activity [117].

3 Structural Studies of Estrogen Receptor/Coactivator Complexes

Numerous crystallography and NMR studies described above shed light on how individual domains or motifs of coactivators interact with transcription factors and/or exert their enzymatic functions. How these domains cooperate with each other in full-length intact proteins and how receptors and coactivators function in the context of large protein complexes are less clear. Most coactivators and transcription factors have intrinsically disordered regions or flexible domains that only fold into a higher-order structure when interacting with their protein partners. Such a property limits structural studies on full-length coactivators since it is nearly impossible to analyze such large complexes using X-ray crystallography and NMR due to limitations in protein molecular size and weight. Recent advances in single-particle electron cryomicroscopy (cryo-EM) now make solving large nuclear receptor/coactivator complex possible.

Cryo-EM is a rapidly expanding methodology that is particularly well suited for studying three-dimensional structures of molecular machines in native solution or under chemically defined conditions without using negative stain or chemical fixatives. This method is ideal for specimens that are difficult to study by X-ray crystallography or NMR. Cryo-EM has been used to study macromolecular complexes of various sizes (50 kD–30 MDa), shapes (spherical, filamentous, or amyloid) and symmetries, or even complexes that completely lack symmetry (e.g., ribosomes). In the last decade, cryo-EM has generated a large increase in the number of published macromolecular structures, as well as an ever-growing user base. This rapid growth, in part, has been due to improvements in instrumentation: particularly in detectors that are able to increase signal-to-noise ratios in the image data and microscopes that have pushed the limits of very stable single-particle cryo-EM to sub-2 Å resolution [121]. This resolvability even enables the derived structural models to become usable for structure-based drug design.

Nuclear receptor coactivators act synergistically with complex partners to activate nuclear receptor-targeted transcription, but the molecular basis of this synergism is not completely understood. Our recent work on cryo-EM structures of large DNA-bound full-length estrogen receptor α (ER) and coactivator complexes provides new information that addresses this issue [21, 120].

Purified recombinant ERα, SRC-3, and p300 proteins were assembled on a biotinylated ERE (estrogen-responsive element) containing DNA in the presence of estrogen. The complex was then separated from unbound coactivators using magnetic streptavidin beads [21]. These purified proteins were intact and shown to activate target reporter transcription synergistically in vitro. The reconstituted cryo-EM structure of the complex is estimated to have a validated 25 Å resolution with a dimension of $220 \times 260 \times 320$ Å. Using individual p300 cryo-EM structure, antibody labeling, and density map segmentation, the complex density was determined and segmented into four components: one ERα dimer, two distinct SRC-3s (SRC-3a and SRC-3b), and one p300. The structure shows that each of the ERα monomers independently recruits one SRC-3 and the two separate SRC-3s in turn lock one p300 in the complex through multiple contact points to form a more stable complex (Fig. 4). The quaternary structure of this full-length protein complex reveals an "adaptation and fit" assembly mechanism for coactivator recruitment by the nuclear receptor. The two SRC-3s adopt slightly different conformations although both interact with ERα and p300. SRC-3a has the strongest interaction with the p300 CID domain. It also appears to contact both the ERα N-terminal AF-1 domain and the C-terminal AF-2 domain. This observation provides a structural basis for cooperativity between AF-1 and AF-2 predicted previously [122–124]. SRC-3b, on the other hand, contacts different regions of p300 and appears to have a weaker interaction with ERα. It needs to adapt to a different conformation in order to fit into the position required to connect it with both ERα and p300.

Recruitment of p300 to the ERα complex is mediated through its association with SRC-3s. A conformational change was observed for p300 upon assembly into the complex. This conformational change not only allows p300 to fit into the center to contact the two SRC-3s but also increases its HAT activity toward histone H3. The intrinsically disordered, highly flexible ERα AF-1 region is mobilized upon binding to SRC-3. Nuclear receptor activates transcription in response to ligand

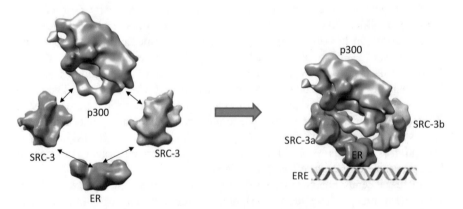

Fig. 4 ERE/ERα/SRC-3/p300 complex structural organization. One ERα dimer recruits two distinct SRC-3s which in turn bring in one p300 through multiple contacts

stimulation and recruits different coactivators at different stages of transcription; transcription activation needs to be turned off when the stimulus is no longer present. The highly flexible and dynamic nature of nuclear receptor and coactivator interactions allow rapid assembly and disassembly of different complexes in response to signal stimulation.

SRC-3 can recruit not only CBP/p300 but also CARM1 to the ER complex. CARM1 recruitment follows later than SRC-3 and CBP/p300 recruitment [120, 125]. A cross talk between CBP/p300-mediated histone acetylation and CARM1-mediated histone methylation has been well documented [113, 125, 126]. Addition of CARM1 to the purified ERα/SRC-3/p300 complex brings in new heterogeneity to the complex structure. Using a multiple refinement algorithm, three different classes of complex structures were found in our analyses [120] (Fig. 5a). Surprisingly none of the classes generates an extra density in the complex upon the addition of CARM1 to the ERα/SRC-3/p300 mixture. One of the classes is essentially the same as the ERα/SRC-3/p300 complex, representing the group without CARM1 binding. Another class shows a CARM1 density replacing the density of SRC-3b; this was confirmed by CARM1-specific antibody labeling and represents the complex now containing CARM1. The third class has only one SRC-3a in the complex, leaving an unoccupied space where SRC-3b or CARM1 is located in the other two classes; this likely reflects a less stable intermediate state.

Consistent with a previous observation [94], CARM1 does not directly interact with ERα. As a result, the density pertaining to the AF-1 region is missing in one of the ER monomers that does not contact SRC-3, probably due to its high mobility. Although CARM1 occupies the position of SRC-3b in the complex, it contacts different regions in p300 compared to SRC-3. Understandably, a further conformational change of p300 was observed to accommodate this change in binding partners (Fig. 5b). This sequentially occurring conformational change significantly increases p300 HAT activity on histone H3K18, which in turn promotes CARM1-mediated H3R17 dimethylation (Fig. 5b). Increased H3R17 methylation has been linked to active gene transcription [127–129]. Several reader proteins, including Tudor domain proteins and PAF1 complex that are involved in transcription elongation, were found to bind arginine-methylated motifs [130–132]. It is likely that CARM1 recruitment to the complex alters the complex structure to functionally prepare transcription transitioning from initiation to elongation. This structural impact of sequential coactivator recruitment also provides a general explanation for the synergistic transcriptional activation observed for different coactivators.

In the X-ray structural study of CARM1, the N-terminal PHD domain was not visible due to high mobility [112]. It was proposed that this domain could be involved in protein-protein interaction [117]. Indeed, the N-terminal domain of CARM1 was found to connect CARM1 and p300 in the complex through N-terminal domain-specific antibody labeling [120]. Two antibodies bind to the CARM1 density in the complex, suggesting that CARM1 may exist as a dimer in the complex. This result is consistent with X-ray structural studies [112, 113]. Deletion of the CARM1 N-terminal domain abolishes the synergism between CBP/p300 and CARM1 [117]

A

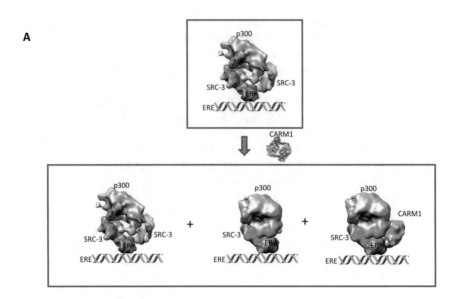

B

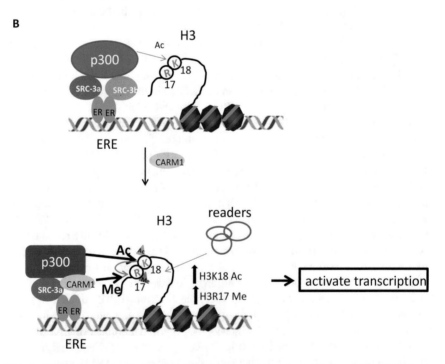

Fig. 5 CARM1 recruitment alters ERα/coactivator complex structural organization (**a**) Three classes of ERα/coactivator complex structures were found in the mixture of ERα, SRC-3, p300, and CARM1. (**b**) Sequential CARM1 recruitment replaces SRC-3b from the complex and alters p300 conformation, leading increased p300-mediated H3K18 acetylation and CARM1-mediated H3R17 methylation to activate transcription (adapted from [120] with modification)

as well as the promotional effect of CARM1 recruitment on p300 HAT activity [120], highlighting the significance of the CARM1 PHD domain in regulating the ERα/coactivator complex function.

4 Future Perspective

With recent advances in cryo-EM technology, we now have made substantial new progress in understanding assembly mechanisms of nuclear receptor and coactivator complexes. However, as pointed above, nuclear receptors and coactivators are highly dynamic and have intrinsic disordered regions that must fit their need to quickly assemble and disassemble into different protein complexes at different stages of transcription. Compositional heterogeneity, conformational flexibility, and dynamism are limiting factors for obtaining high resolutions for these complexes. Recent improvement in cryo-EM in automated large-scale data collection [133–135] and improved image processing workflows will help in part to address the difficulties in dealing with these structurally heterogeneous samples. With large-scale imaging data, usage of unsupervised 3D classification algorithms will be able to categorize data with structural variability or reconstruct structures into multiple functional states that exist dynamically in one dataset, thereby improving the resolution for each state. A prominent structural feature for nuclear receptors and coactivators is that intrinsically disordered structures become structured and flexible regions become mobilized when interaction partners contact each other. In fact, ER/coactivator complexes become very stable (even resistant to urea denaturation) after forming a giant protein complex [136]. Building a much larger protein complex by including more coregulatory proteins in future structural studies might in itself improve resolution by limiting the conformational dynamics occurring in ice on the cryo-EM grid of the nuclear receptor and coactivator complex.

Acknowledgments This work is supported by NIH grants HD8818 and NIDDK59820 to B.W.O.

References

1. Bulynko YA, O'Malley BW (2011) Nuclear receptor coactivators: structural and functional biochemistry. Biochemistry 50(3):313–328. https://doi.org/10.1021/bi101762x
2. Rastinejad F, Huang P, Chandra V, Khorasanizadeh S (2013) Understanding nuclear receptor form and function using structural biology. J Mol Endocrinol 51(3):T1–T21. https://doi.org/10.1530/JME-13-0173
3. Helsen C, Claessens F (2014) Looking at nuclear receptors from a new angle. Mol Cell Endocrinol 382(1):97–106. https://doi.org/10.1016/j.mce.2013.09.009
4. Rastinejad F, Ollendorff V, Polikarpov I (2015) Nuclear receptor full-length architectures: confronting myth and illusion with high resolution. Trends Biochem Sci 40(1):16–24. https://doi.org/10.1016/j.tibs.2014.10.011

5. Meyer ME, Gronemeyer H, Turcotte B, Bocquel MT, Tasset D, Chambon P (1989) Steroid hormone receptors compete for factors that mediate their enhancer function. Cell 57(3):433–442
6. Shemshedini L, Ji JW, Brou C, Chambon P, Gronemeyer H (1992) In vitro activity of the transcription activation functions of the progesterone receptor. Evidence for intermediary factors. J Biol Chem 267(3):1834–1839
7. Onate SA, Tsai SY, Tsai MJ, O'Malley BW (1995) Sequence and characterization of a coactivator for the steroid hormone receptor superfamily. Science 270(5240):1354–1357
8. Voegel JJ, Heine MJ, Zechel C, Chambon P, Gronemeyer H (1996) TIF2, a 160 kDa transcriptional mediator for the ligand-dependent activation function AF-2 of nuclear receptors. EMBO J 15(14):3667–3675
9. Hong H, Kohli K, Trivedi A, Johnson DL, Stallcup MR (1996) GRIP1, a novel mouse protein that serves as a transcriptional coactivator in yeast for the hormone binding domains of steroid receptors. Proc Natl Acad Sci U S A 93(10):4948–4952
10. Anzick SL, Kononen J, Walker RL, Azorsa DO, Tanner MM, Guan XY, Sauter G, Kallioniemi OP, Trent JM, Meltzer PS (1997) AIB1, a steroid receptor coactivator amplified in breast and ovarian cancer. Science 277(5328):965–968
11. Torchia J, Rose DW, Inostroza J, Kamei Y, Westin S, Glass CK, Rosenfeld MG (1997) The transcriptional co-activator p/CIP binds CBP and mediates nuclear-receptor function. Nature 387(6634):677–684. https://doi.org/10.1038/42652
12. Takeshita A, Cardona GR, Koibuchi N, Suen CS, Chin WW (1997) TRAM-1, a novel 160-kDa thyroid hormone receptor activator molecule, exhibits distinct properties from steroid receptor coactivator-1. J Biol Chem 272(44):27629–27634
13. Chen H, Lin RJ, Schiltz RL, Chakravarti D, Nash A, Nagy L, Privalsky ML, Nakatani Y, Evans RM (1997) Nuclear receptor coactivator ACTR is a novel histone acetyltransferase and forms a multimeric activation complex with P/CAF and CBP/p300. Cell 90(3):569–580
14. Li H, Gomes PJ, Chen JD (1997) RAC3, a steroid/nuclear receptor-associated coactivator that is related to SRC-1 and TIF2. Proc Natl Acad Sci U S A 94(16):8479–8484
15. York B, O'Malley BW (2010) Steroid receptor coactivator (SRC) family: masters of systems biology. J Biol Chem 285(50):38743–38750. https://doi.org/10.1074/jbc.R110.193367
16. Szwarc MM, Lydon JP, O'Malley BW (2015) Steroid receptor coactivators as therapeutic targets in the female reproductive system. J Steroid Biochem Mol Biol 154:32–38. https://doi.org/10.1016/j.jsbmb.2015.06.010
17. Dasgupta S, O'Malley BW (2014) Transcriptional coregulators: emerging roles of SRC family of coactivators in disease pathology. J Mol Endocrinol 53(2):R47–R59. https://doi.org/10.1530/JME-14-0080
18. Stashi E, York B, O'Malley BW (2014) Steroid receptor coactivators: servants and masters for control of systems metabolism. Trends Endocrinol Metab 25(7):337–347. https://doi.org/10.1016/j.tem.2014.05.004
19. Kim JH, Li H, Stallcup MR (2003) CoCoA, a nuclear receptor coactivator which acts through an N-terminal activation domain of p160 coactivators. Mol Cell 12(6):1537–1549
20. Chen YH, Kim JH, Stallcup MR (2005) GAC63, a GRIP1-dependent nuclear receptor coactivator. Mol Cell Biol 25(14):5965–5972. https://doi.org/10.1128/MCB.25.14.5965-5972.2005
21. Yi P, Wang Z, Feng Q, Pintilie GD, Foulds CE, Lanz RB, Ludtke SJ, Schmid MF, Chiu W, O'Malley BW (2015) Structure of a biologically active estrogen receptor-coactivator complex on DNA. Mol Cell 57(6):1047–1058. https://doi.org/10.1016/j.molcel.2015.01.025
22. Johnson AB, O'Malley BW (2012) Steroid receptor coactivators 1, 2, and 3: critical regulators of nuclear receptor activity and steroid receptor modulator (SRM)-based cancer therapy. Mol Cell Endocrinol 348(2):430–439. https://doi.org/10.1016/j.mce.2011.04.021
23. Li C, Wu RC, Amazit L, Tsai SY, Tsai MJ, O'Malley BW (2007) Specific amino acid residues in the basic helix-loop-helix domain of SRC-3 are essential for its nuclear localization and proteasome-dependent turnover. Mol Cell Biol 27(4):1296–1308. https://doi.org/10.1128/MCB.00336-06

24. Wu RC, Feng Q, Lonard DM, O'Malley BW (2007) SRC-3 coactivator functional lifetime is regulated by a phospho-dependent ubiquitin time clock. Cell 129(6):1125–1140

25. Spencer TE, Jenster G, Burcin MM, Allis CD, Zhou J, Mizzen CA, McKenna NJ, Onate SA, Tsai SY, Tsai MJ, O'Malley BW (1997) Steroid receptor coactivator-1 is a histone acetyl-transferase. Nature 389(6647):194–198. https://doi.org/10.1038/38304

26. Heery DM, Kalkhoven E, Hoare S, Parker MG (1997) A signature motif in transcriptional co-activators mediates binding to nuclear receptors. Nature 387(6634):733–736. https://doi.org/10.1038/42750

27. Shiau AK, Barstad D, Loria PM, Cheng L, Kushner PJ, Agard DA, Greene GL (1998) The structural basis of estrogen receptor/coactivator recognition and the antagonism of this inter-action by tamoxifen. Cell 95(7):927–937

28. Darimont BD, Wagner RL, Apriletti JW, Stallcup MR, Kushner PJ, Baxter JD, Fletterick RJ, Yamamoto KR (1998) Structure and specificity of nuclear receptor-coactivator interactions. Genes Dev 12(21):3343–3356

29. Nolte RT, Wisely GB, Westin S, Cobb JE, Lambert MH, Kurokawa R, Rosenfeld MG, Willson TM, Glass CK, Milburn MV (1998) Ligand binding and co-activator assembly of the peroxisome proliferator-activated receptor-gamma. Nature 395(6698):137–143. https://doi.org/10.1038/25931

30. Demarest SJ, Martinez-Yamout M, Chung J, Chen H, Xu W, Dyson HJ, Evans RM, Wright PE (2002) Mutual synergistic folding in recruitment of CBP/p300 by p160 nuclear receptor coactivators. Nature 415(6871):549–553

31. Dyson HJ, Wright PE (2016) Role of intrinsic protein disorder in the function and interactions of the transcriptional coactivators CREB-binding protein (CBP) and p300. J Biol Chem 291(13):6714–6722. https://doi.org/10.1074/jbc.R115.692020

32. Chrivia JC, Kwok RP, Lamb N, Hagiwara M, Montminy MR, Goodman RH (1993) Phosphorylated CREB binds specifically to the nuclear protein CBP. Nature 365(6449):855–859. https://doi.org/10.1038/365855a0

33. Stein RW, Corrigan M, Yaciuk P, Whelan J, Moran E (1990) Analysis of E1A-mediated growth regulation functions: binding of the 300-kilodalton cellular product correlates with E1A enhancer repression function and DNA synthesis-inducing activity. J Virol 64(9):4421–4427

34. Eckner R, Ewen ME, Newsome D, Gerdes M, DeCaprio JA, Lawrence JB, Livingston DM (1994) Molecular cloning and functional analysis of the adenovirus E1A-associated 300-kD protein (p300) reveals a protein with properties of a transcriptional adaptor. Genes Dev 8(8):869–884

35. Shiama N (1997) The p300/CBP family: integrating signals with transcription factors and chromatin. Trends Cell Biol 7(6):230–236. https://doi.org/10.1016/S0962-8924(97)01048-9

36. Janknecht R, Hunter T (1996) Transcription. A growing coactivator network. Nature 383(6595):22–23. https://doi.org/10.1038/383022a0

37. Goodman RH, Smolik S (2000) CBP/p300 in cell growth, transformation, and development. Genes Dev 14(13):1553–1577

38. Bedford DC, Kasper LH, Fukuyama T, Brindle PK (2010) Target gene context influences the transcriptional requirement for the KAT3 family of CBP and p300 histone acetyltransferases. Epigenetics 5(1):9–15

39. Giles RH, Peters DJ, Breuning MH (1998) Conjunction dysfunction: CBP/p300 in human disease. Trends Genet 14(5):178–183

40. Dutta R, Tiu B, Sakamoto KM (2016) CBP/p300 acetyltransferase activity in hema-tologic malignancies. Mol Genet Metab 119(1–2):37–43. https://doi.org/10.1016/j.ymgme.2016.06.013

41. Chan HM, La Thangue NB (2001) p300/CBP proteins: HATs for transcriptional bridges and scaffolds. J Cell Sci 114(Pt 13):2363–2373

42. Wang F, Marshall CB, Ikura M (2013) Transcriptional/epigenetic regulator CBP/p300 in tumorigenesis: structural and functional versatility in target recognition. Cell Mol Life Sci 70(21):3989–4008. https://doi.org/10.1007/s00018-012-1254-4

43. Liu X, Wang L, Zhao K, Thompson PR, Hwang Y, Marmorstein R, Cole PA (2008) The structural basis of protein acetylation by the p300/CBP transcriptional coactivator. Nature 451(7180):846–850. https://doi.org/10.1038/nature06546

44. Berndsen CE, Denu JM (2008) Catalysis and substrate selection by histone/protein lysine acetyltransferases. Curr Opin Struct Biol 18(6):682–689. https://doi.org/10.1016/j.sbi.2008.11.004

45. Struhl K (1998) Histone acetylation and transcriptional regulatory mechanisms. Genes Dev 12(5):599–606

46. Turner BM, O'Neill LP (1995) Histone acetylation in chromatin and chromosomes. Semin Cell Biol 6(4):229–236

47. Schiltz RL, Mizzen CA, Vassilev A, Cook RG, Allis CD, Nakatani Y (1999) Overlapping but distinct patterns of histone acetylation by the human coactivators p300 and PCAF within nucleosomal substrates. J Biol Chem 274(3):1189–1192

48. Jin Q, Yu LR, Wang L, Zhang Z, Kasper LH, Lee JE, Wang C, Brindle PK, Dent SY, Ge K (2011) Distinct roles of GCN5/PCAF-mediated H3K9ac and CBP/p300-mediated H3K18/27ac in nuclear receptor transactivation. EMBO J 30(2):249–262. https://doi.org/10.1038/emboj.2010.318

49. Gu W, Roeder RG (1997) Activation of p53 sequence-specific DNA binding by acetylation of the p53 C-terminal domain. Cell 90(4):595–606

50. Lu Q, Hutchins AE, Doyle CM, Lundblad JR, Kwok RP (2003) Acetylation of cAMP-responsive element-binding protein (CREB) by CREB-binding protein enhances CREB-dependent transcription. J Biol Chem 278(18):15727–15734. https://doi.org/10.1074/jbc.M300546200

51. Martinez-Balbas MA, Bauer UM, Nielsen SJ, Brehm A, Kouzarides T (2000) Regulation of E2F1 activity by acetylation. EMBO J 19(4):662–671. https://doi.org/10.1093/emboj/19.4.662

52. Marzio G, Wagener C, Gutierrez MI, Cartwright P, Helin K, Giacca M (2000) E2F family members are differentially regulated by reversible acetylation. J Biol Chem 275(15):10887–10892

53. Boyes J, Byfield P, Nakatani Y, Ogryzko V (1998) Regulation of activity of the transcription factor GATA-1 by acetylation. Nature 396(6711):594–598. https://doi.org/10.1038/25166

54. Imhof A, Yang XJ, Ogryzko VV, Nakatani Y, Wolffe AP, Ge H (1997) Acetylation of general transcription factors by histone acetyltransferases. Curr Biol 7(9):689–692

55. Chen H, Lin RJ, Xie W, Wilpitz D, Evans RM (1999) Regulation of hormone-induced histone hyperacetylation and gene activation via acetylation of an acetylase. Cell 98(5):675–686

56. Sabari BR, Zhang D, Allis CD, Zhao Y (2017) Metabolic regulation of gene expression through histone acylations. Nat Rev Mol Cell Biol 18(2):90–101. https://doi.org/10.1038/nrm.2016.140

57. Sabari BR, Tang Z, Huang H, Yong-Gonzalez V, Molina H, Kong HE, Dai L, Shimada M, Cross JR, Zhao Y, Roeder RG, Allis CD (2015) Intracellular crotonyl-CoA stimulates transcription through p300-catalyzed histone crotonylation. Mol Cell 58(2):203–215. https://doi.org/10.1016/j.molcel.2015.02.029

58. Goudarzi A, Zhang D, Huang H, Barral S, Kwon OK, Qi S, Tang Z, Buchou T, Vitte AL, He T, Cheng Z, Montellier E, Gaucher J, Curtet S, Debernardi A, Charbonnier G, Puthier D, Petosa C, Panne D, Rousseaux S, Roeder RG, Zhao Y, Khochbin S (2016) Dynamic competing histone H4 K5K8 acetylation and butyrylation are hallmarks of highly active gene promoters. Mol Cell 62(2):169–180. https://doi.org/10.1016/j.molcel.2016.03.014

59. Lee JV, Carrer A, Shah S, Snyder NW, Wei S, Venneti S, Worth AJ, Yuan ZF, Lim HW, Liu S, Jackson E, Aiello NM, Haas NB, Rebbeck TR, Judkins A, Won KJ, Chodosh LA, Garcia BA, Stanger BZ, Feldman MD, Blair IA, Wellen KE (2014) Akt-dependent metabolic reprogramming regulates tumor cell histone acetylation. Cell Metab 20(2):306–319. https://doi.org/10.1016/j.cmet.2014.06.004

60. Xie Z, Zhang D, Chung D, Tang Z, Huang H, Dai L, Qi S, Li J, Colak G, Chen Y, Xia C, Peng C, Ruan H, Kirkey M, Wang D, Jensen LM, Kwon OK, Lee S, Pletcher SD, Tan M, Lombard

DB, White KP, Zhao H, Roeder RG, Yang X, Zhao Y (2016) Metabolic regulation of gene expression by histone lysine beta-hydroxybutyrylation. Mol Cell 62(2):194–206. https://doi.org/10.1016/j.molcel.2016.03.036

61. Kaczmarska Z, Ortega E, Goudarzi A, Huang H, Kim S, Marquez JA, Zhao Y, Khochbin S, Panne D (2017) Structure of p300 in complex with acyl-CoA variants. Nat Chem Biol 13(1):21–29. https://doi.org/10.1038/nchembio.2217

62. Thompson PR, Wang D, Wang L, Fulco M, Pediconi N, Zhang D, An W, Ge Q, Roeder RG, Wong J, Levrero M, Sartorelli V, Cotter RJ, Cole PA (2004) Regulation of the p300 HAT domain via a novel activation loop. Nat Struct Mol Biol 11(4):308–315. https://doi.org/10.1038/nsmb740

63. Park S, Stanfield RL, Martinez-Yamout MA, Dyson HJ, Wilson IA, Wright PE (2017) Role of the CBP catalytic core in intramolecular SUMOylation and control of histone H3 acetylation. Proc Natl Acad Sci U S A 114(27):E5335–E5342. https://doi.org/10.1073/pnas.1703105114

64. Delvecchio M, Gaucher J, Aguilar-Gurrieri C, Ortega E, Panne D (2013) Structure of the p300 catalytic core and implications for chromatin targeting and HAT regulation. Nat Struct Mol Biol 20(9):1040–1046. https://doi.org/10.1038/nsmb.2642

65. Das C, Roy S, Namjoshi S, Malarkey CS, Jones DN, Kutateladze TG, Churchill ME, Tyler JK (2014) Binding of the histone chaperone ASF1 to the CBP bromodomain promotes histone acetylation. Proc Natl Acad Sci U S A 111(12):E1072–E1081. https://doi.org/10.1073/pnas.1319122111

66. Plotnikov AN, Yang S, Zhou TJ, Rusinova E, Frasca A, Zhou MM (2014) Structural insights into acetylated-histone H4 recognition by the bromodomain-PHD finger module of human transcriptional coactivator CBP. Structure 22(2):353–360. https://doi.org/10.1016/j.str.2013.10.021

67. Mujtaba S, He Y, Zeng L, Yan S, Plotnikova O, Sachchidanand, Sanchez R, Zeleznik-Le NJ, Ronai Z, Zhou MM (2004) Structural mechanism of the bromodomain of the coactivator CBP in p53 transcriptional activation. Mol Cell 13(2):251–263

68. Kraus WL, Manning ET, Kadonaga JT (1999) Biochemical analysis of distinct activation functions in p300 that enhance transcription initiation with chromatin templates. Mol Cell Biol 19(12):8123–8135

69. Manning ET, Ikehara T, Ito T, Kadonaga JT, Kraus WL (2001) p300 forms a stable, template-committed complex with chromatin: role for the bromodomain. Mol Cell Biol 21(12):3876–3887. https://doi.org/10.1128/MCB.21.12.3876-3887.2001

70. Ragvin A, Valvatne H, Erdal S, Arskog V, Tufteland KR, Breen K, ØYan AM, Eberharter A, Gibson TJ, Becker PB, Aasland R (2004) Nucleosome binding by the bromodomain and PHD finger of the transcriptional cofactor p300. J Mol Biol 337(4):773–788. https://doi.org/10.1016/j.jmb.2004.01.051

71. Rack JG, Lutter T, Kjaereng Bjerga GE, Guder C, Ehrhardt C, Varv S, Ziegler M, Aasland R (2014) The PHD finger of p300 influences its ability to acetylate histone and non-histone targets. J Mol Biol 426(24):3960–3972. https://doi.org/10.1016/j.jmb.2014.08.011

72. Parker D, Ferreri K, Nakajima T, LaMorte VJ, Evans R, Koerber SC, Hoeger C, Montminy MR (1996) Phosphorylation of CREB at Ser-133 induces complex formation with CREB-binding protein via a direct mechanism. Mol Cell Biol 16(2):694–703

73. Radhakrishnan I, Perez-Alvarado GC, Parker D, Dyson HJ, Montminy MR, Wright PE (1997) Solution structure of the KIX domain of CBP bound to the transactivation domain of CREB: a model for activator:coactivator interactions. Cell 91(6):741–752

74. Van Orden K, Giebler HA, Lemasson I, Gonzales M, Nyborg JK (1999) Binding of p53 to the KIX domain of CREB binding protein. A potential link to human T-cell leukemia virus, type I-associated leukemogenesis. J Biol Chem 274(37):26321–26328

75. Zor T, Mayr BM, Dyson HJ, Montminy MR, Wright PE (2002) Roles of phosphorylation and helix propensity in the binding of the KIX domain of CREB-binding protein by constitutive (c-Myb) and inducible (CREB) activators. J Biol Chem 277(44):42241–42248. https://doi.org/10.1074/jbc.M207361200

76. Goto NK, Zor T, Martinez-Yamout M, Dyson HJ, Wright PE (2002) Cooperativity in transcription factor binding to the coactivator CREB-binding protein (CBP). The mixed lineage leukemia protein (MLL) activation domain binds to an allosteric site on the KIX domain. J Biol Chem 277(45):43168–43174. https://doi.org/10.1074/jbc.M207660200

77. Campbell KM, Lumb KJ (2002) Structurally distinct modes of recognition of the KIX domain of CBP by Jun and CREB. Biochemistry 41(47):13956–13964

78. Wang F, Marshall CB, Yamamoto K, Li GY, Gasmi-Seabrook GM, Okada H, Mak TW, Ikura M (2012) Structures of KIX domain of CBP in complex with two FOXO3a transactivation domains reveal promiscuity and plasticity in coactivator recruitment. Proc Natl Acad Sci U S A 109(16):6078–6083. https://doi.org/10.1073/pnas.1119073109

79. Pao GM, Janknecht R, Ruffner H, Hunter T, Verma IM (2000) CBP/p300 interact with and function as transcriptional coactivators of BRCA1. Proc Natl Acad Sci U S A 97(3):1020–1025

80. Oliner JD, Andresen JM, Hansen SK, Zhou S, Tjian R (1996) SREBP transcriptional activity is mediated through an interaction with the CREB-binding protein. Genes Dev 10(22):2903–2911

81. Zhang JJ, Vinkemeier U, Gu W, Chakravarti D, Horvath CM, Darnell JE Jr (1996) Two contact regions between Stat1 and CBP/p300 in interferon gamma signaling. Proc Natl Acad Sci U S A 93(26):15092–15096

82. Ernst P, Wang J, Huang M, Goodman RH, Korsmeyer SJ (2001) MLL and CREB bind cooperatively to the nuclear coactivator CREB-binding protein. Mol Cell Biol 21(7):2249–2258. https://doi.org/10.1128/MCB.21.7.2249-2258.2001

83. Lee CW, Arai M, Martinez-Yamout MA, Dyson HJ, Wright PE (2009) Mapping the interactions of the p53 transactivation domain with the KIX domain of CBP. Biochemistry 48(10):2115–2124. https://doi.org/10.1021/bi802055v

84. De Guzman RN, Wojciak JM, Martinez-Yamout MA, Dyson HJ, Wright PE (2005) CBP/p300 TAZ1 domain forms a structured scaffold for ligand binding. Biochemistry 44(2):490–497. https://doi.org/10.1021/bi048161t

85. Waters L, Yue B, Veverka V, Renshaw P, Bramham J, Matsuda S, Frenkiel T, Kelly G, Muskett F, Carr M, Heery DM (2006) Structural diversity in p160/CREB-binding protein coactivator complexes. J Biol Chem 281(21):14787–14795. https://doi.org/10.1074/jbc.M600237200

86. Lee CW, Martinez-Yamout MA, Dyson HJ, Wright PE (2010) Structure of the p53 transactivation domain in complex with the nuclear receptor coactivator binding domain of CREB binding protein. Biochemistry 49(46):9964–9971. https://doi.org/10.1021/bi1012996

87. Qin BY, Liu C, Srinath H, Lam SS, Correia JJ, Derynck R, Lin K (2005) Crystal structure of IRF-3 in complex with CBP. Structure 13(9):1269–1277. https://doi.org/10.1016/j.str.2005.06.011

88. Ebert MO, Bae SH, Dyson HJ, Wright PE (2008) NMR relaxation study of the complex formed between CBP and the activation domain of the nuclear hormone receptor coactivator ACTR. Biochemistry 47(5):1299–1308. https://doi.org/10.1021/bi701767j

89. Kjaergaard M, Andersen L, Nielsen LD, Teilum K (2013) A folded excited state of ligand-free nuclear coactivator binding domain (NCBD) underlies plasticity in ligand recognition. Biochemistry 52(10):1686–1693. https://doi.org/10.1021/bi4001062

90. Xu W, Chen H, Du K, Asahara H, Tini M, Emerson BM, Montminy M, Evans RM (2001) A transcriptional switch mediated by cofactor methylation. Science 294(5551):2507–2511. https://doi.org/10.1126/science.1065961

91. Chevillard-Briet M, Trouche D, Vandel L (2002) Control of CBP co-activating activity by arginine methylation. EMBO J 21(20):5457–5466

92. Zanger K, Radovick S, Wondisford FE (2001) CREB binding protein recruitment to the transcription complex requires growth factor-dependent phosphorylation of its GF box. Mol Cell 7(3):551–558

93. Zhou XY, Shibusawa N, Naik K, Porras D, Temple K, Ou H, Kaihara K, Roe MW, Brady MJ, Wondisford FE (2004) Insulin regulation of hepatic gluconeogenesis through phosphorylation of CREB-binding protein. Nat Med 10(6):633–637. https://doi.org/10.1038/nm1050

94. Chen D, Ma H, Hong H, Koh SS, Huang SM, Schurter BT, Aswad DW, Stallcup MR (1999) Regulation of transcription by a protein methyltransferase. Science 284(5423):2174–2177

95. Chen D, Huang SM, Stallcup MR (2000) Synergistic, p160 coactivator-dependent enhancement of estrogen receptor function by CARM1 and p300. J Biol Chem 275(52):40810–40816. https://doi.org/10.1074/jbc.M005459200

96. Lee YH, Koh SS, Zhang X, Cheng X, Stallcup MR (2002) Synergy among nuclear receptor coactivators: selective requirement for protein methyltransferase and acetyltransferase activities. Mol Cell Biol 22(11):3621–3632

97. Yadav N, Lee J, Kim J, Shen J, Hu MC, Aldaz CM, Bedford MT (2003) Specific protein methylation defects and gene expression perturbations in coactivator-associated arginine methyltransferase 1-deficient mice. Proc Natl Acad Sci U S A 100(11):6464–6468. https://doi.org/10.1073/pnas.1232272100

98. Schurter BT, Koh SS, Chen D, Bunick GJ, Harp JM, Hanson BL, Henschen-Edman A, Mackay DR, Stallcup MR, Aswad DW (2001) Methylation of histone H3 by coactivator-associated arginine methyltransferase 1. Biochemistry 40(19):5747–5756

99. Casadio F, Lu X, Pollock SB, LeRoy G, Garcia BA, Muir TW, Roeder RG, Allis CD (2013) H3R42me2a is a histone modification with positive transcriptional effects. Proc Natl Acad Sci U S A 110(37):14894–14899. https://doi.org/10.1073/pnas.1312925110

100. Feng Q, Yi P, Wong J, O'Malley BW (2006) Signaling within a coactivator complex: methylation of SRC-3/AIB1 is a molecular switch for complex disassembly. Mol Cell Biol 26(21):7846–7857

101. Lee YH, Coonrod SA, Kraus WL, Jelinek MA, Stallcup MR (2005) Regulation of coactivator complex assembly and function by protein arginine methylation and demethylimination. Proc Natl Acad Sci U S A 102(10):3611–3616. https://doi.org/10.1073/pnas.0407159102

102. Zhao HY, Zhang YJ, Dai H, Zhang Y, Shen YF (2011) CARM1 mediates modulation of Sox2. PLoS One 6(10):e27026. https://doi.org/10.1371/journal.pone.0027026

103. Hein K, Mittler G, Cizelsky W, Kuhl M, Ferrante F, Liefke R, Berger IM, Just S, Strang JE, Kestler HA, Oswald F, Borggrefe T (2015) Site-specific methylation of Notch1 controls the amplitude and duration of the Notch1 response. Sci Signal 8(369):ra30. https://doi.org/10.1126/scisignal.2005892

104. Fujiwara T, Mori Y, Chu DL, Koyama Y, Miyata S, Tanaka H, Yachi K, Kubo T, Yoshikawa H, Tohyama M (2006) CARM1 regulates proliferation of PC12 cells by methylating HuD. Mol Cell Biol 26(6):2273–2285. https://doi.org/10.1128/MCB.26.6.2273-2285.2006

105. Lee J, Bedford MT (2002) PABP1 identified as an arginine methyltransferase substrate using high-density protein arrays. EMBO Rep 3(3):268–273. https://doi.org/10.1093/embo-reports/kvf052

106. Cheng D, Cote J, Shaaban S, Bedford MT (2007) The arginine methyltransferase CARM1 regulates the coupling of transcription and mRNA processing. Mol Cell 25(1):71–83. https://doi.org/10.1016/j.molcel.2006.11.019

107. Kim J, Lee J, Yadav N, Wu Q, Carter C, Richard S, Richie E, Bedford MT (2004) Loss of CARM1 results in hypomethylation of thymocyte cyclic AMP-regulated phosphoprotein and deregulated early T cell development. J Biol Chem 279(24):25339–25344. https://doi.org/10.1074/jbc.M402544200

108. Selvi BR, Swaminathan A, Maheshwari U, Nagabhushana A, Mishra RK, Kundu TK (2015) CARM1 regulates astroglial lineage through transcriptional regulation of Nanog and post-transcriptional regulation by miR92a. Mol Biol Cell 26(2):316–326. https://doi.org/10.1091/mbc.E14-01-0019

109. Yadav N, Cheng D, Richard S, Morel M, Iyer VR, Aldaz CM, Bedford MT (2008) CARM1 promotes adipocyte differentiation by coactivating PPARgamma. EMBO Rep 9(2):193–198. https://doi.org/10.1038/sj.embor.7401151

110. Ito T, Yadav N, Lee J, Furumatsu T, Yamashita S, Yoshida K, Taniguchi N, Hashimoto M, Tsuchiya M, Ozaki T, Lotz M, Bedford MT, Asahara H (2009) Arginine methyltransferase CARM1/PRMT4 regulates endochondral ossification. BMC Dev Biol 9:47. https://doi.org/10.1186/1471-213X-9-47

111. O'Brien KB, Alberich-Jorda M, Yadav N, Kocher O, Diruscio A, Ebralidze A, Levantini E, Sng NJ, Bhasin M, Caron T, Kim D, Steidl U, Huang G, Halmos B, Rodig SJ, Bedford MT, Tenen DG, Kobayashi S (2010) CARM1 is required for proper control of proliferation and differentiation of pulmonary epithelial cells. Development 137(13):2147–2156. https://doi.org/10.1242/dev.037150

112. Troffer-Charlier N, Cura V, Hassenboehler P, Moras D, Cavarelli J (2007) Functional insights from structures of coactivator-associated arginine methyltransferase 1 domains. EMBO J 26(20):4391–4401. https://doi.org/10.1038/sj.emboj.7601855

113. Yue WW, Hassler M, Roe SM, Thompson-Vale V, Pearl LH (2007) Insights into histone code syntax from structural and biochemical studies of CARM1 methyltransferase. EMBO J 26(20):4402–4412. https://doi.org/10.1038/sj.emboj.7601856

114. Rossmann MG, Moras D, Olsen KW (1974) Chemical and biological evolution of nucleotide-binding protein. Nature 250(463):194–199

115. Schluckebier G, O'Gara M, Saenger W, Cheng X (1995) Universal catalytic domain structure of AdoMet-dependent methyltransferases. J Mol Biol 247(1):16–20. https://doi.org/10.1006/jmbi.1994.0117

116. Boriack-Sjodin PA, Jin L, Jacques SL, Drew A, Sneeringer C, Scott MP, Moyer MP, Ribich S, Moradei O, Copeland RA (2016) Structural insights into ternary complex formation of human CARM1 with various substrates. ACS Chem Biol 11(3):763–771. https://doi.org/10.1021/acschembio.5b00773

117. Teyssier C, Chen D, Stallcup MR (2002) Requirement for multiple domains of the protein arginine methyltransferase CARM1 in its transcriptional coactivator function. J Biol Chem 277(48):46066–46072. https://doi.org/10.1074/jbc.M207623200

118. Schapira M, Ferreira de Freitas R (2014) Structural biology and chemistry of protein arginine methyltransferases. Medchemcomm 5(12):1779–1788. https://doi.org/10.1039/c4md00269e

119. Blomberg N, Baraldi E, Nilges M, Saraste M (1999) The PH superfold: a structural scaffold for multiple functions. Trends Biochem Sci 24(11):441–445

120. Yi P, Wang Z, Feng Q, Chou CK, Pintilie GD, Shen H, Foulds CE, Fan G, Serysheva I, Ludtke SJ, Schmid MF, Hung MC, Chiu W, O'Malley BW (2017) Structural and functional impacts of ER coactivator sequential recruitment. Mol Cell 67(5):733–743 e734. https://doi.org/10.1016/j.molcel.2017.07.026

121. Merk A, Bartesaghi A, Banerjee S, Falconieri V, Rao P, Davis MI, Pragani R, Boxer MB, Earl LA, Milne JLS, Subramaniam S (2016) Breaking cryo-EM resolution barriers to facilitate drug discovery. Cell 165(7):1698–1707. https://doi.org/10.1016/j.cell.2016.05.040

122. Onate SA, Boonyaratanakornkit V, Spencer TE, Tsai SY, Tsai MJ, Edwards DP, O'Malley BW (1998) The steroid receptor coactivator-1 contains multiple receptor interacting and activation domains that cooperatively enhance the activation function 1 (AF1) and AF2 domains of steroid receptors. J Biol Chem 273(20):12101–12108

123. Metivier R, Penot G, Flouriot G, Pakdel F (2001) Synergism between ERalpha transactivation function 1 (AF-1) and AF-2 mediated by steroid receptor coactivator protein-1: requirement for the AF-1 alpha-helical core and for a direct interaction between the N- and C-terminal domains. Mol Endocrinol 15(11):1953–1970

124. Dutertre M, Smith CL (2003) Ligand-independent interactions of p160/steroid receptor coactivators and CREB-binding protein (CBP) with estrogen receptor-alpha: regulation by phosphorylation sites in the A/B region depends on other receptor domains. Mol Endocrinol 17(7):1296–1314. https://doi.org/10.1210/me.2001-0316

125. Daujat S, Bauer UM, Shah V, Turner B, Berger S, Kouzarides T (2002) Crosstalk between CARM1 methylation and CBP acetylation on histone H3. Curr Biol 12(24):2090–2097

126. An W, Kim J, Roeder RG (2004) Ordered cooperative functions of PRMT1, p300, and CARM1 in transcriptional activation by p53. Cell 117(6):735–748. https://doi.org/10.1016/j.cell.2004.05.009

127. Ma H, Baumann CT, Li H, Strahl BD, Rice R, Jelinek MA, Aswad DW, Allis CD, Hager GL, Stallcup MR (2001) Hormone-dependent, CARM1-directed, arginine-specific methylation of histone H3 on a steroid-regulated promoter. Curr Biol 11(24):1981–1985

128. Bauer UM, Daujat S, Nielsen SJ, Nightingale K, Kouzarides T (2002) Methylation at arginine 17 of histone H3 is linked to gene activation. EMBO Rep 3(1):39–44. https://doi.org/10.1093/embo-reports/kvf013

129. Denis H, Deplus R, Putmans P, Yamada M, Metivier R, Fuks F (2009) Functional connection between deimination and deacetylation of histones. Mol Cell Biol 29(18):4982–4993. https://doi.org/10.1128/MCB.00285-09

130. Wu J, Xu W (2012) Histone H3R17me2a mark recruits human RNA polymerase-associated factor 1 complex to activate transcription. Proc Natl Acad Sci U S A 109(15):5675–5680. https://doi.org/10.1073/pnas.1114905109

131. Yang Y, Lu Y, Espejo A, Wu J, Xu W, Liang S, Bedford MT (2010) TDRD3 is an effector molecule for arginine-methylated histone marks. Mol Cell 40(6):1016–1023. https://doi.org/10.1016/j.molcel.2010.11.024

132. Gayatri S, Bedford MT (2014) Readers of histone methylarginine marks. Biochim Biophys Acta 1839(8):702–710. https://doi.org/10.1016/j.bbagrm.2014.02.015

133. Suloway C, Pulokas J, Fellmann D, Cheng A, Guerra F, Quispe J, Stagg S, Potter CS, Carragher B (2005) Automated molecular microscopy: the new Leginon system. J Struct Biol 151(1):41–60. https://doi.org/10.1016/j.jsb.2005.03.010

134. Sandberg K, Mastronarde DN, Beylkin G (2003) A fast reconstruction algorithm for electron microscope tomography. J Struct Biol 144(1–2):61–72

135. Mastronarde DN (2005) Automated electron microscope tomography using robust prediction of specimen movements. J Struct Biol 152(1):36–51. https://doi.org/10.1016/j.jsb.2005.07.007

136. Foulds CE, Feng Q, Ding C, Bailey S, Hunsaker TL, Malovannaya A, Hamilton RA, Gates LA, Zhang Z, Li C, Chan D, Bajaj A, Callaway CG, Edwards DP, Lonard DM, Tsai SY, Tsai MJ, Qin J, O'Malley BW (2013) Proteomic analysis of coregulators bound to ERalpha on DNA and nucleosomes reveals coregulator dynamics. Mol Cell 51:185. https://doi.org/10.1016/j.molcel.2013.06.007

The Estrogen-Regulated Transcriptome: Rapid, Robust, Extensive, and Transient

Yasmin M. Vasquez and W. Lee Kraus

Abstract The steroid hormone estrogen has potent effects in a variety of tissues across the body in both females and males. In the nuclear signaling pathway for estrogens, the hormone acts by stimulating the DNA binding and transcriptional activity of estrogen receptors (ERs), transcription factors which robustly and transiently regulate the expression of target genes. More broadly, estrogen signaling controls the ER cistrome, as well as the epigenome and the estrogen-regulated transcriptome. A host of deep sequencing-based genomic assays have provided novel insights into the mechanisms by which ERs regulate transcriptional responses. Estrogen-dependent transcriptional responses have been studied widely in breast cancer cells, primarily in the context of the ER alpha (ERα) isoform. These studies have revealed an intricate cross talk between the estrogen-ERα signaling pathway and other signaling pathways, impacting transcriptional programs and clinical outcomes in breast cancer. This chapter reviews the key features of ERα-regulated transcription and the current technological advances that have allowed for the careful dissection of these mechanisms.

Keywords Cistrome · Epigenome · Enhancer · Estrogen receptor · Transcriptome

1 Estrogen Signaling Through Estrogen Receptors

Many of the biological actions of estrogens are mediated by ERα, which functions primarily as a ligand-regulated, DNA-binding transcription factor (TF) in the nuclei of estrogen-responsive cells [1–3]. Natural estrogens, synthetic agonists, and

Y. M. Vasquez · W. L. Kraus (✉)
Laboratory of Signaling and Gene Regulation, Cecil H. and Ida Green Center for Reproductive Biology Sciences, University of Texas Southwestern Medical Center, Dallas, TX, USA

Division of Basic Research, Department of Obstetrics and Gynecology, University of Texas Southwestern Medical Center, Dallas, TX, USA
e-mail: LEE.KRAUS@utsouthwestern.edu

© Springer Nature Switzerland AG 2019
X. Zhang (ed.), *Estrogen Receptor and Breast Cancer*, Cancer Drug Discovery and Development, https://doi.org/10.1007/978-3-319-99350-8_5

synthetic antagonists promote binding of ERα to the genome. Each of these types of ligands generates distinct and overlapping ERα "cistromes" (i.e., the collection of ERα binding sites across the genome), as well as an "epigenome" (i.e., the collection of chemical modifications on chromatin and genomic DNA) and the estrogen-regulated "transcriptome" (i.e., the collection of all RNA transcripts up- or downregulated by estrogen signaling) (Table 1). Important roles for "non-genomic" or "membrane-initiated" estrogen signaling through ERs have been characterized [4], some of which may ultimately impact the transcriptome [5, 6] (Fig. 1). In this chapter, we will focus on the actions of estrogen signaling through nuclear ERα, and we describe the key concepts and molecular details of estrogen-regulated transcription.

Table 1 Key concepts and molecular components of estrogen-dependent transcriptional regulation: from cistrome to transcriptome

Concept or molecular component	Definition
Cistrome	The collection of TF binding sites across the genome
Coregulator	A protein that interacts with and enhances (or represses) the transcriptional activity of a TF
Enhancer	A regulatory element in the genome that is bound by TFs, nucleates the formation of an active regulatory complex, loops to target gene promoters, and stimulates the expression of target genes
Estrogen response element (ERE)	A DNA element in the genome with a consensus sequence of AGGTCAnnnTGACCT that is bound by ERs
Estrogen receptor (ER)	A ligand-regulated, DNA-binding TF that is responsive to estrogens
Estrogen receptor binding site (ERBS)	Genomic loci that are bound by ERs
Estrogens	A class of steroid hormones synthesized primarily in the ovarian granulosa cells in females
Epigenome	The collection of chemical modifications on chromatin and genomic DNA
Looping	Direct physical interactions between distal regulatory elements and gene promoters or, more broadly, direct physical interactions between any two regions of the genome
Mature transcript	A fully processed RNA transcript. In this case of mRNAs and lncRNAs, a transcript that is 5′-capped, spliced, and polyadenylated
Mutation	An alteration in the sequence of a gene or protein, which may or may not lead to an observable phenotype
Primary transcript	An unprocessed RNA transcript. In this case of mRNAs and lncRNAs, a transcript that is *not* 5′-capped, spliced, and polyadenylated
Promoter	DNA sequences that define where the transcription of a gene by RNA Pol begins
RNA polymerases I, II, and III (RNA Pols I, II, III)	The multiprotein enzymes that transcribe DNA into RNA. RNA Pol I synthesizes rRNA; RNA Pol II synthesizes mRNAs, lncRNAs, and most snRNA and microRNAs; and RNA Pol III synthesizes tRNAs and 5S rRNA
Transcriptome	The collection of all RNA transcripts up- or downregulated by estrogen signaling

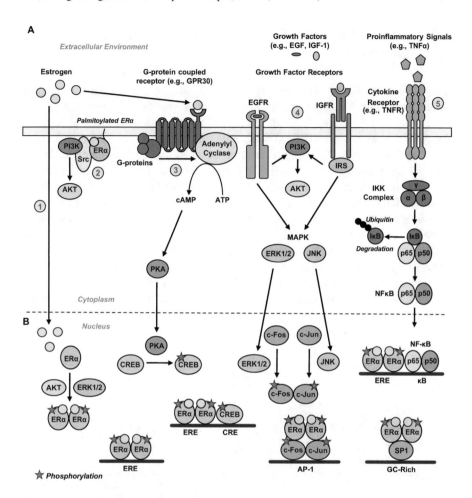

Fig. 1 Cytoplasmic and nuclear signaling pathways converge on nuclear ERα signaling pathways. (**a**) Cytoplasmic and nuclear and signaling pathways originating from the extracellular space or cytoplasmic membrane, including (*from left to right*) (1) direct action of estrogens on ERα in the nucleus; (2) membrane-initiated estrogen signaling through membrane-associated canonical ERα directed to the membrane by palmitoylation [7–9]; (3) membrane-initiated estrogen signaling through GPR30 [a.k.a. G protein-coupled estrogen receptor 1 (GPER-1)], a Gs-coupled heptaheli-cal transmembrane receptor that binds estrogens [10]; (4) growth factor signaling (e.g., EGF and IGF-1) through growth factor receptors; and (5) proinflammatory signaling (e.g., TNFα) through cytokine receptors. The intracellular signaling pathways stimulated by the initiating events described above require kinases (e.g., Src, PI3K, AKT, PKA, JNK1, ERK1/2, IKK). (**b**) The intra-cellular signaling pathways stimulated by the initiating events described in (**a**) require kinases ultimately link to a variety of transcription factors [TFs; e.g., CREB, NF-κB (p65 and p50), AP-1 (Fos and Jun), and SP-1]. Many of these TFs (1) are phosphorylated by the kinases noted in (**a**) (indicated by the red stars) and (2) interact physically and functionally with ERα in the nucleus to promote the formation of estrogen-responsive ERα enhancers across the genome

1.1   ERα Binding Sites, Cistromes, and Transcriptional Enhancers

The binding of ligands to ERα (agonists and antagonists) stimulates receptor dimerization and binding to thousands of sites across the genome, collectively called the ERα "cistrome," within minutes of hormone exposure [11–15]. While many ERα binding sites (ERBSs) contain a DNA sequence motif called the estrogen response element (ERE), the consensus of which is a 13-base pair palindrome with a 3-base pair spacer [2], others lack any semblance of such a motif and may recruit ERα indirectly through other TFs (see below) [16, 17] (Fig. 1b). Direct-binding ERBSs are pre-established and prebound ("marked") by pioneer transcription factors, such as FoxA1 or AP2γ prior to ERα binding [18, 19]. DNA-bound ERα acts as a nucleation site and scaffold for the assembly of multiprotein complexes containing histone-modifying enzymes, ATP-dependent nucleosome-remodeling enzymes, and Mediator, an RNA polymerase II (Pol II)-interacting coregulator [20–23] (Fig. 2 and Table 2). The coordinated recruitment of these coregulator proteins and chromatin-modifying enzymes functions to establish an active transcriptional "enhancer," leading to chromatin looping and target gene

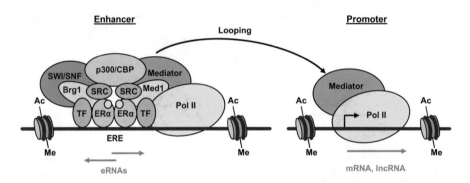

Fig. 2 Features of ERα enhancers. Agonist-bound ERα dimerizes and binds to regulatory regions across the genome to promote the formation of estrogen-regulated enhancers. ERα binds to these regions with assistance from other TFs, such as pioneer factors (e.g., FoxA1) or cooperatively interacting TFs (see Fig. 1). ERα binds to genomic directly DNA through its sequence element [i.e., the estrogen response element (ERE)] or via tethering mechanisms with other DNA-binding transcription factors. ERα nucleates the formation of enhancers by recruiting direct-binding transcriptional coregulators, including members of the SRC family (SRC-1, SRC-2, or SRC-3), the Swi/Snf complex (via its Brg1 subunit), and the Mediator complex (via its Med1 subunit). These, in turn, recruit other coregulators, including histone-modifying enzymes, such as the lysine acetyltransferase p300/CBP. Ultimately, the forming enhancer recruits the RNA Pol II transcriptional machinery, which loops to target gene promoters to promote gene transcription. Enhancers are characterized "active" histone modifications (e.g., H3K27ac and H3K4me1), coregulator recruitment, an open chromatin architecture, and the production of enhancer RNAs (eRNAs). Although not depicted here for simplicity, many of the features and factors shown at the enhancer are also found at the promoter

Table 2 Major classes of coregulators for ERs and other TFs

Class/example	Descriptions
A. *Adapters*	Proteins or RNAs that interact with two or more other proteins to bring them together and promote functional interactions
• Steroid receptor coregulators (SRCs 1, 2, and 3)	LXXLL motif-containing proteins that interact with the AF-2 (helix 12) of ligand-activated ERs and other nuclear receptors to recruit p300 and CBP (as well as other coregulators) to the DNA-bound receptor
Steroid receptor RNA activator (SRA)	A long noncoding RNA that interacts with ER or ER-interacting coregulators to nucleate the formation of coregulator complexes on the DNA-bound receptor
B. *Bridging factors*	Proteins that bind to enhancers and promoters to promote looping
• Mediator	A multipolypeptide complex that interacts with ER and other nuclear receptors through the LXXLL motif-containing subunit Med1. Mediator helps to recruit RNA Pol II to promoters and enhancers and facilitates enhancer-promoter looping, in part through the RNA-binding Med12 subunit
C. *Histone-modifying enzymes*	Proteins with catalytic activities that modify or de-modify histones (or other chromatin- and transcription-related proteins). These enzymes interact directly or indirectly with ER and other nuclear receptors
• p300 and CBP	Protein lysine acetyltransferase enzymes that are recruited to ER and other nuclear receptors through SRC proteins. They modify histone H3 lysine 27 by acetylation, a mark that is associated with active enhancers, as well other histones and transcription factors with acetylation
D. *Nucleosome remodeling enzymes*	Enzymes or enzyme complexes that use the energy from ATP to mobilize, structurally alter, or evict nucleosomes
• Swi/Snf	A nucleosome-remodeling enzyme that interacts with ER and other nuclear receptors through the Brg1 (SMARCA4) ATPase subunit

transcription [24–28] (Fig. 2). The transcriptional effects of estrogen signaling are rapid, on the order of minutes, resulting in transcription at both ERα enhancers and their target genes [25, 29, 30].

1.2   Direct and Indirect ERα Binding Sites

The nuclear actions of ERα occur through both "classical" (direct) and "nonclassical" (indirect) binding of ERα to the genome [31]. In the classical pathway, ERα binds to EREs (short DNA motifs with the consensus AGGTCAnnnTGACCT) [32, 33]. In contrast, the nonclassical genomic pathway does not require the presence of ERE in ERα binding sites. Rather, the binding of ERα to the genome is facilitated by tethering mechanisms with other TFs, such as AP1, NF-κB, CREB, and SP1 [34–37] (Fig. 1b). Variable binding of ERα and other TFs to their genomic binding sites may also be influenced by neighboring sequence or motifs, as well as combinations of different TFs [16, 17, 38, 39]. Notably, many ERα binding sites contain "imperfect" (i.e., non-consensus) EREs, which has led to a reevaluation of the sequence determinants for ERα binding and perhaps a redefinition of the concept of classical and nonclassical binding.

1.3   Features of Active ERα Enhancers

Active ERα enhancers (i.e., those capable of promoting target gene expression) are associated with a variety of features that provide useful "marks" of enhancer activity [40]. These include (1) enrichment of specific histone modifications [e.g., H3 lysine 4 monomethyl (H3K4me1), H3 lysine 27 acetyl (H3K27ac)], coregulators (e.g., p300/CBP, Mediator), and RNA polymerase II (Pol II) [41–43], (2) an open chromatin structure (e.g., DNAse I hypersensitivity, nucleosome depletion by FAIRE-seq) [44, 45], (3) enhancer transcription (enhancer RNA production) [25, 45, 46], and (4) looping to target gene promoters [47] (Figs. 2 and 3). Different classes of enhancers may exhibit differential accumulation of these features in a context-dependent manner to specify distinct gene regulatory mechanisms [48]. Differential enhancer selection and activity result in cell- and context-specific gene expression. While the definition of enhancers continues to evolve, technological advances have revealed new features of enhancer function and generated renewed interest in enhancers as important regulators of tissue-specific gene expression. Some of the remaining questions address challenges in the identification, conservation, and functional annotation of these enhancers [49].

2   Coregulators for Estrogen Receptors

The binding of ERα to genomic regulatory regions promotes the recruitment of a broad array of coregulator proteins and coregulator complexes (Table 2). Some of these coregulators interact directly with ERα (e.g., the steroid receptor coactivators, SRC1, 2, and 3; the Mediator complex via Med1; and the Swi/Snf complex via Brg1), while others interact indirectly through scaffolding coregulators (e.g., p300

Fig. 3 (continued) and distal enhancer in ERα-positive MCF-7 breast cancer cells (*from top to bottom*): (1) GRO-seq measures of actively transcribing RNA polymerases across the genome, shown for a 40 min time course of treatment with 17β-estradiol (E2); (2) RNA-seq measures the steady-state levels of RNAs, including mRNAs; and (3) ChIP-seq for ERα (±E2, 45 min), FoxA1 (+E2, 45 min), H3K4me1 (+E2, 45 min), and H3K27ac (+E2, 45 min) shows the enrichment of these factors and chromatin modifications at various loci. The *P2RY2* gene annotation (with exons and introns) and a size marker (in kb) are shown. Adapted from [25]

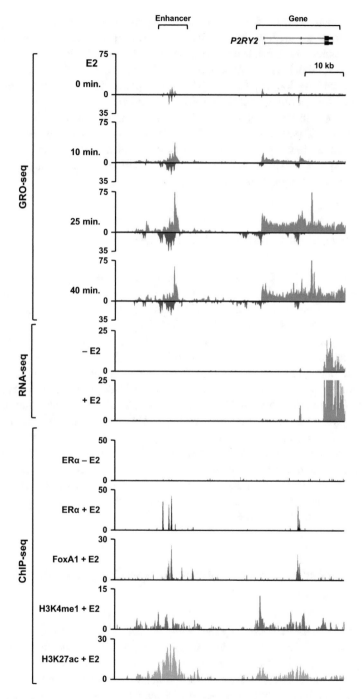

Fig. 3 Visualizing ERα enhancer formation and E2-regulated gene transcription with genomic assays. The use of genomic assays to visualize estrogen-dependent regulation of the *P2RY2* gene

and CBP, which interact with ERα through SRCs proteins) [50–53]. These coregulators serve a variety of functions, including (1) the posttranslational modification of histones and other transcription-related proteins (p300 and CBP, which are protein acetyltransferases) [54], (2) chromatin remodeling (e.g., Swi/Snf complex) [55], and (3) chromatin looping (e.g., Mediator complex) [56–59]. These events ultimately facilitate looping events that associate enhancers to target promoters and induce changes in RNA polymerase II (Pol II) occupancy or activity [60]. While SRCs, p300/CBP (sometimes referred to collectively), Swi/Snf, and Mediator function with ERα, they also support the transcriptional activity of many other TFs. Thus, the ligand activation and specific ERBSs are critical determinants of their function in the estrogen signaling pathway.

2.1   Coregulators and Noncoding RNAs

Details about the specific functions of coregulators, especially as they relate to enhancer formation and activity, are becoming clearer. Some of these functions require interactions with noncoding RNAs. For example, SRC-1 interacts with SRA (steroid receptor RNA activator) to facilitate ERα-dependent transcriptional outcomes [61]. SRA was subsequently found to enhance the activities of the AF-1 and AF-2 domains of ERα [62, 63]. p300/CBP is thought to be the key enzyme that acetylates histone H3 at lysine 27 (H3K27), a mark of active enhancers [42, 64, 65]. Interestingly, interactions with short noncoding RNAs produced from enhancers (i.e., eRNAs) may stimulate p300 catalytic activity at enhancers [66]. Interaction of Mediator with enhancer-derived noncoding RNAs [e.g., long noncoding RNAs (lncRNAs) or eRNAs] via the Med12 subunit promotes enhancer-promoter looping [59]. These are a few of the details about coregulatory functions that have emerged recently, but a number of gaps in our knowledge remain. For example, we still know little about the temporal aspects of coregulator function, although recent studies have shown that coregulators may have distinct and changing roles during the time course of enhancer function [67].

3   Molecular Aspects of Estrogen-Dependent Transcriptional Outcomes

ERα regulates gene expression by increasing or decreasing transcription of its target genes, which include protein-coding mRNA genes, as well as noncoding RNA genes for microRNAs, lncRNAs, transfer RNAs (tRNAs), and ribosomal RNAs (rRNAs) [29]. In turn, the products of these transcriptional targets are involved in various cellular functions, including the regulation of a secondary "wave" of target genes and their RNA products. Ultimately, estrogen-regulated transcriptional responses lead to changes in the transcriptome by altering RNA Pol I, II, and III transcription, as well as the proteome by altering the levels of mRNAs (via microRNAs), ribosome

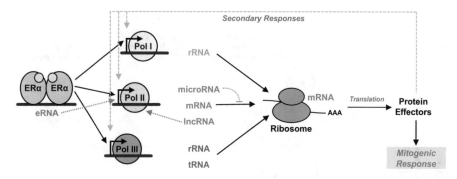

Fig. 4 Broad effects of estrogen signaling on the transcriptome. Estrogen signaling via ERα regulates transcription from all three RNA polymerases (Pols I, II, and III) in ERα-positive MCF-7 breast cancer cells. The products from these estrogen-regulated transcription events include eRNAs, mRNAs, lncRNAs, microRNAs, rRNAs, and tRNAs. Estrogen signaling regulates (1) mRNA expression by controlling Pol II activity at target gene promoters via eRNAs and lncRNAs, as well as mRNA stability via microRNAs; (2) ribosome biogenesis by enhancing the production of rRNAs, as well as mRNAs encoding ribosomal proteins; and (3) protein translation by enhancing the production of tRNAs, as well as promoting ribosome biogenesis as noted above. The functional interactions between the RNA products from estrogen-regulated transcription have profound effects on the cell and collectively promote mitogenic responses [29, 30]

biogenesis (via rRNAs and ribosomal proteins), and translation (via tRNAs and translation regulatory proteins) [29] (Fig. 4).

3.1 Primary and Secondary Transcriptional Responses

Defining the hierarchy of the estrogen transcriptional responses has helped delineate the mechanism of estrogen action. To this end, estrogen transcriptional responsive genes can be categorized as primary response and secondary response genes. Primary response genes are those that are regulated as an immediate response to cellular signaling without the requirement for protein synthesis [68, 69]. Recently, the concept of "direct" target genes has emerged to describe target genes whose promoters are associated with TF binding at proximal or distal enhancers [11, 15, 26]. Secondary response genes are regulated following protein synthesis. The transcriptional regulation of secondary response genes may involve transcriptional cross talk between ERα with the products of the primary response (Fig. 4).

3.2 Pol II Recruitment and Promoter-Proximal Pausing

The concepts of "primary/immediate" and "direct" target genes often describe two distinct aspects of the mechanism of transcriptional regulation and are often incorrectly used synonymously. The distinction arises from the underlying mechanisms

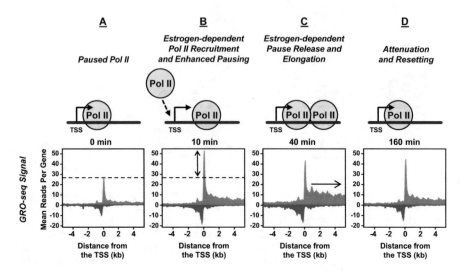

Fig. 5 Robust and transient ERα-regulated transcription. Metaplots showing the average read profiles of GRO-seq data for estrogen-stimulated genes in ERα-positive MCF-7 breast cancer cells over a 160 min time course of E2 treatment. The data are aligned relative to the transcriptional start sites (TSSs) of the genes. For the genes shown here with maximal transcription at 40 min of E2 treatment, the GRO-seq data reveal the following: (**a**) Strong polymerase pause peak immediately downstream of the TSS prior to E2 treatment. (**b**) Additional E2-dependent Pol II recruitment (loading), as well as enhanced pausing, after 10 min of E2 treatment. (**c**) Robust transition from pausing to elongation across the gene body. (**d**) Attenuation of transcriptional activity are resetting to basal levels. Adapted from [29]

of Pol II regulation at ERα target promoters [70]. The prevailing view of the regulation commences with ligand-dependent ERα enhancer formation, which subsequently mediates the recruitment of the Pol II machinery to promoters. The rate-limiting step in this mechanism is the recruitment of Pol II [70, 71] (Fig. 3). However, more recent studies in the fly and mammalian systems have revealed that Pol II is preloaded at many promoters across the genome prior to stimulation, initiating the synthesis of a short transcript and subsequently "pausing" ~20–40 base pairs downstream of the TSS [72] (Fig. 5). This mechanism may allow rapid transcriptional responses to stimuli by bypassing the rate-limiting step of the aforementioned mechanism or possibly generate synchronous transcriptional responses to stimuli for a population of genes or cells. In the context of estrogen-regulated transcription, regulation of Pol II loading and release of Pol II from pause sites can be regulated by nuclear ERα action, as well as membrane-initiated estrogen signaling.

In the subsequent sections, we have summarized the approaches employed to interrogate these aspects of transcriptional regulation and highlight the most significant findings from recent studies of estrogen-dependent transcription through ERα.

4 Overview of Genomic Analyses of Estrogen-Regulated Transcription

The advent of microarray-based genomic technologies in the late 1980s and early 1990s, leading to the groundbreaking paper by Pat Brown and colleagues in 1995 reporting the results of the first microarray expression analysis [73], ushered in the age of genomics. The fields of molecular biology and biomedical sciences have never looked back. The past decade has seen a rapid expansion of "genomic" methods for the analysis of signal-regulated transcription, including estrogen-regulated transcription through ERα. Today, a plethora of genomic technologies, now based on next-generation or deep sequencing technologies, are available to scientists to explore the features of the genome, transcriptome, and cistrome of their favorite biological system in a facile and robust manner. As scientists have learned how to apply these technologies, we have seen how they can be used effectively for discovery-based experiments, as well as to test specific hypotheses on a global scale [74].

4.1 Aspects of Estrogen-Regulated Transcription Queried on a Genomic Scale

Today, nearly every aspect of signal-regulated transcription by a diverse array of TFs, including ERα and other nuclear receptors, can be probed with a genomic approach. These include TF binding, chromatin opening, enhancer assembly, enhancer-promoter looping, and transcriptional outcomes (Table 3). More broadly, downstream actions, such as protein translation, can also be probed as well through Ribo-seq and ribosome profiling [75] (Table 3). Through these approaches, a clearer picture of the molecular details of signal-regulated transcription has emerged.

4.2 Current Challenges and Opportunities in Genomic Analyses of Transcription

While our understanding of the estrogen-regulated transcriptome has advanced quite rapidly in the age of genomics, there are a number of challenges that must be overcome to increase our understanding further. These challenges include (1) single cell analyses of not only the transcriptome, but also of cistromes, chromatin accessibility, and looping, (2) allele-specific transcriptional effects, and (3) analyses in tissues and pathological samples. Overcoming some of these challenges will require the development of new methodologies.

The age of genomics and high-throughput screening (e.g., siRNA, shRNA, or CRISPR screens; [76, 77]) has also brought many new opportunities. The

Table 3 Genomic methods used to interrogate estrogen-dependent transcriptional regulation

Assays	Descriptions
A. Cistrome	
• ChIP-seq	A method used to analyze protein-DNA interactions genome-wide, which combines chromatin immunoprecipitation (ChIP) with next generation DNA sequencing
• ChIP-exo	A ChIP-based method for mapping protein-DNA interactions genome-wide, which has improved resolution compared to ChIP-seq
• RIME	*R*apid *i*mmunoprecipitation *m*ass spectrometry of *e*ndogenous proteins is a method that allows the identification of chromatin and transcription factor complexes by mass spectrometry
B. Chromatin accessibility	
• DNase I-seq	A method used to identify the location of accessible regions in chromatin across the genome, which is based on the genome-wide sequencing of regions sensitive to cleavage by DNase I
• MNase-seq	A method used to identify the location of accessible regions in chromatin across the genome or to map nucleosome positions, which is based on the genome-wide sequencing of regions sensitive to cleavage by MNase
• ATAC-seq	*A*ssay for *t*ransposase-*a*ccessible *c*hromatin using is a technique used to study chromatin accessibility, which aims to identify accessible DNA regions, equivalent to DNase I hypersensitive sites. The assay relies on the action of the transposase Tn5 on genomic DNA
C. Chromatin looping	
• ChIA-PET	*C*hromatin *i*nteraction *a*nalysis by *p*aired-*e*nd *t*ag *s*equencing is a technique that incorporates ChIP-based enrichment, chromatin proximity ligation, paired-end tags, and deep sequencing to determine long-range chromatin interactions genome-wide
• 3C-based sequencing methods	*C*hromosome *c*onformation *c*apture techniques (e.g., 5C and Hi-C) are a set of molecular biology methods used to analyze the spatial organization of chromatin in a cell
D. Transcriptome	
• Expression microarrays	A probe hybridization-based method for monitoring the relative levels of mRNA in a sample
• RNA-seq	A deep sequencing-based method for monitoring the relative levels of mRNAs in a sample and determining the exon-intron structure of those RNAs
• GRO-seq, PRO-seq	Run-on based methods for mapping the position and orientation of actively engaged RNA Pols by monitoring labeled nascent RNAs
• 5′ GRO-seq, PRO-cap	Run-on based methods for mapping the 5′ start sites of RNAs using nascent RNA
E. Translation	
• Ribo-seq	A method for deep sequencing of RNA that is engaged by the ribosome in order to monitor the translation process
• Ribosome profiling	A method for deep sequencing of ribosome-protected mRNA fragments

possibility to conduct perturbation-response experiments and assays of kinetics on a genome-wide scale should bring even greater understanding of the molecular mechanisms of estrogen-regulated transcription. While there has been a predominant focus on upregulation, genomic assays provide an opportunity to explore downregulation or repression on a global scale.

5   Global Views of the Estrogen-Regulated Transcriptome

Numerous studies over the past two decades have examined the mechanisms and outcomes of estrogen-regulated transcription using various genomic approaches, such as gene expression microarrays, as well as genome-wide chromatin immuno-precipitation (ChIP) assays (ChIP-chip and ChIP-seq) [78]. Although they have provided a wealth of knowledge about the biology of estrogen signaling in the nucleus, these studies have not always provided a consistent view of the primary or immediate estrogen-regulated gene set. This information is critical for mechanistic studies when trying to relate estrogen signaling to specific molecular events at target gene promoters. Like expression microarrays, which have produced discrepancies in the numbers of estrogen-regulated genes within a given cell type [78, 79], genomic ChIP assays of ERα and Pol II have not produced a clear picture of the estrogen-regulated gene set. This is due, in part, to the difficulty in assigning ERα binding events to specific gene regulatory outcomes [15, 80]. New technologies for assessing enhancer-promoter looping events (e.g., ChIA-PET) and for measuring nascent transcription (e.g., GRO-seq) have helped to overcome some of these problems [72, 81]. A limitation of many of the earlier analyses is that they focused on the effects of estrogen signaling on the expression of annotated Pol II transcripts (i.e., transcripts encoding proteins and microRNAs), without considering potential effects on unannotated transcripts, or Pol I and Pol III transcripts. In this section, we describe studies that have employed genomic approaches to query the estrogen-regulated transcriptome.

5.1   Expression Microarrays and RNA-seq

The earliest attempts to understand the global effects of estrogen signaling on the transcriptome were performed using microarrays (reviewed in [82]). Microarray expression profiling relies on the hybridization of differentially labeled fluorescent cDNA probes to control/reference samples and experimental samples to determine relative steady-state expression levels of thousands of annotated mRNAs across different conditions and treatments [73]. Breast cancer was one of the first and has been one of the most widely studied, biological models analyzed with this technique [83].

In fact, the expression profiles of breast cancers were used to identify and define a set of distinct molecular subtypes, a classification system that is still used today [84]. Using information from expression microarrays, molecular taxonomy was used to group breast cancers into four major subtypes, luminal A, luminal B, basal-like, and HER2+, related to expressed molecular markers [85]. These breast cancer molecular subtypes exhibit distinct clinical and pathological phenotypes [86].

The most commonly employed model for studying the estrogen-regulated transcriptome is the ERα-positive, luminal A adenocarcinoma cell line, MCF-7. Microarray analyses using these cells helped to provide an initial view of some of the transcriptional responses to estrogen [79]. Expression microarray experiments in MCF-7 cells have been performed with a wide range of estrogen treatment times (e.g., 0, 3, 6, 12, and 24 h). They have yielded estimates for the number of estrogen-responsive target genes ranging from ~100 to ~1500 [12, 78, 79, 87]. In these experiments, the genes regulated at the earliest time points were considered to be immediate, direct, or primary transcriptional targets, while the genes regulated at the later time points were considered to be late, indirect, or secondary targets. Several attempts have been made to define the primary estrogen-regulated transcriptome by employing cycloheximide, a potent mRNA translation inhibitor, to prevent the secondary effects of estrogen-regulated transcription [87]. However, this approach is limited by the toxic effects of cycloheximide and its inability to account for the effects of noncoding transcriptional products, such as microRNAs and lncRNAs. As discussed below, it is likely that even in the earliest of these time points (i.e., 3 h), the regulated genes reported include indirect or secondary effects of estrogen treatment.

Many of the salient features of the results from the experiments with MCF-7 cells are conserved across estrogen-dependent biological systems. However, the results from different studies using the same cell type exhibit variability due to a variety of factors, including the cell growth and estrogen treatment conditions, the subpopulations of MCF-7 clones, and the specific microarray platforms. Moreover, technical limitations associated with the microarray approach, such as relatively high level of noise, low sensitivity for rare or low-abundance transcripts, narrow dynamic range, and biased detection of transcript variants, gene fusions, single nucleotide variants, and indels (small insertions and deletions), have limited the utility of microarrays for gene expression analyses. However, the low cost and facile application of microarray technology have made expression microarrays a useful diagnostic tool for the clinic [88].

More recent developments in next generation sequencing technologies have given way to more powerful techniques for gene expression profiling, including RNA-seq, which overcome many of the limitations encountered by microarrays. RNA expression analyses using RNA-seq allow for sensitive and unbiased profiling of the steady-state estrogen-regulated transcriptome. From the gene expression perspective, many of the conclusions about the estrogen-regulated transcriptome from RNA-seq studies mirror those made using expression microarrays. But, RNA-seq studies have facilitated a greater exploration of the effects of estrogen on noncoding RNA expression, splicing, and ribosome loading, revealing new facets of the molecular response to estrogen signaling.

5.2   GRO-seq and Derivatives

While gene expression profiling with microarrays and RNA-seq have provided an abundance of information regarding estrogen responses, these approaches have fallen short in defining the primary and immediate responses at the genomic level. Microarray and RNA-seq can reveal the steady-state levels of mRNA (or other RNAs) and, therefore, require the accumulation of transcripts over time. Our understanding of estrogen action at the genomic level has expanded with more recent developments in next generation sequencing technologies that measure active or ongoing transcription with higher sensitivity and temporal resolution. One such method, global run-on coupled with massively parallel sequencing (GRO-seq), has been used in breast cancer cells and other biological systems to identify new features of estrogen-regulated transcription [25, 29, 89].

GRO-seq is a direct sequencing method that provides a "map" of the position and orientation of all engaged RNA polymerases (Pols I, II, and III) across the genome at extremely high resolution. It has helped to (1) identify primary response genes, (2) establish a hierarchy of the estrogen-regulated transcriptional network, (3) reveal mechanisms of the estrogen-regulated transcriptional response, and (4) identify novel unannotated and noncoding transcripts. Derivatives of GRO-seq, such as precision run-on sequencing (PRO-seq) and PRO-cap (or 5'-GRO-seq), allow (1) mapping of the 3' end of nascent RNAs in the Pol II active site with nucleotide resolution and (2) mapping of the 5' end of nascent RNAs with nucleotide resolution [90], respectively (Table 3). These methods have revealed new facets of estrogen-regulated transcription, which have not been discerned using other techniques.

Using GRO-seq and short time courses of estrogen treatment in MCF-7 cells, the Kraus lab has made a number of observations about the estrogen-regulated transcriptional response, reported in a series of papers over the past 8 years. Three adjectives that describe this response are rapid, extensive, and transient [29]. Here we summarize some of these findings.

Estrogen-Dependent Transcriptional Responses Are Rapid The initial GRO-seq experiments in MCF-7 cells recalibrated our understanding about the time scale of estrogen-dependent transcription experiments. While the steady-state RNA experiments with expression microarrays and RNA-seq examined responses on the order of hours, and sometime even days, the direct transcriptional readout from GRO-seq experiments showed that the responses occurred on the order of minutes [29] (Fig. 3). In fact, the transcriptional outcomes of nuclear estrogen signaling occur at least as fast, if not faster, than the so-called "rapid" membrane-initiated actions. Using GRO-seq and with detailed time courses of estrogen treatment, we were able to determine the rates of Pol II transcription for estrogen-regulated genes [91]. Elongation rates varied as much as fourfold at different genomic loci. Gene body elongation rates correlated with the density of Pol II on the gene, resulting in higher rates of transcript production at genes with higher Pol II densities. These studies also revealed that estrogen stimulates gene expression by increasing Pol II initiation, whereas other signaling pathways (e.g., TNFα) reduce Pol II residence time at promoter proximal pause sites [91]. Collectively, these studies provided new insights into the mechanisms of estrogen-regulated transcription.

Estrogen-Dependent Transcriptional Responses Are Extensive The early expression microarray and RNA-seq experiments focused on the Pol II mRNA transcriptome or subsets thereof. Given that GRO-seq can readily detect transcription by all three RNA polymerases, it provides an opportunity to explore the transcriptome more broadly. The initial GRO-seq experiments in MCF-7 cells showed that estrogen signaling not only regulates the Pol II transcriptome but also the Pol I and Pol III transcriptomes as well [29]. The expression of every major class of RNA, including rRNAs and tRNAs, is altered by estrogen signaling (Fig. 4). By developing computational tools for analyzing GRO-seq data, such as groHMM [92], we were able to annotate novel transcripts in MCF-7 cells, including previously unannotated lncRNAs and eRNAs (discussed in more detail below) [29, 93].

Estrogen-Dependent Transcriptional Responses Are Transient An additional observation about the estrogen-regulated transcriptome from the initial GRO-seq experiments was that upregulation was generally transient, with the majority of upregulated genes showing maximal transcription at 40 min and then declining thereafter [29]. In contrast, the downregulated genes stayed down for longer periods of time. Together, these results illustrate that estrogen-dependent transcriptional responses are transient and that upregulation and downregulation may occur by fundamentally different mechanisms [29].

6   LncRNAs and eRNAs Revealed by GRO-seq

As noted above, GRO-seq has been a useful tool for annotating new transcription units, including those that produce lncRNAs and eRNAs.

6.1   LncRNAs

We found that a computational approach integrating both GRO-seq and RNA-seq increased the sensitivity for detecting low-abundance lncRNAs [93]. Integration of these data with genomic information about histone modifications and factor binding at lncRNA gene promoters provided new insights about lncRNA gene structure and regulation, as well as lncRNA transcript stability, regulation, and function. For example, we observed that many ERα binding sites occur in lncRNAs gene promoters, which are also marked with histone modifications that are typical of transcriptional enhancers [93]. Functional analysis of selected lncRNAs with altered expression in breast cancers, such as lncRNA67 and lncRNA152, revealed novel roles for these lncRNAs in cell proliferation, regulation of an E2F-dependent cell-cycle gene expression program, and estrogen-dependent mitogenic growth. These studies illustrated the power of GRO-seq data, when combined with appropriate computational tools, to annotate novel transcription units across the genome.

6.2   Enhancer Transcription and eRNAs

Recent studies, including work from the Kraus lab, have shown that many enhancers overlap with sites of Pol II loading and the production of enhancer RNAs ("eRNAs") [29, 94–99]. GRO-seq has been a powerful approach for detecting, analyzing, and annotating enhancer transcription and eRNAs [25, 67]. Enhancer transcription mirrors the kinetics of the emergence of other enhancer features, as well as enhancer activation and target gene transcription [29, 100, 101] (Fig. 3). A common signature of enhancer transcription is the production of short (i.e., ~1–2 kb) eRNAs that are transcribed bidirectionally [95] and can be readily detected by GRO-seq [25, 29, 96–98, 101]. The role of transcription in enhancer function is unknown, but the act of transcription may help to create an open chromatin environment that promotes enhancer function [46, 102]. Alternatively, the stable accumulation of eRNAs may play a functional or structural role and may facilitate gene looping (reviewed in [103]).

7   Integrating the Estrogen-Regulated Transcriptome with Other Aspects of Gene Regulation

In the sections above, we described fundamental aspects of the estrogen-regulated transcriptome and genomic methods to analyze it. The RNA Pol II transcriptome is of particular interest to the study of hormone signaling because it comprises a set of mRNAs that encode the proteome, as well as functional RNAs that can regulate the expression or abundance of mRNAs (e.g., lncRNAs and microRNAs). As noted above, the promoters of the estrogen-regulated genes that produce mRNAs, lncRNAs, and microRNAs are controlled by transcriptional enhancers that nucleate at ERα binding sites and communicate with the promoters through higher-order chromatin looping mechanisms. Thus, a full understanding of the regulation of the RNA Pol II transcriptome requires the integration of transcriptome data with other genomic data (e.g., including cistrome, epigenome, chromatin accessibility, and chromatin looping data), which allows the identification of active enhancers and their target genes.

7.1   Identifying Active Estrogen-Regulated Enhancers from Genomic Data

Deep sequencing technologies used to study transcriptomes and epigenomes have revealed that the genome is pervasively transcribed [29, 104, 105] and that the epigenome is remarkably plastic [41, 106]. These studies have also identified transcriptional enhancers as the key regulatory elements that control the cell type-specific biology of essentially all biological systems examined to date [48, 107]. However, the cistrome for a given TF is not synonymous with the set of active enhancers nucleated by the TF, since many TF binding sites are not functional as enhancers. For ERα, the number of ERE-like sequences is greater than the number of ERBSs, and the number of ERBSs is greater than the number of functionally active ERα enhancers [25]. Thus, identifying active enhancers, rather than TF binding sites, is important for understanding the estrogen-dependent regulation of gene expression.

As discussed above, our current understanding of the features of active enhancers has been derived from an integration of a variety of genomic techniques and complemented with specific mechanistic assays. Active enhancers, including those nucleated by agonist-occupied ERα, share several common features [48, 107, 108]. For example, enhancers are typically (1) located in open regions of chromatin (as assessed by DNase-seq) [109, 110]; (2) enriched with a common set of histone modifications (as assessed by ChIP-seq), including H3K4me1 and H3K27ac [41, 106]; (3) enriched with the coregulators p300 and CBP (as assessed by ChIP-seq) [41–43]; (4) bound by RNA Pol II (as assessed by ChIP-seq); and (5) actively transcribed, producing enhancer RNAs ("eRNAs") (as assessed by RNA-seq, GRO-seq, and derivatives) [29, 94, 95] and loop to target gene promoters (as assessed by 3C-based methods) [47]. Ongoing transcription at enhancers, as assessed by GRO-seq and derivatives, can be used for the prediction of active enhancers [25, 29, 48, 92, 96, 111]. Integration of data from multiple genomic methods using computational pipelines can provide an effective way to identify active enhancers [25, 67, 112]. Of course, these genomic studies should always be followed up with additional locus-specific perturbation studies to mechanistically define the biological functions of selected enhancers that were identified with the genomic approaches.

7.2 Identifying the Target Genes of ERα Enhancers from Genomic Data

The next challenge after identifying active enhancers is to identify the target genes that they regulate. This has been typically done in one of two ways. The first is with a "nearest neighboring gene" approach, which is based on the assumption that genes closest to an active enhancer have the greatest likelihood of being regulated by that enhancer. Although this assumption is not always true and excludes some nuances related to enhancer-promoter communication and regulation, it can be a useful approach that reveals verifiable aspects of target gene regulation. In fact, the nearest neighboring genes of breast cancer subtype-specific enhancers show predictable patterns of expression in human breast cancer patient samples of the same type [25, 67, 112], supporting the biological significance of this approach. The second is by using assays of enhancer-promoter looping, such as 3C-based sequencing approaches or ChIA-PET, which provide an indication of physical communication between enhancers and their target promoters. These approaches have shown that ERα binding sites that loop to target gene promoters are more likely to be enriched for other features of active enhancers than those that do not loop [25].

Although promoters that are looped to by an enhancer are likely to be true targets of the enhancer, looping does not always specify an active transcriptional outcome. For example, the ERα L540Q mutant (leucine 540 mutated to glutamine) [113–115] still promotes enhancer-promoter looping, even though it is transcriptionally impaired [67]. Furthermore, inhibition of enhancer transcription, a mark of active enhancers, by the transcription inhibitor flavopiridol does not prevent enhancer-promoter looping [25]. These results suggest that although definitive detection of enhancer-promoter loops is an effective way to identify bona fide target genes, the functional outcomes of looping may not be straightforward or always lead to productive transcriptional outcomes.

7.3   Enhancer Landscapes and Transcriptional Outcomes in Breast Cancers

Recent studies have explored unbiased approaches for the identification of functional enhancers in breast cancer cells that do not start with a TF cistrome [112]. In this regard, a recent study identified regulatory elements in cell lines representing the five distinct molecular subtypes of breast cancer by characterizing the epigenomic and transcriptomic profiles of the cells. The profiles of histone marks (i.e., H3K27ac and H3K4me1) from ChIP-seq were integrated with a measure enhancer transcription, as defined by GRO-seq. Putative TFs acting on these enhancers were identified by exploring the underlying sequence motifs in the defined enhancer regions and by integrating expression levels of the TFs defined by RNA-seq in each cell line. This integrative analysis produced as its outcome a "total functional score enhancer elements (TFSEE)" which ultimately allowed for the identification of subtype-specific enhancers and their cognate TFs that could play a functional role in biology of breast cancers [112]. One advantage of this approach is that it requires no prior knowledge of the TF of interest in a given cell type. The TFSEE approach can be further employed to evaluate the contribution of subtype-specific enhancers to therapeutic responses for the understanding of clinical outcomes.

8   Plasticity of ERα Transcription: Cross Talk of Nuclear Signaling Through ERα with Membrane-Initiated Signal Pathways

Genomic ERα action is modulated by diverse membrane-initiated signaling cascades. Membrane signaling can initiate from various extracellular stimuli, including growth factors, cytokines, chemokines, and estrogen via membrane-bound receptors (Fig. 1). These membrane receptors stimulate downstream signaling that activates kinase cascades and impacts transcriptional responses by inducing regulatory posttranslation modification of ERα or by stimulating the activation of other TFs. The following sections will describe key features in the cross talk between genomic ERα activity and membrane-initiated signals.

8.1   Estrogen and cAMP Signaling

Cytoplasmic estrogen signaling may be mediated by a small pool of cytoplasmic membrane-associated ERs (Fig. 1). Among these is the G protein-coupled receptor 30 (GPR30) [116]. Estrogen signaling via GPR30 stimulates heterotrimeric G proteins, which in turn activate adenylate cyclase activity to increase intracellular cAMP. Estrogen-dependent increases in cAMP stimulate transcription driven by cAMP response elements (CREs) [117]. In the murine uterine and human breast cancer models, intracellular cAMP stimulates ERα phosphorylation and transcriptional activity [118]. Furthermore, increases in intracellular cAMP activate protein kinase A (PKA), which in turn translocates to the nucleus to activate the cAMP response element-binding protein (CREB). Functional interactions between ERα and CREB induce a transcriptional response involving a complex containing the CREB-binding protein (CBP). Interestingly, transcriptional cross talk between ERα and CREB may not rely on regulatory regions containing the CREs but rather may be dependent on regulatory regions containing EREs [37]. Although this mechanism remains to be fully evaluated on a genomic scale, these studies demonstrated that extensive cross talk between estrogen and cAMP signaling can regulate ERα transcriptional activity.

8.2   Estrogen and Growth Factor Signaling

Growth factors are powerful mitogens that promote cellular proliferation across normal and disease tissues, especially in the breast and the reproductive tract [119–121]. Activation of transmembrane growth factor receptors by ligands, such as the epidermal growth factor (EGF), stimulates receptor dimerization and intracellular kinase activity. The activated downstream signaling kinases include mitogen-activated protein kinase or extracellular-regulated kinase (MAPK/ERK), protein kinase B (PKB/AKT), and c-Jun N-terminal kinases (JNK) [122] (Fig. 1). The EGF signaling pathway is extensively linked with estrogen signaling [123]. The activation of ERα by EGF involves the direct phosphorylation of ERα by MAPK on serine 118. This phosphorylation is required for full activity of the AF-1 and estrogen-mediated transcription [124]. In MCF-7 cells, estrogen stimulation elicits a rapid increase in intracellular calcium, an important intracellular second messenger, which in turn results in the activation of MAPK [125]. Moreover, ERα interacts with ERK2 and JNK1, downstream effectors in the MAPK pathway, across the genome in regulatory regions [5, 126]. The cross regulation between MAPK and ERα can be a critical component of transcriptional regulation in proliferative biological systems.

8.3   Estrogen and Proinflammatory Signaling

Transcriptional regulation by estrogen can be modulated by cross talk with proinflammatory signaling pathways. The contribution of these pathways to estrogen-regulated transcription has significant impact in breast cancer biology and can have either pro-proliferative or antiproliferative effects depending on the tumor context. Activation of proinflammatory pathways can occur by a variety of chemokines and cytokines, including tumor necrosis alpha (TNFα). The effects of proinflammatory signaling on estrogen-regulated transcription were originally attributed to the TNFα-induced downregulation of ERα protein, resulting in the inhibition of ERα-dependent transcription [127]. Activation of proinflammatory signaling results in the activation of NF-κB by the translocation of the p65 and p50 subunits to the nucleus for target gene regulation (Fig. 1). Extensive cross talk between ERα and NF-κB was revealed in genomic experiments, which showed that TNFα and estrogen signaling acts to redistribute ERα and NF-κB across the genome in MCF-7 cells, resulting in altered cistromes [89]. The redistribution of ERα is driven by the redistribution of the pioneer factor FoxA1 in response to TNFα signaling, which brings ERα to new binding sites across the genome that are only revealed in the presence of TNFα signaling. The activation of these latent ERα binding sites into active enhancers in the presence of TNFα regulates a unique set of target genes that are not modulated by either agent alone and are strongly associated with clinical outcomes in breast cancer [89]. These findings suggest an important role for the early and transient effects of proinflammatory signaling on estrogen-regulated transcription.

9   Insights into Aberrant Estrogen-Regulated Transcription in Breast Cancers

Luminal/ER-positive breast cancers are the most heterogeneous subtype according to gene expression, mutation spectrum, copy number mutations, and patient outcomes [85]. Gene amplification of certain loci, such as *ESR1* (encoding ERα) and *NCOA3* (encoding SRC3), has a causal role in tumorigenesis [128–130]. The hypothesis is that amplification of these genes results in an increased dosage of the expressed proteins, which have oncogenic roles. A similar effect has been observed with the gene encoding the EGF transmembrane tyrosine kinase receptor HER2

(*ERBB2*). Amplifications of *ERBB2* resulting in increased HER2 expression are observed in approximately 20% of breast cancers and are associated with poor prognosis, increased risk for disease progression, and decreased overall survival [131]. Notably, HER2-elevated breast cancers exhibit distinct transcriptional signatures in ER-positive and ER-negative breast cancers, suggesting an important modulatory interaction with estrogen signaling and distinct responses to antiestrogen therapy [132]. Other studies have shown that gene amplification events influence other aspects of transcription, ultimately modulating gene expression outcomes. The following sections highlight some notable examples of altered ERα-mediated transcription in breast cancers.

9.1 Genomic Amplification of Regulatory Elements

Copy number gains do not always correlate with upregulated expression of the genes in the amplified loci [85]. Moreover, many amplified or rearranged regions of the cancer genome do not contain protein- or microRNA-encoding genes that are aberrantly expressed in cancers [133]. Recent evidence suggests that the genetic, structural, or epigenetic disruption of DNA regulatory elements, such as enhancers, represents a major contribution to breast cancer initiation and recurrence. Amplification of EREs is found in ER-positive luminal breast cancers. This can result in deregulated transcription via long-range chromatin interactions with target genes outside of the amplified regions, which can lead to cancer development and tamoxifen resistance [134]. Chronic exposure of normal breast progenitor cells to estrogenic chemicals further results in progressive accumulation of these amplified response elements. The amplification of regulatory regions allows for the synchronized transcriptional control of several genes located on distinct chromosomes through long-range chromatin interactions [135]. This model of transcriptional regulation differs from the prevalent models of enhancer-promoter regulation, which typically assume a 1:1 relationship between regulatory elements and their targets. Assessing sufficiency and necessity of regulatory regions for transcriptional outputs in all of these models remains a challenge and an area of active research. The mechanisms underlying these chromosomal alterations and the functional characterization of these aberrations remain to be fully explored. Nonetheless, estrogen-dependent accumulation and modulation of chromatin interactions are thought to be a driving force of genomic instability driving breast cancer tumorigenesis.

9.2 Gain-of-Function ERα Mutations

Mutations in the gene encoding ERα, *ESR1*, are frequently detected in ER-positive metastatic breast cancers. These mutations are clustered in a "hotspot" which produce mutants in the ligand-binding domain of the expressed ERα. The most common of these mutations, Y537S and D538G, which appear as therapy-related mutations, increase association of ERα with coregulators in the absence of ligand by stabilizing the agonist conformation of helix 12 [136, 137]. These mutations lead to ligand-independent and enhanced ligand-dependent ERα activity that promotes tumor growth and partial resistance to endocrine therapy and may potentially enhance metastatic capacity [136, 137]. However, there is still a gap in our understanding of the molecular mechanisms and genomic effects of enhanced transcription by these ERα mutants, which are thought to involve selective interactions with coregulators or other transcription factors that modulate chromatin binding by ERα. The coregulators SRC3 (NCOA3) and p300 are essential for growth of the breast cancer cells expressing the Y537S mutant [138]. Given that recruitment of p300 may be the rate-limiting step for full ERα enhancer activation [67], it is possible that the enhanced transcriptional output of the Y537S involves a stabilization or overactivation of ERα-enhancers. Understanding the relevant mechanisms would help to identify targetable features of these gain-of-function mutants in endocrine-resistant breast cancer tumors with clinical utility.

10 Summary, Conclusions, and Perspectives

Estrogen-regulated transcription through ERα contributes in important ways to the biology breast cancer, as well as other developmental and physiological systems that depend on estrogen signaling. Tumorigenic estrogen-regulated transcription is induced by genetic mutations that affect (1) ERα expression, posttranslational modifications, and coregulator interactions, (2) regulatory element function, or (3) alterations to chromatin conformation that modify the genomic landscape. Our ability to identify these alterations and measure their contribution to the estrogen-regulated transcriptome has greatly improved in the last decade. As discoveries such as these continue to be made, our understanding of the mechanisms governing estrogen-regulated transcriptional responses will continue to evolve.

The historical molecular techniques that have provided valuable insights into the process of estrogen-regulated transcription have been replaced with more robust and sensitive deep sequencing-based genomic technologies. Approaches that interrogate the nascent transcriptional response to cellular stimuli, such as GRO-seq, have uncovered novel insights into the mechanism of estrogen transcriptional responses, as well as the ERα enhancers that control them. These studies have revealed that estrogen regulates transcription by RNA Pol I, II and III at annotated and unannotated genomic regions, controlling the expression of nearly every class of transcript described to date. Notably, intergenic transcripts produced from ERα binding sites (i.e., eRNAs) represent a novel feature of ERα enhancer biology that is shared with enhancers formed by other TFs. ERα enhancer RNAs have been used as measure of enhancer activity to understand the plasticity of the ERα enhancers in the context of various stimuli. Overall, the picture that has emerged of estrogen-regulated transcription is that it is rapid, robust, extensive, and transient.

While our understanding of the estrogen-regulated transcriptome has advanced dramatically with the use of genomics, a number of challenges and gaps in our understanding remain. These include methodological challenges, such as (1) single cell analyses of transcriptomes, cistromes, chromatin accessibility, and looping, (2) assessing allele-specific transcriptional effects, and (3) analyses in tissues and pathological samples. They also include knowledge gaps related to (1) the kinetics of the transcription process (e.g., enhancer formation, looping, target gene activation), (2) the decommissioning of active enhancers as signaling wanes, and (3) active and passive repression by the ERα. Successful resolution of these and other methodological challenges and knowledge gaps will help to advance our understanding of the estrogen-regulated transcriptome and its relevance to human physiology and disease.

Acknowledgments We are grateful for critical comments and suggestions from members of the Kraus lab, including Shino Murakami, Anusha Nagari, and J. Tyler Piazza. We are also thankful for the contributions of past Kraus lab members, whose studies furthering our understanding of the molecular mechanisms of estrogen-regulated transcription are highlighted in this review, including Nasun Hah, Charles Danko, Shino Murakami, Hector Franco, and Anusha Nagari. The estrogen-related studies in the Kraus lab are supported by grants from the NIH/NIDDK and the Cancer Prevention and Research Institute of Texas (CPRIT) to W.L.K. Y.M.V. is supported by a Postdoctoral Research Fellowship from the Lalor Foundation.

References

1. Couse JF, Korach KS (1999) Estrogen receptor null mice: what have we learned and where will they lead us? Endocr Rev 20(3):358–417. https://doi.org/10.1210/edrv.20.3.0370
2. Warner M, Nilsson S, Gustafsson JA (1999) The estrogen receptor family. Curr Opin Obstet Gynecol 11(3):249–254
3. Welboren WJ, Sweep FC, Span PN, Stunnenberg HG (2009) Genomic actions of estrogen receptor alpha: what are the targets and how are they regulated? Endocr Relat Cancer 16(4):1073–1089. https://doi.org/10.1677/ERC-09-0086
4. Fan W, Chang J, Fu P (2015) Endocrine therapy resistance in breast cancer: current status, possible mechanisms and overcoming strategies. Future Med Chem 7(12):1511–1519. https://doi.org/10.4155/fmc.15.93
5. Madak-Erdogan Z, Lupien M, Stossi F, Brown M, Katzenellenbogen BS (2011) Genomic collaboration of estrogen receptor alpha and extracellular signal-regulated kinase 2 in regulating gene and proliferation programs. Mol Cell Biol 31(1):226–236. https://doi.org/10.1128/MCB.00821-10
6. Madak-Erdogan Z, Gong P, Katzenellenbogen BS (2016) Differential utilization of nuclear and extranuclear receptor signaling pathways in the actions of estrogens, SERMs, and a tissue-selective estrogen complex (TSEC). J Steroid Biochem Mol Biol 158:198–206. https://doi.org/10.1016/j.jsbmb.2015.12.008
7. Adlanmerini M, Solinhac R, Abot A, Fabre A, Raymond-Letron I, Guihot AL, Boudou F, Sautier L, Vessieres E, Kim SH, Liere P, Fontaine C, Krust A, Chambon P, Katzenellenbogen JA, Gourdy P, Shaul PW, Henrion D, Arnal JF, Lenfant F (2014) Mutation of the palmitoylation site of estrogen receptor alpha in vivo reveals tissue-specific roles for membrane versus nuclear actions. Proc Natl Acad Sci U S A 111(2):E283–E290. https://doi.org/10.1073/pnas.1322057111

8. Meitzen J, Luoma JI, Boulware MI, Hedges VL, Peterson BM, Tuomela K, Britson KA, Mermelstein PG (2013) Palmitoylation of estrogen receptors is essential for neuronal membrane signaling. Endocrinology 154(11):4293–4304. https://doi.org/10.1210/en.2013-1172

9. Acconcia F, Ascenzi P, Bocedi A, Spisni E, Tomasi V, Trentalance A, Visca P, Marino M (2005) Palmitoylation-dependent estrogen receptor alpha membrane localization: regulation by 17beta-estradiol. Mol Biol Cell 16(1):231–237. https://doi.org/10.1091/mbc.E04-07-0547

10. Filardo EJ, Thomas P (2012) Minireview: G protein-coupled estrogen receptor-1, GPER-1: its mechanism of action and role in female reproductive cancer, renal and vascular physiology. Endocrinology 153(7):2953–2962. https://doi.org/10.1210/en.2012-1061

11. Carroll JS, Liu XS, Brodsky AS, Li W, Meyer CA, Szary AJ, Eeckhoute J, Shao W, Hestermann EV, Geistlinger TR, Fox EA, Silver PA, Brown M (2005) Chromosome-wide mapping of estrogen receptor binding reveals long-range regulation requiring the forkhead protein FoxA1. Cell 122(1):33–43. https://doi.org/10.1016/j.cell.2005.05.008

12. Carroll JS, Meyer CA, Song J, Li W, Geistlinger TR, Eeckhoute J, Brodsky AS, Keeton EK, Fertuck KC, Hall GF, Wang Q, Bekiranov S, Sementchenko V, Fox EA, Silver PA, Gingeras TR, Liu XS, Brown M (2006) Genome-wide analysis of estrogen receptor binding sites. Nat Genet 38(11):1289–1297. https://doi.org/10.1038/ng1901

13. Lin CY, Vega VB, Thomsen JS, Zhang T, Kong SL, Xie M, Chiu KP, Lipovich L, Barnett DH, Stossi F, Yeo A, George J, Kuznetsov VA, Lee YK, Charn TH, Palanisamy N, Miller LD, Cheung E, Katzenellenbogen BS, Ruan Y, Bourque G, Wei CL, Liu ET (2007) Whole-genome cartography of estrogen receptor alpha binding sites. PLoS Genet 3(6):e87. https://doi.org/10.1371/journal.pgen.0030087

14. Hewitt SC, Li L, Grimm SA, Chen Y, Liu L, Li Y, Bushel PR, Fargo D, Korach KS (2012) Research resource: whole-genome estrogen receptor alpha binding in mouse uterine tissue revealed by ChIP-seq. Mol Endocrinol 26(5):887–898. https://doi.org/10.1210/me.2011-1311

15. Welboren WJ, van Driel MA, Janssen-Megens EM, van Heeringen SJ, Sweep FC, Span PN, Stunnenberg HG (2009) ChIP-Seq of ERalpha and RNA polymerase II defines genes differentially responding to ligands. EMBO J 28(10):1418–1428. https://doi.org/10.1038/emboj.2009.88

16. Stender JD, Kim K, Charn TH, Komm B, Chang KC, Kraus WL, Benner C, Glass CK, Katzenellenbogen BS (2010) Genome-wide analysis of estrogen receptor alpha DNA binding and tethering mechanisms identifies Runx1 as a novel tethering factor in receptor-mediated transcriptional activation. Mol Cell Biol 30(16):3943–3955. https://doi.org/10.1128/MCB.00118-10

17. Heldring N, Isaacs GD, Diehl AG, Sun M, Cheung E, Ranish JA, Kraus WL (2011) Multiple sequence-specific DNA-binding proteins mediate estrogen receptor signaling through a tethering pathway. Mol Endocrinol 25(4):564–574. https://doi.org/10.1210/me.2010-0425

18. Tan SK, Lin ZH, Chang CW, Varang V, Chng KR, Pan YF, Yong EL, Sung WK, Cheung E (2011) AP-2gamma regulates oestrogen receptor-mediated long-range chromatin interaction and gene transcription. EMBO J 30(13):2569–2581. https://doi.org/10.1038/emboj.2011.151

19. Hurtado A, Holmes KA, Ross-Innes CS, Schmidt D, Carroll JS (2011) FOXA1 is a key determinant of estrogen receptor function and endocrine response. Nat Genet 43(1):27–33. https://doi.org/10.1038/ng.730

20. Acevedo ML, Kraus WL (2004) Transcriptional activation by nuclear receptors. Essays Biochem 40:73–88

21. Biddie SC, John S, Hager GL (2010) Genome-wide mechanisms of nuclear receptor action. Trends Endocrinol Metab 21(1):3–9. https://doi.org/10.1016/j.tem.2009.08.006

22. Glass CK, Rosenfeld MG (2000) The coregulator exchange in transcriptional functions of nuclear receptors. Genes Dev 14(2):121–141

23. Lonard DM, O'Malley BW (2012) Nuclear receptor coregulators: modulators of pathology and therapeutic targets. Nat Rev Endocrinol 8(10):598–604. https://doi.org/10.1038/nrendo.2012.100
24. Foulds CE, Feng Q, Ding C, Bailey S, Hunsaker TL, Malovannaya A, Hamilton RA, Gates LA, Zhang Z, Li C, Chan D, Bajaj A, Callaway CG, Edwards DP, Lonard DM, Tsai SY, Tsai MJ, Qin J, O'Malley BW (2013) Proteomic analysis of coregulators bound to ERalpha on DNA and nucleosomes reveals coregulator dynamics. Mol Cell 51(2):185–199. https://doi.org/10.1016/j.molcel.2013.06.007
25. Hah N, Murakami S, Nagari A, Danko CG, Kraus WL (2013) Enhancer transcripts mark active estrogen receptor binding sites. Genome Res 23(8):1210–1223. https://doi.org/10.1101/gr.152306.112
26. Fullwood MJ, Liu MH, Pan YF, Liu J, Xu H, Mohamed YB, Orlov YL, Velkov S, Ho A, Mei PH, Chew EG, Huang PY, Welboren WJ, Han Y, Ooi HS, Ariyaratne PN, Vega VB, Luo Y, Tan PY, Choy PY, Wansa KD, Zhao B, Lim KS, Leow SC, Yow JS, Joseph R, Li H, Desai KV, Thomsen JS, Lee YK, Karuturi RK, Herve T, Bourque G, Stunnenberg HG, Ruan X, Cacheux-Rataboul V, Sung WK, Liu ET, Wei CL, Cheung E, Ruan Y (2009) An oestrogen-receptor-alpha-bound human chromatin interactome. Nature 462(7269):58–64. https://doi.org/10.1038/nature08497
27. Levine M, Cattoglio C, Tjian R (2014) Looping back to leap forward: transcription enters a new era. Cell 157(1):13–25. https://doi.org/10.1016/j.cell.2014.02.009
28. Plank JL, Dean A (2014) Enhancer function: mechanistic and genome-wide insights come together. Mol Cell 55(1):5–14. https://doi.org/10.1016/j.molcel.2014.06.015
29. Hah N, Danko CG, Core L, Waterfall JJ, Siepel A, Lis JT, Kraus WL (2011) A rapid, extensive, and transient transcriptional response to estrogen signaling in breast cancer cells. Cell 145(4):622–634. https://doi.org/10.1016/j.cell.2011.03.042
30. Hah N, Kraus WL (2014) Hormone-regulated transcriptomes: lessons learned from estrogen signaling pathways in breast cancer cells. Mol Cell Endocrinol 382(1):652–664. https://doi.org/10.1016/j.mce.2013.06.021
31. McDevitt MA, Glidewell-Kenney C, Jimenez MA, Ahearn PC, Weiss J, Jameson JL, Levine JE (2008) New insights into the classical and non-classical actions of estrogen: evidence from estrogen receptor knock-out and knock-in mice. Mol Cell Endocrinol 290(1–2):24–30. https://doi.org/10.1016/j.mce.2008.04.003
32. Klein-Hitpass L, Schorpp M, Wagner U, Ryffel GU (1986) An estrogen-responsive element derived from the 5′ flanking region of the Xenopus vitellogenin A2 gene functions in transfected human cells. Cell 46(7):1053–1061
33. Klinge CM (2001) Estrogen receptor interaction with estrogen response elements. Nucleic Acids Res 29(14):2905–2919
34. Safe S (2001) Transcriptional activation of genes by 17 beta-estradiol through estrogen receptor-Sp1 interactions. Vitam Horm 62:231–252
35. Ray A, Prefontaine KE, Ray P (1994) Down-modulation of interleukin-6 gene expression by 17 beta-estradiol in the absence of high affinity DNA binding by the estrogen receptor. J Biol Chem 269(17):12940–12946
36. Kushner PJ, Agard DA, Greene GL, Scanlan TS, Shiau AK, Uht RM, Webb P (2000) Estrogen receptor pathways to AP-1. J Steroid Biochem Mol Biol 74(5):311–317
37. Lazennec G, Thomas JA, Katzenellenbogen BS (2001) Involvement of cyclic AMP response element binding protein (CREB) and estrogen receptor phosphorylation in the synergistic activation of the estrogen receptor by estradiol and protein kinase activators. J Steroid Biochem Mol Biol 77(4–5):193–203
38. Deplancke B, Alpern D, Gardeux V (2016) The genetics of transcription factor DNA binding variation. Cell 166(3):538–554. https://doi.org/10.1016/j.cell.2016.07.012
39. Fiorito E, Katika MR, Hurtado A (2013) Cooperating transcription factors mediate the function of estrogen receptor. Chromosoma 122(1–2):1–12. https://doi.org/10.1007/s00412-012-0392-7

40. Pradeepa MM (2017) Causal role of histone acetylations in enhancer function. Transcription 8(1):40–47. https://doi.org/10.1080/21541264.2016.1253529
41. Heintzman ND, Stuart RK, Hon G, Fu Y, Ching CW, Hawkins RD, Barrera LO, Van Calcar S, Qu C, Ching KA, Wang W, Weng Z, Green RD, Crawford GE, Ren B (2007) Distinct and predictive chromatin signatures of transcriptional promoters and enhancers in the human genome. Nat Genet 39(3):311–318. https://doi.org/10.1038/ng1966
42. Creyghton MP, Cheng AW, Welstead GG, Kooistra T, Carey BW, Steine EJ, Hanna J, Lodato MA, Frampton GM, Sharp PA, Boyer LA, Young RA, Jaenisch R (2010) Histone H3K27ac separates active from poised enhancers and predicts developmental state. Proc Natl Acad Sci U S A 107(50):21931–21936. https://doi.org/10.1073/pnas.1016071107
43. Visel A, Blow MJ, Li Z, Zhang T, Akiyama JA, Holt A, Plajzer-Frick I, Shoukry M, Wright C, Chen F, Afzal V, Ren B, Rubin EM, Pennacchio LA (2009) ChIP-seq accurately predicts tissue-specific activity of enhancers. Nature 457(7231):854–858. https://doi.org/10.1038/nature07730
44. Magnani L, Stoeck A, Zhang X, Lanczky A, Mirabella AC, Wang TL, Gyorffy B, Lupien M (2013) Genome-wide reprogramming of the chromatin landscape underlies endocrine therapy resistance in breast cancer. Proc Natl Acad Sci U S A 110(16):E1490–E1499. https://doi.org/10.1073/pnas.1219992110
45. Melgar MF, Collins FS, Sethupathy P (2011) Discovery of active enhancers through bidirectional expression of short transcripts. Genome Biol 12(11):R113. https://doi.org/10.1186/gb-2011-12-11-r113
46. Natoli G, Andrau JC (2012) Noncoding transcription at enhancers: general principles and functional models. Annu Rev Genet 46:1–19. https://doi.org/10.1146/annurev-genet-110711-155459
47. Liu MH, Cheung E (2014) Estrogen receptor-mediated long-range chromatin interactions and transcription in breast cancer. Mol Cell Endocrinol 382(1):624–632. https://doi.org/10.1016/j.mce.2013.09.019
48. Heinz S, Romanoski CE, Benner C, Glass CK (2015) The selection and function of cell type-specific enhancers. Nat Rev Mol Cell Biol 16(3):144–154. https://doi.org/10.1038/nrm3949
49. Pennacchio LA, Bickmore W, Dean A, Nobrega MA, Bejerano G (2013) Enhancers: five essential questions. Nat Rev Genet 14(4):288–295. https://doi.org/10.1038/nrg3458
50. Yi P, Wang Z, Feng Q, Pintilie GD, Foulds CE, Lanz RB, Ludtke SJ, Schmid MF, Chiu W, O'Malley BW (2015) Structure of a biologically active estrogen receptor-coactivator complex on DNA. Mol Cell 57(6):1047–1058. https://doi.org/10.1016/j.molcel.2015.01.025
51. Metivier R, Penot G, Hubner MR, Reid G, Brand H, Kos M, Gannon F (2003) Estrogen receptor-alpha directs ordered, cyclical, and combinatorial recruitment of cofactors on a natural target promoter. Cell 115(6):751–763
52. Kamei Y, Xu L, Heinzel T, Torchia J, Kurokawa R, Gloss B, Lin SC, Heyman RA, Rose DW, Glass CK, Rosenfeld MG (1996) A CBP integrator complex mediates transcriptional activation and AP-1 inhibition by nuclear receptors. Cell 85(3):403–414
53. Acevedo ML, Kraus WL (2003) Mediator and p300/CBP-steroid receptor coactivator complexes have distinct roles, but function synergistically, during estrogen receptor alpha-dependent transcription with chromatin templates. Mol Cell Biol 23(1):335–348
54. Kim MY, Hsiao SJ, Kraus WL (2001) A role for coactivators and histone acetylation in estrogen receptor alpha-mediated transcription initiation. EMBO J 20(21):6084–6094. https://doi.org/10.1093/emboj/20.21.6084
55. Belandia B, Orford RL, Hurst HC, Parker MG (2002) Targeting of SWI/SNF chromatin remodelling complexes to estrogen-responsive genes. EMBO J 21(15):4094–4103
56. Chen W, Roeder RG (2011) Mediator-dependent nuclear receptor function. Semin Cell Dev Biol 22(7):749–758. https://doi.org/10.1016/j.semcdb.2011.07.026
57. Malik S, Roeder RG (2010) The metazoan Mediator co-activator complex as an integrative hub for transcriptional regulation. Nat Rev Genet 11(11):761–772. https://doi.org/10.1038/nrg2901

58. Plaschka C, Nozawa K, Cramer P (2016) Mediator architecture and RNA polymerase II interaction. J Mol Biol 428(12):2569–2574. https://doi.org/10.1016/j.jmb.2016.01.028
59. Lai F, Orom UA, Cesaroni M, Beringer M, Taatjes DJ, Blobel GA, Shiekhattar R (2013) Activating RNAs associate with Mediator to enhance chromatin architecture and transcription. Nature 494(7438):497–501. https://doi.org/10.1038/nature11884
60. Foulds CE, Feng Q, Ding C, Bailey S, Hunsaker TL, Malovannaya A, Hamilton RA, Gates LA, Zhang Z, Li C, Chan D, Bajaj A, Callaway CG, Edwards DP, Lonard DM, Tsai SY, Tsai MJ, Qin J, O'Malley BW (2013) Proteomic analysis of coregulators bound to ERα on DNA and nucleosomes reveals coregulator dynamics. Mol Cell 51(2):185–199. https://doi.org/10.1016/j.molcel.2013.06.007
61. Lanz RB, McKenna NJ, Onate SA, Albrecht U, Wong J, Tsai SY, Tsai MJ, O'Malley BW (1999) A steroid receptor coactivator, SRA, functions as an RNA and is present in an SRC-1 complex. Cell 97(1):17–27
62. Coleman KM, Lam V, Jaber BM, Lanz RB, Smith CL (2004) SRA coactivation of estrogen receptor-alpha is phosphorylation-independent, and enhances 4-hydroxytamoxifen agonist activity. Biochem Biophys Res Commun 323(1):332–338. https://doi.org/10.1016/j.bbrc.2004.08.090
63. Deblois G, Giguere V (2003) Ligand-independent coactivation of ERalpha AF-1 by steroid receptor RNA activator (SRA) via MAPK activation. J Steroid Biochem Mol Biol 85(2–5):123–131
64. Jin Q, Yu LR, Wang L, Zhang Z, Kasper LH, Lee JE, Wang C, Brindle PK, Dent SY, Ge K (2011) Distinct roles of GCN5/PCAF-mediated H3K9ac and CBP/p300-mediated H3K18/27ac in nuclear receptor transactivation. EMBO J 30(2):249–262. https://doi.org/10.1038/emboj.2010.318
65. Tie F, Banerjee R, Stratton CA, Prasad-Sinha J, Stepanik V, Zlobin A, Diaz MO, Scacheri PC, Harte PJ (2009) CBP-mediated acetylation of histone H3 lysine 27 antagonizes Drosophila Polycomb silencing. Development 136(18):3131–3141. https://doi.org/10.1242/dev.037127
66. Bose DA, Donahue G, Reinberg D, Shiekhattar R, Bonasio R, Berger SL (2017) RNA binding to CBP stimulates histone acetylation and transcription. Cell 168(1–2):135–149 e122. https://doi.org/10.1016/j.cell.2016.12.020
67. Murakami S, Nagari A, Kraus WL (2017) Dynamic assembly and activation of estrogen receptor alpha enhancers through coregulator switching. Genes Dev 31(15):1535–1548. https://doi.org/10.1101/gad.302182.117
68. Herschman HR (1991) Primary response genes induced by growth factors and tumor promoters. Annu Rev Biochem 60:281–319. https://doi.org/10.1146/annurev.bi.60.070191.001433
69. Winkles JA (1998) Serum- and polypeptide growth factor-inducible gene expression in mouse fibroblasts. Prog Nucleic Acid Res Mol Biol 58:41–78
70. Kininis M, Isaacs GD, Core LJ, Hah N, Kraus WL (2009) Postrecruitment regulation of RNA polymerase II directs rapid signaling responses at the promoters of estrogen target genes. Mol Cell Biol 29(5):1123–1133. https://doi.org/10.1128/MCB.00841-08
71. Liu X, Kraus WL, Bai X (2015) Ready, pause, go: regulation of RNA polymerase II pausing and release by cellular signaling pathways. Trends Biochem Sci 40(9):516–525. https://doi.org/10.1016/j.tibs.2015.07.003
72. Core LJ, Waterfall JJ, Lis JT (2008) Nascent RNA sequencing reveals widespread pausing and divergent initiation at human promoters. Science 322(5909):1845–1848. https://doi.org/10.1126/science.1162228
73. Schena M, Shalon D, Davis RW, Brown PO (1995) Quantitative monitoring of gene expression patterns with a complementary DNA microarray. Science 270(5235):467–470
74. Kraus WL (2015) Editorial: would you like a hypothesis with those data? Omics and the age of discovery science. Mol Endocrinol 29(11):1531–1534. https://doi.org/10.1210/me.2015-1253
75. Calviello L, Ohler U (2017) Beyond read-counts: Ribo-seq data analysis to understand the functions of the transcriptome. Trends Genet 33(10):728–744. https://doi.org/10.1016/j.tig.2017.08.003

76. Shalem O, Sanjana NE, Zhang F (2015) High-throughput functional genomics using CRISPR-Cas9. Nat Rev Genet 16(5):299–311. https://doi.org/10.1038/nrg3899
77. Root DE, Hacohen N, Hahn WC, Lander ES, Sabatini DM (2006) Genome-scale loss-of-function screening with a lentiviral RNAi library. Nat Methods 3(9):715–719. https://doi.org/10.1038/nmeth924
78. Kininis M, Kraus WL (2008) A global view of transcriptional regulation by nuclear receptors: gene expression, factor localization, and DNA sequence analysis. Nucl Recept Signal 6:e005
79. Cheung E, Kraus WL (2010) Genomic analyses of hormone signaling and gene regulation. Annu Rev Physiol 72:191–218. https://doi.org/10.1146/annurev-physiol-021909-135840
80. Carroll JS, Brown M (2006) Estrogen receptor target gene: an evolving concept. Mol Endocrinol 20(8):1707–1714. https://doi.org/10.1210/me.2005-0334
81. Zhang J, Poh HM, Peh SQ, Sia YY, Li G, Mulawadi FH, Goh Y, Fullwood MJ, Sung WK, Ruan X, Ruan Y (2012) ChIA-PET analysis of transcriptional chromatin interactions. Methods 58(3):289–299. https://doi.org/10.1016/j.ymeth.2012.08.009
82. Welboren WJ, Stunnenberg HG, Sweep FC, Span PN (2007) Identifying estrogen receptor target genes. Mol Oncol 1(2):138–143. https://doi.org/10.1016/j.molonc.2007.04.001
83. Perou CM, Sorlie T, Eisen MB, van de Rijn M, Jeffrey SS, Rees CA, Pollack JR, Ross DT, Johnsen H, Akslen LA, Fluge O, Pergamenschikov A, Williams C, Zhu SX, Lonning PE, Borresen-Dale AL, Brown PO, Botstein D (2000) Molecular portraits of human breast tumours. Nature 406(6797):747–752. https://doi.org/10.1038/35021093
84. Sorlie T, Perou CM, Tibshirani R, Aas T, Geisler S, Johnsen H, Hastie T, Eisen MB, van de Rijn M, Jeffrey SS, Thorsen T, Quist H, Matese JC, Brown PO, Botstein D, Lonning PE, Borresen-Dale AL (2001) Gene expression patterns of breast carcinomas distinguish tumor subclasses with clinical implications. Proc Natl Acad Sci U S A 98(19):10869–10874. https://doi.org/10.1073/pnas.191367098
85. Cancer Genome Atlas N (2012) Comprehensive molecular portraits of human breast tumours. Nature 490(7418):61–70. https://doi.org/10.1038/nature11412
86. van't Veer LJ, Dai H, van de Vijver MJ, He YD, Hart AA, Mao M, Peterse HL, van der Kooy K, Marton MJ, Witteveen AT, Schreiber GJ, Kerkhoven RM, Roberts C, Linsley PS, Bernards R, Friend SH (2002) Gene expression profiling predicts clinical outcome of breast cancer. Nature 415(6871):530–536. https://doi.org/10.1038/415530a
87. Lin CY, Strom A, Vega VB, Kong SL, Yeo AL, Thomsen JS, Chan WC, Doray B, Bangarusamy DK, Ramasamy A, Vergara LA, Tang S, Chong A, Bajic VB, Miller LD, Gustafsson JA, Liu ET (2004) Discovery of estrogen receptor alpha target genes and response elements in breast tumor cells. Genome Biol 5(9):R66. https://doi.org/10.1186/gb-2004-5-9-r66
88. Dai X, Li T, Bai Z, Yang Y, Liu X, Zhan J, Shi B (2015) Breast cancer intrinsic subtype classification, clinical use and future trends. Am J Cancer Res 5(10):2929–2943
89. Franco HL, Nagari A, Kraus WL (2015) TNFalpha signaling exposes latent estrogen receptor binding sites to alter the breast cancer cell transcriptome. Mol Cell 58(1):21–34. https://doi.org/10.1016/j.molcel.2015.02.001
90. Mahat DB, Kwak H, Booth GT, Jonkers IH, Danko CG, Patel RK, Waters CT, Munson K, Core LJ, Lis JT (2016) Base-pair-resolution genome-wide mapping of active RNA polymerases using precision nuclear run-on (PRO-seq). Nat Protoc 11(8):1455–1476. https://doi.org/10.1038/nprot.2016.086
91. Danko CG, Hah N, Luo X, Martins AL, Core L, Lis JT, Siepel A, Kraus WL (2013) Signaling pathways differentially affect RNA polymerase II initiation, pausing, and elongation rate in cells. Mol Cell 50(2):212–222. https://doi.org/10.1016/j.molcel.2013.02.015
92. Chae M, Danko CG, Kraus WL (2015) groHMM: a computational tool for identifying unannotated and cell type-specific transcription units from global run-on sequencing data. BMC Bioinformatics 16:222. https://doi.org/10.1186/s12859-015-0656-3
93. Sun M, Gadad SS, Kim DS, Kraus WL (2015) Discovery, annotation, and functional analysis of long noncoding RNAs controlling cell-cycle gene expression and proliferation in breast cancer cells. Mol Cell 59(4):698–711. https://doi.org/10.1016/j.molcel.2015.06.023

94. De Santa F, Barozzi I, Mietton F, Ghisletti S, Polletti S, Tusi BK, Muller H, Ragoussis J, Wei CL, Natoli G (2010) A large fraction of extragenic RNA pol II transcription sites overlap enhancers. PLoS Biol 8(5):e1000384. https://doi.org/10.1371/journal.pbio.1000384

95. Kim TK, Hemberg M, Gray JM, Costa AM, Bear DM, Wu J, Harmin DA, Laptewicz M, Barbara-Haley K, Kuersten S, Markenscoff-Papadimitriou E, Kuhl D, Bito H, Worley PF, Kreiman G, Greenberg ME (2010) Widespread transcription at neuronal activity-regulated enhancers. Nature 465(7295):182–187. https://doi.org/10.1038/nature09033

96. Wang D, Garcia-Bassets I, Benner C, Li W, Su X, Zhou Y, Qiu J, Liu W, Kaikkonen MU, Ohgi KA, Glass CK, Rosenfeld MG, Fu XD (2011) Reprogramming transcription by distinct classes of enhancers functionally defined by eRNA. Nature 474(7351):390–394. https://doi.org/10.1038/nature10006

97. Lam MT, Cho H, Lesch HP, Gosselin D, Heinz S, Tanaka-Oishi Y, Benner C, Kaikkonen MU, Kim AS, Kosaka M, Lee CY, Watt A, Grossman TR, Rosenfeld MG, Evans RM, Glass CK (2013) Rev-Erbs repress macrophage gene expression by inhibiting enhancer-directed transcription. Nature 498(7455):511–515. https://doi.org/10.1038/nature12209

98. Li W, Notani D, Ma Q, Tanasa B, Nunez E, Chen AY, Merkurjev D, Zhang J, Ohgi K, Song X, Oh S, Kim HS, Glass CK, Rosenfeld MG (2013) Functional roles of enhancer RNAs for oestrogen-dependent transcriptional activation. Nature 498(7455):516–520. https://doi.org/10.1038/nature12210

99. Hsieh CL, Fei T, Chen Y, Li T, Gao Y, Wang X, Sun T, Sweeney CJ, Lee GS, Chen S, Balk SP, Liu XS, Brown M, Kantoff PW (2014) Enhancer RNAs participate in androgen receptor-driven looping that selectively enhances gene activation. Proc Natl Acad Sci U S A 111(20):7319–7324. https://doi.org/10.1073/pnas.1324151111

100. Arner E, Daub CO, Vitting-Seerup K, Andersson R, Lilje B, Drablos F, Lennartsson A, Ronnerblad M, Hrydziuszko O, Vitezic M, Freeman TC, Alhendi AM, Arner P, Axton R, Baillie JK, Beckhouse A, Bodega B, Briggs J, Brombacher F, Davis M, Detmar M, Ehrlund A, Endoh M, Eslami A, Fagiolini M, Fairbairn L, Faulkner GJ, Ferrai C, Fisher ME, Forrester L, Goldowitz D, Guler R, Ha T, Hara M, Herlyn M, Ikawa T, Kai C, Kawamoto H, Khachigian LM, Klinken SP, Kojima S, Koseki H, Klein S, Mejhert N, Miyaguchi K, Mizuno Y, Morimoto M, Morris KJ, Mummery C, Nakachi Y, Ogishima S, Okada-Hatakeyama M, Okazaki Y, Orlando V, Ovchinnikov D, Passier R, Patrikakis M, Pombo A, Qin XY, Roy S, Sato H, Savvi S, Saxena A, Schwegmann A, Sugiyama D, Swoboda R, Tanaka H, Tomoiu A, Winteringham LN, Wolvetang E, Yanagi-Mizuochi C, Yoneda M, Zabierowski S, Zhang P, Abugessaisa I, Bertin N, Diehl AD, Fukuda S, Furuno M, Harshbarger J, Hasegawa A, Hori F, Ishikawa-Kato S, Ishizu Y, Itoh M, Kawashima T, Kojima M, Kondo N, Lizio M, Meehan TF, Mungall CJ, Murata M, Nishiyori-Sueki H, Sahin S, Nagao-Sato S, Severin J, de Hoon MJ, Kawai J, Kasukawa T, Lassmann T, Suzuki H, Kawaji H, Summers KM, Wells C, Consortium F, Hume DA, Forrest AR, Sandelin A, Carninci P, Hayashizaki Y (2015) Transcribed enhancers lead waves of coordinated transcription in transitioning mammalian cells. Science 347(6225):1010–1014. https://doi.org/10.1126/science.1259418

101. Fang B, Everett LJ, Jager J, Briggs E, Armour SM, Feng D, Roy A, Gerhart-Hines Z, Sun Z, Lazar MA (2014) Circadian enhancers coordinate multiple phases of rhythmic gene transcription in vivo. Cell 159(5):1140–1152. https://doi.org/10.1016/j.cell.2014.10.022

102. Mousavi K, Zare H, Dell'orso S, Grontved L, Gutierrez-Cruz G, Derfoul A, Hager GL, Sartorelli V (2013) eRNAs promote transcription by establishing chromatin accessibility at defined genomic loci. Mol Cell 51(5):606–617. https://doi.org/10.1016/j.molcel.2013.07.022

103. Li W, Notani D, Rosenfeld MG (2016) Enhancers as non-coding RNA transcription units: recent insights and future perspectives. Nat Rev Genet 17(4):207–223. https://doi.org/10.1038/nrg.2016.4

104. Lander ES (2011) Initial impact of the sequencing of the human genome. Nature 470(7333):187–197. https://doi.org/10.1038/nature09792

105. Clark MB, Amaral PP, Schlesinger FJ, Dinger ME, Taft RJ, Rinn JL, Ponting CP, Stadler PF, Morris KV, Morillon A, Rozowsky JS, Gerstein MB, Wahlestedt C, Hayashizaki Y, Carninci P, Gingeras TR, Mattick JS (2011) The reality of pervasive transcription. PLoS Biol 9(7):e1000625.; discussion e1001102. https://doi.org/10.1371/journal.pbio.1000625

106. Heintzman ND, Hon GC, Hawkins RD, Kheradpour P, Stark A, Harp LF, Ye Z, Lee LK, Stuart RK, Ching CW, Ching KA, Antosiewicz-Bourget JE, Liu H, Zhang X, Green RD, Lobanenkov VV, Stewart R, Thomson JA, Crawford GE, Kellis M, Ren B (2009) Histone modifications at human enhancers reflect global cell-type-specific gene expression. Nature 459(7243):108–112. https://doi.org/10.1038/nature07829

107. Shlyueva D, Stampfel G, Stark A (2014) Transcriptional enhancers: from properties to genome-wide predictions. Nat Rev Genet 15(4):272–286. https://doi.org/10.1038/nrg3682

108. Calo E, Wysocka J (2013) Modification of enhancer chromatin: what, how, and why? Mol Cell 49(5):825–837. https://doi.org/10.1016/j.molcel.2013.01.038

109. Crawford GE, Holt IE, Whittle J, Webb BD, Tai D, Davis S, Margulies EH, Chen Y, Bernat JA, Ginsburg D, Zhou D, Luo S, Vasicek TJ, Daly MJ, Wolfsberg TG, Collins FS (2006) Genome-wide mapping of DNase hypersensitive sites using massively parallel signature sequencing (MPSS). Genome Res 16(1):123–131. https://doi.org/10.1101/gr.4074106

110. Sheffield NC, Thurman RE, Song L, Safi A, Stamatoyannopoulos JA, Lenhard B, Crawford GE, Furey TS (2013) Patterns of regulatory activity across diverse human cell types predict tissue identity, transcription factor binding, and long-range interactions. Genome Res 23(5):777–788. https://doi.org/10.1101/gr.152140.112

111. Core LJ, Martins AL, Danko CG, Waters CT, Siepel A, Lis JT (2014) Analysis of nascent RNA identifies a unified architecture of initiation regions at mammalian promoters and enhancers. Nat Genet 46(12):1311–1320. https://doi.org/10.1038/ng.3142

112. Franco HL, Nagari A, Malladi VS, Li W, Xi Y, Richardson D, Allton KL, Tanaka K, Li J, Murakami S, Keyomarsi K, Bedford MT, Shi X, Li W, Barton MC, Dent SYR, Kraus WL (2018) Enhancer transcription reveals subtype-specific gene expression programs controlling breast cancer pathogenesis. Genome Res 28(2):159–170. https://doi.org/10.1101/gr.226019.117

113. Ince BA, Zhuang Y, Wrenn CK, Shapiro DJ, Katzenellenbogen BS (1993) Powerful dominant negative mutants of the human estrogen receptor. J Biol Chem 268(19):14026–14032

114. Schodin DJ, Zhuang Y, Shapiro DJ, Katzenellenbogen BS (1995) Analysis of mechanisms that determine dominant negative estrogen receptor effectiveness. J Biol Chem 270(52):31163–31171

115. Acevedo ML, Lee KC, Stender JD, Katzenellenbogen BS, Kraus WL (2004) Selective recognition of distinct classes of coactivators by a ligand-inducible activation domain. Mol Cell 13(5):725–738

116. Prossnitz ER, Arterburn JB, Smith HO, Oprea TI, Sklar LA, Hathaway HJ (2008) Estrogen signaling through the transmembrane G protein-coupled receptor GPR30. Annu Rev Physiol 70:165–190. https://doi.org/10.1146/annurev.physiol.70.113006.100518

117. Aronica SM, Kraus WL, Katzenellenbogen BS (1994) Estrogen action via the cAMP signaling pathway: stimulation of adenylate cyclase and cAMP-regulated gene transcription. Proc Natl Acad Sci U S A 91(18):8517–8521

118. Aronica SM, Katzenellenbogen BS (1993) Stimulation of estrogen receptor-mediated transcription and alteration in the phosphorylation state of the rat uterine estrogen receptor by estrogen, cyclic adenosine monophosphate, and insulin-like growth factor-I. Mol Endocrinol 7(6):743–752. https://doi.org/10.1210/mend.7.6.7689695

119. Ignar-Trowbridge DM, Nelson KG, Bidwell MC, Curtis SW, Washburn TF, McLachlan JA, Korach KS (1992) Coupling of dual signaling pathways: epidermal growth factor action involves the estrogen receptor. Proc Natl Acad Sci U S A 89(10):4658–4662

120. Hayashi S, Sakamoto T, Inoue A, Yoshida N, Omoto Y, Yamaguchi Y (2003) Estrogen and growth factor signaling pathway: basic approaches for clinical application. J Steroid Biochem Mol Biol 86(3–5):433–442

121. Ribeiro JR, Freiman RN (2014) Estrogen signaling crosstalk: implications for endocrine resistance in ovarian cancer. J Steroid Biochem Mol Biol 143:160–173. https://doi.org/10.1016/j.jsbmb.2014.02.010

122. Wee P, Wang Z (2017) Epidermal growth factor receptor cell proliferation signaling pathways. Cancers (Basel) 9(5). https://doi.org/10.3390/cancers9050052

123. Gee JM, Robertson JF, Gutteridge E, Ellis IO, Pinder SE, Rubini M, Nicholson RI (2005) Epidermal growth factor receptor/HER2/insulin-like growth factor receptor signalling and oestrogen receptor activity in clinical breast cancer. Endocr Relat Cancer 12(Suppl 1): S99–S111. https://doi.org/10.1677/erc.1.01005

124. Kato S, Endoh H, Masuhiro Y, Kitamoto T, Uchiyama S, Sasaki H, Masushige S, Gotoh Y, Nishida E, Kawashima H, Metzger D, Chambon P (1995) Activation of the estrogen receptor through phosphorylation by mitogen-activated protein kinase. Science 270(5241):1491–1494

125. Improta-Brears T, Whorton AR, Codazzi F, York JD, Meyer T, McDonnell DP (1999) Estrogen-induced activation of mitogen-activated protein kinase requires mobilization of intracellular calcium. Proc Natl Acad Sci U S A 96(8):4686–4691

126. Sun M, Isaacs GD, Hah N, Heldring N, Fogarty EA, Kraus WL (2012) Estrogen regulates JNK1 genomic localization to control gene expression and cell growth in breast cancer cells. Mol Endocrinol 26(5):736–747. https://doi.org/10.1210/me.2011-1158

127. Lee SH, Nam HS (2008) TNF alpha-induced down-regulation of estrogen receptor alpha in MCF-7 breast cancer cells. Mol Cells 26(3):285–290

128. Holst F (2016) Estrogen receptor alpha gene amplification in breast cancer: 25 years of debate. World J Clin Oncol 7(2):160–173. https://doi.org/10.5306/wjco.v7.i2.160

129. Gutierrez C, Schiff R (2011) HER2: biology, detection, and clinical implications. Arch Pathol Lab Med 135(1):55–62. https://doi.org/10.1043/2010-0454-RAR.1

130. Gojis O, Rudraraju B, Gudi M, Hogben K, Sousha S, Coombes RC, Cleator S, Palmieri C (2010) The role of SRC-3 in human breast cancer. Nat Rev Clin Oncol 7(2):83–89. https://doi.org/10.1038/nrclinonc.2009.219

131. Menard S, Fortis S, Castiglioni F, Agresti R, Balsari A (2001) HER2 as a prognostic factor in breast cancer. Oncology 61(Suppl 2):67–72. https://doi.org/10.1159/000055404

132. Marchio C, Natrajan R, Shiu KK, Lambros MB, Rodriguez-Pinilla SM, Tan DS, Lord CJ, Hungermann D, Fenwick K, Tamber N, Mackay A, Palacios J, Sapino A, Buerger H, Ashworth A, Reis-Filho JS (2008) The genomic profile of HER2-amplified breast cancers: the influence of ER status. J Pathol 216(4):399–407. https://doi.org/10.1002/path.2423

133. Hampton OA, Den Hollander P, Miller CA, Delgado DA, Li J, Coarfa C, Harris RA, Richards S, Scherer SE, Muzny DM, Gibbs RA, Lee AV, Milosavljevic A (2009) A sequence-level map of chromosomal breakpoints in the MCF-7 breast cancer cell line yields insights into the evolution of a cancer genome. Genome Res 19(2):167–177. https://doi.org/10.1101/gr.080259.108

134. Hsu PY, Hsu HK, Lan X, Juan L, Yan PS, Labanowska J, Heerema N, Hsiao TH, Chiu YC, Chen Y, Liu Y, Li L, Li R, Thompson IM, Nephew KP, Sharp ZD, Kirma NB, Jin VX, Huang TH (2013) Amplification of distant estrogen response elements deregulates target genes associated with tamoxifen resistance in breast cancer. Cancer Cell 24(2):197–212. https://doi.org/10.1016/j.ccr.2013.07.007

135. Hsu PY, Hsu HK, Hsiao TH, Ye Z, Wang E, Profit AL, Jatoi I, Chen Y, Kirma NB, Jin VX, Sharp ZD, Huang TH (2016) Spatiotemporal control of estrogen-responsive transcription in ERalpha-positive breast cancer cells. Oncogene 35(18):2379–2389. https://doi.org/10.1038/onc.2015.298

136. Merenbakh-Lamin K, Ben-Baruch N, Yeheskel A, Dvir A, Soussan-Gutman L, Jeselsohn R, Yelensky R, Brown M, Miller VA, Sarid D, Rizel S, Klein B, Rubinek T, Wolf I (2013) D538G mutation in estrogen receptor-alpha: a novel mechanism for acquired endocrine resistance in breast cancer. Cancer Res 73(23):6856–6864. https://doi.org/10.1158/0008-5472.CAN-13-1197

137. Toy W, Shen Y, Won H, Green B, Sakr RA, Will M, Li Z, Gala K, Fanning S, King TA, Hudis C, Chen D, Taran T, Hortobagyi G, Greene G, Berger M, Baselga J, Chandarlapaty S

(2013) ESR1 ligand-binding domain mutations in hormone-resistant breast cancer. Nat Genet 45(12):1439–1445. https://doi.org/10.1038/ng.2822

138. Jeselsohn R, Bergholz JS, Pun M, Cornwell M, Liu W, Nardone A, Xiao T, Li W, Qiu X, Buchwalter G, Feiglin A, Abell-Hart K, Fei T, Rao P, Long H, Kwiatkowski N, Zhang T, Gray N, Melchers D, Houtman R, Liu XS, Cohen O, Wagle N, Winer EP, Zhao J, Brown M (2018) Allele-specific chromatin recruitment and therapeutic vulnerabilities of ESR1 activating mutations. Cancer Cell 33(2):173–186 e175. https://doi.org/10.1016/j.ccell.2018.01.004

Estrogen Receptor Regulation of MicroRNAs in Breast Cancer

Nicholas Pulliam, Jessica Tang, and Kenneth P. Nephew

Abstract MicroRNAs (miRNAs) are short, noncoding RNAs that posttranscriptionally regulate gene expression through altering mRNA translation and stability. Dysregulation of miRNAs has been demonstrated to alter estrogen receptor (ER) biology, through modulation of ER-alpha (ERα) signaling or regulation of ERα itself. Approximately 70% of breast cancers express ERα, and miRNA expression is demonstrated to correlate with disease status in ER-positive breast cancer. Due to the role of ERα in breast cancer development, its interaction and regulation of miRNAs have been of great interest, particularly within the context of ligand specificity and antiestrogen therapies. Here, we review the cross talk between ERα and miRNAs and their involvement in breast cancer progression, as well as resistance to endocrine therapy. We also briefly discuss the interaction of miRNAs with estrogen-related receptors (ERRs) and ERβ in mediating breast tumorigenesis.

Keywords MicroRNA · Estrogen receptor · Breast cancer · Antiestrogen · Endocrine resistance

N. Pulliam
Molecular and Cellular Biochemistry Department, Indiana University, Bloomington, IN, USA

Medical Sciences Program, Indiana University School of Medicine, Bloomington, IN, USA

J. Tang
Medical Sciences Program, Indiana University School of Medicine, Bloomington, IN, USA

K. P. Nephew (✉)
Molecular and Cellular Biochemistry Department, Indiana University, Bloomington, IN, USA

Medical Sciences Program, Indiana University School of Medicine, Bloomington, IN, USA

Department of Cellular and Integrative Physiology and Department of Obstetrics and Gynecology, Indiana University School of Medicine, Indianapolis, IN, USA
e-mail: knephew@indiana.edu

© Springer Nature Switzerland AG 2019
X. Zhang (ed.), *Estrogen Receptor and Breast Cancer*, Cancer Drug Discovery and Development, https://doi.org/10.1007/978-3-319-99350-8_6

1   Introduction

MicroRNAs (miRNA) are short (20–22 nt), noncoding RNAs, which regulate gene expression posttranscriptionally through binding of a target mRNA 3′-untranslated region (UTR) or open reading frame (ORF) [1]. Upon binding, miRNAs regulate their target gene expression through two mechanisms, repression of mRNA translation and degradation of the associated mRNA sequence, the outcome of which is dependent on sequence complementarity of the miRNA [1, 2]. In cancer, altered miRNA gene regulation often results in oncogenic cellular activities such as increased proliferation and metastasis, ultimately promoting tumor progression [3, 4]. However, depending on the target gene, miRNAs may either be tumor suppressing or oncogenic ("oncomirs") [5, 6]. MiRNA dysregulation in cancer is often considered a hallmark of the disease [7, 8]. Furthermore, our group [3], as well as others [8, 9], previously determined that aberrant expression of miRNAs in breast cancer can discriminate between breast tumors of different pathological phenotypes, such as ERα status and tumor grade [3, 10].

Approximately 70% of breast cancers express ERα [11]. The first report correlating ERα levels with miRNA expression in breast cancer was published in 2005 by Iorio et al. demonstrating several miRNAs, including miR-21, to be dysregulated in ER+ breast cancer [8]. In 2007, Adams et al. subsequently demonstrated estrogen (E2) stimulation of ERα negatively regulated miR-206 expression, and overexpression of miR-206 could posttranscriptionally regulate ERα expression [12], creating a negative feedback loop. In addition to E2 regulation of miRNAs, dysregulation of miRNAs has been demonstrated to contribute to the onset of endocrine resistance; therefore, therapeutically targeting miRNAs and utilizing their expression as a breast cancer biomarker have been of great interest [13, 14]. Here, we will summarize the research on ERα regulation of miRNAs in breast cancer.

2   miRNA Biogenesis

Nearly 50% of miRNAs are expressed from the introns of protein-coding genes and may be processed as sense or antisense from transcripts on the same locus [15]. MiRNA biogenesis may occur by either a canonical or noncanonical pathway. Canonical miRNA biogenesis is initiated by transcription of a primary (pri)-miRNA transcript (60–100 nt), via RNA polymerase II. This is accomplished within the context of a co-transcribed gene or as an independent transcription unit [1]. Following 5′-capping and 3′-polyadenylation of the pri-miRNA, it base pairs with itself forming a hairpin structure. The pri-miRNA transcript binds Drosha (RNAse III family endonuclease) co-transcriptionally. The "Drosha microprocessor complex" and its cofactors cleave the pri-miRNA into a precursor (pre)-miRNA to be exported from the nucleus to the cytoplasm for further processing [1, 4]. Once in the cytoplasm, the Dicer (RNAse III) complex removes the pre-miRNA hairpin structure, generating a mature miRNA (~22 nt) product. The mature miRNA is transported to the RNA-induced silencing complex (RISC) by the Dicer complex. Argonaute proteins (Ago1–4) within RISC then unwind the miRNA double-stranded sequence, and the "passenger" strand is degraded. The remaining "guide" strand is further incorporated into RISC, directing the complex to the target mRNA 3'-UTR or open reading frame (ORF). Imperfect base pairing of the miRNA-mRNA complex results in repressed translation of the associated mRNA, yielding decreased protein. If the miRNA perfectly binds the associated mRNA sequence, the transcript is instead degraded [1, 4]. Noncanonical generation of miRNAs bypasses Drosha-directed processing of the pri-miRNA to pre-miRNA and depends on generation of mirtrons, which are short hairpin pre-miRNAs, produced through sequence splicing [16].

3 Estrogen Receptor-α Regulation of miRNAs

Due to the role of ERα in breast cancer development, its interaction and regulation of miRNAs have been of great interest, particularly within the context of ligand specificity and antiestrogen therapies. Furthermore, while ERα is demonstrated to transcriptionally regulate a growing number of miRNAs, miRNAs have conversely been shown to regulate ERα resulting in either a positive or negative feedback loop. A study by Wickramasinghe et al. [17] demonstrated that miR-21 expression was not only higher in ER+ breast cancer, validating a previous study by Mattie et al. [18], but that miR-21 was negatively regulated by ERα upon estrogen treatment, resulting in increased expression of miR-21 target genes including PDCD4, bcl-2, and PTEN [17]. To further demonstrate the dependence of miR-21 expression on ERα, antiestrogens tamoxifen and fulvestrant, as well as ERα knockdown, were utilized. In response to these treatments, miR-21 expression was increased, and target gene expression decreased [17], implicating miR-21 as an ER-dependent oncogenic miRNA ("oncomir"). Concordantly, the oncogenic activity of miR-21 was validated independently by Han et al., who demonstrated re-expression of the miRNA contributed to increased cell migration and invasion, through induction of an EMT program, as well as increased cancer "stemness" marked by increased expression of ALDH1 [19].

Likewise, we and others have demonstrated that overexpression of miR-221/222 in ER+ breast cancer promotes global gene expression changes [3]. Further, we showed upon hormone treatment ERα binds the miR-221/222 cluster, recruits the corepressors NCoR and SMRT, and transcriptionally downregulates expression of the miR-221/222 locus, implicating miR-221/222 as an oncogenic miRNA [3]. Inhibition of ERα by ERBB2 [3] or antiestrogen therapy [20] increased miR-221/miR-222 expression promoting hormone-independent cell growth and increased cell proliferation, phenotypes associated with resistance to antiestrogen therapy [3, 20].

Many studies aim to understand the role of individual miRNAs regulated by ERα; however, more recently, the impact of ERα on the "miRNome" has become of great interest [9, 21]. A study by Ferraro et al. used miRNA microarray profiling and found altered expression of 172 miRNAs in response to E2 in the ER+ MCF7 and ZR75.1 breast cancer cell lines [22]. Between the two cell lines, 52 miRNAs were similarly regulated by addition of E2, including miR-760 and miR-424, and decreased miR-618, miR-570, and miR-107 over time [22, 23]. Another study by Bhat-Nakshatri et al. [24] showed E2-induction of ERα in MCF7 cells resulted in the activation of 21 miRNAs, repressing another 7, with the potential of these differentially expressed miRNAs to regulate greater than 400 E2-dependent genes (mRNA) [24]. Contrasting the study by Ferraro et al., Bhat-Nakshatri demonstrated upregulation of miR-21, in response to estrogen stimulation, rather than decreased expression [22, 24]. This discrepancy, delineated in a review by Manavathi et al., is explained by the biphasic nature of ERα signaling in response to hormone activation [25]. In concordance with the study by Bhat-Nakshatri, increased expression of miR-21 was observed in response to estrogen stimulation in the T47D cell line (ER+) as well; however, this was not observed in the study by Wickramasinghe et al. [17]. Further studies are needed to better understand the complexity of miRNA regulation and ERα interaction [24].

4   ERα Regulation of Oncogenic Phenotypes via miRNA Regulation

The number of miRNAs regulated by ERα-dependent mechanisms continues to increase as our understanding of miRNA and ERα biology improves. Further, the oncogenic phenotypes mediated by ERα-dependent regulation of miRNA increases, including EMT, cancer "stemness" and differentiation, cell proliferation, and endocrine resistance [26]. ERα-miRNA cross talk promoting endocrine therapy resistance in ER+ breast cancer is summarized below and in Fig. 1.

4.1   EMT

Epithelial-to-mesenchymal transition (EMT) is an important mediator of tumor progression. A study by Manavalan et al. demonstrated the miR-200 family (miR-200a, miR-200b, miR-200c) to be downregulated in endocrine-resistant LY2 cells,

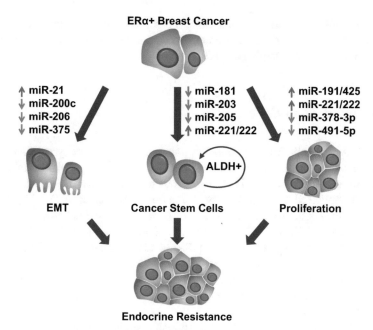

Fig. 1 Summary of the ERα-miRNA cross talk promoting endocrine therapy resistance in ER+ breast cancer. miRNAs associated with ERα-dependent epithelial to mesenchymal transition (EMT), cell proliferation, and cancer stem cell properties resulting in endocrine therapy resistance are shown. The identification and interaction of these miRNAs with ERα are further described in the text

compared to the MCF7 parental (endocrine-responsive) cell line [27]. Decreased expression of the miR-200 family correlated with increased expression of the mesenchymal transcription factor ZEB1, a negative regulator of E-cadherin [27]. Overexpression of miR-200b with or without ectopic expression of miR-200c was sufficient to reverse cell polarity (MET), decrease ZEB1 expression, and increase E-cadherin expression [27, 28]. Additionally, increased expression of these miRNAs sensitized endocrine-resistant LY2 cells to tamoxifen and fulvestrant therapy; however, this was not observed in MCF7 cells (endocrine-sensitive) [27, 28].

Additionally, a study by Ward et al. demonstrated a change in morphology and increased invasiveness of the endocrine-resistant cell line, labeled TamR compared to the MCF7 endocrine-sensitive cell line [29]. Performing a genome-wide microarray analysis, miR-375 was identified to be highly downregulated in the TamR cell line compared to MCF7 parental cells. Re-expression of miR-375 alone was sufficient to resensitize the TamR cells to tamoxifen therapy and at least partially reversed the observed EMT phenotype, indicated by decreased cell invasion and decreased expression of mesenchymal-associated transcription factors, ZEB1 and SNAI2, with a concomitant increase in E-cadherin and ZO-1 expression.

Further bioinformatic analysis and experimental validation identified metadherin (MTDH), widely reported in the literature to mediate breast cancer metastasis [30], as a bona fide miR-375 target gene [29].

4.2   Cancer Stem Cells

The transition of cells from an epithelial state to a more mesenchymal state allows for the development of cancer stem cells (CSC) [31]. ERα regulation of CSC is integral for tumor progression [31]. In this regard, several ERα-dependent miRNAs have been implicated in regulating CSC formation and progression [31, 32]. A study by Li et al. [33] demonstrated miR-221/222 is overexpressed in breast cancer stem cells, denoted by CD44+/CD24− staining and mammosphere formation ability. Ectopic expression of the miR-221/miR-222 cluster resulted in PTEN mRNA degradation and subsequent activation of AKT. The authors showed activation of AKT, mediated by miR-221/miR-222, promotes increased breast cancer self-renewal and proliferation, enhancing cell growth and ultimately hormone-independent growth [33].

Another study by Guttilla et al. independently validated increased expression of miR-221/222 in breast CSC [34]. In MCF7 cells cultured under mammosphere conditions (MCF7$_M$), miR-221/222 targeted ERα mRNA (ESR1) for degradation, promoting hormone-independent growth, EMT, and a CD44+/CD24− stem cell phenotype. The mesenchymal and stemlike phenotype of the MCF7 cells grown under mammosphere (MCF7$_M$) condition was validated by decreased epithelial-associated miRNAs: miR-200c, miR-203, and miR-205. Antisense hairpin targeting of miR-221 was sufficient to promote re-expression of ERα, decreasing the mammosphere formation ability, as well as reverting the cells to a more epithelial (MET) phenotype [34].

The emergence of CSC is recognized as a mechanism to promote cancer cell self-renewal, increased tumorigenicity, and therapeutic resistance. A study by Kastrati et al. revealed an ERα-NFκB regulatory axis, present in ER+ breast cancer, which regulates PHLDA1 gene expression, resulting in increased CSC formation indicated by increased ALDH and CD44+/CD24− cell populations as well as mammosphere formation [35]. Combination of E2 and TNFα, an NFκB activator, promoted increased stability of the PHLDA1 transcript. As miRNAs regulate mRNA stability, potential miRNAs that regulate PHLDA1 expression were identified using TargetScan bioinformatic tool. An exact miR-181 binding site was identified within the 3′-UTR of PHLDA1. Overexpression of miR-181 in MCF7 and T47D ER+ cells was sufficient to decrease PHLDA1 expression and protein levels, as well as stem cell population and mammosphere formation. A PHLDA1 3′-UTR target protector construct demonstrated PHLDA1 as a direct miR-181 target. These data indicate that ERα-NFκB suppression of miR-181 is integral for promoting expression of PHLDA1 and stem cell formation [35].

4.3 Proliferation

Loss or amplification of miRNAs has also been demonstrated to play a role in breast cancer occurrence and development by affecting cell cycle progression and survival programs [8, 36, 37]. Several studies indicate miRNAs may participate in estrogen-driven breast cancer growth; however, little is known about the molecular mechanism of miRNA regulation of ERα in breast cancer. In this regard, many breast cancer patients become resistant to initial chemotherapy treatment, and alternative therapeutic interventions are necessary [38].

Epigenetic therapies like histone deacetylase inhibitors have previously been shown to suppress in vitro clonogenicity and cell proliferation in tamoxifen-resistant MCF7 cells [39]. We have shown histone deacetylase (HDAC) inhibition, by trichostatin A (TSA), to epigenetically regulate miRNA expression. Using a miRNA microarray, we demonstrated 22 miRNAs were found to be upregulated and 10 miRNAs were downregulated in tamoxifen-resistant MCF7 cells after TSA, indicating that tamoxifen resistance is mediated by both epigenetic and miRNA regulation [39]. Another study by Liu et al. demonstrated TSA could increase ERα expression in MCF7 and MDA-MB-231 cells by reducing miR-204 expression [40]. Overexpression of miR-204 reversed TSA-mediated increase in ERα expression. Knockdown of miR-204 enhanced tamoxifen-mediated inhibition of cell growth on ER+ breast cancer cells [40]. Interestingly, Imam et al. found that miR-204 is lost in 28% of breast cancers and that miR-204 directly targets genes involved in tumor growth and chemotherapy response [41]. Additionally, Hui et al. revealed miR-491-5p to be hypermethylated and downregulated in ERα-positive breast cancer and cell lines [42]. Overexpression of miR-491-5p significantly suppressed ERα signaling and estrogen-stimulated proliferation of breast cancer cells. miR-491-5p was demonstrated to be directly targeted by the histone demethylase JMJD2B and ectopic expression of JMJD2B abrogated the phenotypic changes induced by miR-491-5p in breast cancer cells. This data suggests that miR-491-5p may be a novel therapeutic target against ERα-positive breast cancer due to its role as a tumor suppressor in development and progression of breast cancer. ERα-positive breast cancer tissues and cell lines exhibited significantly lower miR-491-5p levels. Estrogen signaling and estrogen-stimulated proliferation of ERα-positive breast cancer cells through induction of cell cycle arrest at G1 phase by directly targeting JMJD2B were suppressed by overexpression of miR-491-5p [42].

With respect to miRNA regulation of cell proliferation, we have previously established the miR-191/425 cluster to regulate breast cancer proliferation in DALRD3-dependent manner [43]. DALRD3 and estrogen control expression of both miR-191/miR-425 and DALRD3 itself. Recruitment of ERα to the regulatory region of the miR-191/425-DALRD3 unit resulted in the accumulation of miR-191 and miR-425 and subsequent decrease in DALRD3 expression levels. miR-191 and miR-425 reduced proliferation and tumorigenesis, providing evidence that ERα recruitment to the miR-191/425-DALRD3 unit can alter miR-191/425 levels and impact breast cancer cell progression [43].

5   MicroRNA and Endocrine Resistance

Due to the fact that 70% of breast cancer patients are ER+, first-line treatment consists of tamoxifen treatment, which targets the receptor, promoting decreased expression of ER-dependent genes [44]. Resistance to tamoxifen therapy frequently develops in the majority of patients even while patients continue to express ERα [3, 45]. Dysregulation of miRNAs has been demonstrated to play a role in endocrine resistance progression, through modulation of ERα signaling or regulating ERα itself [46, 47]. Manavalan et al. identified differentially expressed miRNAs between endocrine-sensitive MCF7 and the derived resistant LY2 cell line [28, 48]. LY2 cells express ERα at levels similar to the parental MCF7 cell line [49] but are resistant to tamoxifen (4-OHT), raloxifene (RAL), and fulvestrant (ICI) [28]. There were 97 differentially expressed miRNAs between the endocrine-sensitive (MCF7) and resistant (LY2) cells. Consistent with previous reports, miR-21 [24, 50] was upregulated in response to tamoxifen treatment in the parental cell line, as well as basally upregulated in the 4-OHT resistant cells. miR-221/miR-222 was likewise overexpressed in the endocrine-resistant cell lines [3, 20, 33], resulting in decreased ESR1 (ERα mRNA) expression.

Numerous miRNAs have been demonstrated to regulate ERα through miRNA binding to the 3′-UTR of ERα mRNA and inducing downstream gene silencing [51–53]. MiRNA targeting of ERα can induce variable effects on breast cancer phenotype and clinical prognosis. For example, miR-221/miR-222 induces endocrine therapy resistance [20] and metastasis, and miR-206 induces antiproliferative and EMT effects [12, 54, 55]. More recently, next-generation sequencing analysis of the MCF7 breast cancer cell line overexpressing miR-335-5p and miR-335-3p resulted in repressed genes involved in ERα signaling pathway and enhanced resistance to the growth inhibitory effects of tamoxifen. Despite its conventional role in tumor suppression, miR-335 can also play an oncogenic role in promoting agonistic estrogen signaling to further promote tumorigenesis [56].

The increasing number of studies demonstrating the vast role of miRNAs in ER biology indicates an opportunity to therapeutically target miRNAs and their potential as breast cancer biomarkers [14, 57]. Numerous studies have described the role that miRNAs play in tamoxifen resistance [4]. Ward et al. using a miRNA microarray identified 67 miRNAs to be upregulated in their derived tamoxifen-resistant (TamR) cell line, compared to the parental MCF7 cell line [58]. Within these significantly upregulated miRNAs, the C19MC cluster, which contains nearly 50 mature miRNAs, was greatly upregulated. Of the 50 miRNAs within the cluster, 18 members showed increased expression consistent with gained tamoxifen resistance. Ectopic expression of miR-519a was sufficient to promote tamoxifen resistance in the parental MCF7 cell line, directly targeting the PI3K signaling and cell cycle regulation pathways [58]. The authors validated CDKN1A as a bona fide miR-519a target, which Gonzalez-Malerva et al. previously identified as a mediator of tamoxifen resistance [59]. In addition to miR-519a, many members of the C19MC miRNA cluster, including miR-520c-3p, miR-520 g, and miR-520 h, have been demonstrated to correlate with gained tamoxifen resistance, increased probability of breast cancer recurrence, and poor disease-free survival [21].

We previously demonstrated by qRT-PCR microarray analysis that ER+ MCF7 cells overexpressing CXCR4 treated with SDF-1 exhibited a distinct miRNA profile compared to non-SDF-1-treated cells, as well as compared to ER cell lines [60]. MiR-222, miR-206, and miR-18b were shown to be upregulated following SDF-1 stimulation. Interestingly, miR-222 overexpression not only regulates ERα expression but also mediates tamoxifen [55] and fulvestrant [20] resistance. These data suggest an SDF-1-CXCR4 axis is able to mediate ERα-dependent endocrine resistance through altered miRNA expression [60].

Due to the continued relevance of ER cross talk with miRNAs, researchers have advanced previous studies recently summarized in a comprehensive review by Klinge et al. in 2015 [47, 61]. Several studies have used miRNA-profiling techniques to elucidate miRNAs dysregulated in breast cancer development and chemoresistance [20, 50]. The majority of studies utilize microarrays to investigate differentially expressed miRNAs in ERα-positive breast cancer [52]. Baran-Gale et al. investigated the global response to estrogen stimulation by analyzing paired mRNA and miRNA measurements over time in MCF7 breast cancer cells by high-throughput sequencing [37], demonstrating miR-503 as a master regulator of estrogen response in breast cancer; in addition, by analyzing temporal expression profiles of MCF7 cells treated with estrogen for 1–24 h, they identified miRNAs and mRNAs that were repressed, induced, or transiently expressed. Analysis of the miRNA expression corresponded to a previous study by Bhat-Nakshatri et al. demonstrating miR-21-5p, miR-200c-3p, miR-93-5p, and the let-7 family of miRNAs to be the most highly expressed in MCF7 cells [24]. Using miRhub, an algorithm to identify candidate master miRNA regulators of gene expression, miR-503 was also identified as the top candidate master regulator, with the largest predicted impact on gene expression response to estrogen stimulation. miR-503 was demonstrated by RNA sequencing to be the most highly expressed miRNA 24 h post-estrogen treatment, and several other genes were identified (CCND1, RET, and ZNF217) as potential miR-503 targets [37]. Interestingly, ZNF217, a known biomarker and oncogene in breast cancer [62, 63], was shown to coordinate estrogen response through binding of estrogen-associated transcriptional binding sites [63, 64], as well as through direct interaction with ERα and recruitment to EREs (estrogen response elements) [63]. Using a ZNF217 3'-UTR reporter assay, miR-503 was demonstrated to directly target and repress ZNF217 expression, resulting in decreased proliferation and increased G1 cell cycle accumulation. Therefore, miR-503 acts as a potent estrogen-induced candidate tumor suppressor miRNA [37]. Based on this work, the authors suggest miR-503 is an oncogenic miRNA and potential therapeutic target.

Cross talk between ERα and mTOR signaling pathways was previously shown as an indicator of hormone receptor status [65]. Deep-sequencing analysis of The Cancer Genome Atlas (TCGA) revealed that expression of a key component of mTOR signaling positively correlated with ERα breast tumor signature, and increased miRNA-155 was also demonstrated to enhance mTORC1 signaling which induced deregulation of ERα signaling [66].

In addition to estrogen-induced expression of miRNAs, many miRNAs are downregulated upon estrogen stimulation. Jiang et al. treated MCF7 with 10 nm estradiol (E2) for 24 h and measured the change in miRNA expression by qRT-PCR [67]. Consistent with previous studies, the authors identified several upregulated miRNAs upon estrogen stimulation, including miR-21 [24], miR-200a [27], and miR-196a [68]. In addition to those estrogen-induced miRNAs, many downregulated miRs were also identified. miR-124 was identified as the most downregulated miRNA post-estrogen treatment (6, 12, and 24 h) in MCF7 cells and not observed in the MDA-MB-231 cell line (TNBC; ER negative). Additionally, knockdown of ERα, and not ERβ, was sufficient to re-express miR-124, demonstrating ERα-dependent regulation of miR-124 [67]. Inhibition of miR-124 promoted cell migration and invasion, indicating miR-124 is an important regulator breast cancer progression, in an ERα-dependent manner [67]. Overexpression of miR-124 decreased MCF7 cell proliferation in response to estradiol treatment. Using an AKT2 3′-UTR reporter assay, AKT2 was validated as a miR-124 target gene, in both MDA-MB-231 and MCF7 cells. Furthermore, AKT2 overexpression was sufficient to overcome miR-124-mediated suppression of cell migration, invasion, and proliferation. Estrogen treatment increased AKT2 expression, consistent with decreased miR-124 expression, while tamoxifen treatment decreased AKT2 expression compared to estradiol-treated cells. In vivo, breast cancer cells overexpressing miR-124 demonstrated both decreased growth, as measured by tumor volume, and angiogenesis, measured by CD31 immunohistochemistry stain. Based on the correlation of ER status and miR-124/AKT2 expression, the authors suggest miR-124 may represent a biomarker of ER+ breast cancer [67].

We previously demonstrated upregulation of 14 miRNAs and downregulation of 2 miRNAs in fulvestrant-resistant MCF7 cells compared to the parental control. Consistent with previous studies, miR-221/222, let7i, and miR-181a were overexpressed in endocrine-resistant cells, while miR-191 and miR199b were downregulated. In this model, miR-222 was predicted to regulate the p27/KIP1 signaling as well as ERBB2, consistent with previous reports by Di Leva et al. and Xin et al. [3, 69].

To identify novel miRNAs associated with endocrine therapy resistance in breast cancer, Ikeda et al. performed high-throughput miRNA sequencing of tamoxifen-resistant MCF7 cells (TamR and LTED) [70]. In the TamR cells, 9 miRNAs were differentially upregulated and 20 in the LTED cells compared to the parental MCF7 cell line. Fifty-five miRNAs were downregulated in both TamR and LTED cells compared to the parental cell line. Ikeda et al. focused on miR-378a-3p whose role in breast cancer has not yet been elucidated. Knockdown of miR-378a-3p in MCF7 cells reduced tamoxifen-mediated suppression of cell growth, while overexpression of miR-378a-3p in the TamR cell line promoted tamoxifen response and subsequent suppression of growth. Additionally, re-expression of miR-378a-3p was observed upon treatment with the DNA methyltransferase inhibitor (DNMTi) 5-aza-2′-deocycytidine (5Aza-dC) in tamoxifen-resistant cells and not the parental cell line [70]. Based on these results, the authors suggested downregulation of miR-378a-3p was epigenetically regulated upon gain of tamoxifen resistance and contributed to breast cancer progression. TargetScan and miRanda target prediction programs identified GOLT1A as a miR-378a-3p target. Overexpression of miR-378a-3p decreased GOLT1A expression measured by qRT-PCR, suggesting miR-378a-3p directly regulates GOLT1A expression. Together these results suggest ER regulation of the miR-378a-3p/GOLT1A signaling axis mediates tamoxifen response in ER+ breast cancer, representing an additional therapeutic target [70].

To identify miRNAs affecting tamoxifen response, Ujihira et al. utilized a lentivirus-based approach expressing 445 miRNA precursors in MCF7 cells. Let-7f, miR-125a, miR-574-3p, and miR-877 were highly repressed, indicating they may function as potential tumor suppressor miRNAs [71]. MiR-574-3p was identified as the most significantly downregulated miRNA and reported to have tumor suppressor function in prostate cancer [72]. Loss of miR-574-3p in tamoxifen-sensitive MCF7 cells decreased tamoxifen-mediated suppression of cell growth, functionally suggesting miR-574-3p contributes to tamoxifen resistance in breast cancer cells. CLTC (clathrin heavy chain 1) was identified (in silico) as a potential miR-574-3p target, which could regulate tamoxifen response [73]. Computational analysis of the CLTC 3'-UTR by miRDB identified a miR-574-3p binding site. Knockdown of miR-574-3p in MCF7 cells resulted in decreased CLTC expression, and CLTC knockdown was sufficient to restore tamoxifen sensitivity in breast cancer cells, representing a potential diagnostic factor for tamoxifen response [71].

The majority of studies demonstrating estrogen-dependent regulation of miRNAs used cell line-based models; however, a study by Cizeron-Clairac et al. measured the expression of 804 miRNAs in 21 ER+ and 10 ER- breast tumors, compared to 8 normal breast tissues using qRT-PCR [74]. Among these miRNAs, 155 were differentially expressed between ER+ and ER- tumors, with 15 upregulated and 140 downregulated. Furthermore, 18 of the most differentially expressed (11 upregulated; 7 downregulated) miRNAs were validated in a larger cohort of 153 tumors, 85 of which were ER+ and 68 ER-, again using the 8 normal breast tissues. MiR-190b was identified as the most upregulated miRNA in the ER+ compared to ER- tumor cohort. MiR-190b expression is not directly regulated by estradiol and does not affect breast cancer cell proliferation. However, miR-190b may be a new clinically relevant biomarker in hormone-dependent breast cancer [74]. Interestingly, miR-190b has been demonstrated to mediate response to androgen therapy in prostate cancer models [75].

ERα regulation of miRNA expression is not only direct as previously demonstrated but may also be indirect, occurring through altered expression of genes which in turn alter miRNA stability [76]. Jin et al. demonstrated that gain of tamoxifen resistance correlated with increased expression of the ERα cofactor HOXB7 [77]. They showed HOXB7 physically interacts with ERα and that the HOXB7-ERα complex enhanced transcription of many ERα target genes, including HER2 [77]. Increased HOXB7 expression was mediated through downregulation of miR-196a, previously demonstrated in malignant melanoma to bind the 3'-UTR of HOXB7 and inhibit HOXB7 expression [78]. Additionally, Manavalan et al. demonstrated miR-196a to be downregulated in endocrine-resistant breast cancer cells [28]. Consistent with previous observations, miR-196a showed decreased expression in the MCF7-TMR (tamoxifen-resistant) cells, and overexpression of miR-196a was sufficient to promote tamoxifen-mediated cell death. MYC, recognized to mediate tamoxifen resistance [79] and able to regulate miRNA expression [76, 77, 80], was identified to be upregulated in tamoxifen-resistant cells. Jin et al. demonstrated EGFR-HER2 signaling phosphorylates MYC and inhibits transcription of miR-196a, a HOXB7 repressor, leading to increased expression of HOXB7, ER target genes, and HER2 [77]. MYC knockdown was sufficient to increase miR-196a expression, decrease HOXB7 expression, and sensitize tamoxifen-resistant cells to tamoxifen therapy, as well as decrease breast cancer xenograft growth. Further, MYC depletion in the presence of a miR-196a luciferase construct, containing the potential MYC binding site, demonstrated MYC directly binds and regulates miR-196a expression to regulate tamoxifen response. These data show inhibiting MYC, as mechanism to target miRNAs, in combination with endocrine therapy may represent a therapeutic strategy in ER+ endocrine-resistant breast cancer [77].

Aromatase inhibitors are widely used in endocrine therapy as a first-line treatment for postmenopausal ERα-positive breast cancer patients [81]. However, resistance to aromatase inhibitors like letrozole and anastrozole that block the biosynthesis of estrogens still develops in patients [82]. Resistance to endocrine therapy is believed to develop in a stepwise fashion where breast cancer cells are converted from an estrogen-dependent phenotype that is responsive to endocrine therapy, to a nonresponsive phenotype, and eventually to an estrogen-independent phenotype. As mentioned above, many miRNAs have been implicated in tamoxifen resistance; however, only a few have been demonstrated to be associated with aromatase inhibitor resistance. Identification of deregulated expression levels of miRNAs in association with aromatase inhibitor resistance is important to provide possible therapeutic targets. In this regard, miR-128a was highly expressed in letrozole-resistant breast cancer cells and targeted the TGF-β signaling pathway [83]. More recently, a miRNA microarray experiment was performed on letrozole-resistant and anastrozole-resistant MCF7 cells [84]. This study identified 33 miRNAs in letrozole-resistant cells and 18 miRNAs in anastrozole-resistant cells were deregulated compared to the anastrozole-sensitive MCF7 cell line [84]. Three miRNAs (miR-125b, miR-205, and miR-424) of interest were similarly deregulated in both aromatase inhibitor-resistant cell lines and found to converge on the AKT/mTOR pathway [84]. Ectopic overexpression of either miR-125b or miR-205, or the silencing of miR-424 expression, in the anastrozole-sensitive MCF7 cell line was sufficient to confer resistance to letrozole and anastrozole, to target and activate the AKT/mTOR pathway, and to increase the formation capacity of stemlike and tumor-initiating cells possessing self-renewing properties. Also, increased miR-125b expression levels were sufficient to confer estrogen-independent growth to anastrozole-sensitive MCF7 cell line [84].

Another strategy for targeting breast cancer is proteasome inhibition, but resistant tumor cells often emerge. Proteasome maturation protein, POMP, can be targeted by miR-101, leading to impaired proteasome assembly and activity and resulting in accumulation of p53 and cyclin-dependent kinase inhibitors, cell cycle arrest, and apoptosis [85]. In ERα-positive breast cancers, miR-101 and

POMP levels are inversely correlated, and high miR-101 expression or low POMP expression associates with prolonged survival. Estrogen-driven transcription was attenuated with miR-101 expression or POMP knockdown. These results suggest that proteasome activity can be regulated endogenously though miR-101, which targets proteasome biogenesis to control overall protein turnover and tumor cell proliferation [85].

6 ERα Regulation of miRNA Procession Machinery

As extensively described throughout this chapter, miRNAs have been shown to be differentially expressed between normal and malignant tissues. Since genomic changes and transcriptional regulation of miRNA expression do not completely explain the differences in miRNA profiles between normal and malignant tissues, the deregulation of miRNA biogenesis was investigated in some cancers [86].

Grelier et al. determined that Dicer protein expression, a ribonuclease required for biogenesis of miRNAs, is significantly associated with hormone receptor status and cancer subtype in breast tumors [87]. However, Dicer mRNA expression appeared to have an independent prognostic impact in metastatic disease. Also, lower Dicer expression was found in cells harboring a mesenchymal phenotype and in metastatic bone derivatives in breast cancer cell lines. These data indicate that Dicer may be involved in breast tumorigenesis by altering miRNA biogenesis [87].

In a similar study by Dedes et al., Drosha and Dicer mRNA levels were reported to be downregulated in 18 and 46% of breast cancer patients ($n = 245$) receiving adjuvant anthracycline-based chemotherapy compared to normal breast tissue. Drosha downregulation was associated with high-grade, high Ki-67, lack of Bcl2 expression, HER3 overexpression, and TOPO2A gene amplification. Dicer downregulation was associated with lack of expression of ER, progesterone receptor, and Bcl2 and with high-grade, high Ki-67, triple-negative, and basal-like phenotypes. These results further suggest that dysregulation of miRNA procession machinery contributes to breast cancer [88].

Little is known about the underlying mechanisms of how altered miRNA expression levels contribute to phenotypic advantages. Martello et al. identified miR-103/107 to be highly expressed in metastatic breast cancer and associated with poor outcome in patients. MiR-103/107 inhibited the expression of Dicer, causing global miRNA downregulation [89]. Functionally, miR-103/107 confers migratory capabilities in vitro by increasing epithelial-to-mesenchymal transition and increase metastatic dissemination of cells in vivo. These results suggest a new pathway by which Dicer inhibition shifts cancer cells toward a less differentiated, mesenchymal state to foster metastasis [89].

The expression of miRNA machinery components could directly influence expression patterns of various genes through the erroneous effects of incompletely matured miRNA. Kwon et al. examined the expression of 4 miRNA machinery components (DGCR8, AGO2, Dicer, and Drosha) in 52 breast tumor tissues and found decreased expression of miRNA machinery components in invasive breast carcinoma, suggesting that miRNA machinery components may be associated with breast pathobiology [90]. In a separate study, AGO2 expression was elevated in ER-breast cancer cell lines and low in ER+ cells, which was dependent upon active ERα/estrogen signaling [91]. Adams et al. demonstrated that AGO2 is upregulated by an EGFR/MAPK signaling pathway in ERα-negative breast cancer cell lines, whereas overexpression of AGO2 is sufficient to drive breast tumor progression in the ERα-positive MCF7 human breast adenocarcinoma cell line [91].

7 ERRs and ERβ Regulation of miRNAs

Additionally, the interaction between ERα and its related receptors (ERR and ERβ) is becoming better appreciated as regulators of breast cancer progression, through cross talk with miRNAs, in the absence of ERα. A study by Han et al. demonstrated overexpression of miR-497 inhibited ERRα expression, as well as MIF levels and MMP9 activity, which led to a significant decrease in cell proliferation, migration, and invasion of ERα-negative breast cancer. Low levels of ERα in ERα-negative breast cancer were shown to reduce miR-497 expression, which promoted ERRα expression enhancing cell proliferation, migration, and invasion by increased MIF expression and MMP9 activity [92]. Additionally, Tribollet et al. demonstrated that miR-135a directly downregulates expression of ERRα through binding of its 3′-UTR, resulting in reduced expression of downstream targets of ERRα, reducing cell invasion [93].

In another study by Lu et al., miR-320a levels were demonstrated to be significantly lower in breast tumor tissues compared with normal breast tissues [94]. In tamoxifen-resistant MCF7 and T47D breast cancer cells, re-expression of miR-320a was sufficient to sensitize these cells to tamoxifen-induced growth inhibition by targeting the cAMP-regulated phosphoprotein (ARPP-19) and ERRγ, as well as their downstream effectors, c-Myc and Cyclin C1. miR-320a levels were increased after progesterone treatment by repressing c-Myc expression, while estrogen exerted the opposite effect. These results suggest a potential therapeutic approach for tamoxifen-resistant breast cancer through restoring miR-320a expression to disrupt ERRγ expression [94].

In addition to estrogen-related receptors (ERRs), ERβ has been demonstrated to regulate miRNA expression in breast cancer. A recent study by Paris et al. demonstrated ERβ overexpression in MCF7 cells resulted in differential expression of 73 miRNAs [95]. Based on the differential expression of miRNAs in ERβ overexpressing cell lines, breast tumors were segregated based on ERβ status and profiled for miRNA expression. Sixty-seven miRNAs were identified which could discriminate between ERβ+ and ERβ−; ten differentially expressed miRNAs correlated with the in vitro data. ERβ was demonstrated to directly regulate several miRNAs based on ERβ binding site alignment in the miRNA regulatory regions. miR-30a was identified as a direct ERβ target and downregulated upon estrogen stimulation in the presence of ERβ and absence of ERα. Interestingly, not only did ERβ directly regulate miRNA transcription, but the receptor also interfered with miRNA biogenesis, disrupting ERα interaction with Drosha. Downregulation of not only miRNA transcriptionally but also biogenesis may explain the less aggressive phenotypes associated with ERβ+ breast cancers. Further ERβ-dependent miRNAs may represent a biomarker for breast cancer progression [95].

8 Endocrine Disruptors and miRNA Regulation

In addition to biological estrogens and endocrine therapies which modulate ERα signaling, environmental agents termed "endocrine disrupting compounds" like DDT and BPA that bind and activate ERα are ubiquitous in our surroundings. We have previously demonstrated that MCF7 cells treated with DDT and BPA potentiate ERα transcriptional activity, resulting in increased expression of ERα target genes. MiRNA microarray revealed that MCF7 cells treated with either DDT plus BPA or estrogen resulted in similar expression of multiple miRNAs, including miR-21. However, DDT and BPA induced differential patterns of miRNA expression compared to estrogen [96]. A recent review by Klinge et al. further describes the role of endocrine disruptors in ERα biology and miRNA regulation [44].

9 Conclusion

The crosstalk between miRNAs and ERα in breast cancer has been of great interest. Here, we have described several studies demonstrating the interaction between ERα and miRNAs, which can mediate cell proliferation, EMT, and differentiation programs, culminating in the onset of endocrine therapy resistance (Fig. 1). While many of these studies characterize the role of miRNAs based on in vitro biology, there is little in vivo support and even less characterization in the clinical setting [45]. Together these studies implicate the role of miRNAs in ER+ breast cancer progression as potential therapeutic targets and biomarkers of the disease. With increased in vivo and clinical studies, a better understanding of the regulatory network involved in ERα regulation of miRNAs in breast cancer will undoubtedly evolve.

Disclosure of Potential Conflicts of Interest None

References

1. Bartel DP (2004) MicroRNAs: genomics, biogenesis, mechanism, and function. Cell 116(2):281–297
2. Ha M, Kim VN (2014) Regulation of microRNA biogenesis. Nat Rev Mol Cell Biol 15(8):509–524. https://doi.org/10.1038/nrm3838
3. Di Leva G, Gasparini P, Piovan C, Ngankeu A, Garofalo M, Taccioli C, Iorio MV, Li M, Volinia S, Alder H, Nakamura T, Nuovo G, Liu Y, Nephew KP, Croce CM (2010) MicroRNA cluster 221-222 and estrogen receptor alpha interactions in breast cancer. J Natl Cancer Inst 102(10):706–721. https://doi.org/10.1093/jnci/djq102
4. Klinge CM (2012) miRNAs and estrogen action. Trends Endocrinol Metab 23(5):223–233. https://doi.org/10.1016/j.tem.2012.03.002
5. Shenouda SK, Alahari SK (2009) MicroRNA function in cancer: oncogene or a tumor suppressor? Cancer Metastasis Rev 28(3–4):369–378. https://doi.org/10.1007/s10555-009-9188-5
6. Kent OA, Mendell JT (2006) A small piece in the cancer puzzle: microRNAs as tumor suppressors and oncogenes. Oncogene 25(46):6188–6196. https://doi.org/10.1038/sj.onc.1209913
7. Garofalo M, Quintavalle C, Romano G, Croce CM, Condorelli G (2012) miR221/222 in cancer: their role in tumor progression and response to therapy. Curr Mol Med 12(1):27–33
8. Iorio MV, Ferracin M, Liu CG, Veronese A, Spizzo R, Sabbioni S, Magri E, Pedriali M, Fabbri M, Campiglio M, Menard S, Palazzo JP, Rosenberg A, Musiani P, Volinia S, Nenci I, Calin GA, Querzoli P, Negrini M, Croce CM (2005) MicroRNA gene expression deregulation in human breast cancer. Cancer Res 65(16):7065–7070. https://doi.org/10.1158/0008-5472.CAN-05-1783
9. Riaz M, van Jaarsveld MT, Hollestelle A, Prager-van der Smissen WJ, Heine AA, Boersma AW, Liu J, Helmijr J, Ozturk B, Smid M, Wiemer EA, Foekens JA, Martens JW (2013) miRNA expression profiling of 51 human breast cancer cell lines reveals subtype and driver mutation-specific miRNAs. Breast Cancer Res 15(2):R33. https://doi.org/10.1186/bcr3415
10. Klinge CM (2015) Estrogen action: receptors, transcripts, cell signaling, and non-coding RNAs in normal physiology and disease. Mol Cell Endocrinol 418(Pt 3):191–192. https://doi.org/10.1016/j.mce.2015.11.028
11. Legare S, Basik M (2016) Minireview: the link between ERalpha corepressors and histone deacetylases in tamoxifen resistance in breast cancer. Mol Endocrinol 30(9):965–976. https://doi.org/10.1210/me.2016-1072
12. Adams BD, Furneaux H, White BA (2007) The micro-ribonucleic acid (miRNA) miR-206 targets the human estrogen receptor-alpha (ERalpha) and represses ERalpha messenger RNA and protein expression in breast cancer cell lines. Mol Endocrinol 21(5):1132–1147. https://doi.org/10.1210/me.2007-0022
13. Lowery AJ, Miller N, McNeill RE, Kerin MJ (2008) MicroRNAs as prognostic indicators and therapeutic targets: potential effect on breast cancer management. Clin Cancer Res 14(2):360–365. https://doi.org/10.1158/1078-0432.CCR-07-0992
14. Muluhngwi P, Klinge CM (2017) Identification of miRNAs as biomarkers for acquired endocrine resistance in breast cancer. Mol Cell Endocrinol 456:76–86. https://doi.org/10.1016/j.mce.2017.02.004
15. Yang JS, Lai EC (2011) Alternative miRNA biogenesis pathways and the interpretation of core miRNA pathway mutants. Mol Cell 43(6):892–903. https://doi.org/10.1016/j.molcel.2011.07.024
16. Ladewig E, Okamura K, Flynt AS, Westholm JO, Lai EC (2012) Discovery of hundreds of mirtrons in mouse and human small RNA data. Genome Res 22(9):1634–1645. https://doi.org/10.1101/gr.133553.111
17. Wickramasinghe NS, Manavalan TT, Dougherty SM, Riggs KA, Li Y, Klinge CM (2009) Estradiol downregulates miR-21 expression and increases miR-21 target gene expression in

MCF-7 breast cancer cells. Nucleic Acids Res 37(8):2584–2595. https://doi.org/10.1093/nar/gkp117

18. Mattie MD, Benz CC, Bowers J, Sensinger K, Wong L, Scott GK, Fedele V, Ginzinger D, Getts R, Haqq C (2006) Optimized high-throughput microRNA expression profiling provides novel biomarker assessment of clinical prostate and breast cancer biopsies. Mol Cancer 5:24. https://doi.org/10.1186/1476-4598-5-24

19. Han M, Liu M, Wang Y, Mo Z, Bi X, Liu Z, Fan Y, Chen X, Wu C (2012) Re-expression of miR-21 contributes to migration and invasion by inducing epithelial-mesenchymal transition consistent with cancer stem cell characteristics in MCF-7 cells. Mol Cell Biochem 363(1–2):427–436. https://doi.org/10.1007/s11010-011-1195-5

20. Rao X, Di Leva G, Li M, Fang F, Devlin C, Hartman-Frey C, Burow ME, Ivan M, Croce CM, Nephew KP (2011) MicroRNA-221/222 confers breast cancer fulvestrant resistance by regulating multiple signaling pathways. Oncogene 30(9):1082–1097. https://doi.org/10.1038/onc.2010.487

21. Lyng MB, Laenkholm AV, Sokilde R, Gravgaard KH, Litman T, Ditzel HJ (2012) Global microRNA expression profiling of high-risk ER+ breast cancers from patients receiving adjuvant tamoxifen mono-therapy: a DBCG study. PLoS One 7(5):e36170. https://doi.org/10.1371/journal.pone.0036170

22. Ferraro L, Ravo M, Nassa G, Tarallo R, De Filippo MR, Giurato G, Cirillo F, Stellato C, Silvestro S, Cantarella C, Rizzo F, Cimino D, Friard O, Biglia N, De Bortoli M, Cicatiello L, Nola E, Weisz A (2012) Effects of oestrogen on microRNA expression in hormone-responsive breast cancer cells. Horm Cancer 3(3):65–78. https://doi.org/10.1007/s12672-012-0102-1

23. Cicatiello L, Mutarelli M, Grober OM, Paris O, Ferraro L, Ravo M, Tarallo R, Luo S, Schroth GP, Seifert M, Zinser C, Chiusano ML, Traini A, De Bortoli M, Weisz A (2010) Estrogen receptor alpha controls a gene network in luminal-like breast cancer cells comprising multiple transcription factors and microRNAs. Am J Pathol 176(5):2113–2130. https://doi.org/10.2353/ajpath.2010.090837

24. Bhat-Nakshatri P, Wang G, Collins NR, Thomson MJ, Geistlinger TR, Carroll JS, Brown M, Hammond S, Srour EF, Liu Y, Nakshatri H (2009) Estradiol-regulated microRNAs control estradiol response in breast cancer cells. Nucleic Acids Res 37(14):4850–4861. https://doi.org/10.1093/nar/gkp500

25. Manavathi B, Dey O, Gajulapalli VN, Bhatia RS, Bugide S, Kumar R (2013) Derailed estrogen signaling and breast cancer: an authentic couple. Endocr Rev 34(1):1–32. https://doi.org/10.1210/er.2011-1057

26. Guttilla IK, Adams BD, White BA (2012) ERalpha, microRNAs, and the epithelial-mesenchymal transition in breast cancer. Trends Endocrinol Metab 23(2):73–82. https://doi.org/10.1016/j.tem.2011.12.001

27. Manavalan TT, Teng Y, Litchfield LM, Muluhngwi P, Al-Rayyan N, Klinge CM (2013) Reduced expression of miR-200 family members contributes to antiestrogen resistance in LY2 human breast cancer cells. PLoS One 8(4):e62334. https://doi.org/10.1371/journal.pone.0062334

28. Manavalan TT, Teng Y, Appana SN, Datta S, Kalbfleisch TS, Li Y, Klinge CM (2011) Differential expression of microRNA expression in tamoxifen-sensitive MCF-7 versus tamoxifen-resistant LY2 human breast cancer cells. Cancer Lett 313(1):26–43. https://doi.org/10.1016/j.canlet.2011.08.018

29. Ward A, Balwierz A, Zhang JD, Kublbeck M, Pawitan Y, Hielscher T, Wiemann S, Sahin O (2013) Re-expression of microRNA-375 reverses both tamoxifen resistance and accompanying EMT-like properties in breast cancer. Oncogene 32(9):1173–1182. https://doi.org/10.1038/onc.2012.128

30. Brown DM, Ruoslahti E (2004) Metadherin, a cell surface protein in breast tumors that mediates lung metastasis. Cancer Cell 5(4):365–374

31. Sreekumar R, Sayan BS, Mirnezami AH, Sayan AE (2011) MicroRNA control of invasion and metastasis pathways. Front Genet 2:58. https://doi.org/10.3389/fgene.2011.00058

32. Volinia S, Nuovo G, Drusco A, Costinean S, Abujarour R, Desponts C, Garofalo M, Baffa R, Aeqilan R, Maharry K, Sana ME, Di Leva G, Gasparini P, Dama P, Marchesini J, Galasso M, Manfrini M, Zerbinati C, Corra F, Wise T, Wojcik SE, Previati M, Pichiorri F, Zanesi N, Alder H, Palatini J, Huebner KF, Shapiro CL, Negrini M, Vecchione A, Rosenberg AL, Croce CM, Garzon R (2014) Pluripotent stem cell miRNAs and metastasis in invasive breast cancer. J Natl Cancer Inst 106(12). https://doi.org/10.1093/jnci/dju324

33. Li B, Lu Y, Wang H, Han X, Mao J, Li J, Yu L, Wang B, Fan S, Yu X, Song B (2016) miR-221/222 enhance the tumorigenicity of human breast cancer stem cells via modulation of PTEN/Akt pathway. Biomed Pharmacother 79:93–101. https://doi.org/10.1016/j.biopha.2016.01.045

34. Guttilla IK, Phoenix KN, Hong X, Tirnauer JS, Claffey KP, White BA (2012) Prolonged mammosphere culture of MCF-7 cells induces an EMT and repression of the estrogen receptor by microRNAs. Breast Cancer Res Treat 132(1):75–85. https://doi.org/10.1007/s10549-011-1534-y

35. Kastrati I, Canestrari E, Frasor J (2015) PHLDA1 expression is controlled by an estrogen receptor-NFkappaB-miR-181 regulatory loop and is essential for formation of ER+ mammospheres. Oncogene 34(18):2309–2316. https://doi.org/10.1038/onc.2014.180

36. Yu Z, Baserga R, Chen L, Wang C, Lisanti MP, Pestell RG (2010) microRNA, cell cycle, and human breast cancer. Am J Pathol 176(3):1058–1064. https://doi.org/10.2353/ajpath.2010.090664

37. Baran-Gale J, Purvis JE, Sethupathy P (2016) An integrative transcriptomics approach identifies miR-503 as a candidate master regulator of the estrogen response in MCF-7 breast cancer cells. RNA 22(10):1592–1603. https://doi.org/10.1261/rna.056895.116

38. Fan M, Yan PS, Hartman-Frey C, Chen L, Paik H, Oyer SL, Salisbury JD, Cheng AS, Li L, Abbosh PH, Huang TH, Nephew KP (2006) Diverse gene expression and DNA methylation profiles correlate with differential adaptation of breast cancer cells to the antiestrogens tamoxifen and fulvestrant. Cancer Res 66(24):11954–11966. https://doi.org/10.1158/0008-5472.CAN-06-1666

39. Rhodes LV, Nitschke AM, Segar HC, Martin EC, Driver JL, Elliott S, Nam SY, Li M, Nephew KP, Burow ME, Collins-Burow BM (2012) The histone deacetylase inhibitor trichostatin A alters microRNA expression profiles in apoptosis-resistant breast cancer cells. Oncol Rep 27(1):10–16. https://doi.org/10.3892/or.2011.1488

40. Liu J, Li Y (2015) Trichostatin A and Tamoxifen inhibit breast cancer cell growth by miR-204 and ERalpha reducing AKT/mTOR pathway. Biochem Biophys Res Commun 467(2):242–247. https://doi.org/10.1016/j.bbrc.2015.09.182

41. Imam JS, Plyler JR, Bansal H, Prajapati S, Bansal S, Rebeles J, Chen HI, Chang YF, Panneerdoss S, Zoghi B, Buddavarapu KC, Broaddus R, Hornsby P, Tomlinson G, Dome J, Vadlamudi RK, Pertsemlidis A, Chen Y, Rao MK (2012) Genomic loss of tumor suppressor miRNA-204 promotes cancer cell migration and invasion by activating AKT/mTOR/Rac1 signaling and actin reorganization. PLoS One 7(12):e52397. https://doi.org/10.1371/journal.pone.0052397

42. Hui Z, Yiling C, Wenting Y, XuQun H, ChuanYi Z, Hui L (2015) miR-491-5p functions as a tumor suppressor by targeting JMJD2B in ERalpha-positive breast cancer. FEBS Lett 589(7):812–821. https://doi.org/10.1016/j.febslet.2015.02.014

43. Di Leva G, Piovan C, Gasparini P, Ngankeu A, Taccioli C, Briskin D, Cheung DG, Bolon B, Anderlucci L, Alder H, Nuovo G, Li M, Iorio MV, Galasso M, Santhanam R, Marcucci G, Perrotti D, Powell KA, Bratasz A, Garofalo M, Nephew KP, Croce CM (2013) Estrogen mediated-activation of miR-191/425 cluster modulates tumorigenicity of breast cancer cells depending on estrogen receptor status. PLoS Genet 9(3):e1003311. https://doi.org/10.1371/journal.pgen.1003311

44. Klinge CM (2015) miRNAs regulated by estrogens, tamoxifen, and endocrine disruptors and their downstream gene targets. Mol Cell Endocrinol 418(Pt 3):273–297. https://doi.org/10.1016/j.mce.2015.01.035

45. Di Leva G, Cheung DG, Croce CM (2015) miRNA clusters as therapeutic targets for hormone-resistant breast cancer. Expert Rev Endocrinol Metab 10(6):607–617. https://doi.org/10.1586/17446651.2015.1099430

46. Nam S, Long X, Kwon C, Kim S, Nephew KP (2012) An integrative analysis of cellular contexts, miRNAs and mRNAs reveals network clusters associated with antiestrogen-resistant breast cancer cells. BMC Genomics 13:732. https://doi.org/10.1186/1471-2164-13-732

47. Muluhngwi P, Klinge CM (2015) Roles for miRNAs in endocrine resistance in breast cancer. Endocr Relat Cancer 22(5):R279–R300. https://doi.org/10.1530/ERC-15-0355

48. Bronzert DA, Greene GL, Lippman ME (1985) Selection and characterization of a breast cancer cell line resistant to the antiestrogen LY 117018. Endocrinology 117(4):1409–1417. https://doi.org/10.1210/endo-117-4-1409

49. Mullick A, Chambon P (1990) Characterization of the estrogen receptor in two antiestrogen-resistant cell lines, LY2 and T47D. Cancer Res 50(2):333–338

50. Zhu S, Wu H, Wu F, Nie D, Sheng S, Mo YY (2008) MicroRNA-21 targets tumor suppressor genes in invasion and metastasis. Cell Res 18(3):350–359. https://doi.org/10.1038/cr.2008.24

51. Li X, Mertens-Talcott SU, Zhang S, Kim K, Ball J, Safe S (2010) MicroRNA-27a indirectly regulates estrogen receptor {alpha} expression and hormone responsiveness in MCF-7 breast cancer cells. Endocrinology 151(6):2462–2473. https://doi.org/10.1210/en.2009-1150

52. de Souza Rocha Simonini P, Breiling A, Gupta N, Malekpour M, Youns M, Omranipour R, Malekpour F, Volinia S, Croce CM, Najmabadi H, Diederichs S, Sahin O, Mayer D, Lyko F, Hoheisel JD, Riazalhosseini Y (2010) Epigenetically deregulated microRNA-375 is involved in a positive feedback loop with estrogen receptor alpha in breast cancer cells. Cancer Res 70(22):9175–9184. https://doi.org/10.1158/0008-5472.CAN-10-1318

53. Spizzo R, Nicoloso MS, Lupini L, Lu Y, Fogarty J, Rossi S, Zagatti B, Fabbri M, Veronese A, Liu X, Davuluri R, Croce CM, Mills G, Negrini M, Calin GA (2010) miR-145 participates with TP53 in a death-promoting regulatory loop and targets estrogen receptor-alpha in human breast cancer cells. Cell Death Differ 17(2):246–254. https://doi.org/10.1038/cdd.2009.117

54. Miller TE, Ghoshal K, Ramaswamy B, Roy S, Datta J, Shapiro CL, Jacob S, Majumder S (2008) MicroRNA-221/222 confers tamoxifen resistance in breast cancer by targeting p27Kip1. J Biol Chem 283(44):29897–29903. https://doi.org/10.1074/jbc.M804612200

55. Zhao JJ, Lin J, Yang H, Kong W, He L, Ma X, Coppola D, Cheng JQ (2008) MicroRNA-221/222 negatively regulates estrogen receptor alpha and is associated with tamoxifen resistance in breast cancer. J Biol Chem 283(45):31079–31086. https://doi.org/10.1074/jbc.M806041200

56. Martin EC, Conger AK, Yan TJ, Hoang VT, Miller DF, Buechlein A, Rusch DB, Nephew KP, Collins-Burow BM, Burow ME (2017) MicroRNA-335-5p and -3p synergize to inhibit estrogen receptor alpha expression and promote tamoxifen resistance. FEBS Lett 591(2):382–392. https://doi.org/10.1002/1873-3468.12538

57. Heneghan HM, Miller N, Kerin MJ (2010) MiRNAs as biomarkers and therapeutic targets in cancer. Curr Opin Pharmacol 10(5):543–550. https://doi.org/10.1016/j.coph.2010.05.010

58. Ward A, Shukla K, Balwierz A, Soons Z, Konig R, Sahin O, Wiemann S (2014) MicroRNA-519a is a novel oncomir conferring tamoxifen resistance by targeting a network of tumour-suppressor genes in ER+ breast cancer. J Pathol 233(4):368–379. https://doi.org/10.1002/path.4363

59. Gonzalez-Malerva L, Park J, Zou L, Hu Y, Moradpour Z, Pearlberg J, Sawyer J, Stevens H, Harlow E, LaBaer J (2011) High-throughput ectopic expression screen for tamoxifen resistance identifies an atypical kinase that blocks autophagy. Proc Natl Acad Sci U S A 108(5):2058–2063. https://doi.org/10.1073/pnas.1018157108

60. Rhodes LV, Bratton MR, Zhu Y, Tilghman SL, Muir SE, Salvo VA, Tate CR, Elliott S, Nephew KP, Collins-Burow BM, Burow ME (2011) Effects of SDF-1-CXCR4 signaling on microRNA expression and tumorigenesis in estrogen receptor-alpha (ER-alpha)-positive breast cancer cells. Exp Cell Res 317(18):2573–2581. https://doi.org/10.1016/j.yexcr.2011.08.016

61. Klinge CM (2009) Estrogen regulation of microRNA expression. Curr Genomics 10(3):169–183. https://doi.org/10.2174/138920209788185289

62. Cohen PA, Donini CF, Nguyen NT, Lincet H, Vendrell JA (2015) The dark side of ZNF217, a key regulator of tumorigenesis with powerful biomarker value. Oncotarget 6(39):41566–41581. https://doi.org/10.18632/oncotarget.5893

63. Nguyen NT, Vendrell JA, Poulard C, Gyorffy B, Goddard-Leon S, Bieche I, Corbo L, Le Romancer M, Bachelot T, Treilleux I, Cohen PA (2014) A functional interplay between ZNF217 and estrogen receptor alpha exists in luminal breast cancers. Mol Oncol 8(8):1441–1457. https://doi.org/10.1016/j.molonc.2014.05.013

64. Frietze S, O'Geen H, Littlepage LE, Simion C, Sweeney CA, Farnham PJ, Krig SR (2014) Global analysis of ZNF217 chromatin occupancy in the breast cancer cell genome reveals an association with ERalpha. BMC Genomics 15:520. https://doi.org/10.1186/1471-2164-15-520

65. Alayev A, Salamon RS, Berger SM, Schwartz NS, Cuesta R, Snyder RB, Holz MK (2016) mTORC1 directly phosphorylates and activates ERalpha upon estrogen stimulation. Oncogene 35(27):3535–3543. https://doi.org/10.1038/onc.2015.414

66. Martin EC, Rhodes LV, Elliott S, Krebs AE, Nephew KP, Flemington EK, Collins-Burow BM, Burow ME (2014) microRNA regulation of mammalian target of rapamycin expression and activity controls estrogen receptor function and RAD001 sensitivity. Mol Cancer 13:229. https://doi.org/10.1186/1476-4598-13-229

67. Jiang CF, Li DM, Shi ZM, Wang L, Liu MM, Ge X, Liu X, Qian YC, Wen YY, Zhen LL, Lin J, Liu LZ, Jiang BH (2016) Estrogen regulates miRNA expression: implication of estrogen receptor and miR-124/AKT2 in tumor growth and angiogenesis. Oncotarget 7(24):36940–36955. https://doi.org/10.18632/oncotarget.9230

68. Yuan Y, Anbalagan D, Lee LH, Samy RP, Shanmugam MK, Kumar AP, Sethi G, Lobie PE, Lim LH (2016) ANXA1 inhibits miRNA-196a in a negative feedback loop through NF-kB and c-Myc to reduce breast cancer proliferation. Oncotarget 7(19):27007–27020. https://doi.org/10.18632/oncotarget.8875

69. Xin F, Li M, Balch C, Thomson M, Fan M, Liu Y, Hammond SM, Kim S, Nephew KP (2009) Computational analysis of microRNA profiles and their target genes suggests significant involvement in breast cancer antiestrogen resistance. Bioinformatics 25(4):430–434. https://doi.org/10.1093/bioinformatics/btn646

70. Ikeda K, Horie-Inoue K, Ueno T, Suzuki T, Sato W, Shigekawa T, Osaki A, Saeki T, Berezikov E, Mano H, Inoue S (2015) miR-378a-3p modulates tamoxifen sensitivity in breast cancer MCF-7 cells through targeting GOLT1A. Sci Rep 5:13170. https://doi.org/10.1038/srep13170

71. Ujihira T, Ikeda K, Suzuki T, Yamaga R, Sato W, Horie-Inoue K, Shigekawa T, Osaki A, Saeki T, Okamoto K, Takeda S, Inoue S (2015) MicroRNA-574-3p, identified by microRNA library-based functional screening, modulates tamoxifen response in breast cancer. Sci Rep 5:7641. https://doi.org/10.1038/srep07641

72. Chiyomaru T, Yamamura S, Fukuhara S, Hidaka H, Majid S, Saini S, Arora S, Deng G, Shahryari V, Chang I, Tanaka Y, Tabatabai ZL, Enokida H, Seki N, Nakagawa M, Dahiya R (2013) Genistein up-regulates tumor suppressor microRNA-574-3p in prostate cancer. PLoS One 8(3):e58929. https://doi.org/10.1371/journal.pone.0058929

73. Tung KH, Lin CW, Kuo CC, Li LT, Kuo YH, Lin CW, Wu HC (2013) CHC promotes tumor growth and angiogenesis through regulation of HIF-1alpha and VEGF signaling. Cancer Lett 331(1):58–67. https://doi.org/10.1016/j.canlet.2012.12.001

74. Cizeron-Clairac G, Lallemand F, Vacher S, Lidereau R, Bieche I, Callens C (2015) MiR-190b, the highest up-regulated miRNA in ERalpha-positive compared to ERalpha-negative breast tumors, a new biomarker in breast cancers? BMC Cancer 15:499. https://doi.org/10.1186/s12885-015-1505-5

75. Xu S, Wang T, Song W, Jiang T, Zhang F, Yin Y, Jiang SW, Wu K, Yu Z, Wang C, Chen K (2015) The inhibitory effects of AR/miR-190a/YB-1 negative feedback loop on prostate cancer and underlying mechanism. Sci Rep 5:13528. https://doi.org/10.1038/srep13528

76. Kim T, Jeon YJ, Cui R, Lee JH, Peng Y, Kim SH, Tili E, Alder H, Croce CM (2015) Role of MYC-regulated long noncoding RNAs in cell cycle regulation and tumorigenesis. J Natl Cancer Inst 107(4). https://doi.org/10.1093/jnci/dju505

77. Jin K, Park S, Teo WW, Korangath P, Cho SS, Yoshida T, Gyorffy B, Goswami CP, Nakshatri H, Cruz LA, Zhou W, Ji H, Su Y, Ekram M, Wu Z, Zhu T, Polyak K, Sukumar S (2015) HOXB7 is an ERalpha cofactor in the activation of HER2 and multiple ER target genes leading to endocrine resistance. Cancer Discov 5(9):944–959. https://doi.org/10.1158/2159-8290. CD-15-0090

78. Braig S, Mueller DW, Rothhammer T, Bosserhoff AK (2010) MicroRNA miR-196a is a central regulator of HOX-B7 and BMP4 expression in malignant melanoma. Cell Mol Life Sci 67(20):3535–3548. https://doi.org/10.1007/s00018-010-0394-7

79. Zheng L, Meng X, Li X, Zhang Y, Li C, Xiang C, Xing Y, Xia Y, Xi T (2018) miR-125a-3p inhibits ERalpha transactivation and overrides tamoxifen resistance by targeting CDK3 in estrogen receptor-positive breast cancer. FASEB J 32(2):588–600. https://doi.org/10.1096/fj.201700461RR

80. Barros-Silva D, Costa-Pinheiro P, Duarte H, Sousa EJ, Evangelista AF, Graca I, Carneiro I, Martins AT, Oliveira J, Carvalho AL, Marques MM, Henrique R, Jeronimo C (2018) MicroRNA-27a-5p regulation by promoter methylation and MYC signaling in prostate carcinogenesis. Cell Death Dis 9(2):167. https://doi.org/10.1038/s41419-017-0241-y

81. Riemsma R, Forbes CA, Kessels A, Lykopoulos K, Amonkar MM, Rea DW, Kleijnen J (2010) Systematic review of aromatase inhibitors in the first-line treatment for hormone sensitive advanced or metastatic breast cancer. Breast Cancer Res Treat 123(1):9–24. https://doi.org/10.1007/s10549-010-0974-0

82. Vilquin P, Villedieu M, Grisard E, Ben Larbi S, Ghayad SE, Heudel PE, Bachelot T, Corbo L, Treilleux I, Vendrell JA, Cohen PA (2013) Molecular characterization of anastrozole resistance in breast cancer: pivotal role of the Akt/mTOR pathway in the emergence of de novo or acquired resistance and importance of combining the allosteric Akt inhibitor MK-2206 with an aromatase inhibitor. Int J Cancer 133(7):1589–1602. https://doi.org/10.1002/ijc.28182

83. Masri S, Liu Z, Phung S, Wang E, Yuan YC, Chen S (2010) The role of microRNA-128a in regulating TGFbeta signaling in letrozole-resistant breast cancer cells. Breast Cancer Res Treat 124(1):89–99. https://doi.org/10.1007/s10549-009-0716-3

84. Vilquin P, Donini CF, Villedieu M, Grisard E, Corbo L, Bachelot T, Vendrell JA, Cohen PA (2015) MicroRNA-125b upregulation confers aromatase inhibitor resistance and is a novel marker of poor prognosis in breast cancer. Breast Cancer Res 17:13. https://doi.org/10.1186/s13058-015-0515-1

85. Zhang X, Schulz R, Edmunds S, Kruger E, Markert E, Gaedcke J, Cormet-Boyaka E, Ghadimi M, Beissbarth T, Levine AJ, Moll UM, Dobbelstein M (2015) MicroRNA-101 suppresses tumor cell proliferation by acting as an endogenous proteasome inhibitor via targeting the proteasome assembly factor POMP. Mol Cell 59(2):243–257. https://doi.org/10.1016/j.molcel.2015.05.036

86. Zhang L, Huang J, Yang N, Greshock J, Megraw MS, Giannakakis A, Liang S, Naylor TL, Barchetti A, Ward MR, Yao G, Medina A, O'Brien-Jenkins A, Katsaros D, Hatzigeorgiou A, Gimotty PA, Weber BL, Coukos G (2006) microRNAs exhibit high frequency genomic alterations in human cancer. Proc Natl Acad Sci U S A 103(24):9136–9141. https://doi.org/10.1073/pnas.0508889103

87. Grelier G, Voirin N, Ay AS, Cox DG, Chabaud S, Treilleux I, Leon-Goddard S, Rimokh R, Mikaelian I, Venoux C, Puisieux A, Lasset C, Moyret-Lalle C (2009) Prognostic value of Dicer expression in human breast cancers and association with the mesenchymal phenotype. Br J Cancer 101(4):673–683. https://doi.org/10.1038/sj.bjc.6605193

88. Dedes KJ, Natrajan R, Lambros MB, Geyer FC, Lopez-Garcia MA, Savage K, Jones RL, Reis-Filho JS (2011) Down-regulation of the miRNA master regulators Drosha and Dicer is associated with specific subgroups of breast cancer. Eur J Cancer 47(1):138–150. https://doi.org/10.1016/j.ejca.2010.08.007

89. Martello G, Rosato A, Ferrari F, Manfrin A, Cordenonsi M, Dupont S, Enzo E, Guzzardo V, Rondina M, Spruce T, Parenti AR, Daidone MG, Bicciato S, Piccolo S (2010) A microRNA

targeting dicer for metastasis control. Cell 141(7):1195–1207. https://doi.org/10.1016/j. cell.2010.05.017

90. Kwon SY, Lee JH, Kim B, Park JW, Kwon TK, Kang SH, Kim S (2014) Complexity in regulation of microRNA machinery components in invasive breast carcinoma. Pathol Oncol Res 20(3):697–705. https://doi.org/10.1007/s12253-014-9750-5

91. Adams BD, Claffey KP, White BA (2009) Argonaute-2 expression is regulated by epidermal growth factor receptor and mitogen-activated protein kinase signaling and correlates with a transformed phenotype in breast cancer cells. Endocrinology 150(1):14–23. https://doi.org/10.1210/en.2008-0984

92. Han L, Liu B, Jiang L, Liu J, Han S (2016) MicroRNA-497 downregulation contributes to cell proliferation, migration, and invasion of estrogen receptor alpha negative breast cancer by targeting estrogen-related receptor alpha. Tumour Biol 37(10):13205–13214. https://doi.org/10.1007/s13277-016-5200-1

93. Tribollet V, Barenton B, Kroiss A, Vincent S, Zhang L, Forcet C, Cerutti C, Perian S, Allioli N, Samarut J, Vanacker JM (2016) miR-135a inhibits the invasion of cancer cells via suppression of ERRalpha. PLoS One 11(5):e0156445. https://doi.org/10.1371/journal.pone.0156445

94. Lu M, Ding K, Zhang G, Yin M, Yao G, Tian H, Lian J, Liu L, Liang M, Zhu T, Sun F (2015) MicroRNA-320a sensitizes tamoxifen-resistant breast cancer cells to tamoxifen by targeting ARPP-19 and ERRgamma. Sci Rep 5:8735. https://doi.org/10.1038/srep08735

95. Paris O, Ferraro L, Grober OM, Ravo M, De Filippo MR, Giurato G, Nassa G, Tarallo R, Cantarella C, Rizzo F, Di Benedetto A, Mottolese M, Benes V, Ambrosino C, Nola E, Weisz A (2012) Direct regulation of microRNA biogenesis and expression by estrogen receptor beta in hormone-responsive breast cancer. Oncogene 31(38):4196–4206. https://doi.org/10.1038/onc.2011.583

96. Tilghman SL, Bratton MR, Segar HC, Martin EC, Rhodes LV, Li M, McLachlan JA, Wiese TE, Nephew KP, Burow ME (2012) Endocrine disruptor regulation of microRNA expression in breast carcinoma cells. PLoS One 7(3):e32754. https://doi.org/10.1371/journal.pone.0032754

The First Targeted Therapy to Treat Cancer: The Tamoxifen Tale

Balkees Abderrahman and V. Craig Jordan

Abstract The chance discovery of a new group of medicines called nonsteroidal anti-estrogens opened the door to new opportunities in therapeutics. Ethamoxytriphetol (MER25) was the first. However, based on studies in rats and mice, initial hopes were that nonsteroidal anti-estrogens would be new "morning after pills." However, the discovery that clomiphene and tamoxifen induced ovulation in subfertile women would produce only a niche market in the 1960s. The treatment of metastatic breast cancer was an obvious choice as endocrine ablative surgery, i.e., oophorectomy, adrenalectomy, or hypophysectomy, was standard of care. Over a decade, in the 1970s, numerous nonsteroidal anti-estrogens were tested, but only tamoxifen went forward for the treatment of all stages of breast cancer, ductal carcinoma in situ, and male breast cancer and the reduction of risk for breast cancer in high-risk pre- and postmenopausal women.

Keywords Nonsteroidal anti-estrogens · Nafoxidine · Clomiphene · Tamoxifen · Estrogen receptor · Breast cancer therapy and prevention

1 Introduction

In 1958, Lerner and coworkers [1] described the anti-estrogenic properties of the first nonsteroidal anti-estrogen ethamoxytriphetol (MER25) (Fig. 1). The compound was discovered by accident. Lerner was scanning the structures of compounds that were being tested in the cardiovascular program at William S. Merrell, in Cincinnati. He was the new young leader of their synthetic estrogen program. Lerner noted that MER25 had a structure similar to the triphenylethylene estrogens [2] used clinically. He asked to test MER25 as an estrogen.

Unexpectedly, MER25 was found to be an anti-estrogen in all species tested and had little or no estrogenic actions at estrogen target tissues [1]. Although numerous

B. Abderrahman · V. C. Jordan (✉)
Department of Breast Medical Oncology, University of Texas,
MD Anderson Cancer Center, Houston, TX, USA
e-mail: bhabderrahman@mdanderson.org; vcjordan@mdanderson.org

© Springer Nature Switzerland AG 2019
X. Zhang (ed.), *Estrogen Receptor and Breast Cancer*, Cancer Drug Discovery and Development, https://doi.org/10.1007/978-3-319-99350-8_7

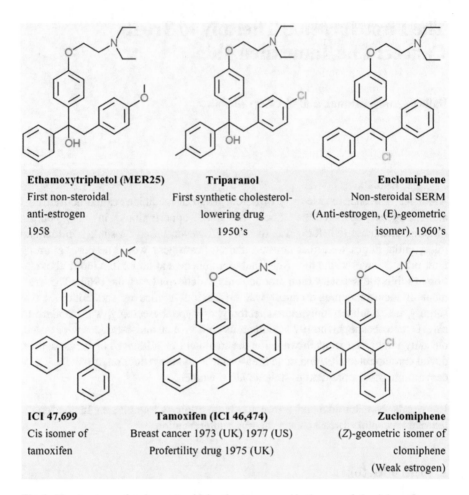

Fig. 1 The structures of early nonsteroidal anti-estrogens and in the case of clomiphene the separated geometric isomers and tamoxifen's estrogenic *cis*-isomer. Triparanol, a cholesterol lowering drug used clinically, is included to demonstrate structural similarities with the nonsteroidal anti-estrogens

applications were suggested for an anti-estrogen in therapeutics [2], it was the finding [3] that MER25 was an antifertility agent in animals that seized the enthusiasm of the pharmaceutical industry. This was because the oral contraceptive, which had recently been successfully tested in clinical trial, had revolutionized the approach to therapeutics. For the first time, individuals were being treated who had no disease. Naturally, Merrell moved forward with MER25, but it was found to be too toxic and of low potency for human use. MER25, however, was valuable as a research tool to study the mechanism of action of estrogen at estrogen target tissues. Dr. Elwood Jensen was the first to show that pretreatment of immature rats with MER25 prevented the uptake of administered [^{3}H] estradiol in the immature rat uterus (noted in the discussion of Emmens, Cox, and Martin "anti-estrogens" [4]).

Lerner was involved in Merrell's second anti-estrogen MRL41 or clomiphene [5] (Fig. 1). However, clomiphene is a mixture of cis- and trans-geometric isomers of a substituted triphenylethylene. Antifertility activity was noted in animals [5], but clinical testing demonstrated the induction of ovulation in subfertile women [6].

Clomiphene is only used in short 5-day courses for the induction of ovulation in subfertile women. This is because clomiphene interrupts cholesterol metabolism and increases the circulating levels of desmosterol. Merrell did not continue clinical testing for indications like breast cancer therapy because of the known link between high circulating levels of desmosterol and early cataract formation [7].

Earlier in the 1950s, Merrell had marketed a medicine called triparanol (Fig. 1) for individuals who needed to reduce their high circulating levels of cholesterol. Triparanol caused an increase in cataracts in young patients [8], and this was linked to increases in circulating desmosterol levels [7]. This litigious history mandated that Merrell would not market any agent that increased circulating desmosterol. Nevertheless, scientist at Merrell separated the cis- and trans-isomers of clomiphene [9] to determine whether they could improve the toxicology of clomiphene (Fig. 1). Unfortunately, they mislabeled the isomers: the trans-isomer was identified as an estrogen with no anti-estrogen actions, and the cis-isomer was misidentified as the anti-estrogenic isomer. None of this would have mattered had not other pharmaceutical companies rigorously investigated the structure function relationships of nonsteroidal anti-estrogens. The goal was to find the clinical use for a safe anti-estrogen.

The UpJohn Company mounted a huge investigation of the structure function relationships of fixed ring naphthalene-based antifertility agents. ICI Pharmaceuticals Division (now AstraZeneca) would follow but with a study of the antifertility properties of the separated isomers of substituted triphenylethylenes [10] (Fig. 1).

Nafoxidine derivatives established structure function relationships for the required position of the "anti-estrogenic side chain." Figure 2 summarizes the extensive structure functions relationship studies conducted on the 3-methoxy naphthalene core as experimental antifertility agents. The substitution on the p-phenyl ethoxyamine side chain is critical for antifertility activity in laboratory animals [11]. Similarly, the length of the para-substituted amino side chain of nafoxidine is critical for anti-estrogenic activity in animals [11, 12]. Indeed, Lednicer [11] suggested that a basic group, at a given position in space is required to obtain a molecule with estrogen antagonist activity. All compounds with a short side chain are estrogens. Indeed, the substitution of two methyl groups ortho to the anti-estrogenic side chain of MER25 [13] and tamoxifen [14] completely reduces anti-estrogenic actions in vivo. The movement of the anti-estrogenic side chain is restricted and cannot rotate and position itself correctly in the estrogen receptor (ER) binding domain.

It is important to appreciate the scale of these extensive animal studies on the antifertility properties of test compounds. In the early 1960s, studies to discover compounds of clinical relevance were only performed in vivo with an antifertility or

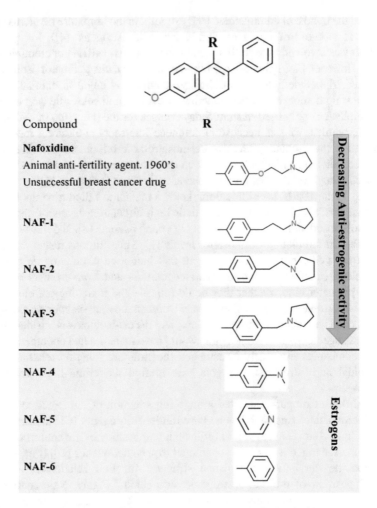

Fig. 2 The critical importance of the anti-estrogenic side chain R of nafoxidine to program anti-estrogenic activity of the steroidal anti-estrogen nafoxidine

anti-estrogenic endpoint in rats or mice. There was no reference to mechanisms of action via the ER as the work of Jensen [15, 16] and Gorski [17, 18] was only just starting and the notion of an ER was not universally accepted as the mechanism of estrogen action. Only the pharmacology of anti-estrogens would verify receptor status for the ER as a mediator of female physiology.

Nafoxidine entered clinical trials for the treatment of metastatic breast cancer (MBC) [19], but the ubiquitous side effects of photophobia and skin rashes caused industry to abandon clinical studies. The husband and wife Katzenellenbogen team pursued an analog U23,469 as a tool to understand the metabolic activation of nafoxidine derivatives through demethylation [20]. In addition, the change in the alkylaminoethoxy side chain was thought to reduce side effects noted with nafoxidine. Despite all of the setbacks with nafoxidine, this molecular scaffold proved to be important for medicinal chemist to create lasofoxifene [21], 30 years later. This molecule will be discussed in the companion chapter, "A Novel Strategy to Improve Women's Health: Selective Estrogen Receptor Modulators" (SERMs). The clinical pharmacology of lasofoxifene exhibits all the properties predicted for SERMs in the original vision statement [2]. The new clinical strategy was based on the early clinical studies with tamoxifen and laboratory studies with keoxifene which would subsequently be reinvented as raloxifene.

2   Tamoxifen Moves Forward Alone but with a Strategic Plan

Imperial Chemical Industry (ICI), now AstraZeneca, has a long history in the synthesis of novel nonsteroidal estrogens. The first chemical therapy for the successful treatment of any cancer was the use of high-dose synthetic estrogens for the treatment of MBC [22]. A response rate of 30% was observed in patients more than 5 years postmenopause [23]. The synthetic estrogens (Fig. 3) were synthesized by ICI Pharmaceuticals Division. Dr. Arthur Walpole, who would become the head of the fertility control program in the new facilities at Alderley Park [26], had an interest in determining which tumors would respond to high-dose estrogen therapy [24]. He was unsuccessful, but the clinical collaboration at the Christie Hospital in Manchester would be critical for the advance of ICI46,474 to become tamoxifen [27].

Harper and Walpole [10] first described the unusual pharmacological properties of the *cis*- and *trans*-isomers of a substituted triphenylethylene. ICI47,699 (*cis*) was estrogenic, but ICI46,474 (*trans*) was anti-estrogen in rats, but both compounds were estrogens in mouse vaginal cornification and uterine weight tests (Fig. 1). Synthesis, isomer separation, and X-ray crystallography proved isomer structure related to biology [28, 29]. The controversy concerning the reverse pharmacology [30] of the separated clomiphene isomers was settled appropriately by the Merrell company changing their isomer names to enclomiphene (*trans*) and zuclomiphene (*cis*) after the German entgegen (opposite) and zusammen (together) referring to the unsubstituted phenyls at the double bond of the ethylene scaffold (Fig. 1).

All laboratory efforts at Alderley Park focused entirely on the antifertility properties of ICI46,474 as a postcoital contraceptive [31–36]. Clinical testing, however, demonstrated that tamoxifen induced ovulation in subfertile women [37, 38]. Tamoxifen is approved for the induction of ovulations in some countries. The details of the design and development of a clinical plan for tamoxifen are documented in the personal postscript. The clinical strategy [39, 40] that was stated and translated was the following: (1) only use tamoxifen to treat ER-positive breast cancer patients, (2) use it long term (forever but starting with 5 years), and (3) tamoxifen can prevent mammary cancer in rats and (subsequently) in mice [41]. Chemoprevention was a possibility for women at high risk. However, very little was known about the clinical pharmacology of tamoxifen during long-term therapy, and there was no information about the metabolism and pharmacology of tamoxifen metabolites.

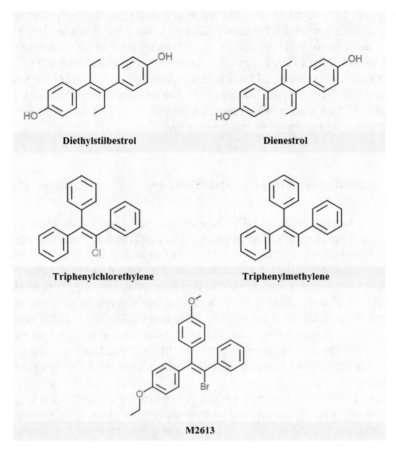

Fig. 3 Formulae of nonsteroidal estrogens used by Dr. A. L. Walpole in clinical studies with Edith Paterson at the Christie Hospital for the treatment of advanced breast cancer [24]. The compounds originally used by Haddow and coworkers (diethylstilbestrol, triphenylchlorethylene, triphenyl-methylethylene) [25] are illustrated for comparison

An examination of the metabolism of tamoxifen and the structure function relationships of nonsteroidal anti-estrogens will be addressed first, followed by a summary of the clinical advance with tamoxifen. Both aspects of the pharmacology of tamoxifen combined advanced the discovery of a new group of medicine referred to as SERMs.

3   The Metabolism of Tamoxifen

The original investigation of the metabolism of tamoxifen was conducted at Alderley Park [26] and published in 1973 [42, 43]. Administration of ^{14}C-labeled tamoxifen to rats, mice, monkeys, and dog demonstrated that the major route of excretion was via the feces. Dog and rat studies demonstrated that over 50% of the radioactivity was excreted via the bile duct and 70% was reabsorbed. There was enterohepatic recirculation. The hydroxylated metabolites were glucuronidated prior to biliary excretion, but there was no information about the biological properties of the three metabolites (Fig. 4) [42, 43]. The hydroxylated metabolites of tamoxifen were 4-hydroxytamoxifen and 3,4-dihydroxytamoxifen, and in the dog, a phenolic metabolite of tamoxifen formed by cutting off the dimethylaminoethyl side chain at the ether link to its phenyl group (metabolite E). A study in four women identified 4-hydroxytamoxifen as the primary metabolite [43]. However, the original technique of thin layer chromatography used to identify 4-hydroxytamoxifen was flawed [44], and N-desmethyltamoxifen was subsequently identified as the major metabolite of tamoxifen [45]. The side chain of tamoxifen was further metabolized (Fig. 5) to N-didesmethyltamoxifen (metabolite Z) [46] and deaminated to metabolite Y, a glycol derivative of tamoxifen [47, 48]. The next surprise, at the end of the 1980s, was the identification of 4-hydroxy-N-desmethyltamoxifen [49, 50]. The current status of tamoxifen metabolism is noted in Fig. 5; there is now evidence that two estrogenic metabolites of tamoxifen occur: metabolite E formed from tamoxifen and bisphenol formed from 4-hydroxytamoxifen [51].

The evaluation of the estrogenic and anti-estrogenic actions of the metabolites of tamoxifen provided a breakthrough for understanding estrogen and anti-estrogen

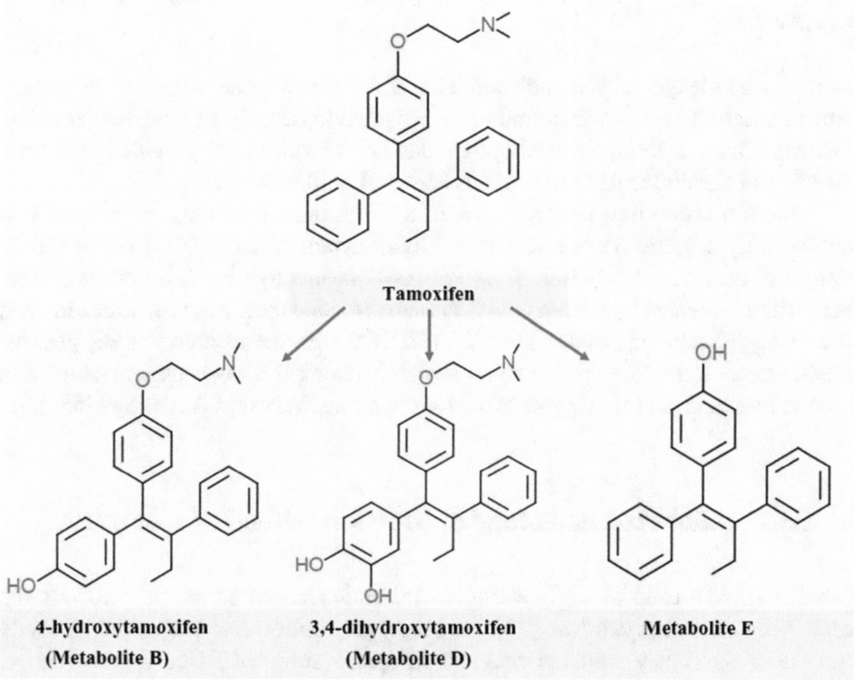

Fig. 4 The original hydroxylated metabolites of tamoxifen noted in animals [42]

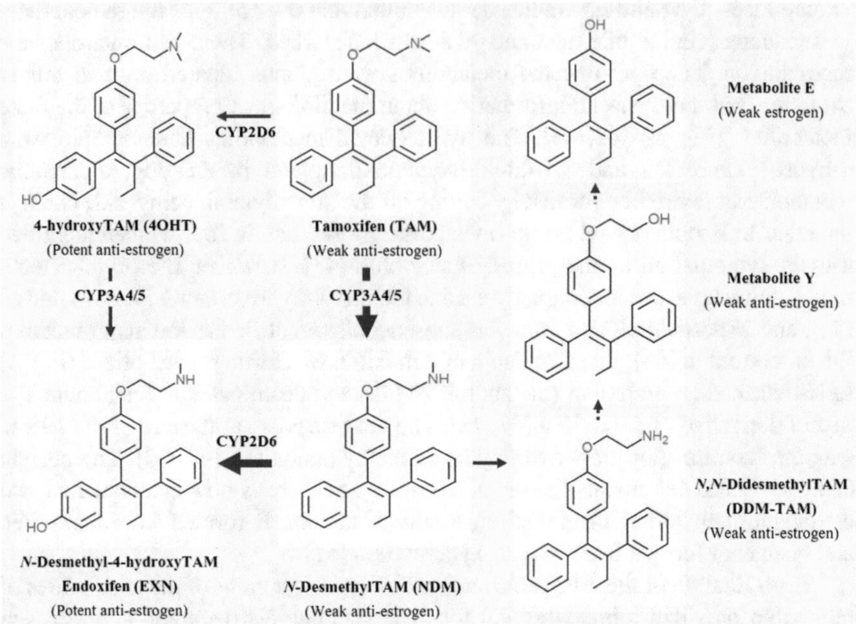

Fig. 5 The metabolic activation of tamoxifen to phenolic metabolites that have a high binding activity for the human estrogen receptor. Both 4-hydroxytamoxifen and endoxifen are potent anti-estrogens in vitro

action. Knowledge of the metabolites were the backbone structure to initiate structure-activity relationship studies investigated to develop new medicines called SERMs. Overall, these early investigations and clarifications provided an under-standing of the molecular mechanisms action of anti-estrogens.

Although tamoxifen possesses weak anti-estrogenic action, the molecule is activated by 4-hydroxylation to either 4-hydroxytamoxifen [52, 53] or the activa-tion of N-desmethyltamoxifen to 4-hydroxy-N-desmethyltamoxifen or endoxifen. Endoxifen is created by the enzyme CYP2D6 [54], and there has been much interest in linking the genomic mutation of the *CYP2D6* with the response of ER-positive breast cancer to tamoxifen treatment. Recently endoxifen has been reinvented as a second line of cancer therapy in MBC following the failure of AI therapy [55, 56].

4 Molecular Pharmacology of the Tamoxifen ER Complex

The first model used to study estrogen and anti-estrogen action in vitro was the MCF7 breast cancer cell line [57]. However, the results were perplexing. Despite the use of rigorously prepared charcoal-stripped serum, MCF7 cells grew with or without added estrogen [58]. Tamoxifen treatment alone caused a decline in cell growth that could be reversed by estrogen. Indeed, a comparison of MCF7 cells in vitro with MCF7 cell inoculated into ovariectomized athymic mice and treated with estrogen demonstrated estrogen-stimulated tumor growth in vivo but not in vitro [59]. This observation led to the idea that estrogen was stimulating a second messenger molecule in the athymic mouse that actually caused tumors to grow. A decade later the Katzenellenbogens discovered [60–62] that culture media indicator (phenol red) contained an estrogenic impurity and MCF7 cells were already growth-stimulated before adding estradiol. Their discovery opened the door to molecular studies of estrogen/anti-estrogen action in breast cancer. Nevertheless, studies in vitro of estrogen-stimulated prolactin synthesis [63], in disrupted anterior pituitary gland cells from immature mice, set the scene to understand estrogen/anti-estrogen action at the level of the ER complex. Cancer cell sensitivity to estrogen as a growth stimulus is extraordinarily low in the range of 10^{-12} M for estradiol. Protein synthesis is regulated at 10–100 logs higher concentration.

5 The Molecular Modulation of Prolactin Synthesis via the ER

Studies in vitro avoid the complications of metabolism in vivo and identify the actions of each metabolite or compound as an estrogen, anti-estrogen, or partial agonist. Studies, in vitro with tamoxifen, its metabolites, and tamoxifen derivatives that could not be metabolically activated to high affinity for 4-hydroxytamoxifen, established a direct and reversible inhibition of estrogen-stimulated prolactin synthesis via the ER [64]. Additionally, ER binding ligands were predictably classified into agonist, partial agonist, and antagonist based upon structure [65–68]. A hypothetical pharmacological model (Fig. 6) of the ER binding domain/ligand interaction could predictably convert an agonist ligand to antagonist based on the length and positioning of the bulky anti-estrogenic side chain of triphenylethylene derivatives [66, 70].

A parallel collaborative study, using both monoclonal antibodies and a goat polyclonal antibody to the human ER, provided valuable supporting evidence for the molecular models developed by the modulation of prolactin synthesis. The [^{3}H] labeled 4-hydroxytamoxifen and [^{3}H] estradiol were compared and contrasted in human breast cancer and rat pituitary tumor ER [71, 72]. The monoclonal antibodies did not detect differences in the ligand ER complex [73]. By contrast, preincubation of the polyclonal antibody with human breast or rat pituitary tumor ER prevented [^{3}H] estradiol binding, but [^{3}H] 4-hydroxytamoxifen binding was unaffected by preincubation. A model was proposed, whereby estradiol binds and is locked into the ER complex with the ligand sealed within the protein complex. By contrast, the anti-estrogen binds within the ligand-binding domain, but the bulky anti-estrogenic side chain ensures that the ligand remains wedged within the receptor (Fig. 7). The mechanism was referred [74] to as "the crocodile model": planar estradiol is sealed within the jaws of the crocodile, but 4-hydroxytamoxifen binds

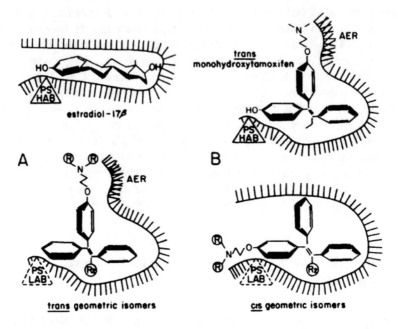

Fig. 6 Hypothetical models for estrogenic and anti-estrogenic ligands binding to the estrogen receptor. Estradiol-17β is anchored at a phenolic site (PS) with high affinity binding (HAB). *Trans*-monohydroxytamoxifen has the same high affinity binding, but this anti-estrogenic ligand binds to the receptor site so that the alkylaminoethoxy side chain can interact with a hypothetical anti-estrogen region (AER) on the protein. Compounds without a phenolic hydroxyl have low affinity binding (LAB). The *trans*- and *cis*-geometric isomers refer to (**a**) tamoxifen (R1 = CH₃, R₂, = C₂H₅) and enclomiphene (R = C₂H₅, R₂ = Cl) and (**b**) ICI 47,699 (R = CH₃, R = C₂H₅) and zuclomiphene (R = C₂H₅, R₂ = Cl). Reproduced with permission from [69]

with high affinity, but the bulky side chain is like "a stick in the jaws of the crocodile" to prevent closure. Indeed, Lieberman and coworkers [70] (Fig. 6) predicted that there was an "anti-estrogenic region" that interacts with the dimethylalkylaminoethoxyphenyl side chain of 4-hydroxytamoxifen. This "anti-estrogenic region" was subsequently identified as amino acid 351 [75] (Fig. 8), evaluated in molecular pharmacology studies [77–81], and physically identified by comparing and contrasting the molecular fit of 4-hydroxytamoxifen and raloxifene by X-ray crystallography [82, 83]. Amino acid asp351 is important for interaction with the anti-estrogenic side chain of SERMs to modulate the estrogen-like actions of the SERM-ER complex. Extensive studies of the relationship of the nitrogen-containing side chain of SERMs with different amino acids at asp351 are informative [77–81]. This interaction is important to prevent helix 12 appropriately sealing the ligand within the ER complex. Modulation with agonists, partial agonists, and antagonist creates the range of SERM/agonist/antagonist action. Indeed, the essential nature of this well-studied amino acid asp351 [77–81] has recently been identified as a significant form of acquired resistance in aromatase inhibitor therapy. Amino acid

Proposed Model

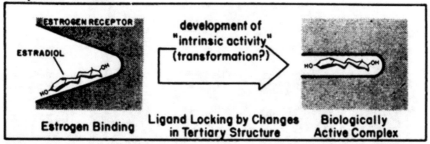

Effect of Ab Preincubation

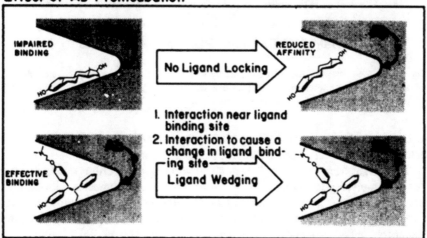

Effect of Ab After Ligand Binding

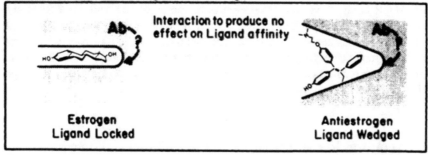

Fig. 7 Effect of goat polyclonal antibody (Ab) on the binding of estradiol and monohydroxy-tamoxifen to the ligand-binding site on the ER. Reproduced with permission from [71]

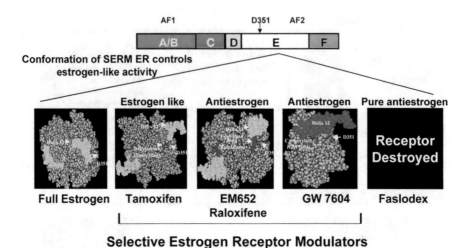

Fig. 8 The modulation of the ERα complex by interaction of the anti-estrogenic side chain of SERMs with surface amino acid D351. Data adapted from X-ray crystallography and the biology of complexes. Reproduced with permission from [76]

asp351 seals the unoccupied ER by binding to mutant amino acids at 537, 538 in helix 12 [84]. This unoccupied complex stimulates tumor growth.

The insight from Lednicer [11], some 50 years ago, is worth restating "a basic group, at a given position in space, is required to obtain a molecule with estrogen antagonist activity." The aforementioned events illustrate the continuum of research into ER-regulated events that traveled to a successful conclusion from (1) medicinal chemistry applied to define anti-estrogen action in vivo [11, 12, 85], (2) the discovery of a mutant amino acid asp351tyr in a natural model of drug resistance to tamoxifen in breast cancer [75, 77] that modulates estrogenic/anti-estrogenic action of the SERM-ER complex via a conversation of amino acids 351 with the SERM side chain [77–81], (3) the actual identification and proof of the "crocodile model" of estrogen/anti-estrogen side chain interacting with amino acid 351 revealed by X-ray crystallography (Fig. 8) (4) to the present with the autostimulation of AI-resistant breast cancer recurrence with mutant ER at amino acids 537/538 closing the empty ER with helix 12 at amino acid 351 [84].

6 Acquired Resistance to Tamoxifen, Clinical Endocrinology, and Long-Term Clinical Pharmacology

The use of models to determine mechanisms of tamoxifen action provides an insight into tamoxifen metabolism in various animal species and patients [86, 87]. The proposal, in the 1970s, to deploy long-term, i.e., 5 years or indefinite, adjuvant tamoxifen therapy, mandated an evaluation of tamoxifen treatment in patients over time [88]. One concern, based on studies of acquired resistance to tamoxifen in athymic mice [89], was that long-term therapy might encourage the induction of metabolic pathways that produced estrogenic metabolites to simulate tumor growth. Tamoxifen was known to have a species-specific pharmacology, i.e., tamoxifen is an estrogen in mice [10], an anti-estrogen with partial estrogen-like properties in rats [31], and anti-estrogenic properties in chickens [90].

A standard model to study the actions of tamoxifen in vivo was the athymic mouse inoculated with breast cancer cells [57]. Continuous tamoxifen treatment of athymic mice transplanted with MCF-7 breast tumors, eventually results, demonstrates that tamoxifen cannot prevent breast cancer growth during a year of tamoxifen treatment [91]. This was important. One possibility was hormone-independent growth during tamoxifen treatment. Acquired resistance to treatment would then occur if the mouse model had amplification of metabolic enzymes that convert tamoxifen to high levels of estrogenic metabolites. The issue was clarified when tamoxifen-treated tumors were retransplanted tumors into a fresh generation of athymic mice. The discovery that tumors grew because of either tamoxifen or low-dose estrogen, not despite tamoxifen treatment, was unique. Molecular mechanisms have subsequently been deciphered [92, 93] and are summarized in Fig. 9. Additionally, studies [94] were conducted in athymic rats, where the pharmacology of tamoxifen is predominantly anti-estrogenic. Tamoxifen-stimulated tumor growth occurred in athymic rats. Therefore, it was the direct effect of the tamoxifen on the tumor rather than the host that was important.

These studies, and the successful testing of the first selective ER disrupter [95] SERD ICI 164,384 in the model of acquired resistance to tamoxifen, led to the development of fulvestrant [96] and the clinical evaluation of second-line treatments following the development of acquired tamoxifen resistance in MBC. Clinical trials, a decade later, demonstrated that either an aromatase inhibitor (anastrozole) or fulvestrant was equally effective second-line treatments [97, 98]. Tamoxifen-stimulated tumor growth has been demonstrated with a withdrawal response in the clinic [99].

Tamoxifen acts as an anti-estrogen to interfere with the hypothalamo-pituitary-ovarian access in premenopausal patients. There is an increase in ovarian secretion of estradiol and its metabolites [100]. Ovulation is triggered as evidenced by rises in progesterone secretion [101]. In postmenopausal patients, there are partial decreases in luteinizing hormone (LH) and follicle-stimulating hormone (FSH). Additionally, there are increases in antithrombin III and sex hormone binding globulin as an indication of the estrogen-like activity of tamoxifen and its metabolites [102]. At this point, it was important to establish whether the induction of tamoxifen-metabolizing enzymes occurs during long-term adjuvant therapy. Patients were monitored for up to 10 years, but no estrogenic metabolites were observed [88]. Results demonstrated stability for tamoxifen and its metabolites over this time period.

In the final sections, the clinical applications of tamoxifen will be summarized. Tamoxifen pioneered long-term anti-estrogen therapy for breast cancer. Additionally tamoxifen was successfully tested as a chemopreventative in high-risk pre- and postmenopausal women to reduce the incidence of breast cancer.

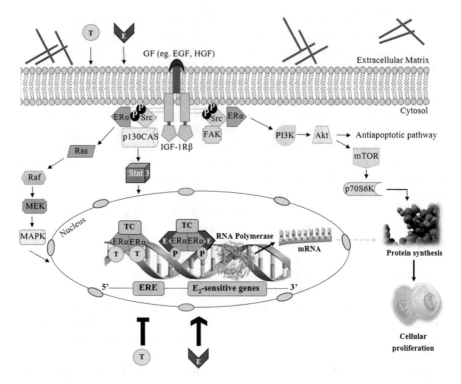

Fig. 9 Genomic and nongenomic signal transduction pathways in tamoxifen-resistant model. E_2 and TAM exert differential functions on nuclear ER. E_2 activates classical ER-target genes, but TAM acts to block gene activation. Both E_2 and TAM increase the nongenomic activity of ER through membrane-associated molecules such as c-Src, IGF-1Rβ, and FAK to enhance downstream signaling cascades. *IGF-1Rβ* insulin-like growth factor-1 receptor beta, *FAK* focal adhesion kinase, *c-Src* proto-oncogene tyrosine-protein kinase, *T* tamoxifen, *E* estrogen, *ERE* estrogen response element, *TC* transcription complex, *GF* growth factor, *MAPK* mitogen-activated protein kinase, *PI3K* phosphatidylinositol-4,5-bisphosphate 3-kinase

7 Long-Term Adjuvant Tamoxifen Therapy: The Prelude to Prevention

The initial testing of adjuvant tamoxifen therapy was cautious with a duration of 1 or 2 years [103]. This cautious approach, by the clinical community, was based upon their knowledge that tamoxifen was only effective for the treatment of MBC in 30% of patients for 2–3 years. However, the effectiveness of adjuvant tamoxifen therapy was based upon the fact that tamoxifen was preventing the estrogen-stimulated growth of micrometastatic disease and not the high tumor burden and mutational plasticity of MBC. The paradox with increases in survival with adjuvant tamoxifen was that tamoxifen is not a cytotoxic therapy. Clinical trials demonstrated long-term benefit following long-term adjuvant tamoxifen therapy [104, 105]. This is referred to as "the carryover effect." To explain decreases in recurrences and mortality, after tamoxifen therapy stops, it is proposed that tamoxifen exerts continuous selection pressure on ER-positive populations of breast cancer cells which become resistant and ultimately sensitive to estrogen to initiate apoptosis [106].

There was initial caution about advancing adjuvant tamoxifen therapy beyond 5 years. This decision was made by building extension upon results from the 5-year NSABP node-negative trial B14 [107]. The new trial design was to compare and contrast women with node-negative disease who received either 5 years of tamoxifen or 10 years of tamoxifen [108]. The results demonstrated that patients receiving 10 years of tamoxifen had a higher increase in side effects but no therapeutic benefit was noted.

The EBCTCG lead the way with extrapolation of the benefits of tamoxifen. A recent evaluation of 15 years of follow-up of the efficacy of 5 years of adjuvant tamoxifen therapy demonstrates that despite the "carryover effect," recurrences occur relentlessly. These recurrences are predictable, with more recurrences occurring for patients that had a large primary tumor and large numbers of lymph nodes involved [109]. This begs the question: Is longer going to be better than shorter adjuvant therapy if 5 years is extended to 10 years of tamoxifen treatment?

Initial analysis of the Adjuvant Tamoxifen: Longer Against Shorter (ATLAS) trial demonstrates both a decrease in recurrences for longer tamoxifen treatment and mortality decreases between 5 and 10 years of tamoxifen. However, the effect on mortality is only evident in the 5 years after 10 years of tamoxifen is completed [110]. A similar trial referred to as adjuvant Tamoxifen Treatment offers more (aTTom) has only been reported in abstract form. Nevertheless, data has been pooled [111] for ATLAS and aTTom demonstrating high significance for longer against shorter in recurrence and decreases in mortality. Nevertheless, it is important to ensure that strategies are devised to identify and treat only those patients at high risk of recurrence. It should not be forgotten that the rules of acquired resistance to tamoxifen treatment are relentless and consistent with all antihormone therapies. Rather than continuing adjuvant tamoxifen, in the words of author Basil A. Stoll "as a mindless exercise" [112], we need to develop an algorithm for who to treat and for how long.

The change in clinical care with a cheap and proven adjuvant treatment strategy for ER-positive breast cancer naturally caused an interest in the prevention of breast cancer in women at high risk. Three critical pieces of information all indicated that tamoxifen could reduce the risk of developing primary breast cancer. (1) Animal models demonstrated that tamoxifen could prevent chemical carcinogenesis in rats and spontaneous mammary carcinogenesis in high [113]- risk strains of mice [41]. (2) Tamoxifen prevented contralateral breast cancer during adjuvant therapy administered to prevent recurrence after the first breast cancer had been removed surgically [114]. (3) Clinical trials demonstrated the safety of tamoxifen during the treatment of node-negative breast cancer. There is only a 15–20% recurrence rate for node-negative ER-positive breast cancer, so the majority of patients treated in trials remain cancer-free for decades. In effect, these node-negative clinical trials acted as an evaluation of tamoxifen in women without cancer.

8   The Chemoprevention of Breast Cancer: A Flawed Strategy

The prevention of breast cancer in women is not a new idea. Professor Antoine Lacassagne stated at the American Association for Cancer Research in 1936 [115]:

> "If one accepts the consideration of adenocarcinoma of the breast as the consequence of special hereditary sensibility to the proliferative actions of estrone, one is led to imagine a therapeutic preventive for subjects predisposed by their heredity to this cancer. It would consist-perhaps in the very near future when the knowledge and use of hormones will be better understood – in the suitable use of a hormone antagonist or excretory, to prevent the stagnation of estrone in the ducts of the breast."

Some 50 years later, it was possible to consider chemoprevention as a realistic clinical opportunity. Dr. Trevor Powels took the first bold step at the Royal Marsden Hospital to initiate a pilot study of tamoxifen in women with known risk factors for breast cancer. The results of the pilot study, published in 1989 [116], justified the strategy based on two facts: (1) tamoxifen prevents rat mammary carcinogenesis [113]. (2) Short-term (2 years) adjuvant tamoxifen treatment for breast cancer caused a decrease in contralateral breast cancer [116].

Four large randomized clinical trials were initiated during the 1990s: (1) the Royal Marsden Study, (2) the NSABP P-1 Study, (3) the Italian Study, and (4) the International Breast Cancer Intervention Study (IBIS). The studies as a whole can be summarized (Table 1). The NSABP P-1 trial [117] demonstrated an approximate 50% decrease in breast cancer incidence for both pre- and postmenopausal high-risk women. There were no significant reductions in breast cancer incidence in the Italian study [118], but this was to be expected as the women were of normal risk and there was an added complication of allowing women to take hormone replacement therapy.

The overall value of chemoprevention with tamoxifen is limited. The public health strategy failed for two main reasons: (1) a thousand high-risk women need to

Table 1 Comparison of the tamoxifen randomized chemoprevention trials

Characteristics	Royal Marsden	NSABP	Italian	IBIS
Patient population	2471	13,388	5408	7152
Women/years of follow-up	12,355	46,856	5408	29,800
Women <50 years old (%)	62	40	36	52
Breast cancer incidence per 1000				
Tamoxifen	4.7	3.4	2.1	4.7
Placebo	6.7	5.5	2.3	6.7
Side effects				
Endometrial cancer[a]	13/5	36/15	–	13/5
Tamoxifen/placebo	14/9	35/22	–	64/38
Pulmonary embolism	Not reported	18/6	–	44/32

[a]Endometrial cancer was only significantly evaluated in postmenopausal women

be treated to benefit two or three individuals annually. (2) The side effects of tamoxifen are great enough to convince high-risk women not to engage in this strategy.

Despite the fact that tamoxifen is the first FDA-approved preventive, the strategy is both unrealistic and imprecise. Indeed, physicians themselves discount chemo-prevention, and recent studies show there is a remarkable lack to knowledge by general practitioners concerning the potential benefits for select high-risk women [119]. The solution for society was the discovery of SERMs, which will be considered in the companion chapter.

9 Conclusion

Tamoxifen is a successful lifesaving drug because of the translational research strategy of targeting the breast tumor ER and applying long-term adjuvant therapy. There were initial faltering steps toward development of the clinical strategy. Most importantly, an anti-estrogenic medicine was an unlikely path to progress competing in a world dominated by cytotoxic chemotherapy that was predicted to cure cancer. Nevertheless, individuals working together in concerts made the medicine become a pioneer, as the first of a new group of medicines called SERMs.

Personal Postscript V. Craig Jordan

Dr. Elwood Jensen dedicated his career to describe the target for successful therapeutics in breast tumor—the ER. His basic work in the early 1960s established the presence of ER in estrogen target tissues, e.g., uterus, vagina, and pituitary gland of laboratory rats [15, 16]. His collaborative team of clinicians then translated the laboratory research to patients [120] with metastatic breast cancer. The team found a positive correlation between ER in MBA and adrenalectomy. Breast cancer that was ER-negative was less likely to respond. This work catalyzed efforts to create the ER assay in breast tumors in order to predict whether patients would respond to ablative endocrine therapy, i.e., oophorectomy, adrenalectomy, or hypophysectomy [121].

The nonsteroidal anti-estrogen ICI46,474 was discovered in the 1960s in the fertility control program at Alderley Park, the research headquarters of ICI Pharmaceuticals Division in Cheshire, England [26]. The description in the patent was: "The alkene derivatives of the invention are useful for the modification of the endocrine status in man and animals and they may be useful for the control of hormone dependent tumors or for the management of the sexual cycle and aberrations thereof. They also have useful hypocholesterolaemic activity." The patent history of tamoxifen is unique. The United Kingdom patent was published in 1965 but denied in the United States until 1985. Merrell had defensive patenting of triphenylethylenes. By the time patent protection was lost everywhere in the world but America, where there was no patent, the 17-year patent life started. This was just as the NCI recommended adjuvant tamoxifen therapy as standard of care [122].

In the 1960s, the team of Dr. Dora Richardson (chemist) had synthesized the substituted triphenylethylene (Fig. 10) and separated the product into pure *cis-* and

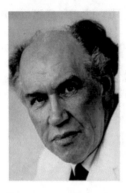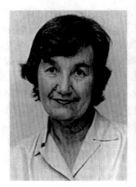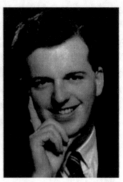

Fig. 10 The principal players in the discovery of ICI 46,474 at ICI Pharmaceuticals Division, Cheshire, UK, in the 1960s that eventually evolved into tamoxifen a decade later. Arthur Walpole (Walop) (left) was the head of the fertility control program tasked with the mission to discover safer compounds to "regulate the sexual cycle." Dora Richardson (center), the team organic chemist who synthesized all of the isomers of the triphenylethylene derivatives that would be tested as antifertility agents in rats by Mike Harper, the team reproductive endocrinologist. Arthur Walpole would be VCJ's PhD examiner, scientific supporter, and administrative link to ICI until his untimely death on July 2, 1977. Dora Richardson would provide the metabolites of tamoxifen to the author to be tested as anticancer agents, and Mike Harper would offer the author a 2-year BTA (Been to America) at the Worcester Foundation, MA. Each individual was generous with important opportunities, investment, and support for a young investigator starting their adventure to investigate "failed morning after pills" as future important therapeutic agents in women's health

trans-isomers [28]; Dr. MJK Harper (reproductive biologist) and Walpole had described the *cis*-isomer, ICI 47,699, as an estrogen in rats and mice and the *trans*-isomer ICI 46,474 as an anti-estrogen in rats but with weak estrogen-like actions [10]. Strangely enough ICI 46,474 was classified as an estrogen both in mouse vaginal cornification assays [10] and in immature mouse uterine weight tests [123]. This biological knowledge was pivotal for the subsequent discovery of SERMs some 20 years later at the University of Wisconsin, Madison.

However, by 1972, all clinical data was reviewed at ICI Pharmaceuticals Division and the decision made to terminate development [124]. The product was not predicted to recover sufficient revenues to support marketing in the niche area of the induction of ovulation in subfertile women and the treatment of metastatic breast cancer. In the case of MBC, only one in three tumors responded, and responses were only for a year or 2. The head of the fertility control program at ICI Pharmaceuticals Division in 1972 was Dr. Arthur Walpole [125]. He chose to take early retirement if ICI 46,474 was abandoned for clinical development as a drug to treat breast cancer.

In 1972, I was completing my PhD at Leeds University, Department of Pharmacology, on the structure function relationships and contraceptive properties of nonsteroidal anti-estrogens in mice. However, no academic faculty member in the United Kingdom would agree to examine my thesis on "A study of the oestrogenic and anti-oestrogenic activities of some substituted triphenylethylene and ethane's" (or failed contraceptive for short!), but this is how life takes an unpredictable turn.

The research facility for ICI Pharmaceuticals in Cheshire, Alderley Park [26], was 10 miles from my home. In 1967, I had wanted to be a summer student at Alderley Park, but how could I get an interview. I had read Dr. Steven Carter's publications in Nature [126]. He was a cell biologist at Alderley Park studying mouse cancer cells. Cancer research is what I wanted to do. I decided to take a bus to Alderley Park and phoned Dr. Carter from the phone box outside the research facility. I was connected to Dr. Carter through the Alderley Park Operator—"Hello Dr. Carter, my name is Craig Jordan and I am a student at the University of Leeds, but I live nearby Alderley Park in Bramhall. I have read your publications in Nature on cytochalasins and I wonder whether you had room in your laboratory for me as a summer student?" He replied "Next time you are home in Bramhall, arrange to have an interview with me." I told him I was calling from outside the front gate of Alderley Park. He invited me in immediately and I got the job!

I was excited, as a pharmacology student at the University of Leeds, to be witnessing research and discovery first hand. I learned electron microscopy, listened to all of their weekly research lectures, and spent hours in their library. I was in heaven! By strange coincidence, years later, cytochalasins were used in rat pituitary tumors GH_3 cells to demonstrate that the unoccupied ER was located in the nucleus [127]. The same technique was used in my laboratory using MCF-7 breast cancer cells [128].

In the cardiovascular laboratory next door to Dr. Carter's laboratory was Dr. Michael Barrett. He was head of the β-blocker program at Alderley Park. Dr. Walpole's fertility control group had laboratories opposite to Dr. Carters'. Dr. Walpole had just published his papers on ICI46,474 [10, 31]. I went out for lunch in Alderley Edge each Friday with all of his laboratory staff. All the scientists who would later influence my life surrounded me that summer in 1967.

In 1971, Professor Michael Barrett became head of the Department of Pharmacology at the University of Leeds. He recruited me to be a lecturer in pharmacology and convinced the university authorities that Dr. Walpole would be an appropriate examiner for my PhD thesis despite the fact that he was "from industry." Professor Barrett and Dr. Walpole secured a 2-year visiting scientist position for me working at the Worcester Foundation for Experimental Biology (WFEB) in America. Their friend and former colleague Dr. Michael Harper was working to produce a once-a-month contraceptive based on the emerging pharmacology of prostaglandins. Therefore, off to the WFEB, I went to immerse myself in contraception research.

The WFEB is the "home of the oral contraceptive," but what I really wanted to do, as a pharmacologist, was to devise medicines to treat cancer. However, this was considered a very high-risk enterprise. Few were interested, in new therapeutic methods of treating cancer, as the favored approach was to use combination cytotoxic chemotherapy. Numerous toxic side effects for patients were life threatening. Nevertheless, cytotoxic chemotherapy was predicted to cure all cancers despite the fact that the therapy also targeted normal dividing cells.

When I arrived at the WFEB, I was shocked to discover that my supervisor, Dr. Michael Harper, had planned to leave immediately as he had secured a position at the World Health Organization heading their contraception program. My new boss Dr. Edward Klaiber (Fig. 11) was most generous, allowing my family to stay at his home in Princeton, MA, while he and his wife Jennie were in Austria for 2 weeks. He even lent me his car, an unheard event in England! Dr. Klaiber said that I should plan my 2 years of work on prostaglandins. He had inherited the large contraception program grant awarded by the USAID to Dr. Harper, and that grant was paying my salary. Other than that, I was free to study anything I liked as long as I got funding. That was the WFEB way. By lucky chance, in 1971, President Nixon had signed the National Cancer Act. The goal was to take treatment strategies and new medicines from the bench to the bedside. Now was my opportunity to work on cancer.

I was unaware that ICI46,474 was not planning to develop ICI46,474 despite having low toxicity and showing modest activity in MBC [27]. The advantage of tamoxifen compared with other endocrine therapies was reduced side effects. Clomiphene had been successfully tested earlier [129] so the approach was not new. A phone call to Dr. Walpole secured his support to study ICI46,474 in the laboratory, but he had to arrange with Stuart Pharmaceuticals, ICI's new acquisition in Wilmington, Delaware, to provide funding. He succeeded and I met the drug monitor for ICI46,474 Lois Trench (Fig. 12). She was tasked with initiating clinical studies, and she claimed I was just what she needed, a scientist who knew the literature on anti-estrogens. I had knowledge of current thinking about the ER and would

Fig. 11 The award of an honorary Doctor of Science degree from the University of Massachusetts (2001) for laboratory work started at the WFEB that resulted in the evaluations of tamoxifen for the prevention of breast cancer in high-risk women. On the right of Dr. Jordan is Dr. Edward Klaiber and his wife Jeannie (far right). Dr. Klaiber was Dr. Jordan's "boss" at the WFEB

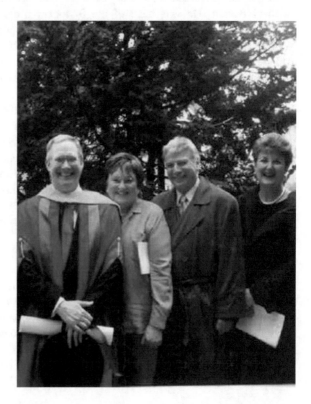

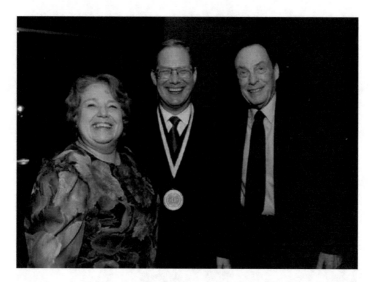

Fig. 12 Lois Trench and Dr. Elwood Jensen on the occasion of Dr. Jordan's investiture as the Diana, Princess of Wales, Professor of Cancer Research at Northwestern University (1999). Lois Trench the energetic and committed clinical monitor for ICI America for tamoxifen clinical trials in North America. She accomplished the FDA approval of tamoxifen in America in record time on December 30, 1977. Lois is the godmother of Dr. Jordan's daughter Alexandra

subsequently speak to clinicians from the Eastern Cooperative Oncology Group (ECOG) and the National Surgical Breast and Bowel Project (NSABP). However, the problem I was tasked with by Dr. Walpole was (to paraphrase) "we will put tamoxifen on the market, your task is to devise a strategy how best to use the medicine." Even to me it was obvious that treating MBC with tamoxifen was futile; everybody died. I planned first to train myself in methods in cancer research pertaining to breast cancer but how? That problem was solved for me by the signing of the National Cancer Act in 1971 and now being free to do research at the WFEB.

Dr. Elwood V. Jensen (Figs. 12 and 13), Director of the Ben May Laboratory for Cancer Research at the University of Chicago, had been appointed, to the Scientific Advisory Board of the WFEB. He was asked to encourage the exploitation of the rich knowledge of endocrinology at the foundation but now to apply it to cancer research and treatment. Dr. Jensen was to visit the WFEB in late 1972. I, as the only person with in-depth knowledge of estrogen and anti-estrogen action, was asked to make myself available to meet Dr. Jensen.

I was invited to go out to dinner in Worcester with a small group of faculty to entertain Dr. Jensen. During the following day, Dr. Jensen and I were to meet for scientific discussions. I explained my ideas for ICI46,474 and showed him my thesis on "failed contraceptives." Later in the afternoon, he gave a major presentation before the whole of the WFEB. Imagine my surprise when he mentioned our discussion about ICI46,474 and my plans for new strategies to treat breast cancer.

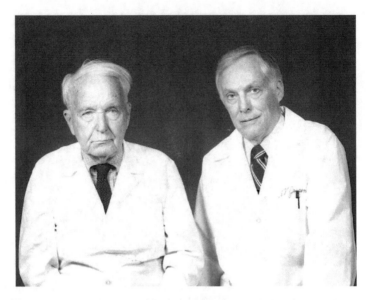

Fig. 13 Professor Charles Huggins (left) and Elwood Jensen, the founding Director and subsequent Director of the Ben May Laboratory for Cancer Research at the University of Chicago. Huggins was to receive the Nobel Prize in Physiology and Medicine for his work on androgen action and Jensen the Lasker Award for estrogen action

Following our meeting in late 1972, Dr. Jensen (Fig. 12) invited me to Chicago to learn ER assays on breast tumors. I was taught by Sylvia Smith and Elwood's staff at the Ben May Laboratory for Cancer Research. Additionally, I met the Nobel Laureate and former Director, Professor Charles Huggins (Fig. 13). At the Ben May Laboratory, Dr. Gene DeSombre taught me the DMBA-induced rat mammary carcinoma model (aka the "Huggins model") [130].

The WFEB had secured a contract from the NCI to measure ER in breast cancer. To expand our knowledge, Drs. Chris Longcorpe, David Kupfer, and I went off to San Antonio to learn ER measurement techniques in Dr. Bill McGuire's laboratory. Some of our analytical results on endometrial cancers were subsequently published [131]. Armed with all this cutting-edge technology and the DMBA model, I set about my task to initiate a systematic study of the anticancer actions of tamoxifen (still ICI46,474 at the time). My first experiment, and my first paper, replicated a study of high-dose subcutaneous injections of H774 and H1076, in ovariectomized mice [132, 133] published by Professor Cliff Emmens in Australia. These nonsteroidal anti-estrogens were similar to tamoxifen, so I used tamoxifen instead. Initial estrogenic effect on ovariectomized mouse vagina occurred for about a week, but then the vagina became refractory to estrogen stimulation for 6 weeks thereafter [134]. This, my first publication (single author as I did all the work), was accepted with two minor spelling changes. Well that never happened again! I was, however, formulating an idea that perhaps depot injections of tamoxifen might be the way to prevent breast cancer in women. First, I chose to address a controversy that some investigators could not demonstrate that tamoxifen blocked estrogen binding to the ER. This was addressed using sucrose density gradient analysis at the WFEB using the technique and equipment provided by Dr. Jensen. The result was clear. In both breast and endometrial tumors, tamoxifen blocked the binding of [³H] estradiol to the 8S estrogen receptor [135]. So if the ER was a drug target, could a couple of tamoxifen injections prevent DMBA-induced rat mammary carcinogenesis? Again, the results were clear; two consecutive peanut oil sc injections of 5 mg tamoxifen given simultaneously with 20 mg of DMBA to 50-day-old female Sprague-Dawley rats inhibited rat mammary carcinogenesis by 95%! News traveled fast at the foundation, and Dr. Ferdinand Peron came into my lab exclaiming "My God, you have cured cancer; tell me about it!" I explained it was obvious. If oophorectomy prevents rat mammary carcinogenesis, then an "anti-estrogen" should accomplish the same result. I wrote up my work for the European Journal of Cancer and sent it off. The three referees recommended rejection, but one referee (I suspect Dr. Walpole) made a list of good suggestions, which I followed when I returned to Leeds. I did additional well-controlled experiments, and my paper was rewritten, resubmitted, and accepted [113].

I also submitted an abstract to the International Congress of Steroid Endocrinology in Mexico City. This abstract was accepted and presented orally. Dr. Marc Lippman then at the National Cancer Institute, heading their Breast Cancer Program, asked several questions because he too was seduced into tamoxifen research by Lois Trench. He subsequently published an important paper in Nature [58] in 1975. Indeed, it was that paper and the statement "the phenomenon of tamoxifen killing is invariably reversible if estradiol is added to the medium by 48 hours even though the anti-estrogen remains in the medium." That observation led me to address the issue of adjuvant therapy with tamoxifen. How long was long enough to control recurrence if tamoxifen was used as an adjuvant therapy? Did tamoxifen destroy breast cancer cells in vivo? At that time, the clinical community had selected 1 year of tamoxifen after mastectomy because they knew that tamoxifen only controls MBC for a year or 2 [103]. Maybe this strategy would work if tamoxifen did kill breast cancer cells.

Back at the Department of Pharmacology, at the University of Leeds, we chose to complete a study of dose escalation for 1 month of treatment starting at 1 month after the oral administration of 20 mg DMBA dissolved in peanut oil. The scientific goal was to determine whether tamoxifen could kill the micro-foci of precancerous and early microscopic mammary cancer.

Karen Allen (now Porter) and my PhD student Clive Dix showed that increasing daily sc doses of tamoxifen administered for a month caused a dose-dependent delay in mammary carcinogenesis [136–138]. Knowledge that the injections of the lipophilic compound ICI46,474 formed a depot for slow release, and the fact that tamoxifen has a long half-life in animals and humans [42, 43], led to the conclusion that continuous treatment was necessary to suppress rat mammary carcinogenesis completely [137, 138]. So it proved to be.

These data were obtained because of the financial investment of Dr. Arthur Walpole, Roy Cotton (the initial physician at ICI Pharmaceuticals Division responsible for initiating the clinical development of tamoxifen), and Brian Newbold (Research Director) into the laboratory of a young scientist with a plan "to target the ER in breast cancer, to use long-term adjuvant tamoxifen therapy (my battle cry was 'tamoxifen forever'), and open the door for chemoprevention studies with tamoxifen." On July 2, 1977, Arthur Walpole died suddenly. This was only 6 months after his recruitment. I attended the church service with the ICI pharmaceuticals staff, and at the time, the Research Director, Dr. Brian Newbold, reassured me that Alderley Park would maintain its support for my progress at the University of Leeds. We were now making enormous progress with my new strategy, but Dr. Walpole, my friend and supporter, would never see the results of his discovery of ICI46,474.

In 1978, the Pharmaceuticals Division was to receive the Queen's Award for Technological Achievement (Fig. 14a–c). At the luncheon, I discovered I was the only nonmember of Alderley Park to be invited. I sat with Drs. Sandy Todd and Roy Cotton, both who were so supportive at the beginning and remain lifelong friends. However, laboratory data and scientific publications are all fine. The good news was that the strategies proposed were proposed on solid data. These data were facts not opinions. The path to progress in medical oncology, however, is by convincing the medical establishment to change!

In September 1977, I was invited to present a talk at a clinical meeting for physicians at King College, Cambridge. The meeting was sponsored annually by ICI Pharmaceuticals Division to educate physicians (Fig. 15a–c). I presented my new adjuvant therapy strategy. Resistance was vigorous with objections that the animal model did not replicate human breast cancer. Indeed, it was dangerous because to paraphrase "we know that tamoxifen is effective only for a year or 2 in the treatment of metastatic breast cancer, so your approach will encourage early resistance to tamoxifen. We will have wasted a valuable palliative medicine to use at the end of life. In fact your approach is dangerous for patients!"

Later that month, in 1977, I traveled to the University of Wisconsin Clinical Cancer Center in Madison, as Lois Trench was trying to get them to recruit me to come to America. I presented the expanded talk and included the new chemoprevention data. Dr. Harold Rusch, then Director of the UWCCC, and Dr. Paul Carbone, Chairman of the Department of Human Oncology, decided to offer me a job on the spot [139]. I had a plan, and they had an embryonic Clinical Cancer Center funded 6 years earlier as a result of the National Cancer Act. By contrast, in Britain there was continuing medical resistance to the use of the ER assay to select patients for tamoxifen treatment. This was based on poor ER/patient response data in the NATO trial and the Scottish trial [140, 141]. Indeed much laboratory work was focused on the biological rational of why tamoxifen was an anticancer agent in ER-negative breast cancer [142]. Indeed, during the 1980s, I was informed that at some hospitals all patients were given tamoxifen.

Through a multitude of clinical trials worldwide, but most importantly the Early Breast Cancer Trials Collaborative Group (EBCTCG) in Oxford, solid conclusions were made about the veracity of the translational research: the ER is the essential

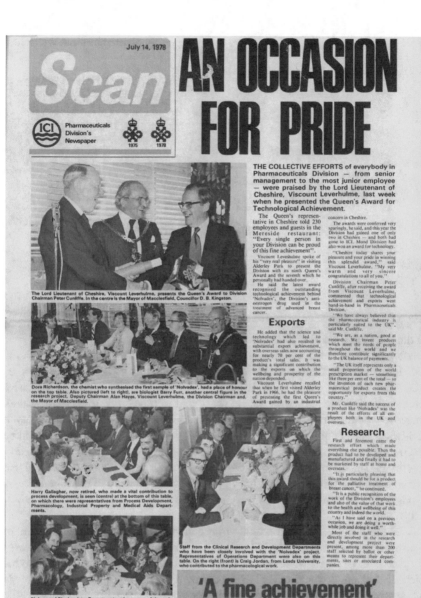

Fig. 14 The Queen's Award for Industry is the highest recognition possible. It recognizes outstanding achievement by industry to aid the country's economy. The award made by the Lord Lieutenant of Cheshire, Viscount Leverhulme, the Queen's representative, in July 1978, was celebrated by 230 handpicked employees, who were recognized for their role in the drug development of tamoxifen. Dr. Walpole, the team leader and champion of tamoxifen development, had died the year earlier and never saw the success of his invention. Dr. Roy Cotton (sitting opposite from Dr. Jordan in panel **c**) was the initial clinical monitor for tamoxifen development. He was advised not to spend too much time on tamoxifen as it was not predicted to be a successful product. However, Fig. 14 (continued) Dr. Jordan's strategy that came out of their investment at the WFEB and Leeds University for 7 years proved successful. Dr. Jordan (his personal invite as 14b) was the only one for a person not working for Pharmaceuticals Division

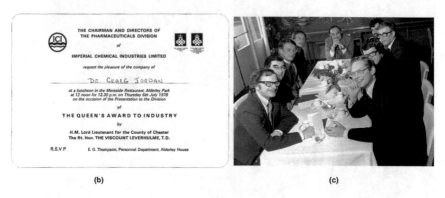

THE CHAIRMAN AND DIRECTORS OF
THE PHARMACEUTICALS DIVISION

of

IMPERIAL CHEMICAL INDUSTRIES LIMITED

request the pleasure of the company of

DR. CRAIG JORDAN

at a luncheon in the Mereside Restaurant, Alderley Park
at 12 noon for 12.30 p.m. on Thursday 6th July 1978
on the occasion of the Presentation to the Division

of

THE QUEEN'S AWARD TO INDUSTRY

by

H.M. Lord Lieutenant for the County of Chester
The Rt. Hon. THE VISCOUNT LEVERHULME, T.D.

R.S.V.P.   E. G. Thompson, Personnel Department, Alderley House

(b)   (c)

Fig. 14 (continued)

marker for tamoxifen activity; lives are saved [143]. Those lives saved depend upon the duration of tamoxifen administration; longer is better [110].

After an interlude in Switzerland (1979–1980) designing and building a new Ludwig Institute for Cancer Research in Bern, I was to find myself in the right place at the right time and closer to Dr. Elwood Jensen, the Director of Ben May Cancer Laboratories in Chicago. However, he was about to travel to Zurich, Switzerland, where he would be the Director of all the Ludwig Institutes for Cancer Research worldwide. Never could I have imagined that 20 years later, Elwood and I would be the co-recipients of the then highest award from the AACR. This is the inaugural Dorothy P. Landon award for translational cancer research in 2002 (Fig. 16a–c). He defined the tumor target, and I provided the lifesaving strategy to use tamoxifen as a long-term adjuvant treatment for patients with ER-positive primary breast cancer.

Over the decades, Elwood would write numerous letters of support for me to receive awards or promotions. At the start of my journey with tamoxifen, never would I have believed we would both be members of the national Academy of Sciences. Indeed, it would never have occurred to me that the University of Leeds and AstraZeneca would co-nominate me for consideration for an Order of the British Empire (OBE) for my role in the "tamoxifen tale." It was the late Barry Furr (Fig. 17a, b), the Chief Scientist at AstraZeneca, who wrote my citation based on not only my laboratory studies funded by ICI Pharmaceuticals Division in the 1970s but also my role as an expert witness for AstraZeneca to defend their patents in the United States during repeated challenges in the 1990s. The Smalkin decision in Baltimore in 1996 was a true education. I found this a unique experience. It turned out that not only did Judge Smalkin have an interest in British military history but also discovered that I was a Regular Army Reserve Officer in the British Special Air Service (SAS). This is the premier Special Forces regiment in the world. He spoke to me directly from the bench during my testimony, about matters pertaining to the SAS members, much to the confusion of the lawyers! Subsequently, I discovered

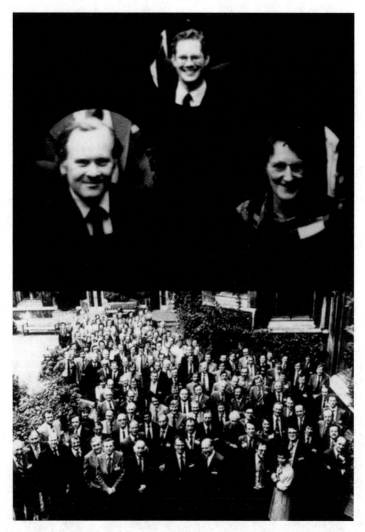

Fig. 15 (**a**) Participants at a Breast Cancer Symposium in September 1977 at Kings College, Cambridge, England. The concept of extended adjuvant tamoxifen treatment was first proposed at this meeting. Clinical studies of a 1-year adjuvant tamoxifen were in place; regrettably, a decade later this approach was shown to produce little survival benefit for patients. In the insets (top), the author, who presented the new concept (bottom left); Professor Michael Baum, the session chairman who was about to launch the Nolvadex Adjuvant Trial Organization (NATO) 2-year adjuvant tamoxifen trial; and (bottom right) Dr. Helen Stewart, who was a participant at the conference. She would initiate a pilot trial in 1978 and, led by Sir Patrick Forest, would later guide the full randomized Scottish trial of 5 years' adjuvant tamoxifen treatment vs. control in the 1980s. Both clinical trials were later proven to produce survival advantages for patients. The concept of longer tamoxifen treatment producing more survival benefits for patients was eventually established indirectly by the Oxford Overview Analysis in 1992 and directly by the Swedish group led by Dr. Lars Rutqvist. (**b**) The front of the program for the symposium. (**c**) The closing statement that by targeting the ER-positive breast cancers with long-term adjuvant tamoxifen therapy would be an appropriate clinical trials strategy

as the drug is cleared from the body. Therefore in this case Tamoxifen would appear to have a suppressive effect rather than a tumour specific killing effect.

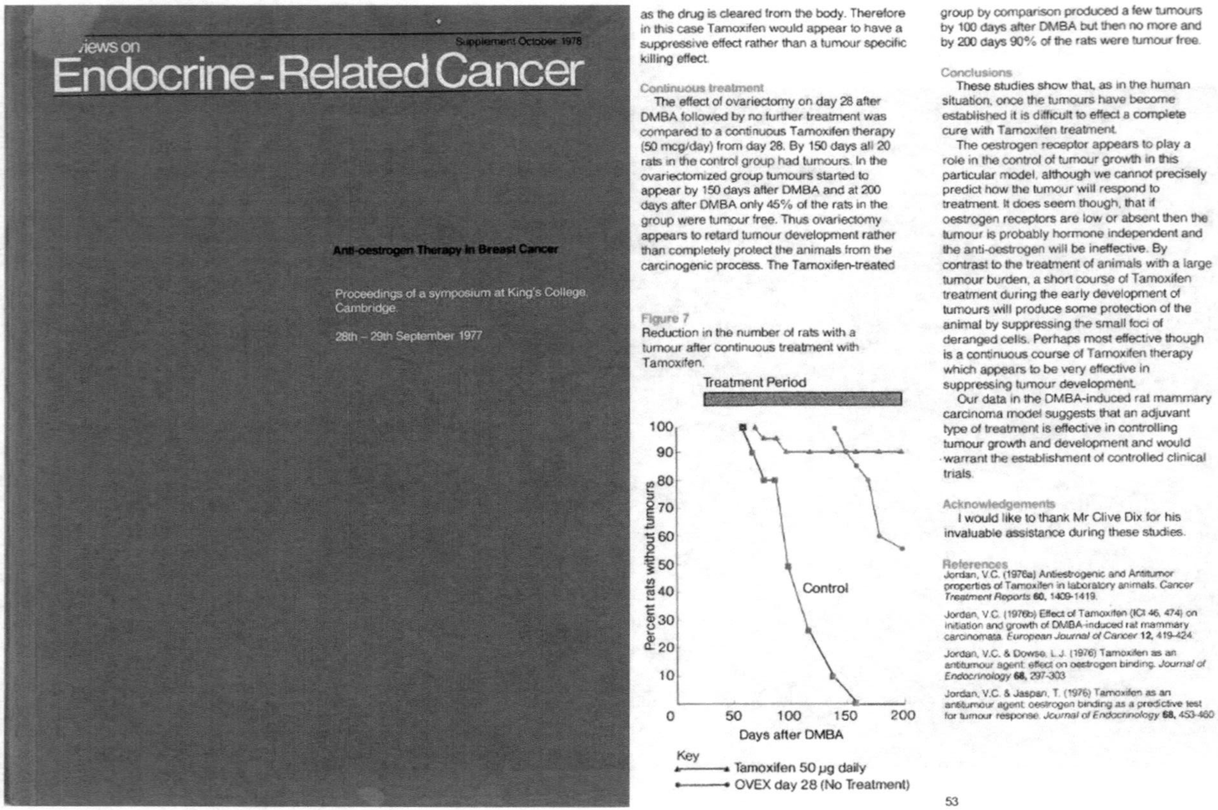

Continuous treatment

The effect of ovariectomy on day 28 after DMBA, followed by no further treatment was compared to a continuous Tamoxifen therapy (50 mcg/day) from day 28. By 150 days all 20 rats in the control group had tumours. In the ovariectomized group tumours started to appear by 150 days after DMBA, and at 200 days after DMBA only 45% of the rats in the group were tumour free. Thus ovariectomy appears to retard tumour development rather than completely protect the animals from the carcinogenic process. The Tamoxifen-treated group by comparison produced a few tumours by 100 days after DMBA but then no more and by 200 days 90% of the rats were tumour free.

Conclusions

These studies show that, as in the human situation, once the tumours have become established it is difficult to effect a complete cure with Tamoxifen treatment.

The oestrogen receptor appears to play a role in the control of tumour growth in this particular model, although we cannot precisely predict how the tumour will respond to treatment. It does seem though, that if oestrogen receptors are low or absent then the tumour is probably hormone independent and the anti-oestrogen will be ineffective. By contrast to the treatment of animals with a large tumour burden, a short course of Tamoxifen treatment during the early development of tumours will produce some protection of the animal by suppressing the small foci of deranged cells. Perhaps most effective though is a continuous course of Tamoxifen therapy which appears to be very effective in suppressing tumour development.

Our data in the DMBA-induced rat mammary carcinoma model suggests that an adjuvant type of treatment is effective in controlling tumour growth and development and would warrant the establishment of controlled clinical trials.

Acknowledgements

I would like to thank Mr Clive Dix for his invaluable assistance during these studies.

References

Jordan, V.C. (1976a) Antiestrogenic and Antitumor properties of Tamoxifen in laboratory animals. Cancer Treatment Reports 60, 1409-1419.

Jordan, V.C. (1976b) Effect of Tamoxifen (ICI 46, 474) on initiation and growth of DMBA-induced rat mammary carcinomas. European Journal of Cancer 12, 419-424.

Jordan, V.C. & Dowse, L.J. (1976) Tamoxifen as an antitumour agent: effect on oestrogen binding. Journal of Endocrinology 68, 297-303.

Jordan, V.C. & Jaspan, T. (1976) Tamoxifen as an antitumour agent: oestrogen binding as a predictive test for tumour response. Journal of Endocrinology 68, 453-460

Views on
Endocrine-Related Cancer
Supplement October 1978

Anti-oestrogen Therapy in Breast Cancer

Proceedings of a symposium at King's College Cambridge.

28th - 29th September 1977

Figure 7
Reduction in the number of rats with a tumour after continuous treatment with Tamoxifen.

Treatment Period

Control

Percent rats without tumours — Days after DMBA

Key: Tamoxifen 50 µg daily; OVEX day 28 (No Treatment)

Fig. 15 (continued)

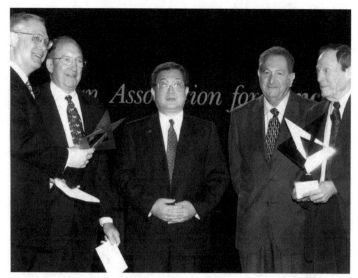

Fig. 16 (**a**) The presentation of the inaugural Dorothy P. Landon/AACR Award for Translational Research by AACR President Ki Hong, MD, and the Chairman of the Landon Prize evaluation committee Dr. Joseph Bertino in 2002 to Dr. Elwood V. Jensen and Dr. V. Craig Jordan. (**b**) The letter of the inaugural Dorothy P. Landon/AACR Award for Translational Research award with citations for Dr. Elwood V. Jensen and Dr. V. Craig Jordan

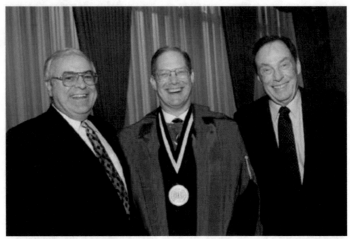

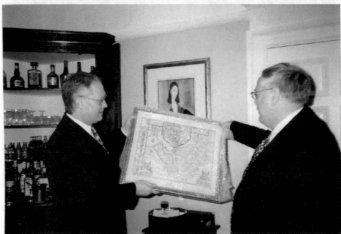

Fig. 17 (**a**) Dr. Barry Furr, Chief Scientist at AstraZeneca, at the investiture of Dr. Jordan as the Diana, Princess of Wales, Professor of Cancer Research. Both Dr. Furr (left) and Dr. Jordan (right) were presenters in the symposium in Dr. Jordan's honor. (**b**) The day following Dr. Jordan's investiture as Officer of the Most Excellent Order of the British Empire by her Majesty Queen Elizabeth II, senior staff held a celebration dinner in Alderley Edge near ICI Pharmaceuticals Division Alderley Park. There Dr. Jordan was presented with an antique map of Cheshire by the pioneering historian and mapmaker, John Speed. Speed was a Cheshire man. Craig Jordan's maternal family (Mottram) and Alderley Park are all in Cheshire within 10 miles of each other. The framed map is from Speed's original collection from 1611. The map is from his book, *The Theatre of the Empire of Great Britain*, which was signed on the back by all the guests from the original Alderley Park team in the 1970s

that Judge Smalkin mentioned me by name in his ruling for the veracity of my cross-examination of the stand. I am told this usually doesn't happen for expert witnesses. AstraZeneca earned many billions of dollars, as a result of exclusive tamoxifen sales, in the United States.

I thank the late Arthur Walpole (PhD examiner and academic supporter), the late Barry Furr (early friend in the 1970s and subsequently Chief Scientist), Dr. Roy Cotton, Lois Trench, and Dr. Brian Newbold for taking a chance on a young scientist with a plan to realize the full potential of tamoxifen.

Acknowledgments We thank the benefactors of the Dallas/Ft. Worth Living Legend Professorship in Cancer Research, the George and Barbra Bush Foundation for Innovative Cancer Research grant, and the CCSG P30 CA-016672 to the University of Texas MD Anderson Cancer Center.

References

1. Lerner LJ, Holthaus FJ Jr, Thompson CR (1958) A non-steroidal estrogen antagonist 1-(p-2-diethylaminoethoxyphenyl)-1-phenyl-2-p-methoxyphenyl ethanol. Endocrinology 63(3):295–318. https://doi.org/10.1210/endo-63-3-295
2. Lerner LJ, Jordan VC (1990) Development of antiestrogens and their use in breast cancer: eighth Cain memorial award lecture. Cancer Res 50(14):4177–4189
3. Segal SJ, Nelson WO (1958) An orally active compound with anti-fertility effects in rats. Proc Soc Exp Biol Med 98(2):431–436
4. Emmens CW, Cox RI, Martin L (1962) Antioestrogens. Recent Prog Horm Res 18:415
5. Holtkamp DE, Greslin JG, Root CA, Lerner LJ (1960) Gonadotrophin inhibiting and anti-fecundity effects of chloramiphene. Proc Soc Exp Biol Med 105:197–201
6. Greenblatt RB, Barfield WE, Jungck EC, Ray AW (1961) Induction of ovulation with MRL/41. Preliminary report. JAMA 178:101–104
7. Avigan J, Steinberg D, Vroman HE, Thompson MJ, Mosettig E (1960) Studies of cholesterol biosynthesis. I. The identification of desmosterol in serum and tissues of animals and man treated with MER-29. J Biol Chem 235:3123–3126
8. Laughlin RC, Carey TF (1962) Cataracts in patients treated with triparanol. JAMA 181:339–340
9. Palopoli FP, Feil VJ, Allen RE, Holtkamp DE, Richardson A Jr (1967) Substituted aminoalkoxytriarylhaloethylenes. J Med Chem 10(1):84–86
10. Harper MJ, Walpole AL (1966) Contrasting endocrine activities of cis and trans isomers in a series of substituted triphenylethylenes. Nature 212(5057):87
11. Lednicer D, Lyster SC, Duncan GW (1967) Mammalian antifertility agents. IV. Basic 3,4-dihydronaphthalenes and 1,2,3,4-tetrahydro-1-naphthols. J Med Chem 10(1):78–84
12. Lednicer D, Lyster SC, Aspergren BD, Duncan GW (1966) Mammalian antifertility agents. 3. 1-Aryl-2-phenyl-1,2,3,4-tetrahydro-1-naphthols, 1-aryl-2-phenyl-3,4-dihydronaphthalenes, and their derivatives. J Med Chem 9(2):172–176
13. Clark ER, Jordan VC (1976) Oestrogenic, anti-oestrogenic and fertility effects of some triphenylethanes and triphenylethylenes related to ethamoxytriphetol (MER 25). Br J Pharmacol 57(4):487–493
14. Abbott AC, Clark ER, Jordan VC (1976) Inhibition of oestradiol binding to oestrogen receptor proteins by a methyl-substituted analogue of tamoxifen. J Endocrinol 69(3):445–446
15. Jensen EV, Suzuki T, Kawashima T, Stumpf WE, Jungblut PW, DeSombre ER (1968) A two-step mechanism for the interaction of estradiol with rat uterus. Proc Natl Acad Sci U S A 59(2):632–638
16. Jensen EV, Suzuki T, Numata M, Smith S, DeSombre ER (1969) Estrogen-binding substances of target tissues. Steroids 13(4):417–427
17. Toft D, Gorski J (1966) A receptor molecule for estrogens: isolation from the rat uterus and preliminary characterization. Proc Natl Acad Sci U S A 55(6):1574–1581

18. Toft D, Shyamala G, Gorski J (1967) A receptor molecule for estrogens: studies using a cell-free system. Proc Natl Acad Sci U S A 57(6):1740–1743
19. Legha SS, Slavik M, Carter SK (1976) Nafoxidine--an antiestrogen for the treatment of breast cancer. Cancer 38(4):1535–1541
20. Tatee T, Carlson KE, Katzenellenbogen JA, Robertson DW, Katzenellenbogen BS (1979) Antiestrogens and antiestrogen metabolites: preparation of tritium-labeled (+/−)-cis-3-[p-(1,2,3,4-tetrahydro-6-methoxy-2-phenyl-1-naphthyl)phenoxyl]-1,2-propanediol (U-23469) and characterization and synthesis of a biologically important metabolite. J Med Chem 22(12):1509–1517
21. Rosati RL, Da Silva Jardine P, Cameron KO, Thompson DD, Ke HZ, Toler SM, Brown TA, Pan LC, Ebbinghaus CF, Reinhold AR, Elliott NC, Newhouse BN, Tjoa CM, Sweetnam PM, Cole MJ, Arriola MW, Gauthier JW, Crawford DT, Nickerson DF, Pirie CM, Qi H, Simmons HA, Tkalcevic GT (1998) Discovery and preclinical pharmacology of a novel, potent, non-steroidal estrogen receptor agonist/antagonist, CP-336156, a diaryltetrahydronaphthalene. J Med Chem 41(16):2928–2931. https://doi.org/10.1021/jm980048b
22. Haddow A, Watkinson JM, Paterson E, Koller PC (1944) Influence of synthetic oestrogens on advanced malignant disease. Br Med J 2(4368):393–398
23. Haddow A (1970) David A. Karnofsky memorial lecture. Thoughts on chemical therapy. Cancer 26(4):737–754
24. Walpole AL, Paterson E (1949) Synthetic oestrogens in mammary cancer. Lancet 2(6583):783–786
25. Haddow A, Watkinson JM, Paterson E, Koller PC (1944) Influence of synthetic oestrogens upon advanced malignant disease. Br Med J 1944:393–398
26. Hill GB (2016) Alderley Park discovered. Palatine Books, Lancaster
27. Cole MP, Jones CT, Todd ID (1971) A new anti-oestrogenic agent in late breast cancer. An early clinical appraisal of ICI46474. Br J Cancer 25(2):270–275
28. Bedford GR, Richardson DN (1966) Preparation and identification of cis and trans isomers of a substituted triarylethylene. Nature 212:733–734. https://doi.org/10.1038/212733b0
29. Kilbourn BT, Mais RHB, Owston PG (1968) Identification of isomers of a substituted triaryle-thylene: the crystal structure of 1-p-(2-dimethylaminoethoxyphenyl)-1,2-cis-diphenylbut-1-ene hydrobromide. Chem Commun:291
30. DiPietro DL, Sanders FJ, Goss DA (1969) Effect of cis and trans isomers of clomiphene citrate on uterine hexokinase activity. Endocrinology 84(6):1404–1408. https://doi.org/10.1210/endo-84-6-1404
31. Harper MJ, Walpole AL (1967) A new derivative of triphenylethylene: effect on implantation and mode of action in rats. J Reprod Fertil 13(1):101–119
32. Harper MJ, Walpole AL (1967) Mode of action of I.C.I. 46,474 in preventing implantation in rats. J Endocrinol 37(1):83–92
33. Labhsetwar AP (1970) Role of oestrogen in spontaneous ovulation demonstrated by use of an antagonist of oestrogen, ICI 46,474. Nature 225(5227):80–81
34. Labhsetwar AP (1970) Role of estrogens in ovulation: a study using the estrogen-antagonist, I.C.I. 46,474. Endocrinology 87(3):542–551. https://doi.org/10.1210/endo-87-3-542
35. Labhsetwar AP (1971) Effects of an antioestrogen on the corpus luteum of rabbits and rats. J Reprod Fertil 25(2):295–297
36. Labhsetwar AP (1972) Role of estrogens in spontaneous ovulation: evidence for the positive feedback in hamsters. Endocrinology 90(4):941–946. https://doi.org/10.1210/endo-90-4-941
37. Klopper A, Hall M (1971) New synthetic agent for the induction of ovulation: preliminary trials in women. Br Med J 1(5741):152–154
38. Williamson JG, Ellis JD (1973) The induction of ovulation by tamoxifen. J Obstet Gynaecol Br Commonw 80(9):844–847
39. Jordan VC (2014) Tamoxifen as the first targeted long-term adjuvant therapy for breast cancer. Endocr Relat Cancer 21(3):R235–R246. https://doi.org/10.1530/ERC-14-0092
40. Jordan VC (2008) Tamoxifen: catalyst for the change to targeted therapy. Eur J Cancer 44(1):30–38. https://doi.org/10.1016/j.ejca.2007.11.002

41. Jordan VC, Lababidi MK, Langan-Fahey S (1991) Suppression of mouse mammary tumorigenesis by long-term tamoxifen therapy. J Natl Cancer Inst 83(7):492–496
42. Fromson JM, Pearson S, Bramah S (1973) The metabolism of tamoxifen (I.C.I. 46,474). I. In laboratory animals. Xenobiotica 3(11):693–709. https://doi.org/10.3109/00498257309151594
43. Fromson JM, Pearson S, Bramah S (1973) The metabolism of tamoxifen (I.C.I. 46,474). II. In female patients. Xenobiotica 3(11):711–714. https://doi.org/10.3109/00498257309151595
44. Adam HK, Gay MA, Moore RH (1980) Measurement of tamoxifen in serum by thin-layer densitometry. J Endocrinol 84(1):35–42
45. Adam HK, Douglas EJ, Kemp JV (1979) The metabolism of tamoxifen in human. Biochem Pharmacol 28(1):145–147
46. Kemp JV, Adam HK, Wakeling AE, Slater R (1983) Identification and biological activity of tamoxifen metabolites in human serum. Biochem Pharmacol 32(13):2045–2052
47. Bain RR, Jordan VC (1983) Identification of a new metabolite of tamoxifen in patient serum during breast cancer therapy. Biochem Pharmacol 32(2):373–375
48. Jordan VC, Bain RR, Brown RR, Gosden B, Santos MA (1983) Determination and pharmacology of a new hydroxylated metabolite of tamoxifen observed in patient sera during therapy for advanced breast cancer. Cancer Res 43(3):1446–1450
49. Lien EA, Solheim E, Kvinnsland S, Ueland PM (1988) Identification of 4-hydroxy-N-desmethyltamoxifen as a metabolite of tamoxifen in human bile. Cancer Res 48(8):2304–2308
50. Lien EA, Solheim E, Lea OA, Lundgren S, Kvinnsland S, Ueland PM (1989) Distribution of 4-hydroxy-N-desmethyltamoxifen and other tamoxifen metabolites in human biological fluids during tamoxifen treatment. Cancer Res 49(8):2175–2183
51. Johanning J, Kroner P, Thomas M, Zanger UM, Norenberg A, Eichelbaum M, Schwab M, Brauch H, Schroth W, Murdter TE (2018) The formation of estrogen-like tamoxifen metabolites and their influence on enzyme activity and gene expression of ADME genes. Arch Toxicol 92(3):1099–1112. https://doi.org/10.1007/s00204-017-2147-y
52. Jordan VC, Collins MM, Rowsby L, Prestwich G (1977) A monohydroxylated metabolite of tamoxifen with potent antioestrogenic activity. J Endocrinol 75(2):305–316
53. Allen KE, Clark ER, Jordan VC (1980) Evidence for the metabolic activation of non-steroidal antioestrogens: a study of structure-activity relationships. Br J Pharmacol 71(1):83–91
54. Dehal SS, Kupfer D (1997) CYP2D6 catalyzes tamoxifen 4-hydroxylation in human liver. Cancer Res 57(16):3402–3406
55. Goetz MP, Suman VJ, Reid JM, Northfelt DW, Mahr MA, Ralya AT, Kuffel M, Buhrow SA, Safgren SL, McGovern RM, Black J, Dockter T, Haddad T, Erlichman C, Adjei AA, Visscher D, Chalmers ZR, Frampton G, Kipp BR, Liu MC, Hawse JR, Doroshow JH, Collins JM, Streicher H, Ames MM, Ingle JN (2017) First-in-human phase I study of the tamoxifen metabolite Z-endoxifen in women with endocrine-refractory metastatic breast cancer. J Clin Oncol 35(30):3391–3400. https://doi.org/10.1200/JCO.2017.73.3246
56. Jordan VC (2017) Endoxifen: the end, or are we at the beginning? J Clin Oncol 35(30):3378–3379. https://doi.org/10.1200/JCO.2017.74.9325
57. Levenson AS, Jordan VC (1997) MCF-7: the first hormone-responsive breast cancer cell line. Cancer Res 57(15):3071–3078
58. Lippman ME, Bolan G (1975) Oestrogen-responsive human breast cancer in long term tissue culture. Nature 256(5518):592–593
59. Shafie SM (1980) Estrogen and the growth of breast cancer: new evidence suggests indirect action. Science 209(4457):701–702
60. Berthois Y, Katzenellenbogen JA, Katzenellenbogen BS (1986) Phenol red in tissue culture media is a weak estrogen: implications concerning the study of estrogen-responsive cells in culture. Proc Natl Acad Sci U S A 83(8):2496–2500
61. Bindal RD, Carlson KE, Katzenellenbogen BS, Katzenellenbogen JA (1988) Lipophilic impurities, not phenolsulfonphthalein, account for the estrogenic activity in commercial preparations of phenol red. J Steroid Biochem 31(3):287–293

62. Bindal RD, Katzenellenbogen JA (1988) Bis(4-hydroxyphenyl)[2-(phenoxysulfonyl)phenyl] methane: isolation and structure elucidation of a novel estrogen from commercial preparations of phenol red (phenolsulfonphthalein). J Med Chem 31(10):1978–1983

63. Lieberman ME, Maurer RA, Gorski J (1978) Estrogen control of prolactin synthesis in vitro. Proc Natl Acad Sci U S A 75(12):5946–5949

64. Lieberman ME, Jordan VC, Fritsch M, Santos MA, Gorski J (1983) Direct and reversible inhibition of estradiol-stimulated prolactin synthesis by antiestrogens in vitro. J Biol Chem 258(8):4734–4740

65. Jordan VC, Koch R, Langan S, McCague R (1988) Ligand interaction at the estrogen receptor to program antiestrogen action: a study with nonsteroidal compounds in vitro. Endocrinology 122(4):1449–1454. https://doi.org/10.1210/endo-122-4-1449

66. Jordan VC, Koch R, Mittal S, Schneider MR (1986) Oestrogenic and antioestrogenic actions in a series of triphenylbut-1-enes: modulation of prolactin synthesis in vitro. Br J Pharmacol 87(1):217–223

67. Jordan VC, Lieberman ME (1984) Estrogen-stimulated prolactin synthesis in vitro. Classification of agonist, partial agonist, and antagonist actions based on structure. Mol Pharmacol 26(2):279–285

68. Jordan VC, Lieberman ME, Cormier E, Koch R, Bagley JR, Ruenitz PC (1984) Structural requirements for the pharmacological activity of nonsteroidal antiestrogens in vitro. Mol Pharmacol 26(2):272–278

69. Jordan VC (1984) Biochemical pharmacology of antiestrogen action. Pharmacol Rev 36(4):245–276

70. Lieberman ME, Gorski J, Jordan VC (1983) An estrogen receptor model to describe the regulation of prolactin synthesis by antiestrogens in vitro. J Biol Chem 258(8):4741–4745

71. Tate AC, Greene GL, DeSombre ER, Jensen EV, Jordan VC (1984) Differences between estrogen- and antiestrogen-estrogen receptor complexes from human breast tumors identified with an antibody raised against the estrogen receptor. Cancer Res 44(3):1012–1018

72. Tate AC, Lieberman ME, Jordan VC (1984) The inhibition of prolactin synthesis in GH3 rat pituitary tumor cells by monohydroxytamoxifen is associated with changes in the properties of the estrogen receptor. J Steroid Biochem 20(1):391–395

73. Tate AC, DeSombre ER, Greene GL, Jensen EV, Jordan VC (1983) Interaction of [3H] estradiol- and [3H] monohydroxytamoxifen-estrogen receptor complexes with a monoclonal antibody. Breast Cancer Res Treat 3(3):267–277

74. Jordan VC (1987) Laboratory models of breast cancer to aid the elucidation of antiestrogen action. J Lab Clin Med 109(3):267–277

75. Wolf DM, Jordan VC (1994) The estrogen receptor from a tamoxifen stimulated MCF-7 tumor variant contains a point mutation in the ligand binding domain. Breast Cancer Res Treat 31(1):129–138

76. Jordan VC (2001) Selective estrogen receptor modulation: a personal perspective. Cancer Res 61(15):5683–5687

77. Levenson AS, Catherino WH, Jordan VC (1997) Estrogenic activity is increased for an antiestrogen by a natural mutation of the estrogen receptor. J Steroid Biochem Mol Biol 60(5–6):261–268

78. Levenson AS, Jordan VC (1998) The key to the antiestrogenic mechanism of raloxifene is amino acid 351 (aspartate) in the estrogen receptor. Cancer Res 58(9):1872–1875

79. Liu H, Lee ES, Deb Los Reyes A, Zapf JW, Jordan VC (2001) Silencing and reactivation of the selective estrogen receptor modulator-estrogen receptor alpha complex. Cancer Res 61(9):3632–3639

80. Liu H, Park WC, Bentrem DJ, McKian KP, Reyes Ade L, Loweth JA, Schafer JM, Zapf JW, Jordan VC (2002) Structure-function relationships of the raloxifene-estrogen receptor-alpha complex for regulating transforming growth factor-alpha expression in breast cancer cells. J Biol Chem 277(11):9189–9198. https://doi.org/10.1074/jbc.M108335200

81. MacGregor Schafer J, Liu H, Bentrem DJ, Zapf JW, Jordan VC (2000) Allosteric silencing of activating function 1 in the 4-hydroxytamoxifen estrogen receptor complex is induced by substituting glycine for aspartate at amino acid 351. Cancer Res 60(18):5097–5105

82. Brzozowski AM, Pike AC, Dauter Z, Hubbard RE, Bonn T, Engstrom O, Ohman L, Greene GL, Gustafsson JA, Carlquist M (1997) Molecular basis of agonism and antagonism in the oestrogen receptor. Nature 389(6652):753–758. https://doi.org/10.1038/39645

83. Shiau AK, Barstad D, Loria PM, Cheng L, Kushner PJ, Agard DA, Greene GL (1998) The structural basis of estrogen receptor/coactivator recognition and the antagonism of this interaction by tamoxifen. Cell 95(7):927–937

84. Fanning SW, Mayne CG, Dharmarajan V, Carlson KE, Martin TA, Novick SJ, Toy W, Green B, Panchamukhi S, Katzenellenbogen BS, Tajkhorshid E, Griffin PR, Shen Y, Chandarlapaty S, Katzenellenbogen JA, Greene GL (2016) Estrogen receptor alpha somatic mutations Y537S and D538G confer breast cancer endocrine resistance by stabilizing the activating function-2 binding conformation. elife 5. https://doi.org/10.7554/eLife.12792

85. Lednicer D, Babcock JC, Marlatt PE, Lyster SC, Duncan GW (1965) Mammalian antifertility agents. I. Derivatives of 2,3-diphenylindenes. J Med Chem 8:52–57

86. Robinson SP, Langan-Fahey SM, Johnson DA, Jordan VC (1991) Metabolites, pharmacodynamics, and pharmacokinetics of tamoxifen in rats and mice compared to the breast cancer patient. Drug Metab Dispos 19(1):36–43

87. Robinson SP, Langan-Fahey SM, Jordan VC (1989) Implications of tamoxifen metabolism in the athymic mouse for the study of antitumor effects upon human breast cancer xenografts. Eur J Cancer Clin Oncol 25(12):1769–1776

88. Langan-Fahey SM, Tormey DC, Jordan VC (1990) Tamoxifen metabolites in patients on long-term adjuvant therapy for breast cancer. Eur J Cancer 26(8):883–888

89. Gottardis MM, Jordan VC (1988) Development of tamoxifen-stimulated growth of MCF-7 tumors in athymic mice after long-term antiestrogen administration. Cancer Res 48(18):5183–5187

90. Sutherland R, Mester J, Baulieu EE (1977) Tamoxifen is a potent "pure" anti-oestrogen in chick oviduct. Nature 267(5610):434–435

91. Osborne CK, Coronado EB, Robinson JP (1987) Human breast cancer in the athymic nude mouse: cytostatic effects of long-term antiestrogen therapy. Eur J Cancer Clin Oncol 23(8):1189–1196

92. Fan P, Agboke FA, Cunliffe HE, Ramos P, Jordan VC (2014) A molecular model for the mechanism of acquired tamoxifen resistance in breast cancer. Eur J Cancer 50(16):2866–2876. https://doi.org/10.1016/j.ejca.2014.08.011

93. Fan P, Cunliffe HE, Griffith OL, Agboke FA, Ramos P, Gray JW, Jordan VC (2014) Identification of gene regulation patterns underlying both oestrogen- and tamoxifen-stimulated cell growth through global gene expression profiling in breast cancer cells. Eur J Cancer 50(16):2877–2886. https://doi.org/10.1016/j.ejca.2014.08.010

94. Gottardis MM, Wagner RJ, Borden EC, Jordan VC (1989) Differential ability of antiestrogens to stimulate breast cancer cell (MCF-7) growth in vivo and in vitro. Cancer Res 49(17):4765–4769

95. Gottardis MM, Jiang SY, Jeng MH, Jordan VC (1989) Inhibition of tamoxifen-stimulated growth of an MCF-7 tumor variant in athymic mice by novel steroidal antiestrogens. Cancer Res 49(15):4090–4093

96. Wakeling AE, Dukes M, Bowler J (1991) A potent specific pure antiestrogen with clinical potential. Cancer Res 51(15):3867–3873

97. Howell A, Robertson JF, Quaresma Albano J, Aschermannova A, Mauriac L, Kleeberg UR, Vergote I, Erikstein B, Webster A, Morris C (2002) Fulvestrant, formerly ICI 182,780, is as effective as anastrozole in postmenopausal women with advanced breast cancer progressing after prior endocrine treatment. J Clin Oncol 20(16):3396–3403. https://doi.org/10.1200/JCO.2002.10.057

98. Osborne CK, Pippen J, Jones SE, Parker LM, Ellis M, Come S, Gertler SZ, May JT, Burton G, Dimery I, Webster A, Morris C, Elledge R, Buzdar A (2002) Double-blind, randomized trial comparing the efficacy and tolerability of fulvestrant versus anastrozole in postmenopausal women with advanced breast cancer progressing on prior endocrine therapy: results of a North American trial. J Clin Oncol 20(16):3386–3395. https://doi.org/10.1200/JCO.2002.10.058

99. Howell A, Dodwell DJ, Anderson H, Redford J (1992) Response after withdrawal of tamoxifen and progestogens in advanced breast cancer. Ann Oncol 3(8):611–617

100. Ravdin PM, Fritz NF, Tormey DC, Jordan VC (1988) Endocrine status of premenopausal node-positive breast cancer patients following adjuvant chemotherapy and long-term tamoxifen. Cancer Res 48(4):1026–1029

101. Jordan VC, Fritz NF, Langan-Fahey S, Thompson M, Tormey DC (1991) Alteration of endocrine parameters in premenopausal women with breast cancer during long-term adjuvant therapy with tamoxifen as the single agent. J Natl Cancer Inst 83(20):1488–1491

102. Jordan VC, Fritz NF, Tormey DC (1987) Long-term adjuvant therapy with tamoxifen: effects on sex hormone binding globulin and antithrombin III. Cancer Res 47(16):4517–4519

103. Jordan VC (1990) Long-term adjuvant tamoxifen therapy for breast cancer. Breast Cancer Res Treat 15(3):125–136

104. Early Breast Cancer Trialists' Collaborative Group (1998) Tamoxifen for early breast cancer: an overview of the randomised trials. Lancet 351(9114):1451–1467

105. Early Breast Cancer Trialists' Collaborative Group (2005) Effects of chemotherapy and hormonal therapy for early breast cancer on recurrence and 15-year survival: an overview of the randomised trials. Lancet 365(9472):1687–1717. https://doi.org/10.1016/S0140-6736(05)66544-0

106. Jordan VC (2014) Linking estrogen-induced apoptosis with decreases in mortality following long-term adjuvant tamoxifen therapy. J Natl Cancer Inst 106(11):dju296. https://doi.org/10.1093/jnci/dju296

107. Fisher B, Costantino J, Redmond C, Poisson R, Bowman D, Couture J, Dimitrov NV, Wolmark N, Wickerham DL, Fisher ER et al (1989) A randomized clinical trial evaluating tamoxifen in the treatment of patients with node-negative breast cancer who have estrogen-receptor-positive tumors. N Engl J Med 320(8):479–484. https://doi.org/10.1056/NEJM198902233200802

108. Fisher B, Dignam J, Bryant J, DeCillis A, Wickerham DL, Wolmark N, Costantino J, Redmond C, Fisher ER, Bowman DM, Deschenes L, Dimitrov NV, Margolese RG, Robidoux A, Shibata H, Terz J, Paterson AH, Feldman MI, Farrar W, Evans J, Lickley HL (1996) Five versus more than five years of tamoxifen therapy for breast cancer patients with negative lymph nodes and estrogen receptor-positive tumors. J Natl Cancer Inst 88(21):1529–1542

109. Pan H, Gray R, Braybrooke J, Davies C, Taylor C, McGale P, Peto R, Pritchard KI, Bergh J, Dowsett M, Hayes DF, EBCTCG (2017) 20-year risks of breast-cancer recurrence after stopping endocrine therapy at 5 years. N Engl J Med 377(19):1836–1846. https://doi.org/10.1056/NEJMoa1701830

110. Davies C, Pan H, Godwin J, Gray R, Arriagada R, Raina V, Abraham M, Medeiros Alencar VH, Badran A, Bonfill X, Bradbury J, Clarke M, Collins R, Davis SR, Delmestri A, Forbes JF, Haddad P, Hou MF, Inbar M, Khaled H, Kielanowska J, Kwan WH, Mathew BS, Mittra I, Muller B, Nicolucci A, Peralta O, Pernas F, Petruzelka L, Pienkowski T, Radhika R, Rajan B, Rubach MT, Tort S, Urrutia G, Valentini M, Wang Y, Peto R, Adjuvant Tamoxifen: Longer Against Shorter Collaborative G (2013) Long-term effects of continuing adjuvant tamoxifen to 10 years versus stopping at 5 years after diagnosis of oestrogen receptor-positive breast cancer: ATLAS, a randomised trial. Lancet 381(9869):805–816. https://doi.org/10.1016/S0140-6736(12)61963-1

111. Schiavon G, Smith IE (2014) Status of adjuvant endocrine therapy for breast cancer. Breast Cancer Res 16(2):206

112. Jordan VC (1991) Prolonged adjuvant tamoxifen: a beginning not the end. Ann Oncol 2(7):481–484

113. Jordan VC (1976) Effect of tamoxifen (Ici 46,474) on initiation and growth of Dmba-induced rat mammary carcinomata. Eur J Cancer 12(6):419–424. https://doi.org/10.1016/0014-2964(76)90030-X
114. Cuzick J, Baum M (1985) Tamoxifen and contralateral breast cancer. Lancet 2(8449):282
115. Lacassagne A (1936) Hormonal pathogenesis of adenocarcinoma of the breast. Am J Cancer 27(2):217–228. https://doi.org/10.1158/ajc.1936.217
116. Powles TJ, Hardy JR, Ashley SE, Farrington GM, Cosgrove D, Davey JB, Dowsett M, McKinna JA, Nash AG, Sinnett HD et al (1989) A pilot trial to evaluate the acute toxicity and feasibility of tamoxifen for prevention of breast cancer. Br J Cancer 60(1):126–131
117. Fisher B, Costantino JP, Wickerham DL, Cecchini RS, Cronin WM, Robidoux A, Bevers TB, Kavanah MT, Atkins JN, Margolese RG, Runowicz CD, James JM, Ford LG, Wolmark N (2005) Tamoxifen for the prevention of breast cancer: current status of the National Surgical Adjuvant Breast and Bowel Project P-1 study. J Natl Cancer Inst 97(22):1652–1662. https://doi.org/10.1093/jnci/dji372
118. Veronesi U, Maisonneuve P, Costa A, Sacchini V, Maltoni C, Robertson C, Rotmensz N, Boyle P (1998) Prevention of breast cancer with tamoxifen: preliminary findings from the Italian randomised trial among hysterectomised women. Italian tamoxifen prevention study. Lancet 352(9122):93–97
119. Smith SG, Foy R, McGowan JA, Kobayashi LC, DeCensi A, Brown K, Side L, Cuzick J (2017) Prescribing tamoxifen in primary care for the prevention of breast cancer: a national online survey of GPs' attitudes. Br J Gen Pract 67(659):e414–e427. https://doi.org/10.3399/bjgp17X689377
120. Jensen EV, Block GE, Smith S, Kyser K, DeSombre ER (1971) Estrogen receptors and breast cancer response to adrenalectomy. Natl Cancer Inst Monogr 34:55–70
121. McGuire W, Carbone P, Sears M, Escher G (1975) Estrogen receptors in human breast cancer: an overview. In: WL MG, Carbone PP, Vollmer EP (eds) Estrogen receptors in human breast cancer. Raven Press, New York
122. Consensus conference. Adjuvant chemotherapy for breast cancer (1985) JAMA 254(24):3461–3463
123. Terenius L (1971) Structure-activity relationships of anti-oestrogens with regard to interaction with 17-beta-oestradiol in the mouse uterus and vagina. Acta Endocrinol 66(3):431–447
124. Jordan VC (2006) Tamoxifen (ICI46,474) as a targeted therapy to treat and prevent breast cancer. Br J Pharmacol 147(Suppl 1):S269–S276. https://doi.org/10.1038/sj.bjp.0706399
125. Jordan VC (1988) The development of tamoxifen for breast cancer therapy: a tribute to the late Arthur L. Walpole. Breast Cancer Res Treat 11(3):197–209
126. Carter SB (1967) Effects of cytochalasins on mammalian cells. Nature 213(5073):261–264
127. Welshons WV, Lieberman ME, Gorski J (1984) Nuclear localization of unoccupied oestrogen receptors. Nature 307(5953):747–749
128. Welshons WV, Grady LH, Judy BM, Jordan VC, Preziosi DE (1993) Subcellular compartmentalization of MCF-7 estrogen receptor synthesis and degradation. Mol Cell Endocrinol 94(2):183–194
129. Herbst AL, Griffiths CT, Kistner RW (1964) Clomiphene citrate (Nsc-35770) in disseminated mammary carcinoma. Cancer Chemother Rep 43:39–41
130. Huggins C, Grand LC, Brillantes FP (1961) Mammary cancer induced by a single feeding of polymucular hydrocarbons, and its suppression. Nature 189:204–207
131. Hunter RE, Longcope C, Jordan VC (1980) Steroid hormone receptors in adenocarcinoma of the endometrium. Gynecol Oncol 10(2):152–161
132. Emmens CW (1971) Compounds exhibiting prolonged antioestrogenic and antifertility activity in mice and rats. J Reprod Fertil 26(2):175–182
133. Emmens CW, Carr WL (1973) Further studies of compounds exhibiting prolonged antioestrogenic and antifertility activity in the mouse. J Reprod Fertil 34(1):29–40
134. Jordan VC (1975) Prolonged antioestrogenic activity of ICI 46, 474 in the ovariectomized mouse. J Reprod Fertil 42(2):251–258

135. Jordan VC, Koerner S (1975) Tamoxifen (ICI 46,474) and the human carcinoma 8S oestrogen receptor. Eur J Cancer 11(3):205–206
136. Jordan VC, Allen KE (1980) Evaluation of the antitumour activity of the non-steroidal anti-oestrogen monohydroxytamoxifen in the DMBA-induced rat mammary carcinoma model. Eur J Cancer 16(2):239–251
137. Jordan VC, Allen KE, Dix CJ (1980) Pharmacology of tamoxifen in laboratory animals. Cancer Treat Rep 64(6–7):745–759
138. Jordan VC, Dix CJ, Allen KE (1979) The effectiveness of long term tamoxifen treatment in a laboratory model for adjuvant hormone therapy of breast cancer. In: Salmon SE, Jones SE (eds) Adjuvant therapy of cancer II. Grune and Stratton, New York, pp 19–26
139. Jordan VC (2016) A retrospective: on clinical studies with 5-fluorouracil. Cancer Res 76(4):767–768. https://doi.org/10.1158/0008-5472.CAN-16-0150
140. Controlled trial of tamoxifen as single adjuvant agent in management of early breast cancer. Analysis at six years by Nolvadex Adjuvant Trial Organisation (1985) Lancet 1(8433):836–840
141. Adjuvant tamoxifen in the management of operable breast cancer: the Scottish Trial. Report from the Breast Cancer Trials Committee, Scottish Cancer Trials Office (MRC), Edinburgh (1987) Lancet 2(8552):171–175
142. Colletta AA, Benson JR, Baum M (1994) Alternative mechanisms of action of anti-oestrogens. Breast Cancer Res Treat 31(1):5–9
143. Early Breast Cancer Trialists' Collaborative G, Davies C, Godwin J, Gray R, Clarke M, Cutter D, Darby S, McGale P, Pan HC, Taylor C, Wang YC, Dowsett M, Ingle J, Peto R (2011) Relevance of breast cancer hormone receptors and other factors to the efficacy of adjuvant tamoxifen: patient-level meta-analysis of randomised trials. Lancet 378(9793):771–784. https://doi.org/10.1016/S0140-6736(11)60993-8

A Novel Strategy to Improve Women's Health: Selective Estrogen Receptor Modulators

Balkees Abderrahman and V. Craig Jordan

Abstract Tamoxifen is the first selective estrogen receptor modulator. The extensive clinical and laboratory testing during the 1980s and 1990s raised questions about why there is target site specificity of tamoxifen in different species, i.e., tamoxifen is an estrogen in mice but a complete anti-estrogen in chicks. Additionally, tamoxifen has estrogen-like effects to lower circulating cholesterol, build postmenopausal bone in women, and stimulate the uterus and endometrial cancer growth but paradoxically prevents breast tumor growth. These observations lead to the SERM solution to prevent osteoporosis with a safe SERM but to prevent breast cancer at the same time. Raloxifene is the result with no increase in endometrial cancer incidence. There are now five FDA-approved SERMS available for use: tamoxifen, raloxifene, bazedoxifene, toremifene, and ospemifene. All have connections with discovery and basic research in Jordan's laboratory.

Keywords Selective estrogen receptor modulators · Women's health · Bazedoxifene · Ospemifene · Toremifene · Raloxifene · Lasofoxifene

1 Introduction

The clinical evaluation of tamoxifen in the 1970s for the treatment of metastatic breast cancer (MBC) and during the 1980s for the long-term adjuvant therapy of breast cancer [1] created a therapeutic benchmark to be improved. Numerous new nonsteroidal anti-estrogens were evaluated to treat MBC (Fig. 1), but only one toremifene was successful in achieving a market. By a lucky set of circumstances, tamoxifen, a nonsteroidal anti-estrogen, was to dominate the endocrine therapy and prevention of breast cancer for 35 years.

During the 1970s and early 1980s, the unusually species-specific pharmacology of tamoxifen and indeed other nonsteroidal anti-estrogens [2] was perplexing.

B. Abderrahman · V. C. Jordan (✉)
Department of Breast Medical Oncology, University of Texas, MD Anderson Cancer Center, Houston, TX, USA
e-mail: bhabderrahman@mdanderson.org; vcjordan@mdanderson.org

© Springer Nature Switzerland AG 2019
X. Zhang (ed.), *Estrogen Receptor and Breast Cancer*, Cancer Drug Discovery and Development, https://doi.org/10.1007/978-3-319-99350-8_8

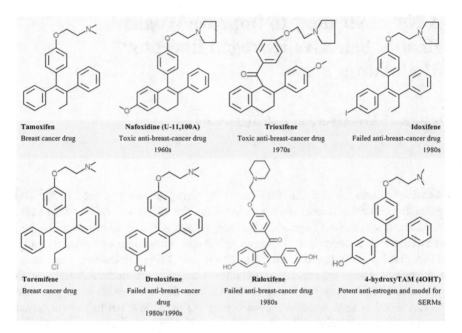

Fig. 1 Compounds that were evaluated in clinical trials but failed as competitors for tamoxifen 1960s–1990s. The exception was toremifene that is used for MBC. The tamoxifen metabolite, 4OHT, became the key drug discovery with high binding affinity for the ER. This was the new model for SERM discoveries (Fig. 5)

Tamoxifen was classified as an estrogen in short-term mouse uterine weight or vaginal cornification assays [2]. Tamoxifen was a partial agonist in the rat uterine weight test but an anti-estrogen in rat vaginal cornification assays [3]. Tamoxifen was a complete anti-estrogen in the chick oviduct [4]. In the dog, tamoxifen is an estrogen, and metabolite E, tamoxifen without the dimethylamine-ethane anti-estrogenic side chain, is observed [5]. One possible explanation considered for the species-specific estrogen target site, estrogenic actions of tamoxifen was the species-specific metabolism of tamoxifen to nonsteroidal estrogens.

This hypothesis was addressed in vivo and in vitro [6] with liver microsomes using [³H] tamoxifen. It was first proven that tamoxifen was metabolically activated to the more potent uterotrophic agent, 4-hydroxytamoxifen, in ovariectomized mice. This was achieved by using 4-chlorotamoxifen, which cannot be hydroxylated at the four position [7]; the tamoxifen derivative was a weak uterotrophic agent. Tamoxifen was ten times more potent as a uterotrophic agent than 4-chlorotamoxifen [6]. 4-Hydroxytamoxifen is more potent than tamoxifen in the ovariectomized mouse uterus [6]. This confirmed previous work in the immature rat [7] where 4-hydroxytamoxifen and 4-chlorotamoxifen exhibited potent and weak partial uterotrophic effects, respectively. The candidate nonsteroidal estrogenic metabolites of tamoxifen as estrogen are metabolite E (tamoxifen with the dimethylamino-ethyl side chain severed at the ether link) and bisphenol, the equivalent metabolite of 4-hydroxytamoxifen. The principal metabolite of tamoxifen 4-hydroxytamoxifen comprised 27%, 14%, and 17% of radio activity from mouse, rat, and chicken livers [6]. Bisphenol and metabolite E were not detected. A similar conclusion was reported in a comparison of athymic mice and human sera [8].

In 1980, Sutherland and coworkers [9] reported a new class of binding sites in uterine tissue that bound anti-estrogens with high affinity and specificity but did not bind estradiol. This was called the anti-estrogen-binding protein (AEBP). It was proposed that the AEBP independently binds nonsteroidal anti-estrogens and blocks estrogen action [9]. This hypothesis was addressed by using mouse uterine weight assays to compare and contrast tamoxifen, an estrogen in the mouse, with MER25, a complete anti-estrogen, which binds to ER but has little interaction AEBS. Additionally, a broad range of ligands that bound with different binding affinities for AEBS were used to explore the modulation of anti-uterotrophic action in the mouse [10]. The study by Lyman reported that (1) MER25 completely inhibits the uterotrophic response of tamoxifen and 4-hydroxytamoxifen as well as estradiol and (2) the panel AEBS ligands did not correlate with biological properties in mice [10]. In related studies, the Katzenellenbogen group found no evidence for the role of the AEBS in anti-estrogen action [11, 12]. Simultaneously, Lieberman and coworkers [13] demonstrated that estrogen/anti-estrogen action was dependent upon a direct and reversible interaction of nonsteroidal anti-estrogens with the ER. The shape of the resulting ER complexes resulted in agonist, partial agonist, and antagonist actions [14–17]. However, it was the biology of nonsteroidal anti-estrogens in vivo that was to result in the new group of medicines referred to as SERMs. A recognition of the unusual species-specific actions of tamoxifen at estrogen target tissues was essential to advance therapeutics.

2   The Athymic Rodent Model in Breast Cancer Research

The description of the immune-deficient mouse [18] and its development for the hetero-transplantation and growth of human cancer cells [19] was an important new laboratory model to investigate human cancer therapeutics. The MCF-7 cell line grows into solid tumors if inoculated into estrogen-treated athymic mice [20]. This is necessary because athymic mice have a hypothalamus pituitary lesion [21] resulting in very low estradiol levels and no estrous cycles.

3   Pharmacology of Tamoxifen in the Athymic Mouse Model Transplanted with ER-Positive Tumors

The fact that estrogen-stimulated growth of human breast tumor MCF-7 is blocked by tamoxifen in athymic mice was unexplained because the mouse uterus was simultaneously stimulated to grow [22, 23]. Administration of [^{3}H] tamoxifen to investigate the radiolabeled metabolites of tamoxifen in either human ER-positive breast tumors or mouse uterus revealed no differences [23]. The conclusion was "these studies strongly support the concept that the drug can selectively stimulate or inhibit events in the target tissues of different species without metabolic intervention. We propose that the species differences observed with tamoxifen are the result of differences in the interpretation of the drug-ER complex by the cell. The drug ER complex is perceived as either a stimulatory or an inhibitory signal in the different target tissue from different species."

Taken one step further, Satyaswaroop and coworkers [24] first described that a transplanted human ER-positive endometrial cancer could be stimulated to grow with tamoxifen. This laboratory report received little clinical attention, as it was not focused on the clinical community and patient care. In a later collaborative study, athymic mice were bitransplanted with either a human endometrial tumor or a breast cancer and the two anterior axillae [25]. The results demonstrated that tamoxifen blocked the growth of estrogen-stimulated breast cancer, but endometrial cancer grew with tamoxifen, estrogen, or the combination (Fig. 2). These data were presented at a symposium to celebrate the 800th anniversary of the University of Bologna. There was an immediate but unexpected response from the clinical community through letters to the Lancet [26–28]. However, proof was needed that there was a correlation between tamoxifen treatment and an increased incidence of

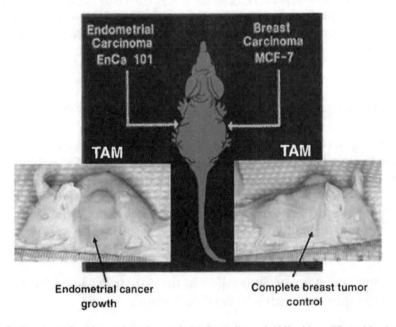

Fig. 2 The pioneering bitransplantation study by Gottardis et al. [25] with an ER-positive breast tumor MCF-7 implanted in one axilla and an ER-positive endometrial tumor (EnCa101) in the other axilla. Tamoxifen blocks estrogen-stimulated growth of the breast tumor, but tamoxifen encourages the growth of the endometrial cancer

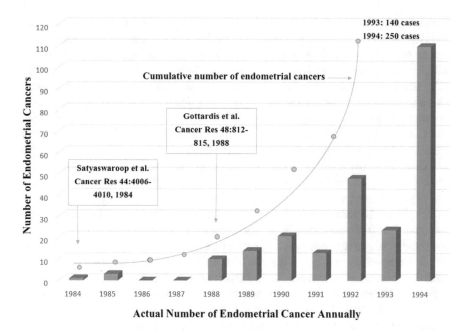

Fig. 3 Reporting of endometrial carcinomas in tamoxifen-treated patients per annum. Cumulative number of cases is plotted; two major studies [24, 25] that led the medical community to focus on the issue are highlighted (Reproduced with permission from [30])

endometrial cancer in randomized clinical trials. Proof was provided by Fornander and coworkers [29], who compared a contrasted 2 and 5 years of adjuvant tamoxifen therapy vs placebo in postmenopausal patients following surgery. Longer adjuvant tamoxifen treatment caused an increase in the detection of endometrial cancer. This chain of events triggered enormous interest by the clinical community summarized in Fig. 3 [31]. Standards of clinical care were changed based on the target tissue-specific actions of tamoxifen around a patient's body. However, the question was subsequently posed: "If tamoxifen is an estrogen, in mouse estrogen target tissues, would tamoxifen be an antitumor agent during mouse mammary carcinogenesis in high incidence strains?" Results of 2-year experiments showed that long-term tamoxifen therapy was superior to ovariectomy in causing mammary tumor chemoprevention in mice. There was tissue site modulation of target tissues in mice where tamoxifen is classified as an estrogen! [32, 33].

4   The Target Site Specificity of Tamoxifen and Keoxifene (Now Known as Raloxifene) in Rats and Humans

The clinical utilization of tamoxifen expanded in the 1980s from its original focus on the treatment of early breast cancer by extending adjuvant therapy [34] to a strategic application to prevent the development of breast cancer in high-risk women [35]. However, not only is estrogen action necessary to cause the development and growth of breast cancer [36] but also to maintain bone density and reduce circulating low-density lipoprotein cholesterol. Presaged by animal studies which showed that tamoxifen and keoxifene (a failed breast cancer drug from Eli Lilly that became raloxifene) could maintain bone density in ovariectomized rats [37] and lower circulating cholesterol [3], tamoxifen was shown to do the same in postmenopausal women [38, 39]. These laboratory and clinical data with tamoxifen and laboratory data with keoxifene were used as evidence to develop the SERM solution. This was simply stated [40] as a roadmap for the pharmaceutical industry to follow. This they did! "Is this the end of the possible applications for anti-estrogens? Certainly not, we have obtained valuable clinical information about this group of drugs that can be applied in other disease states. Research does not travel in straight lines and observations in one field of science often become major discoveries in another. Important clues have been garnered about the effects of tamoxifen on bone and lipids so it is possible that derivatives could find targeted applications to retard osteoporosis or atherosclerosis. The ubiquitous application of novel compounds to prevent diseases associated with the progressive changes after menopause may, as a side effect, significantly retard the development of breast cancer. The target population would be postmenopausal women in general, thereby avoiding the requirement to select a high-risk group to prevent breast cancer."

Subsequent work with tamoxifen [41] and raloxifene [42] in laboratory animals confirmed the bone-sparing properties of these "anti-estrogens" as did the clinical studies published subsequently. The SERM solution was validated by effective translation to clinical practice. A new group of medicines was created and new applications of SERMs advanced.

The development of SERMs not only promised to improve on tamoxifen to prevent breast cancer but also provided the first multifunctional medicines to prevent multiple diseases in aging women. Hormone replacement therapy (HRT) had promised eternal youth for women but numerous problems occurred (Fig. 4), and potentially there was a better way to prevent multiple diseases in postmenopausal women. Indeed, as we will show, SERMs and HRT coalesced after 20 years of trial and error with a SERM plus conjugated equine estrogen (CEE) as an HRT.

5 The Development of SERMs from Laboratory Leads

Interestingly enough, the new SERMs all had origins in earlier publications in the refereed literature. The discovery that tamoxifen is metabolically activated as a prodrug to 4-hydroxytamoxifen [7, 43] was important to create the new group of medicines now referred to as SERMs. Although 4-hydroxytamoxifen was not developed itself as a SERM because the tamoxifen metabolite is rapidly excreted [44], the structural modification and high binding characteristics for the ER were key to future SERM design [45]. The SERMs that were evaluated in clinical trial with a strategic hydroxyl group are raloxifene, bazedoxifene, arzoxifene, and lasofoxifene (Fig. 5).

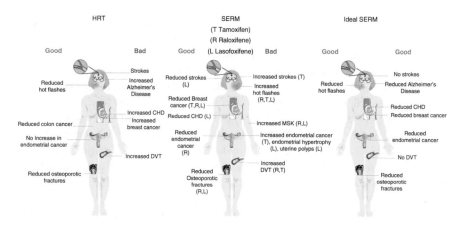

Fig. 4 Current status of available SERMs and progress toward an ideal SERM. The overall good or bad aspects of administering hormone replacement therapy to postmenopausal women compared with the observed site-specific actions of the selective estrogen receptor modulators tamoxifen and raloxifene. The known beneficial or negative actions of SERMs have opened the door for drug discovery to create the ideal SERM or targeted SERMs to either improve quality of life or prevent diseases associated with aging in women. *CHD* cardiovascular heart diseases, *DVT* deep vein thrombosis, *MSK* musculoskeletal symptoms

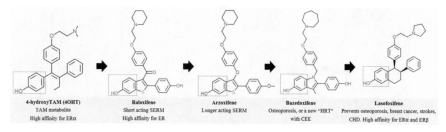

Fig. 5 The value of the early clue from 4OHT that the strategically placed phenolic hydroxyl will result in high binding affinity for prospective SERMs

The SERMs arzoxifene and lasofoxifene were not advanced successfully for FDA approval. Arzoxifene was designed as a "longer-acting raloxifene derivative." In this way it was predicted that arzoxifene would prove to be useful for the treatment of breast cancer [46]. However, the phase III breast cancer trial was stopped because "arzoxifene was statistically significantly inferior to tamoxifen with regard to progression-free survival and other time-to-event parameters, although tumor response was comparable between the treatments" [46]. Nevertheless, in a phase III trial [47], arzoxifene treatment increased spine and hip bone density in postmenopausal women. Other trials support the conclusion that arzoxifene is effective only at preventing vertebral fractures. Further development of arzoxifene was abandoned.

Lasofoxifene is a remarkable molecule and a miracle of medicinal chemistry. The molecule uses the core structure of nafoxidine, the failed contraceptive and failed breast cancer drug (Fig. 6). In laboratory test, lasofoxifene exhibits no uterotrophic actions in either immature or aged female rats [48]. Additionally lasofoxifene preserves bone density and lowers serum cholesterol in ovariectomized rats [49, 50]. There are no stimulatory effects of lasofoxifene on the growth of estrogen-deprived MCF-7 cells in vitro [48]. Lasofoxifene prevents rat mammary carcinogenesis induced by N-nitrosomethylurea [51]. Drug excretion of lasofoxifene is reported [52] to be 95% via the biliary route as a glucuronidated conjugate.

Lasofoxifene is the levorotatory (*l*) enantiomer which is more potent at binding to the ER than the dextrorotatory (*d*) isomer. The (*l*) enantiomer is also resistant to glucuronidation thereby improving bioavailability [48]. Increased potency was confirmed in humans using 0.017, 0.05, 0.15, and 0.5 mg/day which was shown to be effective at maintaining lumbar bone density over a 1-year period [53].

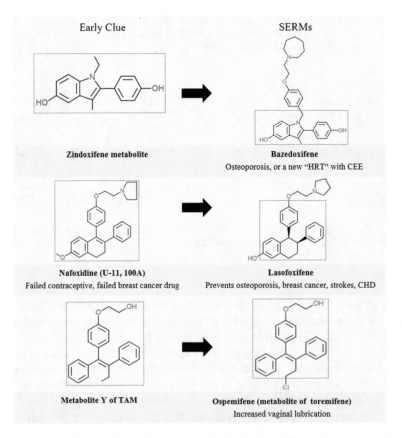

Fig. 6 The laboratory or literature clues that provided the rationale for the development of new SERMs

There are results from three phase III clinical trials with lasofoxifene: (1) Postmenopausal Evaluation and Risk Reduction with Lasofoxifene (PEARL), (2) Osteoporosis Prevention and Lipid Lowering (OPAL), and (3) the study and the Comparison of Raloxifene and Lasofoxifene (CORAL). The PEARL Study noted that lumbar spine and femoral neck bone mineral density were increased at 3 years [54]. The OPAL trial tested three doses of lasofoxifene versus placebo [55, 56]. All three doses showed improved lumbar spine and hip bone mineral density compared to placebo. CORAL noted that lasofoxifene maintained bone mineral density in the lumbar spine better than raloxifene and lowered cholesterol better than raloxifene [56].

Overall lasofoxifene is not only the most potent SERM to date, being a 100 times more potent than raloxifene used at 60 mg daily, but also comes the closest to the therapeutics properties of the ideal SERM [40]. Lasofoxifene reduces breast cancer incidence, producing no increase in endometrial cancer, reduces lumbar fractures, reduces strokes, and reduces coronary heart disease. The medicine is approved in the European Union, and plans are in place for a European marketing plan.

Bazedoxifene has its origins in the failed breast cancer drug zindoxifene (Fig. 6). A study of the metabolites of zindoxifene [57] found them to be estrogens, one of which was extremely potent at the ER. This metabolite, with an appropriately positioned anti-estrogenic side chain, became bazedoxifene [58].

Bazedoxifene has been successfully tested as an agent to improve bone density and bone turnover [59] without negative effects upon the reproductive track [60]. Vertebral fractures are reduced compared to placebo, and in high-risk women, bazedoxifene lowers the risk of non-vertebral fractures significantly relative to placebo and raloxifene [61]. Nevertheless, bazedoxifene is not available in the United States as a treatment for osteoporosis. The innovation that is preferred is to substitute bazedoxifene in HRT instead of medroxyprogesterone acetate (MPA).

Women have used HRT in the United States for the past 40 years. Originally, CEE was used alone, but a small but significant increase in endometrial cancer was noted in the mid-1970s [62, 63]. It was reasoned that a combination of CEE with a progestin would prevent unopposed estrogen-stimulated uterine proliferation that resulted in endometrial cancer. Despite the conviction that HRT would not only create a strong skeleton but also reduce the risk of coronary disease following menopause, the Women's Health Initiative (WHI) put the theory to the test by selecting women over their 60s to enter trials of HRT versus placebo in women with a uterus and CEE versus placebo in hysterectomized women. The results were interesting. The trial of HRT versus placebo was stopped once a predetermined incidence of breast cancer was observed in the HRT arm [64]. This was anticipated. However, the CEE versus placebo was stopped not for an increased risk of breast cancer but an increase incidence of strokes [65]. There was an unanticipated persistent decrease in breast cancer in the CEE group. Though surprising to the medical community, these data for CEE in long-term estrogen-deprived women followed biological rules established through clinical trials over the previous 60 years. The first therapy to treat any cancer successfully was high-dose synthetic estrogen treatment of metastatic breast cancer in postmenopausal women [66, 67]. No mechanisms were known at the time (1950–1975); the biology of estrogen-killing breast cancer cells in patients was established by experimental medicine and observations. However, this was a paradox as oophorectomy with estrogen withdrawal was standard of care for premenopausal patients with MBC. Response rates were about 30%. Paradoxically high-dose estrogen therapy was only effective in 30% of patients if administered 5 years after menopause [67]. If estrogen was administered earlier, breast tumors grew. It is interesting to note that 5 years of adjuvant tamoxifen therapy became the standard of care for 20 years at the end of the twentieth century. However, there was an unexplained phenomenon, the "carryover effect."

Tamoxifen is a competitive inhibitor of estrogen action at the ER. It is a rule of pharmacology that if tamoxifen was not being given to block the ER, a woman's own estrogen would reactivate tumor growth. In the case of 5 years adjuvant tamoxifen therapy, this did not occur, and in fact mortality decreased after the drug was stopped! [68]. The key was the consistent 5-year rule of LTED in breast cancer. It is proposed that there is clonal selection pressure for survival of breast cancer cells in micrometastases during LTED [69]. Discovery of mechanisms started with the finding that the serial transplantation of MCF-7 breast tumors with acquired tamoxifen resistance into new generations of athymic mice treated with tamoxifen actually sensitized the tumors to the tumoricidal actions of low-dose estrogen [70, 71]. Estrogen-induced apoptosis has been noted to occur [72, 73], and this experimental biology has been advanced as the reason for the "carryover effect" after adjuvant antihormone therapy is stopped [69] and for the tumoricidal action of CEE alone in hysterectomized woman in the WHI [74].

The idea of combining CEE with a SERM was first proposed in 1998 [75]. To paraphrase, "there are concerns that site-specific anti-estrogens used for the long-term treatment of postmenopausal women may not produce estrogenic effects in the CNS." In fact, the main problem with long-term anti-estrogen therapy is menopausal side effects. "Indeed, the combination of an appropriate compound with Premarin would provide the benefits in the CNS and the benefits of a targeted anti-estrogen in the periphery" [75]. The combination of CEE and bazedoxifene is available for the amelioration of postmenopausal symptoms. The anti-estrogen bazedoxifene blocks breast and endometrial tumor ER, thereby preventing an increase in breast and endometrial cancer [76].

The question has to be asked: "If an anti-estrogen prevents estrogen-stimulated breast cancer growth with a bazedoxifene/CEE combination, why does MPA increase breast cancer when combined with CEE?" The answer lies in the modulation of estrogen-induced apoptosis by glucocorticoids [77–79]. It is well known that MPA has glucocorticoid activity at the glucocorticoid receptor and has been proven to block estrogen-induced apoptosis in LTED breast cancer cells [78]. As a result, microscopic early breast cancer has the potential to grow into invasive breast cancer during HRT. By contrast, CEE alone causes apoptosis in LTED breast cancer thereby reducing the incidence of breast cancer.

Finally, there is the interesting application of ospemifene, a known metabolite of the tamoxifen derivative of toremifene (Fig. 6). The discovery of metabolite Y of tamoxifen [80, 81] was found to be a step during the systematic metabolism of the anti-estrogenic side chain of tamoxifen. The molecule has a low binding affinity for the ER, but the innovation was the identification of the equivalent metabolite for toremifene and the use of the metabolite for dyspareunia. The trick was knowing that tamoxifen causes increase vaginal secretions in women [82]. The metabolite now called ospemifene does the same.

The extensive investigation of tamoxifen and related nonsteroidal anti-estrogens in the 1980s [40, 83] created the incentive to commercialize the new group of medicines now referred to as SERMs [45]. This resulted in multiple advances in women's health [84]. In the next section, we will describe the new knowledge pertaining to the molecular biology of estrogen action that provides an insight into the mechanisms of SERM action.

6   Mechanism of SERM Action

Studies of the pharmacology of the metabolites of tamoxifen provided the laboratory tools to explore mechanisms of action of anti-estrogens in modulating prolactin synthesis in normal cells [13, 14, 16, 17] and the replication of breast cancer cells in culture [85, 86]. The resulting hypothetical "crocodile model" [17, 87] informed what was occurring inside of the ER and led to the identification of the "anti-estrogen region" [17] that is required by anti-estrogenic action for both 4-hydroxytamoxifen and raloxifene to create an anti-estrogenic mechanism. The target for the bulky anti-estrogen side chain is asp351 [88–91]. The subsequent x-ray crystallography of raloxifene and 4-hydroxytamoxifen demonstrated that the anti-estrogenic side chain of raloxifene neutralized and shielded asp351 [92], whereas the anti-estrogenic side chain of 4-hydroxytamoxifen was positioned further away from asp 351 which was not adequately shielded [93]. Indeed, these data illustrated the reason for the more promiscuous estrogen-like action of tamoxifen compared to raloxifene. This mechanism can be traced back to the imperfect closing of helix 12 in the tamoxifen ER complex. Subsequent, structure-activity relationships of asp351 and the anti-estrogens side chain of either tamoxifen or raloxifene confirmed the pivotal role of asp351 as an anchor to helix 12 closure [94–99].

Hypothetical models were advanced to aid in the explanation of agonist (crocodile jaws closed), antagonist (crocodile jaws open by the anti-estrogenic side chain), and partial agonist (a proportional mixture of estrogen/anti-estrogen complexes) [83]. However, advances in technology and the molecular biology of estrogen action facilitated an understanding of SERM action.

Differences between estrogen and anti-estrogen actions are based on the change in the conformation of the ER complex (Fig. 7). There are three complementary mechanisms that modulate the ligand ER complex:

(1) The ligand shape alters the shape of the external surface of the ER complex [101, 102]. Selective estrogen receptor modulators each induce distinct conformational changes in ER alpha and ER beta [102, 103] that attract either coactivators or

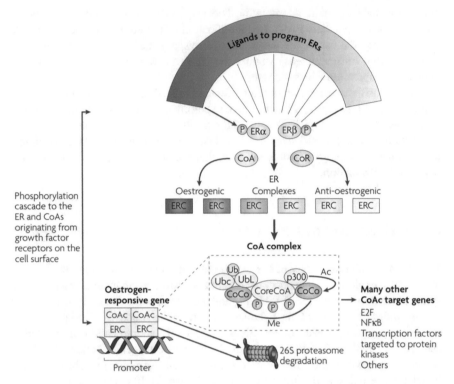

Fig. 7 Molecular networks potentially influence the expression of SERM action in a target tissue. The shape of the ligands that bind to the estrogen receptors (ERs)α and β programs the complex to become an estrogenic or anti-estrogenic signal. The context of the ER complex (ERC) can influence the expression of the response through the numbers of corepressors (CoR) or coactivators (CoA). In simple terms, a site with few CoAs or high levels of CoRs might be a dominant antiestrogenic site. However, the expression of estrogenic action is not simply the binding of the receptor complex to the promoter of the estrogen-responsive gene but a dynamic process of CoA complex assembly and destruction. A core CoA, for example, steroid receptor coactivator protein 3 (SRC3), and the ERC are influenced by phosphorylation cascades that phosphorylate target sites on both complexes. The core CoA then assembles an activated multiprotein complex containing specific co-coactivators (CoCo) that might include p300, each of which has a specific enzymatic activity to be activated later. The CoA complex (CoAc) binds to the ERC at the estrogen-responsive gene promoter to switch on transcription. The CoCo proteins then perform methylation (Me) or acetylation (Ac) to activate dissociation of the complex. Simultaneously, ubiquitylation by the bound ubiquitin-conjugating enzyme (Ubc) targets ubiquitin ligase (UbL) destruction of protein members of the complex through the 26S proteasome. The ERs are also ubiquitylated and destroyed in the 26S proteasome. Therefore, a regimented cycle of assembly, activation, and destruction occurs on the basis of the preprogrammed ER complex. However, the coactivator, specifically SRC3, has ubiquitous action and can further modulate or amplify the ligand-activated trigger through many modulating genes 101 that can consolidate and increase the stimulatory response of the ERC in a tissue. Therefore, the target tissue is programmed to express a spectrum of responses between full estrogen action and anti-estrogen action on the basis of the shape of the ligand and the sophistication of the tissue-modulating network. *NFκB* nuclear factor κB (Reproduced with permission from [100])

corepressors. Indeed, peptide antagonist of the human estrogen receptor can block SERM actions [104, 105].

(2) Allosteric regulation of ER structure and function by different estrogen response elements [106].

(3) The turnover of the SERM ER complex whose stability is regulated by agonist, antagonist, and SERM complexes by the ubiquitinylation and destruction of the complex via the 26S proteasome.

The discovery of coactivators [107] that bind to the estrogen ER complex and corepressors that bind to the anti-estrogen ER complex provided a new dimension in the understanding of the complexities of SERM action [108, 109]. Now it is documented that not only is the ER complex with the SERM modulated through destruction, but also the coactivators are independently destroyed thereby emasculating signal transduction pathway. These events are all summarized in Fig. 7.

7   Summary and Selective Nuclear Receptor Modulators

Blockbuster success, i.e., revenues over a billion dollars annually with tamoxifen, the first SERM, and raloxifene, the first truly multifunctional SERM, has naturally raised the possibility that modulators for all members of the nuclear receptor super family can be discovered. This prospect could result in the treatment of diseases never before believed to be possible. Additionally, steroid therapies could be safer, e.g., a selective glucocorticoid could be found with anti-inflammatory action but without the problem of promoting bone resorption.

The full range of experimental compounds is selective ER modulators (SERMs), selective androgen receptor modulators (SARMs), selective progesterone receptor modulators (SPRMs), selective glucocorticoid receptor modulators (SGRMs), selective mineralocorticoid receptor modulators (SMRMs), selective thyroid receptor modulators (STRMs), and selective peroxisome proliferator-activated receptor modulators (SPPARMs), which has recently been reviewed [110].

At the beginning of the journey to SERMs in the 1980s, once the foundation had been laid with the first SERM tamoxifen in the 1970s, one could not have immediately predicted the success of the concept with the enhancement of women's health nor the survival of millions of women with breast cancer or, in the case of raloxifene for the treatment of osteoporosis, fewer breast cancer. Nevertheless, search continues for the ideal SERM. This search is achieving successes (Fig. 4) and especially if the plans to market lasofoxifene in Europe come to fruition.

Personal Postscript of V. Craig Jordan

In 1980, I was recruited to the University of Wisconsin Clinical Cancer Center (UWCCC), Madison. At this one campus, there was excellence in basic and clinical cancer research. The University of Wisconsin-Madison was perfect for me.

The University of Wisconsin was then unique in America as it had two cancer centers. The McArdle Laboratory for Cancer Research focused on basic research for the causes of cancer. This remarkable cancer research unit was created by its inaugural Director Harold Rusch, MD. Harold went on to create the UWCCC following the signing of the National Cancer Act in 1971. It was Harold that recruited Paul P. Carbone, MD, from the National Cancer Institute in Washington to be his successor upon his retirement. The goal was to build a team of staff to translate discoveries in the laboratory that would accelerate progress in cancer care.

The UWCCC, at that time, had no graduate program, but the faculty at the McArdle laboratory generously permitted Anna C. Tate, a Fulbright Hays Scholar (see Fig. 8b Anna Riegel (née Tate)), to be my PhD student in their program. I was permitted to be her PhD supervisor for a McArdle PhD but with her work conducted in the Department of Human Oncology, UWCCC. She had already been awarded a BSc with first class honors in Pharmacology and a Master's of Science degree with distinction in Steroid Endocrinology, both from the University of Leeds. She successfully defended her thesis at the end of the 3 years in my laboratory at UWCCC. Her thesis work built upon my earlier connections with Elwood Jensen in Chicago who introduced me to his postdoctoral fellow Geoffrey Greene (see Fig. 8c). We became collaborators then, and we have an active collaboration today. During his fellowship with Elwood Jensen, Geoff created the first polyclonal antibodies to the human ER [111] and the first monoclonal antibodies [112, 113]. This work was critical to make the subsequent cloning and sequencing of the human ER possible [114]. However, I had a different idea: to understand the molecular interaction of anti-estrogens with the ligand binding domain of the ER.

My collaboration with Geoff Greene and Elwood Jensen (who then had moved to Switzerland) resulted in numerous publications using polyclonal and monoclonal antibodies to the human ER. The hypothesis was that there would be differences in the estradiol and 4-hydroxytamoxifen ER complexes. The fact that I had received the first synthetic $[^3H]$4-hydroxytamoxifen (4OHT) from ICI pharmaceuticals in Cheshire was a plus [115]. A difference in antibody binding to reconfigured epitope might be informative for estrogen and anti-estrogen ER complexes. The monoclonal antibodies did not detect differences in the estrogen or anti-estrogen receptor complex from rat pituitary tumor GH3 cells, MCF-7 breast cancer cells, or breast tumor cytosols. By contrast, the polyclonal goat antibody raised to the calf uterine ER [116] discriminated radiolabeled E_2 or radiolabeled 4-OHT binding to human breast cancer ER. Preincubation of the unoccupied human ER with the polyclonal antibodies prevented radiolabel E_2 from being locked into the ER. Estrogen rapidly dissociated from the paralyzed ER. The "crocodile jaws" remained open with polyclonal antibody binding to the ER. By contrast, the $[^3H]$ 4-OHT wedged into the ER complex whether the polyclonal antibody was preincubated with ER or the complex was incubated subsequently [116]. Anti-estrogens worked by preventing the jaws from closing. Subsequently, the jaws would be identified as helix 12, a dozen years later.

During my 3-month recruitment visit to Madison in 1977, I was lucky to become friends with Jack Gorski. This was during the worst winter in living memory as snow started the week we arrived in October and continued for 4 months after we left in January 1978. Jack introduced me to Mara Lieberman in his laboratory who showed me her unpublished data on estradiol-stimulated prolactin synthesis in

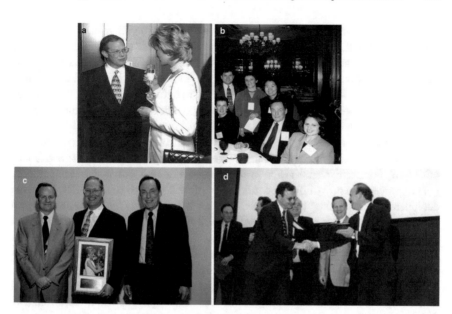

Fig. 8 Multiple photographs from the 2 days of celebrations in 1999 for Dr. Jordan's investiture as the Inaugural Diana, Princess of Wales, Professor of Cancer Research at Northwestern University in Chicago. (**a**) Dr. Jordan with Diana, Princess of Wales, at a private reception given by the President of Northwestern University. Dr. Jordan had organized the program of a symposium on women's health. Diana, Princess of Wales, had agreed to deliver the keynote address and accepting the invitation to visit Chicago's Northwestern University June 4–6, 1996. (**b**) Elwood V. Jensen keynote speaker in the symposium honoring Dr. Jordan during the celebrations surrounding his investiture as the Inaugural Diana, the Princess of Wales, Professor for Cancer Research. Their positions in the tamoxifen teams when they were in training followed by their current positions. From left to right clockwise: Anna T. Riegel (née Tate), PhD student, today Cecilia Fisher Rudman Professor Department of Oncology and Pharmacology Director of Research Education. William H. Catherino, MD PhD student, today Professor and Research Head, Department of Obstetrics and Gynecology, Uniformed Services University of the Health Sciences Associate Program Director. Anna Levenson, MD, PhD, postdoctoral fellow, today Associate Dean for Research and Graduate Studies. Eun-Sook Lee, visiting Faculty, today Director of the Cancer Research Center of South Korea. Dr. Elwood Jensen. Dr. Debra Tonetti, postdoctoral fellow, today Department Head, Professor of Pharmacology at the University of Illinois, Chicago. (**c**) Dr. Geoffrey Greene and Dr. Elwood Jensen, participants in the symposium honoring Dr. Jordan during the 2-day celebration with his investiture as the Diana, Princess of Wales, Professor of Cancer Research. (**d**) The symposium speakers at the event to honor Dr. Jordan upon his investiture as the Diana, Princess of Wales, Professor of Cancer Research. Dr. Marco Gottardis, who was Dr. Jordan's PhD student at Wisconsin in the Tamoxifen Team, is receiving his commemorative plaque from Dr. Steven Rosen, the Director of the Robert H. Lurie Cancer Center in Chicago

isolated immature rat pituitary cells in short-term culture. She published it a year later in the Proceedings of the National Academy of Sciences [117]. Here was a new and, at the time, the only model we could use to address the structure function relationships of nonsteroidal anti-estrogens! This was an essential first step toward our discovery of the pharmacology of SERMs, as we had just published our work on the metabolic activation of tamoxifen to 4-hydroxytamoxifen [43].

The discovery that an anti-estrogen could have this same affinity for the ER as an estrogen was revolutionary. Up to that point, it was reasoned that since anti-estrogens had only weak binding affinity to the ER, the complex would easily dissociate and full estrogen action would be impossible [118]. If low affinity to the ER did not predict anti-estrogen action, the hypothesis evolved to become the shape of the complex that predicted pharmacological activity. Based upon the shape of the resulting ligand, ER complex partial agonist or complete antagonist could be predicted [83].

The modulation of estrogen-stimulated synthesis of prolactin in vitro resulted in the publication of the "crocodile model": the bulky alkyl aminoethoxy side chain of 4OHT (or later raloxifene) needs to interact with an anti-estrogen binding region [17] to prevent closure of the crocodile's jaw (now known to be helix 12). This was deciphered and validated by the UWCCC Tamoxifen Team. This advance was told in our companion chapter: the Tamoxifen Tale. It required a multifaceted team of PhD students to create models to decipher mechanisms that paralleled the essential work of others to crystallize the ligand binding domain of the human ER with estrogens and the SERMs 4-hydroxytamoxifen and raloxifene.

An understanding of the species differences of the pharmacology of nonsteroidal anti-estrogens was pivotal for progress in human therapeutics with tamoxifen. The development of athymic animals that were immune deficient now allowed human breast cancer cell lives to be inoculated and therapy evaluated in vivo. We were fortunate in the new facilities at UWCCC to have state-of-the-art athymic animal suites. Marco Gottardis (Fig. 8d) and Doug Wolf, both PhD students on the UWCCC T32 training grant (Doug was also a recipient of a Komen scholarship), deserve credit for their skill using the new research model. Marco was the pioneer. He developed the model of acquired resistance to tamoxifen using MCF-7 breast cancer cells inoculated into athymic mice. He proved that acquired resistance to tamoxifen in athymic mice was tamoxifen-stimulated growth [119]. He used athymic rats to demonstrate that metabolism was not critical for tamoxifen-stimulated tumor growth [120]. Furthermore, he was the first to test a new pure steroidal anti-estrogen in the mouse model to show that a "pure anti-estrogen" would be suitable second-line therapy in patients when acquired resistance to tamoxifen occurred [121]. Today fulvestrant is used routinely in the treatment of MBC.

Most importantly, Marco was an essential investigator in the SERM story. He used the athymic mouse model bitransplanted with a human ER-positive endometrial cancer with a human ER-positive breast cancer transplanted in the contralateral axilla. The question to be addressed was: "Is tamoxifen an anti-estrogen in both target tissue tumors from women?" The answer was that tamoxifen prevented breast tumor growth, but the endometrial cancer grew robustly [25]. Following much correspondence in the Lancet [26–28], a link was established between long-term adjuvant tamoxifen use to treat breast cancer, and a small but significant increase in an increased incidence in endometrial cancer was noted. As a result, gynecologists were involved in screening women for occult endometrial cancer prior to tamoxifen therapy. Patient care was changed.

Most importantly, tamoxifen and, a failed breast cancer drug, keoxifene were tested in the laboratory to determine the extent of bone loss in ovariectomized old breeder rats [37]. This line of research came about by accident but was an essential step to progress with chemoprevention in healthy women. Without this study [37], there would not have been the SERM solution, as it would not have been proposed in 1990 [40]. If estrogen is essential to build bones in women, it would be a disaster to prevent breast cancer in planned chemoprevention trials but at the same time increase the incidence of osteoporosis for all who took the anti-estrogen tamoxifen. If estrogen prevents osteoporosis, then an anti-estrogen by definition would make osteoporosis worse. This was the pivotal laboratory clue that drove all subsequent clinical work at Wisconsin on tamoxifen, and, eventually, after several years, the baton in the relay race for SERMs was picked up by Eli Lilly.

Dr. Urban Lindgren was a visiting scientist from the Karlinska Institute in Stockholm who was now working at the University of Wisconsin, Madison, in the Biochemistry Department. He approached me to consider using nonsteroidal anti-estrogens to create an enhanced laboratory model of osteoporosis. He wanted to test vitamin D analogs to prevent osteoporosis. He reasoned if estrogen is good to build bone, then an anti-estrogen would make osteoporosis worse. This did not seem like an unreasonable hypothesis. We used as our study design a prior study by Beall and coworkers [122], who determined the action of the nonsteroidal anti-estrogen clomiphene on bone density of ovariectomized retired breeder rats. The study [122] paradoxically showed that clomiphene maintained bone density. But I noticed the authors had made a fatal error with their choice of an anti-estrogen. Clomiphene is a mixture of estrogenic and anti-estrogenic geometric isomers. I reasoned that the estrogenic zuclomiphene might be bone specific and that could prevent osteoporosis. By contrast, our study tested tamoxifen, the pure anti-estrogenic *trans* isomer, and keoxifene (LY156758), a high-affinity anti-estrogen that had been abandoned by Eli Lilly as a breast cancer drug. Fortunately, they had allowed me to keep a large quantity of their anti-estrogen keoxifene. Eric Phelps a summer student in our Wisconsin Tamoxifen Team analyzed the data. He showed that both tamoxifen and keoxifene were estrogen-like on ovariectomized rat bone density. All osteoporosis journals rejected our manuscript with the opinion that our data could not be correct, as an anti-estrogen cannot build bone! However, Breast Cancer Research and Treatment and Bill McGuire, the editor, embraced our findings. The bone density data in rats with tamoxifen was confirmed by others [41], but no animal bone studies with keoxifene were published after the original Jordan study in 1987 [37]. This study [37] became the translational research foundation for the whole of the Wisconsin tamoxifen study [38, 39]. In 1987, my Cancer Center Director Paul Carbone appointed me to be the Director of his Breast Cancer Research and Treatment Breast Program (1987–1993). As a full professor, appointed in 1985, I was a member of Dr. Richard Love's promotion committee along with Drs. Ernest Borden and Tom Davis. Dick was an assistant professor, but Paul was keen to ensure that Dick appropriately advanced up the professional ladder. However, up to this point, Dick's strong academic suit was teaching rather than translational research. He was, however, enthusiastic about chemoprevention and had previously struck up a collaboration with Dr. Ray Brown, who was enthusiastic about the application of retinoids, as chemopreventive agents. Much clinical work in this area was then being conducted by Professor Umberto Veronesi's group in Milan. However, this strategy changed very rapidly after Paul and I attended a meeting in New York that was planning to address chemoprevention. This meeting was held because of the announcement by Dr. Trevor Powles in the United Kingdom that he was about to start a pilot clinical trial of tamoxifen. These preliminary data were published in 1989 [123]. We now saw tamoxifen as top of the international clinical agenda. Indeed, it was of such importance that my mother rang me up and declared that "somebody in England is planning to use your drug to prevent breast cancer – do something about it!" So, at Wisconsin we did.

I became the Head of the Breast Cancer Research and Treatment program, and Dick started to plan clinical studies with tamoxifen. Dick's assets at Wisconsin were Polly Newcome, an excellent epidemiologist; Dave DeMets, an exceptional biostatistician from NIH; and my Tamoxifen Team which was considered the world's center of tamoxifen research at that time. This was a most fortuitous mix of talent at one place. Dick advanced the laboratory data on tamoxifen and bone density we had produced [37]. He threw the dice to get a quick positive paper comparing and contrasting patients taking tamoxifen, but this was, regrettably, a negative finding [124]. He, then, chose to go the clinical trial route with funding for him from the American Cancer Society and support for our program from AstraZeneca. The rat bone data with tamoxifen became the translational rationale for the Wisconsin Tamoxifen Study of bones and lipids in node-negative patients treated with tamoxifen or placebo for 2 years.

Keoxifene was reinvented as raloxifene by changing the salt of the compound from LY156758 mesylate (keoxifene) to LY139481 HCl (raloxifene). There were no patents for the use of either keoxifene or raloxifene in the late 1980s for osteoporosis, only a breast cancer indication, and that was abandoned after 1987. Black and coworkers [42] confirmed that the molecule keoxifene (raloxifene) was able to reduce circulating cholesterol and build bone in laboratory rats. Patents were awarded [125], and raloxifene went forward to become a blockbuster medicine (i.e., a billion dollar a year sales).

Raloxifene went to clinical trials to test the hypothesis that the compound would prevent osteoporosis and reduce the incidence of breast cancer at the same time. Marco had already demonstrated that tamoxifen and keoxifene would prevent rat mammary carcinogenesis. However, keoxifene was less effective [126].

The Multiple Outcome of Raloxifene Evaluation (MORE) trial demonstrated that raloxifene reduced spinal fractures by 50% compared to placebo. A separate analysis of breast cancer incidence demonstrated a 76% decrease in the incidence of ER-positive breast cancer over a 3-year period [127]. At the Robert H. Lurie Comprehensive Cancer Center of Northwestern University, I was the Director of the Breast Cancer Research Program and because of my previous interactions with Diana, Princess of Wales, I was appointed the Diana, Princess of Wales, Professor of Cancer Research (Fig. 8a) after her untimely death. I (VCJ) was the chair of the breast cancer adjudication committee of the MORE trial. This translational work was an exceptional, though unconventional, team effort between a university (Wisconsin/Northwestern) investigator and the pharmaceutical industry. The SERM concept [40] worked!

References

1. Furr BJ, Jordan VC (1984) The pharmacology and clinical uses of tamoxifen. Pharmacol Ther 25(2):127–205
2. Terenius L (1971) Structure-activity relationships of anti-oestrogens with regard to interaction with 17-beta-oestradiol in the mouse uterus and vagina. Acta Endocrinol 66(3):431–447
3. Harper MJ, Walpole AL (1967) A new derivative of triphenylethylene: effect on implantation and mode of action in rats. J Reprod Fertil 13(1):101–119
4. Sutherland R, Mester J, Baulieu EE (1977) Tamoxifen is a potent pure anti-oestrogen in chick oviduct. Nature 267(5610):434–435. https://doi.org/10.1038/267434a0
5. Fromson JM, Pearson S, Bramah S (1973) The metabolism of tamoxifen (I.C.I. 46,474). I. In laboratory animals. Xenobiotica 3(11):693–709. https://doi.org/10.3109/00498257309151594
6. Lyman SD, Jordan VC (1985) Metabolism of tamoxifen and its uterotrophic activity. Biochem Pharmacol 34(15):2787–2794
7. Allen KE, Clark ER, Jordan VC (1980) Evidence for the metabolic activation of non-steroidal antioestrogens: a study of structure-activity relationships. Br J Pharmacol 71(1):83–91
8. Robinson SP, Langan-Fahey SM, Jordan VC (1989) Implications of tamoxifen metabolism in the athymic mouse for the study of antitumor effects upon human breast cancer xenografts. Eur J Cancer Clin Oncol 25(12):1769–1776
9. Sutherland RL, Murphy LC, San Foo M, Green MD, Whybourne AM, Krozowski ZS (1980) High-affinity anti-oestrogen binding site distinct from the oestrogen receptor. Nature 288(5788):273–275
10. Lyman SD, Jordan VC (1985) Possible mechanisms for the agonist actions of tamoxifen and the antagonist actions of MER-25 (ethamoxytriphetol) in the mouse uterus. Biochem Pharmacol 34(15):2795–2806
11. Katzenellenbogen BS, Miller MA, Eckert RL, Sudo K (1983) Antiestrogen pharmacology and mechanism of action. J Steroid Biochem 19(1A):59–68
12. Miller MA, Katzenellenbogen BS (1983) Characterization and quantitation of antiestrogen binding sites in estrogen receptor-positive and -negative human breast cancer cell lines. Cancer Res 43(7):3094–3100
13. Lieberman ME, Jordan VC, Fritsch M, Santos MA, Gorski J (1983) Direct and reversible inhibition of estradiol-stimulated prolactin synthesis by antiestrogens in vitro. J Biol Chem 258(8):4734–4740
14. Jordan VC, Lieberman ME, Cormier E, Koch R, Bagley JR, Ruenitz PC (1984) Structural requirements for the pharmacological activity of nonsteroidal antiestrogens in vitro. Mol Pharmacol 26(2):272–278
15. Jordan VC, Lieberman ME (1984) Estrogen-stimulated prolactin synthesis in vitro. Classification of agonist, partial agonist, and antagonist actions based on structure. Mol Pharmacol 26(2):279–285
16. Jordan VC, Koch R, Mittal S, Schneider MR (1986) Oestrogenic and antioestrogenic actions in a series of triphenylbut-1-enes: modulation of prolactin synthesis in vitro. Br J Pharmacol 87(1):217–223
17. Lieberman ME, Gorski J, Jordan VC (1983) An estrogen receptor model to describe the regulation of prolactin synthesis by antiestrogens in vitro. J Biol Chem 258(8):4741–4745
18. Pantelouris EM (1968) Absence of thymus in a mouse mutant. Nature 217(5126):370–371
19. Rygaard J, Povlsen CO (1969) Heterotransplantation of a human malignant tumour to "nude" mice. Acta Pathol Microbiol Scand 77(4):758–760
20. Soule HD, McGrath CM (1980) Estrogen responsive proliferation of clonal human breast carcinoma cells in athymic mice. Cancer Lett 10(2):177–189
21. Weinstein Y (1978) Impairment of the hypothalamo-pituitary-ovarian axis of the athymic "nude" mouse. Mech Ageing Dev 8(1):63–68

22. Shafie SM, Grantham FH (1981) Role of hormones in the growth and regression of human breast cancer cells (MCF-7) transplanted into athymic nude mice. J Natl Cancer Inst 67(1):51–56

23. Jordan VC, Robinson SP (1987) Species-specific pharmacology of antiestrogens: role of metabolism. Fed Proc 46(5):1870–1874

24. Satyaswaroop PG, Zaino RJ, Mortel R (1984) Estrogen-like effects of tamoxifen on human endometrial carcinoma transplanted into nude mice. Cancer Res 44(9):4006–4010

25. Gottardis MM, Robinson SP, Satyaswaroop PG, Jordan VC (1988) Contrasting actions of tamoxifen on endometrial and breast tumor growth in the athymic mouse. Cancer Res 48(4):812–815

26. Hardell L (1988) Tamoxifen as risk factor for carcinoma of corpus uteri. Lancet 2(8610):563

27. Jordan VC (1989) Tamoxifen and endometrial cancer. Lancet 1(8640):733–734

28. Jordan VC (1988) Tamoxifen and endometrial cancer. Lancet 2(8618):1019

29. Fornander T, Rutqvist LE, Cedermark B, Glas U, Mattsson A, Silfversward C, Skoog L, Somell A, Theve T, Wilking N et al (1989) Adjuvant tamoxifen in early breast cancer: occurrence of new primary cancers. Lancet 1(8630):117–120

30. Assikis VJ, Jordan VC (1995) A realistic assessment of the association between tamoxifen and endometrial cancer. Endocr Relat Cancer 2(3):235–241. https://doi.org/10.1677/erc.0.0020235

31. Jordan VC, Assikis VJ (1995) Endometrial carcinoma and tamoxifen: clearing up a controversy. Clin Cancer Res 1(5):467–472

32. Jordan VC, Lababidi MK, Mirecki DM (1990) Anti-oestrogenic and anti-tumour properties of prolonged tamoxifen therapy in C3H/OUJ mice. Eur J Cancer 26(6):718–721

33. Jordan VC, Lababidi MK, Langan-Fahey S (1991) Suppression of mouse mammary tumorigenesis by long-term tamoxifen therapy. J Natl Cancer Inst 83(7):492–496

34. Jordan VC (1990) Long-term adjuvant tamoxifen therapy for breast cancer. Breast Cancer Res Treat 15(3):125–136

35. Jordan VC (2007) Chemoprevention of breast cancer with selective oestrogen-receptor modulators. Nat Rev Cancer 7(1):46–53. https://doi.org/10.1038/nrc2048

36. Yager JD, Davidson NE (2006) Mechanisms of disease: estrogen carcinogenesis in breast cancer. N Engl J Med 354(3):270–282. https://doi.org/10.1056/NEJMra050776

37. Jordan VC, Phelps E, Lindgren JU (1987) Effects of anti-estrogens on bone in castrated and intact female rats. Breast Cancer Res Treat 10(1):31–35

38. Love RR, Mazess RB, Barden HS, Epstein S, Newcomb PA, Jordan VC, Carbone PP, DeMets DL (1992) Effects of tamoxifen on bone mineral density in postmenopausal women with breast cancer. N Engl J Med 326(13):852–856. https://doi.org/10.1056/NEJM199203263261302

39. Love RR, Wiebe DA, Newcomb PA, Cameron L, Leventhal H, Jordan VC, Feyzi J, DeMets DL (1991) Effects of tamoxifen on cardiovascular risk factors in postmenopausal women. Ann Intern Med 115(11):860–864

40. Lerner LJ, Jordan VC (1990) Development of antiestrogens and their use in breast cancer: eighth Cain memorial award lecture. Cancer Res 50(14):4177–4189

41. Turner RT, Wakley GK, Hannon KS, Bell NH (1988) Tamoxifen inhibits osteoclast-mediated resorption of trabecular bone in ovarian hormone-deficient rats. Endocrinology 122(3):1146–1150. https://doi.org/10.1210/endo-122-3-1146

42. Black LJ, Sato M, Rowley ER, Magee DE, Bekele A, Williams DC, Cullinan GJ, Bendele R, Kauffman RF, Bensch WR et al (1994) Raloxifene (LY139481 HCI) prevents bone loss and reduces serum cholesterol without causing uterine hypertrophy in ovariectomized rats. J Clin Invest 93(1):63–69. https://doi.org/10.1172/JCI116985

43. Jordan VC, Collins MM, Rowsby L, Prestwich G (1977) A monohydroxylated metabolite of tamoxifen with potent antioestrogenic activity. J Endocrinol 75(2):305–316

44. Jordan VC, Allen KE (1980) Evaluation of the antitumour activity of the non-steroidal antioestrogen monohydroxytamoxifen in the DMBA-induced rat mammary carcinoma model. Eur J Cancer 16(2):239–251

45. Jordan VC (2003) Antiestrogens and selective estrogen receptor modulators as multifunctional medicines. 2. Clinical considerations and new agents. J Med Chem 46(7):1081–1111. https://doi.org/10.1021/jmj020450x

46. Deshmane V, Krishnamurthy S, Melemed AS, Peterson P, Buzdar AU (2007) Phase III double-blind trial of arzoxifene compared with tamoxifen for locally advanced or metastatic breast cancer. J Clin Oncol 25(31):4967–4973. https://doi.org/10.1200/JCO.2006.09.5992

47. Kendler DL, Palacios S, Cox DA, Stock J, Alam J, Dowsett SA, Zanchetta J (2012) Arzoxifene versus raloxifene: effect on bone and safety parameters in postmenopausal women with osteoporosis. Osteoporos Int 23(3):1091–1101. https://doi.org/10.1007/s00198-011-1587-0

48. Rosati RL, Da Silva Jardine P, Cameron KO, Thompson DD, Ke HZ, Toler SM, Brown TA, Pan LC, Ebbinghaus CF, Reinhold AR, Elliott NC, Newhouse BN, Tjoa CM, Sweetnam PM, Cole MJ, Arriola MW, Gauthier JW, Crawford DT, Nickerson DF, Pirie CM, Qi H, Simmons HA, Tkalcevic GT (1998) Discovery and preclinical pharmacology of a novel, potent, non-steroidal estrogen receptor agonist/antagonist, CP-336156, a diaryltetrahydronaphthalene. J Med Chem 41(16):2928–2931. https://doi.org/10.1021/jm980048b

49. Ke HZ, Paralkar VM, Grasser WA, Crawford DT, Qi H, Simmons HA, Pirie CM, Chidsey-Frink KL, Owen TA, Smock SL, Chen HK, Jee WS, Cameron KO, Rosati RL, Brown TA, Dasilva-Jardine P, Thompson DD (1998) Effects of CP-336,156, a new, nonsteroidal estrogen agonist/antagonist, on bone, serum cholesterol, uterus and body composition in rat models. Endocrinology 139(4):2068–2076. https://doi.org/10.1210/endo.139.4.5902

50. Ke HZ, Qi H, Crawford DT, Chidsey-Frink KL, Simmons HA, Thompson DD (2000) Lasofoxifene (CP-336,156), a selective estrogen receptor modulator, prevents bone loss induced by aging and orchidectomy in the adult rat. Endocrinology 141(4):1338–1344. https://doi.org/10.1210/endo.141.4.7408

51. Cohen LA, Pittman B, Wang CX, Aliaga C, Yu L, Moyer JD (2001) LAS, a novel selective estrogen receptor modulator with chemopreventive and therapeutic activity in the N-nitroso-N-methylurea-induced rat mammary tumor model. Cancer Res 61(24):8683–8688

52. Prakash C, Johnson KA, Schroeder CM, Potchoiba MJ (2008) Metabolism, distribution, and excretion of a next generation selective estrogen receptor modulator, lasofoxifene, in rats and monkeys. Drug Metab Dispos 36(9):1753–1769. https://doi.org/10.1124/dmd.108.021808

53. Moffett A, Ettinger M, Bolognese M (2004) Lasofoxifene, a next generation SERM, is effective in preventing loss of BMD and reducing LDL-C in postmenopausal women. J Bone Miner Res 19:S96

54. Cummings SR, Ensrud K, Delmas PD, LaCroix AZ, Vukicevic S, Reid DM, Goldstein S, Sriram U, Lee A, Thompson J, Armstrong RA, Thompson DD, Powles T, Zanchetta J, Kendler D, Neven P, Eastell R, Investigators PS (2010) Lasofoxifene in postmenopausal women with osteoporosis. N Engl J Med 362(8):686–696. https://doi.org/10.1056/NEJMoa0808692

55. Davidson M, Moffett A, Welty F (2005) Extraskeletal effects of lasofoxifene on postmenopausal women. J Bone Miner Res 20:S173

56. McClung MR, Siris E, Cummings S, Bolognese M, Ettinger M, Moffett A, Emkey R, Day W, Somayaji V, Lee A (2006) Prevention of bone loss in postmenopausal women treated with lasofoxifene compared with raloxifene. Menopause 13(3):377–386. https://doi.org/10.1097/01.gme.0000188736.69617.4f

57. Robinson SP, Koch R, Jordan VC (1988) In vitro estrogenic actions in rat and human cells of hydroxylated derivatives of D16726 (zindoxifene), an agent with known antimammary cancer activity in vivo. Cancer Res 48(4):784–787

58. Miller CP, Collini MD, Tran BD, Harris HA, Kharode YP, Marzolf JT, Moran RA, Henderson RA, Bender RH, Unwalla RJ, Greenberger LM, Yardley JP, Abou-Gharbia MA, Lyttle CR, Komm BS (2001) Design, synthesis, and preclinical characterization of novel, highly selective indole estrogens. J Med Chem 44(11):1654–1657

59. Miller PD, Chines AA, Christiansen C, Hoeck HC, Kendler DL, Lewiecki EM, Woodson G, Levine AB, Constantine G, Delmas PD (2008) Effects of bazedoxifene on BMD and bone turnover in postmenopausal women: 2-yr results of a randomized, double-blind, placebo-, and active-controlled study. J Bone Miner Res 23(4):525–535. https://doi.org/10.1359/jbmr.071206

60. Pinkerton JV, Archer DF, Utian WH, Menegoci JC, Levine AB, Chines AA, Constantine GD (2009) Bazedoxifene effects on the reproductive tract in postmenopausal women at risk for osteoporosis. Menopause 16(6):1102–1108. https://doi.org/10.1097/gme.0b013e3181a816be

61. Silverman SL, Christiansen C, Genant HK, Vukicevic S, Zanchetta JR, de Villiers TJ, Constantine GD, Chines AA (2008) Efficacy of bazedoxifene in reducing new vertebral fracture risk in postmenopausal women with osteoporosis: results from a 3-year, randomized, placebo-, and active-controlled clinical trial. J Bone Miner Res 23(12):1923–1934. https://doi.org/10.1359/jbmr.080710

62. Smith DC, Prentice R, Thompson DJ, Herrmann WL (1975) Association of exogenous estrogen and endometrial carcinoma. N Engl J Med 293(23):1164–1167. https://doi.org/10.1056/NEJM197512042932302

63. Ziel HK, Finkle WD (1975) Increased risk of endometrial carcinoma among users of conjugated estrogens. N Engl J Med 293(23):1167–1170. https://doi.org/10.1056/NEJM197512042932303

64. Chlebowski RT, Hendrix SL, Langer RD, Stefanick ML, Gass M, Lane D, Rodabough RJ, Gilligan MA, Cyr MG, Thomson CA, Khandekar J, Petrovitch H, McTiernan A, Investigators WHI (2003) Influence of estrogen plus progestin on breast cancer and mammography in healthy postmenopausal women: the Women's Health Initiative randomized trial. JAMA 289(24):3243–3253. https://doi.org/10.1001/jama.289.24.3243

65. Anderson GL, Limacher M, Assaf AR, Bassford T, Beresford SA, Black H, Bonds D, Brunner R, Brzyski R, Caan B, Chlebowski R, Curb D, Gass M, Hays J, Heiss G, Hendrix S, Howard BV, Hsia J, Hubbell A, Jackson R, Johnson KC, Judd H, Kotchen JM, Kuller L, LaCroix AZ, Lane D, Langer RD, Lasser N, Lewis CE, Manson J, Margolis K, Ockene J, O'Sullivan MJ, Phillips L, Prentice RL, Ritenbaugh C, Robbins J, Rossouw JE, Sarto G, Stefanick ML, Van Horn L, Wactawski-Wende J, Wallace R, Wassertheil-Smoller S, Women's Health Initiative Steering C (2004) Effects of conjugated equine estrogen in postmenopausal women with hysterectomy: the Women's Health Initiative randomized controlled trial. JAMA 291(14):1701–1712. https://doi.org/10.1001/jama.291.14.1701

66. Haddow A, Watkinson JM, Paterson E, Koller PC (1944) Influence of synthetic oestrogens upon advanced malignant disease. Br Med J 2:393–398

67. Haddow A (1970) David A. Karnofsky memorial lecture. Thoughts on chemical therapy. Cancer 26(4):737–754

68. Early Breast Cancer Trialists' Collaborative G, Davies C, Godwin J, Gray R, Clarke M, Cutter D, Darby S, McGale P, Pan HC, Taylor C, Wang YC, Dowsett M, Ingle J, Peto R (2011) Relevance of breast cancer hormone receptors and other factors to the efficacy of adjuvant tamoxifen: patient-level meta-analysis of randomised trials. Lancet 378(9793):771–784. https://doi.org/10.1016/S0140-6736(11)60993-8

69. Jordan VC (2014) Linking estrogen-induced apoptosis with decreases in mortality following long-term adjuvant tamoxifen therapy. J Natl Cancer Inst 106(11):dju296. https://doi.org/10.1093/jnci/dju296

70. Yao K, Lee ES, Bentrem DJ, England G, Schafer JI, O'Regan RM, Jordan VC (2000) Antitumor action of physiological estradiol on tamoxifen-stimulated breast tumors grown in athymic mice. Clin Cancer Res 6(5):2028–2036

71. Wolf DM, Jordan VC (1993) A laboratory model to explain the survival advantage observed in patients taking adjuvant tamoxifen therapy. Recent Results Cancer Res 127:23–33

72. Song RX, Mor G, Naftolin F, McPherson RA, Song J, Zhang Z, Yue W, Wang J, Santen RJ (2001) Effect of long-term estrogen deprivation on apoptotic responses of breast cancer cells to 17beta-estradiol. J Natl Cancer Inst 93(22):1714–1723

73. Jordan VC (2015) The new biology of estrogen-induced apoptosis applied to treat and prevent breast cancer. Endocr Relat Cancer 22(1):R1–R31. https://doi.org/10.1530/ERC-14-0448

74. Abderrahman B, Jordan VC (2016) The modulation of estrogen-induced apoptosis as an interpretation of the Women's Health Initiative trials. Expert Rev Endocrinol Metab 11:81–86. https://doi.org/10.1586/17446651.2016.1128324

75. MacGregor JI, Jordan VC (1998) Basic guide to the mechanisms of antiestrogen action. Pharmacol Rev 50(2):151–196
76. Kharode Y, Bodine PV, Miller CP, Lyttle CR, Komm BS (2008) The pairing of a selective estrogen receptor modulator, bazedoxifene, with conjugated estrogens as a new paradigm for the treatment of menopausal symptoms and osteoporosis prevention. Endocrinology 149(12):6084–6091. https://doi.org/10.1210/en.2008-0817
77. Ariazi EA, Cunliffe HE, Lewis-Wambi JS, Slifker MJ, Willis AL, Ramos P, Tapia C, Kim HR, Yerrum S, Sharma CG, Nicolas E, Balagurunathan Y, Ross EA, Jordan VC (2011) Estrogen induces apoptosis in estrogen deprivation-resistant breast cancer through stress responses as identified by global gene expression across time. Proc Natl Acad Sci U S A 108(47):18879–18886. https://doi.org/10.1073/pnas.1115188108
78. Sweeney EE, Fan P, Jordan VC (2014) Molecular modulation of estrogen-induced apoptosis by synthetic progestins in hormone replacement therapy: an insight into the women's health initiative study. Cancer Res 74(23):7060–7068. https://doi.org/10.1158/0008-5472.CAN-14-1784
79. Obiorah IE, Fan P, Jordan VC (2014) Breast cancer cell apoptosis with phytoestrogens is dependent on an estrogen-deprived state. Cancer Prev Res 7(9):939–949. https://doi.org/10.1158/1940-6207.Capr-14-0061
80. Bain RR, Jordan VC (1983) Identification of a new metabolite of tamoxifen in patient serum during breast cancer therapy. Biochem Pharmacol 32(2):373–375
81. Jordan VC, Bain RR, Brown RR, Gosden B, Santos MA (1983) Determination and pharmacology of a new hydroxylated metabolite of tamoxifen observed in patient sera during therapy for advanced breast cancer. Cancer Res 43(3):1446–1450
82. Jordan VC (2017) Concerns about methodology of a trial investigating vaginal health during aromatase inhibitor therapy for breast cancer. JAMA Oncol 3(8):1141–1141. https://doi.org/10.1001/jamaoncol.2017.2074
83. Jordan VC (1984) Biochemical pharmacology of antiestrogen action. Pharmacol Rev 36(4):245–276
84. Jordan VC (2013) Estrogen action, selective estrogen receptor modulators and women's health: progress and promise. Imperial College Press, London
85. Murphy CS, Langan-Fahey SM, McCague R, Jordan VC (1990) Structure-function relationships of hydroxylated metabolites of tamoxifen that control the proliferation of estrogen-responsive T47D breast cancer cells in vitro. Mol Pharmacol 38(5):737–743
86. Murphy CS, Parker CJ, McCague R, Jordan VC (1991) Structure-activity relationships of nonisomerizable derivatives of tamoxifen: importance of hydroxyl group and side chain positioning for biological activity. Mol Pharmacol 39(3):421–428
87. Jordan VC (1987) Laboratory models of breast cancer to aid the elucidation of antiestrogen action. J Lab Clin Med 109(3):267–277
88. Wolf DM, Jordan VC (1994) The estrogen receptor from a tamoxifen stimulated MCF-7 tumor variant contains a point mutation in the ligand binding domain. Breast Cancer Res Treat 31(1):129–138
89. Jiang SY, Jordan VC (1992) Growth regulation of estrogen receptor-negative breast cancer cells transfected with complementary DNAs for estrogen receptor. J Natl Cancer Inst 84(8):580–591
90. Catherino WH, Wolf DM, Jordan VC (1995) A naturally occurring estrogen receptor mutation results in increased estrogenicity of a tamoxifen analog. Mol Endocrinol 9(8):1053–1063. https://doi.org/10.1210/mend.9.8.7476979
91. Levenson AS, Catherino WH, Jordan VC (1997) Estrogenic activity is increased for an antiestrogen by a natural mutation of the estrogen receptor. J Steroid Biochem Mol Biol 60(5–6):261–268
92. Brzozowski AM, Pike AC, Dauter Z, Hubbard RE, Bonn T, Engstrom O, Ohman L, Greene GL, Gustafsson JA, Carlquist M (1997) Molecular basis of agonism and antagonism in the oestrogen receptor. Nature 389(6652):753–758. https://doi.org/10.1038/39645

93. Shiau AK, Barstad D, Loria PM, Cheng L, Kushner PJ, Agard DA, Greene GL (1998) The structural basis of estrogen receptor/coactivator recognition and the antagonism of this interaction by tamoxifen. Cell 95(7):927–937

94. Levenson AS, Jordan VC (1998) The key to the antiestrogenic mechanism of raloxifene is amino acid 351 (aspartate) in the estrogen receptor. Cancer Res 58(9):1872–1875

95. MacGregor Schafer J, Liu H, Bentrem DJ, Zapf JW, Jordan VC (2000) Allosteric silencing of activating function 1 in the 4-hydroxytamoxifen estrogen receptor complex is induced by substituting glycine for aspartate at amino acid 351. Cancer Res 60(18):5097–5105

96. Schafer JI, Liu H, Tonetti DA, Jordan VC (1999) The interaction of raloxifene and the active metabolite of the antiestrogen EM-800 (SC 5705) with the human estrogen receptor. Cancer Res 59(17):4308–4313

97. Bentrem D, Dardes R, Liu H, MacGregor-Schafer J, Zapf J, Jordan V (2001) Molecular mechanism of action at estrogen receptor alpha of a new clinically relevant antiestrogen (GW7604) related to tamoxifen. Endocrinology 142(2):838–846. https://doi.org/10.1210/endo.142.2.7932

98. Liu H, Lee ES, Deb Los Reyes A, Zapf JW, Jordan VC (2001) Silencing and reactivation of the selective estrogen receptor modulator-estrogen receptor alpha complex. Cancer Res 61(9):3632–3639

99. Liu H, Park WC, Bentrem DJ, McKian KP, Reyes Ade L, Loweth JA, Schafer JM, Zapf JW, Jordan VC (2002) Structure-function relationships of the raloxifene-estrogen receptor-alpha complex for regulating transforming growth factor-alpha expression in breast cancer cells. J Biol Chem 277(11):9189–9198. https://doi.org/10.1074/jbc.M108335200

100. Jordan VC (2003) Tamoxifen: a most unlikely pioneering medicine. Nat Rev Drug Discov 2(3):205–213. https://doi.org/10.1038/nrd1031

101. McDonnell DP, Clemm DL, Hermann T, Goldman ME, Pike JW (1995) Analysis of estrogen receptor function in vitro reveals three distinct classes of antiestrogens. Mol Endocrinol 9(6):659–669. https://doi.org/10.1210/mend.9.6.8592512

102. Paige LA, Christensen DJ, Gron H, Norris JD, Gottlin EB, Padilla KM, Chang CY, Ballas LM, Hamilton PT, McDonnell DP, Fowlkes DM (1999) Estrogen receptor (ER) modulators each induce distinct conformational changes in ER alpha and ER beta. Proc Natl Acad Sci U S A 96(7):3999–4004

103. Norris JD, Fan D, Stallcup MR, McDonnell DP (1998) Enhancement of estrogen receptor transcriptional activity by the coactivator GRIP-1 highlights the role of activation function 2 in determining estrogen receptor pharmacology. J Biol Chem 273(12):6679–6688

104. Norris JD, Paige LA, Christensen DJ, Chang CY, Huacani MR, Fan D, Hamilton PT, Fowlkes DM, McDonnell DP (1999) Peptide antagonists of the human estrogen receptor. Science 285(5428):744–746

105. Wijayaratne AL, Nagel SC, Paige LA, Christensen DJ, Norris JD, Fowlkes DM, McDonnell DP (1999) Comparative analyses of mechanistic differences among antiestrogens. Endocrinology 140(12):5828–5840. https://doi.org/10.1210/endo.140.12.7164

106. Hall JM, McDonnell DP, Korach KS (2002) Allosteric regulation of estrogen receptor structure, function, and coactivator recruitment by different estrogen response elements. Mol Endocrinol 16(3):469–486. https://doi.org/10.1210/mend.16.3.0814

107. Onate SA, Tsai SY, Tsai MJ, O'Malley BW (1995) Sequence and characterization of a coactivator for the steroid hormone receptor superfamily. Science 270(5240):1354–1357

108. Smith CL, O'Malley BW (2004) Coregulator function: a key to understanding tissue specificity of selective receptor modulators. Endocr Rev 25(1):45–71. https://doi.org/10.1210/er.2003-0023

109. Jordan VC, O'Malley BW (2007) Selective estrogen-receptor modulators and antihormonal resistance in breast cancer. J Clin Oncol 25(36):5815–5824. https://doi.org/10.1200/JCO.2007.11.3886

110. Fan P, Jordan VC (2013) An emerging principle: selective nuclear receptor modulators. In: Jordan VC (ed) Estrogen action, selective estrogen receptor modulators and women's health: progress and promise. Imperial College Press, London, pp 431–456

111. Greene GL, Closs LE, Fleming H, DeSombre ER, Jensen EV (1977) Antibodies to estrogen receptor: immunochemical similarity of estrophilin from various mammalian species. Proc Natl Acad Sci U S A 74(9):3681–3685
112. Greene GL, Fitch FW, Jensen EV (1980) Monoclonal antibodies to estrophilin: probes for the study of estrogen receptors. Proc Natl Acad Sci U S A 77(1):157–161
113. Greene GL, Nolan C, Engler JP, Jensen EV (1980) Monoclonal antibodies to human estrogen receptor. Proc Natl Acad Sci U S A 77(9):5115–5119
114. Greene GL, Gilna P, Waterfield M, Baker A, Hort Y, Shine J (1986) Sequence and expression of human estrogen receptor complementary DNA. Science 231(4742):1150–1154
115. Jordan VC, Bowser-Finn RA (1982) Binding of [3H]monohydroxytamoxifen by immature rat tissues in vivo. Endocrinology 110(4):1281–1291. https://doi.org/10.1210/endo-110-4-1281
116. Tate AC, Greene GL, DeSombre ER, Jensen EV, Jordan VC (1984) Differences between estrogen- and antiestrogen-estrogen receptor complexes from human breast tumors identified with an antibody raised against the estrogen receptor. Cancer Res 44(3):1012–1018
117. Lieberman ME, Maurer RA, Gorski J (1978) Estrogen control of prolactin synthesis in vitro. Proc Natl Acad Sci U S A 75(12):5946–5949
118. Bouton MM, Raynaud JP (1979) The relevance of interaction kinetics in determining biological response to estrogens. Endocrinology 105(2):509–515. https://doi.org/10.1210/endo-105-2-509
119. Gottardis MM, Jordan VC (1988) Development of tamoxifen-stimulated growth of MCF-7 tumors in athymic mice after long-term antiestrogen administration. Cancer Res 48(18):5183–5187
120. Gottardis MM, Wagner RJ, Borden EC, Jordan VC (1989) Differential ability of antiestrogens to stimulate breast cancer cell (MCF-7) growth in vivo and in vitro. Cancer Res 49(17):4765–4769
121. Gottardis MM, Jiang SY, Jeng MH, Jordan VC (1989) Inhibition of tamoxifen-stimulated growth of an MCF-7 tumor variant in athymic mice by novel steroidal antiestrogens. Cancer Res 49(15):4090–4093
122. Beall PT, Misra LK, Young RL, Spjut HJ, Evans HJ, LeBlanc A (1984) Clomiphene protects against osteoporosis in the mature ovariectomized rat. Calcif Tissue Int 36(1):123–125
123. Powles TJ, Hardy JR, Ashley SE, Farrington GM, Cosgrove D, Davey JB, Dowsett M, McKinna JA, Nash AG, Sinnett HD et al (1989) A pilot trial to evaluate the acute toxicity and feasibility of tamoxifen for prevention of breast cancer. Br J Cancer 60(1):126–131
124. Love RR, Mazess RB, Tormey DC, Barden HS, Newcomb PA, Jordan VC (1988) Bone mineral density in women with breast cancer treated with adjuvant tamoxifen for at least two years. Breast Cancer Res Treat 12(3):297–302
125. Lewis JS, Meeke K, Osipo C, Ross EA, Kidawi N, Li TY, Bell E, Chandel NS, Jordan VC (2005) Intrinsic mechanism of estradiol-induced apoptosis in breast cancer cells resistant to estrogen deprivation. J Natl Cancer Inst 97(23):1746–1759. https://doi.org/10.1093/jnci/dji400
126. Gottardis MM, Jordan VC (1987) Antitumor actions of keoxifene and tamoxifen in the N-nitrosomethylurea-induced rat mammary carcinoma model. Cancer Res 47(15):4020–4024
127. Cummings SR, Eckert S, Krueger KA, Grady D, Powles TJ, Cauley JA, Norton L, Nickelsen T, Bjarnason NH, Morrow M, Lippman ME, Black D, Glusman JE, Costa A, Jordan VC (1999) The effect of raloxifene on risk of breast cancer in postmenopausal women: results from the MORE randomized trial. Multiple outcomes of raloxifene evaluation. JAMA 281(23):2189–2197

Endocrine Therapy in Clinical Practice

Tomas Reinert, Ryoichi Matsunuma, Airi Han, and Matthew J. Ellis

Abstract Endocrine therapy (ET) is the mainstay of treatment of estrogen receptor-positive (ER+) breast cancer both in the early-stage as in the advanced disease settings. ET targets the ER pathway by blocking the body's ability to produce estrogen or by directly modulating the ER. Since the estrogens are produced by the ovaries in premenopausal women and by some other tissues such as fat and skin in both premenopausal and postmenopausal women, ET for premenopausal women is different from for postmenopausal women. Needless to say, therapeutic options for early breast cancer are different to metastatic setting where more drugs are approved. This chapter will mainly review the clinical use of ET through all stages of breast cancer, with special considerations on recent advances in this field like ovarian function suppression in premenopausal patients with higher-risk early-stage tumors and the incorporation of targeted therapies that aim to circumvent mechanisms of endocrine resistance in metastatic ER+ breast cancer.

Keywords Breast neoplasm · Endocrine therapy · Estrogen receptor · Aromatase inhibitors

T. Reinert
Programa de Pós-Graduação em Ciências Médicas, Universidade Federal do Rio Grande do Sul, Porto Alegre, Brazil

R. Matsunuma
Lester and Sue Smith Breast Center, Baylor College of Medicine, Houston, TX, USA

First Department of Surgery, Hamamatsu University School of Medicine, Hamamatsu, Shizuoka, Japan

Hamamatsu Oncology Center, Hamamatsu, Shizuoka, Japan

A. Han
Lester and Sue Smith Breast Center, Baylor College of Medicine, Houston, TX, USA

Department of Surgery, Yonsei University Wonju College of Medicine, Wonju, South Korea

M. J. Ellis (✉)
Lester and Sue Smith Breast Center, Baylor College of Medicine, Houston, TX, USA
e-mail: mjellis@bcm.edu

© Springer Nature Switzerland AG 2019
X. Zhang (ed.), *Estrogen Receptor and Breast Cancer*, Cancer Drug Discovery and Development, https://doi.org/10.1007/978-3-319-99350-8_9

1   Introduction

Estrogen receptor-positive (ER+) breast cancer is the most frequent form of this disease and remains a major cause of cancer death in women. Ever since Beatson's historical observation that breast tumors can regress following oophorectomy, endocrine therapy (ET) plays a pivotal role in the prevention and treatment of breast cancer at all stages of its pathogenesis [1].

The estrogen receptor (ER) pathway has been targeted for breast cancer treatment for several decades, but many challenges persist. The expression of ER by breast cancer cells identifies the largest breast cancer group, and ER-directed therapies prolong survival and improve symptoms in breast cancer patients with a favorable side effect profile. ET may target directly the ER with the use of selective ER modulators (SERMs) or selective ER degrader (SERDs), or it may block estrogen synthesis, with the use of aromatase inhibitors (AIs) in postmenopausal women or ovarian function suppression (OFS) in premenopausal women, preventing estrogen-mediated signaling that leads to cell proliferation and tumor evolution. Even though ET is associated with significant clinical benefits for breast cancer patients, approximately one-third of patients with early-stage ER+ breast cancer treated with curative intent locoregional and systemic therapies develop disease recurrence. In the metastatic setting, even though the majority of patients obtain benefits in terms of prolongation of progression-free survival (PFS) and symptom palliation, clinical resistance and progression of disease will invariably develop, and metastatic breast cancer remains a systemic, incurable, and lethal disease [2].

Recent advances in the ability to understand the molecular biology of ER pathway and its interactions with important growth factor, metabolic and cell division pathways have brought the possibility of improving therapeutic results by modulating endocrine signaling and interfering with a variety of mechanisms of endocrine resistance (see our published reviews on this subject [2, 3] and Chapter "Molecular Mechanisms of Endocrine Resistance"). CDK4/CDK6 inhibitors and mTOR inhibitors that address ET-resistant disease have been incorporated into clinical practice (see Chapter "Emerging Therapeutic Approaches to Overcome Breast Cancer Endocrine Resistance"). Nonetheless, important questions remain about patient selection, optimal treatment algorithm, unavailability of predictive biomarkers, and lack of adequate information about how to sequence available ET agents in the advanced disease setting [1, 4].

In this chapter we will review the contemporary use of endocrine therapy in clinical practice. We will focus the discussion on the most recent trials of ET in the treatment of ER+ breast cancer across all disease stages, including prevention strategies in in situ disease, current (neo)adjuvant therapy recommendations, and an update on recent advances and remaining challenges in the treatment of patients with advanced disease.

2 Current Endocrine Agent Armamentarium

The current armamentarium of endocrine agents is summarized in Table 1. Tamoxifen was approved by the FDA in 1977 for the treatment of patients with advanced breast cancer and several years later for adjuvant treatment of early-stage disease. For decades, tamoxifen has been the gold standard for ET of all stages of estrogen receptor-positive breast cancer, and the WHO lists tamoxifen as an essential drug for the treatment of breast cancer. Tamoxifen is a SERM, a class of drugs with mixed agonist/antagonist action on the ER in different tissues (see Chapters "The First Targeted Therapy to Treat Cancer: The Tamoxifen Tale" and "A Novel Strategy to Improve Women's Health: Selective Estrogen Receptor Modulators"). The antagonistic proprieties are responsible for the therapeutic effect in breast cancer; on the other hand, the agonist characteristics are responsible for the side effect profile and are illustrated occasionally in patients with advanced disease when "flare reactions" and withdrawal responses occur. Tamoxifen is used for the treatment of ER+ invasive breast cancer in the neoadjuvant, adjuvant, and metastatic settings. Tamoxifen is also used in the treatment of ductal carcinoma in situ and for breast cancer prevention in high-risk patients.

At menopause, the production of ovarian hormones ceases. Still, estrogen continues to be converted from androgens by aromatase, an enzyme from the CYP superfamily. This biologic pathway was the basis for the development of the aromatase inhibitors (AIs) class of compounds. AIs markedly suppress circulating estrogen

Table 1 Current endocrine therapy armamentarium

• Selective endocrine receptor modulators (SERM)
Tamoxifen
• Aromatase inhibitors
Anastrozole
Letrozole
Exemestane
• Selective endocrine receptor degrader/downregulators (SERD)
Fulvestrant
• CDK4/CDK6 inhibitors
Palbociclib
Ribociclib
Abemaciclib
• MTOR inhibitors
Everolimus
• Hormone receptor agonists
Progestins (megestrol acetate)
Diethylstilbestrol and estradiol
Testosterone

levels in postmenopausal women by inhibiting or inactivating aromatase, the enzyme responsible for the synthesis of estrogens from androgenic substrates. Unlike tamoxifen, AIs have no partial agonist activity. AIs are currently the mainstay of ET in mostly all setting of breast cancer. AIs have shown superior efficacy in comparison with tamoxifen in both early-stage and advanced disease. AIs are also used as the endocrine backbone in therapeutic strategies combining endocrine resistance modulators like mTOR inhibitors and CDK4/CDK6 inhibitors.

Fulvestrant, the prototypic SERD, is a pure ER antagonist that binds competitively to the ER and exerts selective ER downregulation though receptor degradation. Fulvestrant has a binding affinity 100 times greater than tamoxifen. However, in contrast to tamoxifen, binding of fulvestrant to the ER induces a rapid degradation making the receptor unavailable or unresponsive to estrogen; consequently the drug strongly attenuates the ability of the ER to activate gene transcription [5]. A key characteristic of fulvestrant, that distinguishes its mechanism of action from that of SERMs, is that fulvestrant consistently reduces estrogen and progesterone receptor levels in the tumor and endometrium as well, without having agonist effects. Fulvestrant has been proved effective in the treatment of advanced breast cancer as both first-line [6] and second-line [7] therapy, and it is currently used as the endocrine backbone for combination with CDK4/CDK6 inhibitors in patients with AI-refractory disease [4]. Fulvestrant is not an approved treatment for early-stage breast cancer, and its used as (neo)adjuvant therapy should not be considered outside a clinical trial.

Several alternative hormone therapies have been utilized with variable success over the last decades and remain as options to be considered with the goal of delaying chemotherapy as long as possible. Megestrol acetate and intermediate dose estradiol (2 mg tid) represent cheaper options that need to be taken into consideration. Ideal patients for these agents are those that have experienced long-term disease control with an AI and/or tamoxifen before disease progression [8, 9].

Over the last decade, targeted therapies that modulate mechanisms of ET resistance have been developed with varying levels of success. Some of them, like CDK4/CDK6 and mTOR inhibitors, have been associated with significant benefits in patients with hormone-resistant disease and are now the standard treatment of ER+ MBC in both first- and second-line. These agents are also under investigation in the (neo)adjuvant setting. A variety of different classes of agents, such as PI3K, HDAC, and SRC inhibitors, are also been evaluated in a variety of clinical trials, and the treatment algorithm of ER+ MBC probably will change significantly over the next years (see Chapter "Emerging Therapeutic Approaches to Overcome Breast Cancer Endocrine Resistance").

3   Chemoprevention Strategies Using Endocrine Therapy

Risk factors of breast cancer include advanced age, a strong family history of breast cancer, and have precancerous lesions in the breast, such as ductal carcinoma in situ (DCIS), lobular carcinoma in situ (LCIS), or atypical hyperplasia. Breast Cancer

Risk Assessment Tool is available (https://www.cancer.gov/bcrisktool/) for an individual patient who is interested in assessing her own risk. This tool is based on a statistical model known as the "Gail model" [10]. Based upon a careful risk assessment, women at a high risk of breast cancer may take therapy with medications into consideration. These medications include SERMs [11] and AIs [12, 13], which have been shown to be effective for breast cancer prevention. However, in general these medications only work to prevent hormone receptor-positive tumors. The overall barrier to the use of these agents has been the side effect profile. For tamoxifen major concerns have been venous thrombosis and endometrial cancer. For AI's vaginal atrophy, poor tolerability is due to AI musculoskeletal syndrome and osteoporosis. Thus the use of these agents for prevention has proven problematic and adoption rates low. Of all agents, the SERD raloxifene may have the best risk/benefit ratio as this agent treats osteoporosis, and in terms of patient selection, the presence of high-risk pathology (LCIS or ADH) is the best candidate, followed by patients with high-risk alleles such as deleterious BRCA1 or BRCA2 as well as other lower penetrance genes such as ATM, CHK2, and PALB2. Since the efficacy of chemoprevention is not a settled question in patients with high-risk genetics, mastectomy is ultimately the most definitive approach usually resorted to. Specialist high-risk clinics and genetic counseling are the preferred management approaches for these patients.

4   Endocrine Therapy for In Situ Tumors

For women with ER-positive DCIS treated with breast-conserving surgery (BCS) with or without RT, endocrine therapy rather than observation is recommended. For women who are suitable for treatment, the choice between anastrozole and tamoxifen should be individualized based on the side effect profile of each medication, menopausal status, and the preferences of the patient.

Arguably for women who underwent mastectomy for ER-positive DCIS, the use of endocrine therapy should be considered as "chemoprevention" and not as "treatment" to prevent recurrence for this diagnosis.

For women with ER-negative DCIS, endocrine therapy likely does not reduce the risk of recurrence of the incident DCIS. Some women may opt to take tamoxifen, however, to decrease the risk of developing a new hormone receptor-positive DCIS or invasive breast cancer.

For women treated with BCS, multiple trials have demonstrated that postoperative tamoxifen is more effective than placebo in reducing the risk of invasive ipsilateral breast cancer recurrence, although there is no apparent benefit for survival [14–17]. A meta-analysis of two randomized trials, NSABP B-24 and UK/ANZ DCIS, showed tamoxifen treatment for the patients who got BCT due to DCIS which reduced the recurrence risk of ipsilateral DCIS (hazard ratio [HR] 0.75, 95% CI 0.61–0.92) and contralateral DCIS (relative risk [RR] 0.50, 95% CI 0.28–0.87) and showed tendency of lower risk in recurrent ipsilateral invasive carcinoma (HR 0.79, 95% CI 0.61–1.01) and contralateral invasive carcinoma (RR 0.57, 95% CI 0.39–0.83) and no benefit in all-cause mortality (RR 1.11, 95% CI 0.89–1.39) [18].

Aromatase inhibitors are reasonable alternatives to tamoxifen in postmenopausal women with ER-positive DCIS. The NRG Oncology/NSABP B-35 trial, which enrolled over 3100 postmenopausal women with hormone receptor-positive DCIS who underwent BCT, demonstrated that anastrozole resulted in a decreased rate of breast cancer events compared with tamoxifen, but no significant difference in either disease-free survival (DFS, 235 versus 260 events; HR 0.89, 95% CI 0.75–1.07) or overall survival (OS, 98 versus 88 deaths; HR 1.11, 95% CI 0.83–1.48) [19].

5   Adjuvant Endocrine Therapy

There are several meta-analyses that shows endocrine therapy improves overall survival for women with ER-positive early breast cancer [20]. Therefore, there is wide consensus that these patients should receive adjuvant endocrine therapy.

The agents used in this setting are the following:

- The selective estrogen receptor modulator (SERM), e.g., tamoxifen
- Aromatase inhibitors, e.g., anastrozole, letrozole, and exemestane
- Ovarian suppression or ablation

5.1   Adjuvant Endocrine Therapy for Premenopausal Women

The standard option is 5 years of tamoxifen with or without ovarian suppression or 5 years of exemestane plus ovarian suppression. For those who remain premenopausal after the initial 5 years of tamoxifen, continuing up to 10 years of tamoxifen therapy should be considered. For women who became postmenopausal during the 5 years of initial treatment, extended therapy with aromatase inhibitor up to 5 years should be considered, or based on the data from ATLAS trial, additional tamoxifen for 5 years (up to 10 years totally) should be considered as well. The long-term (greater than 5 years) safety and efficacy of aromatase inhibitor are still under investigation.

The decision whether patients will have adjuvant endocrine therapy is usually made based on a risk criteria of recurrence. Even though there is no formal or standard criteria to define such risk, a reasonable approach with endocrine therapy can be made based on the criteria for chemotherapy indication, such as patients with metastasis axillary lymph node(s), tumor size larger than 2 cm, high tumor grade, lymphovascular invasion, and/or high risk of recurrence based on a genomic assay (e.g., Recurrence Score [RS] >31 on the 21-gene recurrence assay). In addition, women at a younger age such as younger than 35 years also can be considered as higher risk of recurrence [21].

Table 2 Endocrine therapy and ovarian function suppression

Study	Patients	Detail	Primary endpoint	Follow-up (months)	Outcome
TEXT [22]	2672	– EXE and OFS – TAM and OFS	DFS	68	EXE and OFS improve DFS
SOFT [23]	3066	– EXE and OFS – TAM and OFS – TAM	DFS	67	No diff between TAM and OFS vs TAM alone EXE and OFS: further improvement
TEXT and SOFT	4690	– EXE and OFS – TAM and OFS	DFS	68	EXE and OFS improve DFS. OS: not significance (HR 0.72; 95% CI, 0.60–0.85; $P < 0.001$)

For women with high-risk breast cancer, ovarian suppression plus exemestane rather than tamoxifen as single-agent therapy is provided (Table 2). This recommendation is based on the results of the Suppression of Ovarian Function Trial (SOFT) and the Tamoxifen and Exemestane Trial (TEXT). Despite the overall negative results of the SOFT, exploratory and subgroup, analyses suggested that patients with a higher risk of relapse may derive a benefit over tamoxifen alone with ovarian suppression plus either aromatase inhibition or tamoxifen [22–24]. Given the results of the combined analyses of SOFT and Tamoxifen and Exemestane Trial (TEXT), our preference is for aromatase inhibition rather than tamoxifen when combining with ovarian suppression for patients with high-risk disease [22].

Ovarian suppression with either tamoxifen or aromatase inhibition does not provide a significant benefit over tamoxifen alone for most premenopausal patients (Table 2) [4–6]. Tamoxifen therapy without ovarian suppression is a reasonable option for premenopausal patient with lower risk of recurrence or metastasis.

5.2 Adjuvant Endocrine Therapy for Postmenopausal Women

An aromatase inhibitor is a better option than tamoxifen as adjuvant endocrine treatment for postmenopausal patients. For women who wish to discontinue an AI, it would be reasonable to switch to tamoxifen.

Options: Aromatase inhibitor as an initial adjuvant therapy for 5 years. Tamoxifen 2–3 years followed by one of the following options: an aromatase inhibitor to complete 5 years of adjuvant endocrine therapy or 5 years of aromatase inhibitor therapy. Tamoxifen 4.5–6 years followed by 5 years of an aromatase inhibitor or consideration of tamoxifen for up to 10 years.

Aromatase inhibitors showed more substantial reduction in recurrence rates and lower breast cancer mortality in postmenopausal women comparing to tamoxifen (Table 3).

Table 3 Adjuvant AI monotherapy in the adjuvant setting

	Patients	Detail	Primary endpoint	Follow-up	Outcome
ATAC [25]	9366	– ANA 5y – TAM 5y	DFS	120 months	ANA improved DFS. OS: not significant [HR] 0.91, 95% CI 0.8.99; $p = 0.04$
BIG 1-98 [26, 27]	8010	– LET 5y – TAM 5y – LET to TAM – TAM to LET	DFS	8.1 years	LET improved DFS. OS: significant HR 0.82 [95% CI 0.74–0.92]
TEAM [28]	9779	– TAM to EXE – EXE 5y	DFS	5.1 years	No sig diff between switching and EXE alone
EBCTCG Meta-analysis [29]	9885	– AI 5y – TAM 5y	–	–	Recurrence and mortality were both significantly reduced

There are numerous randomized trials and meta-analyses demonstrating that aromatase inhibitor showed better efficacy in postmenopausal women with early breast cancer patients in terms of tumor recurrence and mortality. EBCTCG undertook meta-analyses of individual data on 9885 postmenopausal women with ER-positive early breast cancer in the randomized trials of 5 years of aromatase inhibitor versus 5 years of tamoxifen as one of the cohorts [29], showing aromatase inhibitor reduced breast cancer recurrence, particularly during years 0–1 (RR 0.64, 95% CI 0.52–0.78) and years 2–4 (RR 0.80, 95% CI 0.68–0.93), and lower 10-year breast cancer mortality (RR 0.85, 95% CI 0.75–0.96).

Patients with hormone receptor-positive breast cancer are treated for a minimum of 5 years with adjuvant endocrine therapy. Extended adjuvant endocrine therapy beyond 5 years should be considered for all patients with hormone receptor-positive breast cancer since longer durations of endocrine therapy can improve DFS [30–34]. While there is no clear consensus on which patients should receive extended therapy, the original prognosis, the presence of ongoing side effects, and the potentials for toxicity must be taken into consideration. Patients with larger tumors or node-positive disease may be reasonable to receive extended endocrine treatment. The benefits are unclear for breast cancer patients with smaller tumors or node-negative disease. General idea of extended therapy is usually divided into two groups based on which endocrine therapy, tamoxifen or aromatase inhibitor, will be given as extended treatment.

5.3 Which Patients Should Receive Extended Therapy?

Since there is no clear consensus on which patients will get extended therapy, decisions should be made based on recurrence risk, symptomatic side effects, and toxicities such as thrombosis and endometrial cancer.

In the meta-analysis of the results of 88 trials involving 62,923 women with ER-positive breast cancer who were disease-free after 5 years of scheduled endocrine therapy, the associations of tumor size, nodal status, tumor grade, and other factors with patients' outcomes were assessed during the period from 5 to 20 years. The risk of distant recurrence was strongly correlated with the original tumor size, nodal status, and tumor grade [35].

Retrospective evaluations of several adjuvant endocrine trials incorporating multi-parameter gene and protein expression assays have suggested that such assays may identify patients who need extended endocrine therapy to acquire better outcome. The TransATAC trial evaluated the ability of various genomic signatures in identifying patients at risk for late recurrence [36]. While it appeared that all assays were effective at identifying node-negative patients at low risk for late recurrence, models integrating clinical information with genomic data (i.e., PAM50/Prosigna and EndoPredict) were more effective at identifying node-positive disease at low risk for recurrence than assays relying on genomics only (i.e., Oncotype DX Recurrence Score or Breast Cancer Index). Other data support the Clinical Treatment Score post-5 years (CTS5), which relies on nodal status, tumor size and grade, and age, as a tool to guide the use of extended therapy [37]. However, none of these has been well validated in other data sets, and the American Society of Clinical Oncology (ASCO) Tumor Marker Guidelines for Early Breast Cancer Panel has not recommended using any of these to guide the decision about extended endocrine therapy at this time.

5.3.1 Tamoxifen for Extended Therapy and Sequential Therapy

Support for extended endocrine therapy for the patients who were treated with tamoxifen comes from ATLAS and aTTom trials (Table 4) [31–33, 39, 40]. ATLAS trial randomly allocated 12,894 women to continue up to 10 years or stop tamoxifen at 5 years. The outcome analyses of 6846 women with ER-positive early breast cancer showed that by extending adjuvant treatment to 10 years, the risk of recurrence and breast cancer-related mortality was reduced. Patients receiving tamoxifen beyond 10 years of treatment had a greater reduction in risk of progression, possibly due to a "carry-over effect." There were also decreases in the incidence of

Table 4 Extended tamoxifen adjuvant therapy

Study	Patients	Detail	Primary endpoint	Follow-up	Outcome
ATLAS [30]	6846	– TAM 10y – TAM 5y	DFS	7.6 years after entry at year 5	TAM 10y reduced the risk of breast cancer recurrence ($p = 0.002$) and reduced overall mortality ($p = 0.01$)
aTTom [38]	6953	– TAM 10y – TAM 5y	DFS		TAM 10y reduced the risk of breast cancer recurrence ($p = 0.003$) and reduced breast cancer mortality ($p = 0.05$)

contralateral breast cancer [39]. Preliminary results of the aTTom trial also demonstrated decreased recurrences and a reduction in breast cancer mortality (392 versus 443 deaths) with 10 versus 5 years of tamoxifen [40]. In these studies, extended tamoxifen increased incidences of endometrial cancer and pulmonary embolus but reduced the rate of ischemic heart disease [39, 40].

The Breast International Group 1-98 (BIG 1-98) trial randomized 8010 women to 5 years of tamoxifen or letrozole monotherapy or sequential treatment with 2 years of one of these drugs followed by 3 years of the other [27]. While breast cancer outcomes, such as disease free survival or overall survival, were better for letrozole compared with tamoxifen monotherapy, there was no significant difference in either disease-free or overall survival (OS) between the sequential therapies and letrozole monotherapy.

5.3.2 Aromatase Inhibitor for Extended Therapy and Sequential Therapy

MA17 showed improved DFS given extended letrozole after completing 5 years of adjuvant tamoxifen compared with placebo control. MA.17R was originally designed to randomize women who had received 5 years of tamoxifen and 5 years of an aromatase inhibitor on MA17 into extended placebo or extended letrozole. The number of patients was not enough to power the trial appropriately. So they allowed patients who had taken 5 years of an aromatase inhibitor as up-front therapy to be randomized for the trial. Among 1918 postmenopausal women who had completed 4.5–6 years of therapy with an aromatase inhibitor after any duration of prior tamoxifen, letrozole for an additional 5 years improved DFS relative to those who received placebo (HR 0.66; $P = 0.01$) (Table 5). An overview of trials comparing the toxicities of extended versus shorter aromatase inhibitor therapy demonstrated a higher rate of osteoporotic fractures and trend toward increased cardiovascular events in the group that received longer aromatase inhibitor therapy [46].

For postmenopausal patient who received adjuvant tamoxifen treatment for 2–3 years, an additional aromatase inhibitor is recommended to complete 5 years of adjuvant endocrine therapy (Table 6).

In the IES 031 trial, 4724 postmenopausal patients who were disease-free on 2–3 years of tamoxifen were randomly assigned to switch to exemestane or to continue tamoxifen for the remainder of a 5-year adjuvant endocrine treatment. The result suggests exemestane group improved DFS (HR, 0.76; 95% CI, 0.66–0.88) [52].

In the meta-analysis of ABCSG 8, ARNO 95, and ITA trial, patients who switched to anastrozole had fewer disease recurrences and deaths than did those who remained on tamoxifen, resulting in significant improvements in disease-free survival (hazard ratio 0.59 [95% CI 0.48–0.74]; $p < 0.0001$) and overall survival (0.71 [0.52–0.98]; $p = 0.04$) [53].

In EBCTCG meta-analysis in which women ($n = 11,798$) were randomly assigned to 5 years of tamoxifen versus 2–3 years of tamoxifen followed by an

Table 5 Extended AI adjuvant therapy

Study	Patients	Detail	Primary endpoint	Follow-up	Outcome
MA17 [32, 33]	5187	– TAM 4.5–6y to LET 5y – TAM 4.5–6y to placebo	DFS	64 months	LET improved DFS (HR 0.52, 95% CI, 0.45–0.61; $P < 0.001$) and OS (HR 0.61, 95% CI, 0.52–0.71; $P < 0.001$)
DATA [41]	1912	– TAM 2–3y to ANA 3y – TAM 2–3y to ANA 6y	DFS	4.2 years	No difference in DFS
IDEAL [42]	1824	– Any ET 5y to LET 2.5y – Any ET 5y to LET 5y	DFS	6.6 years	No difference in DFS and OS
NSABP B-42 [43]	3966	– ET 5y to LET 5y – ET 5y to placebo (ET:AI or TAM -> AI)	DFS	6.9 years	No difference in DFS and OS
MA17R [44]	1918	– AI 4.5–6y to LET 5y – AI 4.5–6y to placebo (prior TAM use, 79.3%)	DFS	6.3 years	LET improved DFS (HR 0.66; $P = 0.01$). No difference n OS
ABCSG-6a [45]	856	– TAM 5y – TAM 5y to ANA 3y	RFS	62.3 months	Extended ANA improved RFS
NSABP-33 [34]	1598	– TAM 5y to EXE 5y – TAM 5y to placebo	DFS	30 months	Extended EXE improved DFS

Table 6 Sequential AI therapy in adjuvant trials

Study	Patients	Detail	Primary endpoint	Follow-up	Outcome
IES [47]	4724	– TAM 2y to EXE 3y – TAM 5y	DFS	91 months	Switch improved DFS
ARNO 95 [48, 49]	979	– TAM 2y to ANA 3y – TAM 5y	DFS	30.1 months	Switch improved DFS
ABCSG-8 [48]	3714	– TAM 2y to ANA 3y – TAM 5y	RFS	60 months	Switch improved RFS
ITA [50]	448	– TAM 2–3y to ANA 5y – TAM 5y	RFS	128 months	Switch improved RFS
BIG 1-98 [51]	8010	– LET 5y – TAM 5y – TAM to LET – LET to TAM	DFS	8.1 years	No sig diff between switching and LET alone
TEAM [28]	9779	– EXE 5y – TAM 2.5–3y to EXE	DFS	5.1 years	No sig diff between switching and EXE alone
EBCTCG [29] Meta-analysis	11,798	– TAM to AI – TAM	–	–	Recurrence and mortality were both significantly reduced

aromatase inhibitor for 5 years of total endocrine therapy, switching to an aromatase inhibitor resulted in reduced breast cancer recurrence during years 2–4 (RR 0.56, 95% CI 0.46–0.67) and fewer deaths from breast cancer (RR 0.84, 95% CI 0.72–0.96) [29].

6   Neoadjuvant Endocrine Therapy

Neoadjuvant endocrine therapy (NET) is, a logical alternative to neoadjuvant chemotherapy for ER-positive tumors as it is well tolerated, simple to deliver and has proven benefits. The potential of NET is being increasingly explored, not only to allow less extensive surgery but also as a scientific tool, generating biomarkers to predict outcomes both for individual patients and in adjuvant clinical trials [36]. Nevertheless, it has been timidly evaluated in clinical trials and even more so implemented in clinical practice. According to the National Cancer Database in the USA, only 3% of the eligible patients receive this therapy [37].

It is known that in patients with early-stage luminal tumors, the use of cytotoxic chemotherapy remains controversial. In neoadjuvant therapy, it is associated with lower pathological complete response rates in comparison with triple-negative and HER2-positive tumors [54], whereas in the adjuvant treatment, a variety of evidences suggest that the absolute OS benefit in unselected postmenopausal women is no more than 3–4% [55]. NET has additional potential benefits such as favorable toxicity profile (especially in comparison with anthracycline- and taxane-based chemotherapy), low cost, and easy translatability to clinical practice in areas of the world with limited healthcare resources where the most frequent presentation of breast cancer is a breast mass. These factors are especially relevant as approximately 70% of breast cancer deaths now occur in women from low-income and middle-income countries [56].

Modern NET approaches have two major objectives: tumor down-staging in order to allow breast-conserving surgery (BCS) and to provide an in vivo evaluation of the pattern of resistance or sensitivity to ET. The ideal candidates are postmenopausal women with stage II and III ER-positive HER2-negative breast cancer with endocrine-sensitive characteristics such as low-grade, low-Ki67 expression, and high ER expression. The AIs are the preferred agents based on trials that demonstrated that they have superior ORR and eligibility for breast conservation in comparison with tamoxifen [57]. Recently, the American College of Surgeons Oncology Group (ACOSOG) Z1031 study confirmed that for patients who are told they need a mastectomy, about half could undergo successful breast-conserving surgery after 16–18 weeks of AI treatment [58]. This trial compared NET with exemestane, letrozole, and anastrozole head to head and demonstrated that the effectiveness of the three agents is equivalent. The optimal duration of NET has been studied in some studies that reported that the ORR and conversion to BCS increased after 6 months of treatment, with approximately one-third of patients achieving maximal reduction

Table 7 Randomized trials comparing different endocrine agents in the neoadjuvant setting

Trial (ref) phase	Treatment arm (N)	Duration	Primary endpoint	ORR	BCS
IMPACT [61] III	A: anastrozole (113) B: tamoxifen (108) C: anastrozole + tamoxifen (109)	3 months	OR by ultrasound	A: 37% B: 36% C: 39%	A: 44% B: 31% C: 29%
PO24 [62] III	A: letrozole (162) B: tamoxifen (223)	4 months	OR by clinical palpation	A: 55%* B: 36% $P < 0.001$	A: 45%* B: 35% P 0.02
PROACT [63] III	A: anastrozole (228) B: tamoxifen (223)	3 months	OR by ultrasound	A: 39% B: 35%	A: 43%* B: 31% P 0.04
ACOSOG Z1011 [58] II	A: exemestane (124) B: letrozole (128) C: anastrozole (125)	4 months	OR by clinical palpation	A: 63% B: 75% C: 69%	A: 48% B: 41% C: 64%
STAGE [64] III	A: anastrozole (+goserelin) (98) B: tamoxifen (+goserelin) (98)	6 months	OR by ultrasound	A: 70%* B: 50% P: 0.004	A: 86% B: 68%
RUSSIAN TRIAL [65] II	A: exemestane (76) B: tamoxifen (75)	3 months	OR by clinical palpation	A: 76%* B: 40% P 0.05	A: 37% B: 25% P 0.05
CARMINA [66] II	A: anastrozole (57) B: fulvestrant 500 mg (59)	4–6 months	OR by clinical palpation	A: 62% B: 46%	A: 59% B: 49%
Semiglazov et al. [67]	A: chemotherapy (118) (doxorubicin + paclitaxel) B: endocrine therapy (121) (anastrozole 61) (exemestane 60)	3 months	OR by clinical palpation	A: 63% B: 64%	A: 24% B: 33% P 0.058
GEICAM 2006-03 [68]	A: chemotherapy (EC → docetaxel) B: exemestane (plus goserelin if premenopausal)		Response rate by MRI	A: 66% B: 48%	A: 47% B: 56%
NEOCENT [69]	A: chemotherapy (22) B: letrozole (22)	18–23 weeks	Recruitment feasibility and tissue collection	A: 54% B: 59%	
UNICANCER-NEOPAl [70]	A: chemotherapy (53) B: letrozole/ palbociclib (53)	20 weeks	Residual cancer burden index (RCB)	A: 76% B: 75%	A: 69% B: 69%

* = statistically significant difference

in tumor volume after this period [59, 60]. Selected trials of NET are summarized in Table 7. Most of the published trials have compared different endocrine agents, and there is only a limited amount of data comparing NET with neoadjuvant chemotherapy.

NET has been increasingly used as a scientific instrument as it can lead to the identification of patterns of ET resistance or sensitivity based on tools like the pre-operative endocrine prognostic index (PEPI) that can help identify a subgroup of extreme responders with excellent prognosis, therefore avoiding chemotherapy [71]. On the other hand, NET may identify, within a window of curability, a subgroup of patients with primary endocrine resistance who might benefit from additional forms of systemic therapy. Finally, tumor samples from patients treated with NET are providing valuable insights into the molecular basis for intrinsic resistance to ET, and promise a more rational basis and precise approach to the systemic treatment of ER+ breast cancer. A variety of translational and clinical trials combining NET with targeted therapies, such as CDK4/CDK6 inhibitors, are ongoing with promising initial results.

7   Endocrine Therapy for Metastatic Breast Cancer

ET is an active therapeutic strategy and has been used for the treatment of ER+ MBC for several decades with significant efficacy and limited toxicity. The clinical paradigms that guide our treatment recommendations to these patients are the indication of ET whenever there is no visceral crisis or suspected endocrine resistance and the use of available endocrine agents in a sequential manner [72]. Nowadays, breast cancer patients have an unprecedented number of endocrine-based treatment alternatives that can palliate symptoms and improve long-term outcomes and that can be used before the need of cytotoxic chemotherapy. Unfortunately, even after many decades of translational and clinical research, there are no validated predictive biomarkers to help the clinician to distinguish between those patients who may be adequately managed with endocrine monotherapy and those who are more likely to benefit from the combination of ET and targeted therapies. Moreover, there is still a lack of definitive recommendations about the optimal strategy for sequencing endocrine agents in this patient population [73]. Overall survival reports are highly awaited as well as future trials addressing sequencing strategies. Furthermore, biomarkers for patient selection as well as cost-effectiveness analysis are awaited and should be considered a research priority in this field.

Several factors need to be considered when selecting the optimal ET agent for the treatment of ER+ MBC. These factors include patient's characteristics (i.e., menopausal status, comorbidities, adherence) as well as tumor and disease characteristics like the site of metastasis, tumor burden, need for rapid symptom control, disease-free interval, and response to previous ET. Nonetheless, an assortment of additional factors such as cost, access to innovative drugs, availability of clinical research, as well as financial and social hardships can make this decision even more challenging. Individual breast tumors have different patterns of response and resistance to each ET strategy, and the ability to select which endocrine agent an individual patient's cancer is most sensitive to is a realistic, as well as a clinically, worthwhile goal [1].

7.1 First-Line Endocrine Therapy for Metastatic Breast Cancer

Patients who are ET naïve and present with de novo metastatic breast cancer are candidates for first-line ET. Therapeutic options in the first-line setting include endocrine monotherapy or the combination of endocrine agents and CDK4/CDK6 inhibitors. The most important phase III trials are summarized in Table 8.

Up-front use of CDK4/CDK6 was analyzed in phase III trials that compared the combination of three available agents (palbociclib, ribociclib, and abemaciclib) with an AI versus AI plus placebo. The PALOMA-2 trial randomized 666 postmenopausal patients without previous ET for advanced disease for treatment with palbociclib in combination with letrozole versus letrozole monotherapy. Treatment with palbociclib was associated with a statistically significant benefit in terms of PFS (24.8 months vs 14.5 months; HR, 0.58; 95% CI, 0.46–0.72; $p > 0.001$) [78]. This data confirmed the results from the phase II trial PALOMA-1, which served as the basis for the approval of palbociclib in the first-line setting by the FDA in 2015 [79]. In a similar population of patients, the MONALEESA-2 trial compared ribociclib, a different CDK4/CDK6 inhibitor, in association with letrozole versus letrozole monotherapy in 668 patients. A preplanned interim analysis showed a significant benefit regarding PFS favoring the ribociclib arm (median PFS: NR vs 14.7 months, HR 0.56, $p < 0.0001$) [80] and led to FDA approval in 2017. The third CDK4/CDK6 inhibitor called abemaciclib was tested in the first-line setting in the MONARCH-3 trial that reported similar benefits in terms of PFS prolongation (HR 0.54; $p < 0.0001$) and a different toxicity profile of abemaciclib with higher rates of diarrhea and

Table 8 Selected first-line phase III clinical trials

Trial	Experimental arm	Control arm	PFS	OS
PALOMA-2 [74]	Palbociclib + letrozole	Letrozole	PFS 24.8 (95% CI 22.1–not reached) vs 14.5 (12.9–17.1); HR 0.58 (0.46–0.72); $p < 0.001$	NM
MONALEESA-2 [75]	Ribociclib + letrozole	Letrozole	PFS NR (19.3–NR) vs 14.7 (13.0–16.5)	NM
MONARCH-3 [76]	Abemaciclib + anastrozole or letrozole	Anastrozole or letrozole	PFS: NR vs 14.7 HR 0.54 (0.41–0.72) $p < 0.00001$	NM
FALCON [6]	Fulvestrant 500 mg	Anastrozole	PFS 16.6 (13.8–20.9) vs 13.8 (11.9–16.5) HR 0.797 (0.637–0.999); $p = 0.0486$	NM
MONALEESA-7 [77]	Ribociclib + goserelin with tamoxifen or NSAI	Goserelin with tamoxifen or NSAI	PFS = 23.8 (19.2–not reached) vs 13.0 (11.0–16.4), HR 0.553 (95% CI: 0.441–0.694; $p < 0.0000001$)	NM

fatigue and an inferior rate of hematological toxicity in comparison with ribociclib and palbociclib [81]. The MONALEESA-7 evaluated the same question specifically in the premenopausal patient and found that the addition of a CDK4/CDK6 inhibitor, in this case ribociclib, to standard ET with a GnRH analogue and an AI or tamoxifen, was associated with a similar benefit in terms of PFS (median PFS 23.8 vs 13.0; HR 0.55; $p < 0.00001$) and side effect profile as compared to the trials with postmenopausal patients [77].

In summary, these studies demonstrated significant statistical and clinical benefits in terms of improved PFS and time to chemotherapy with a tolerable toxicity profile. It is important to emphasize that, so far, no OS benefit has been demonstrated. Nonetheless, first-line treatment with CDK4/CDK6 inhibitors in combination with a NSAI is being increasingly adopted as the preferential strategy, especially in the USA and Western Europe [82].

The first-line trials of CDK4/CDK6 inhibitors enrolled patients with "de novo" MBC and patients that experienced recurrence after a long DFI following the completion of adjuvant ET, therefore, representing a population with potentially highly endocrine-sensitive tumors. Endocrine-naïve patients presenting with MBC are increasingly rare in regions of the globe where breast cancer screening programs allow detection of cancers at an early stage and treatment with adjuvant ET is commonly prescribed in the vast majority of patients. Nevertheless, for this subgroup of patients, the use of first-line fulvestrant is a valid approach based on the FALCON trial, especially in patients without visceral metastasis [6]. This recommendation is based on the phase III FALCON trial, a study that randomized 462 postmenopausal patients with endocrine-naïve (no exposure to any kind of ET in the adjuvant setting) ER+ HER2-negative advanced breast cancer to first-line treatment with anastrozole versus fulvestrant 500 mg. A significant benefit in terms of PFS was seen in the fulvestrant arm (16.6 versus 13.8; HR 0.79; CI 0.63–0.99; $p = 0.04$). A preplanned subgroup analysis identified patients without visceral disease as the only subgroup with superior PFS outcomes in the fulvestrant arm.

7.2 Second-Line Endocrine Therapy for Metastatic Breast Cancer

Patients with disease resistance to first-line treatment and patients who progress during adjuvant ET or within the initial 12 months after the completion of adjuvant ET are candidates for second-line ET. As previously described, several factors should be considered while selecting the optimal second-line strategy. Subsequent use of endocrine agents should always take into considerations what were the previous lines of treatment as well as the type and duration of response to previous ET. Two major patterns of endocrine resistance are recognized clinically: "intrinsic resistance" whereby ER+ cancers never respond adequately to ET and "acquired resistance" which occurs following an initial response [83]. An arbitrary cutoff of 2 years for relapse (in the early-stage setting) or 6 months for progression (in the

Table 9 Selected second-line phase III clinical trials

Trial	Experimental arm	Control arm	PFS	OS
BOLERO-2 [84, 85]	Everolimus + exemestane	Exemestane	7.8 versus 3.2; HR 0.45 (0.38–0.54); $p < 0.0001$	31.0 versus 26.6; HR 0.89 (0.73–1.10); $p = 0.143$
PALOMA-3 [86]	Palbociclib + fulvestrant	Fulvestrant	9.5 versus 4.6 HR 0.46 (0.36–0.59); $p < 0.0001$	NM
MONARCH 2 [87]	Abemaciclib + fulvestrant	Fulvestrant	16.4 vs 9.3 months; HR, 0.553; 95% CI, 0.449–0.681; $P < 0.001$	NM
CONFIRM [7, 88]	Fulvestrant 500 mg	Fulvestrant 250 mg	6.5 versus 5.5; HR 0.80 (0.68–0.94); $p = 0.006$	26.4 versus 22.3; HR 0.81 (0.69–0.96); $p = 0.02$

metastatic setting) has been used to define intrinsic versus acquired resistance in clinical trials. However, these distinctions are somewhat arbitrary, and the underlying mechanisms between intrinsic and acquired resistance are likely to overlap. In addition, resistance to ET may be agent-selective. For example, after failure of AI therapy, tumors can respond to other ET approaches such as another AI, ER modulators (tamoxifen) or downregulators (fulvestrant) and even estradiol [9].

Important trials of second-line ET are reviewed in Table 9. In AI-refractory disease, the use of combination of endocrine agents with targeted therapies aiming to modulate mechanisms of endocrine resistance has been incorporated into clinical practice initially with the mTOR inhibitor everolimus and more recently with the use of CDK4/CDK6 inhibitors in combination with fulvestrant (see Chapter "Emerging Therapeutic Approaches to Overcome Breast Cancer Endocrine Resistance"). The CDK4/CDK6 inhibitors palbociclib and abemaciclib have also shown significant clinical benefits and prolongation of median PFS when used in combination with fulvestrant in the PALOMA-3 [89] and MONARCH 2 [87] phase III trials, respectively. These studies included patients who relapsed during first-line treatment with AI for MBC as well as patients that recurred during adjuvant AI or experienced a short DFI after completion of adjuvant ET. The PALOMA-3 trial randomized 521 patients (including premenopausal patients undergoing OFS and postmenopausal women) to receive the combination of palbociclib and fulvestrant versus fulvestrant monotherapy. Approximately one-third have been treated for MBC with chemotherapy. The study reached the primary endpoint and reported an increase in PFS (9.2 months vs 3.8 months; HR = 0.42; $p < 0.001$) [89]. Abemaciclib was evaluated in the second-line setting in the MONARCH 2 trial where postmenopausal patients without previous treatment for MBC treated with abemaciclib and fulvestrant had superior PFS in comparison with patients treated with fulvestrant alone (16.4 months vs 9.3 months; HR = 0.55; $p < 0.001$) [87]. Also, in a similar population with NSAI refractory tumors, the BOLERO-2 trial showed better outcomes with treatment with everolimus in combination with exemestane, in comparison with exemestane monotherapy.

As previously discussed, the contemporary unavailability of predictive biological markers leaves us with clinical factors such as type of previous ET exposure and timing of disease progression as the only elements to help us define the optimal therapeutic strategy. In patients with long PFS (as a surrogate of endocrine sensitivity), the sequential use of endocrine agents can be considered a valid option. Despite limited data, drug treatment withdrawal in selected patients with progressive advanced ER+ breast cancer may eventually be utilized [90]. Tamoxifen, megestrol acetate, estradiol, and androgens also remain potential treatment options in those patients with long-lasting ER-sensitive disease as well as in limited resources settings, where drug availability is limited.

In premenopausal patients with HR+ advanced breast cancer, for decades the standard ET has been tamoxifen or ovarian function suppression. Studies that compared tamoxifen with surgical castration have shown similar efficacy [91, 92]. In a meta-analysis the combination of a GnRH agonist with tamoxifen resulted in a significant increase in median PFS and OS in comparison with either agent alone [93]. The use of AI monotherapy in premenopausal patients is not recommended since these women have estrogen production by the functioning ovaries. Therefore, AIs can only be administered in combination with OFS that can be achieved by the use of a GnRH analog or by surgical castration. After progression on tamoxifen and with the indication of further ET, the NCCN guideline and a limited amount of clinical data [94–96] suggest that premenopausal and perimenopausal patients with ER+ MBC should be treated with OFS and treated in the same manner as postmenopausal patients. As mentioned above, the recently presented MONALEESA-7 trial was designed to evaluate the role of the CDK4/CDK6 inhibitor ribociclib specifically in the premenopausal population and demonstrated similar benefits regarding PFS and response rates as seen in the trials with postmenopausal patients [77].

8   Future Perspectives

While we can claim a degree of progress over the last several decades since the introduction of tamoxifen, ER+ breast cancer remains a frustrating disease to treat with a high relapse rate for higher-stage and higher-grade disease. Aromatase inhibitors have brought improvements in relapse-free survival but not marked gains in overall survival. Despite the molecular promise of SERD therapy and some gains in overall survival in the advanced disease setting, fulvestrant was never measured as an adjuvant treatment in large part because of difficulties in establishing the correct dose and schedule for intramuscular drug delivery. The approval of everolimus and three CDK4/CDK6 inhibitors in the advanced disease setting has come to a number of trials examining these agents as adjuvant treatment. However at a molecular level, ER+ breast cancer shows remarkable inter- and intra-tumoral genomic heterogeneity which is clearly responsible for the evolution of resistance mechanism [2, 83, 97–99]. Continued study of the relationships between outcomes for endocrine therapy and genomic characteristics of ER+ breast cancer is likely to drive new insights into treatment selections that will propel the next wave of therapeutic advances.

References

1. Reinert T, Barrios C (2015) Optimal management of hormone receptor positive metastatic breast cancer in 2016. Ther Adv Med Oncol 7(6):304–320
2. Ma C, Reinert T, Chmielewska I, Ellis M (2015) Mechanisms of aromatase inhibitors resistance. Nat Rev Cancer 15:261–275
3. Goncalves RWW, Luo J, Ellis MJ (2014) New concepts in breast cancer genomics and genetics. Breast Cancer Res 16:460
4. Reinert T, Barrios C (2017) Overall survival and progression-free survival with endocrine therapy for hormone receptor-positive, HER2-negative advanced breast cancer: review. Ther Adv Med Oncol 9:693–709
5. Ciruelos EPT, Vozmediano MLA et al (2014) The therapeutic role of fulvestrant in the management of patients with hormone receptor-positive breast cancer. Breast 23:201–208
6. RObertson J, Bondarenko I, Trishkina E et al (2016) Fulvestrant 500 mg versus anastrozole 1 mg for hormone receptor-positive advanced breast cancer (FALCON): an international, randomised, double-blind, phase 3 trial. Lancet 388:2997
7. Di Leo A, Jerusalem G, Petruzelka L et al (2010) Results of the CONFIRM phase III trial comparing fulvestrant 250mg with fulvestrant 500mg in postmenopausal women with estrogen receptor-positive advanced breast cancer. J Clin Oncol 28(30):4594–4600
8. Bines JDR, Obadia RM et al (2014) Activity of megestrol acetate in postmenopausal women with advanced breast cancer after nonsteroidal aromatase inhibitor failure: a phase II trial. Ann Oncol 25(4):831–836
9. Ellis MJ, Gao F, Dehdashti F, Jeffe DB, Marcom PK, Carey LA, Dickler MN, Silverman P, Fleming GF, Kommareddy A, Jamalabadi-Majidi S, Crowder R, Siegel BA (2009) Lowerdose vs high-dose oral estradiol therapy of hormone receptor-positive, aromatase inhibitorresistant advanced breast cancer: a phase 2 randomized study. JAMA 302(7):774–780. https://doi.org/10.1001/jama.2009.1204
10. Gail MH, Brinton LA, Byar DP, Corle DK, Green SB, Schairer C, Mulvihill JJ (1989) Projecting individualized probabilities of developing breast cancer for white females who are being examined annually. J Natl Cancer Inst 81(24):1879–1886
11. Visvanathan K, Chlebowski RT, Hurley P, Col NF, Ropka M, Collyar D, Morrow M, Runowicz C, Pritchard KI, Hagerty K, Arun B, Garber J, Vogel VG, Wade JL, Brown P, Cuzick J, Kramer BS, Lippman SM (2009) American society of clinical oncology clinical practice guideline update on the use of pharmacologic interventions including tamoxifen, raloxifene, and aromatase inhibition for breast cancer risk reduction. J Clin Oncol 27(19):3235–3258. https://doi.org/10.1200/jco.2008.20.5179
12. Goss PE, Ingle JN, Ales-Martinez JE, Cheung AM, Chlebowski RT, Wactawski-Wende J, McTiernan A, Robbins J, Johnson KC, Martin LW, Winquist E, Sarto GE, Garber JE, Fabian CJ, Pujol P, Maunsell E, Farmer P, Gelmon KA, Tu D, Richardson H (2011) Exemestane for breast-cancer prevention in postmenopausal women. N Engl J Med 364(25):2381–2391. https://doi.org/10.1056/NEJMoa1103507
13. Cuzick J, Sestak I, Forbes JF, Dowsett M, Knox J, Cawthorn S, Saunders C, Roche N, Mansel RE, von Minckwitz G, Bonanni B, Palva T, Howell A (2014) Anastrozole for prevention of breast cancer in high-risk postmenopausal women (IBIS-II): an international, double-blind,

randomised placebo-controlled trial. Lancet (London, England) 383(9922):1041–1048. https://doi.org/10.1016/s0140-6736(13)62292-8

14. Wapnir IL, Dignam JJ, Fisher B, Mamounas EP, Anderson SJ, Julian TB, Land SR, Margolese RG, Swain SM, Costantino JP, Wolmark N (2011) Long-term outcomes of invasive ipsilateral breast tumor recurrences after lumpectomy in NSABP B-17 and B-24 randomized clinical trials for DCIS. J Natl Cancer Inst 103(6):478–488. https://doi.org/10.1093/jnci/djr027

15. Cuzick J, Sestak I, Pinder SE, Ellis IO, Forsyth S, Bundred NJ, Forbes JF, Bishop H, Fentiman IS, George WD (2011) Effect of tamoxifen and radiotherapy in women with locally excised ductal carcinoma in situ: long-term results from the UK/ANZ DCIS trial. Lancet Oncol 12(1):21–29. https://doi.org/10.1016/s1470-2045(10)70266-7

16. Fisher B, Dignam J, Wolmark N, Mamounas E, Costantino J, Poller W, Fisher ER, Wickerham DL, Deutsch M, Margolese R, Dimitrov N, Kavanah M (1998) Lumpectomy and radiation therapy for the treatment of intraductal breast cancer: findings from National Surgical Adjuvant Breast and Bowel Project B-17. J Clin Oncol 16(2):441–452. https://doi.org/10.1200/jco.1998.16.2.441

17. Fisher B, Dignam J, Wolmark N, Wickerham DL, Fisher ER, Mamounas E, Smith R, Begovic M, Dimitrov NV, Margolese RG, Kardinal CG, Kavanah MT, Fehrenbacher L, Oishi RH (1999) Tamoxifen in treatment of intraductal breast cancer: National Surgical Adjuvant Breast and Bowel Project B-24 randomised controlled trial. Lancet (London, England) 353(9169):1993–2000. https://doi.org/10.1016/s0140-6736(99)05036-9

18. Staley H, McCallum I, Bruce J (2012) Postoperative tamoxifen for ductal carcinoma in situ. Cochrane Database Syst Rev 10:Cd007847. https://doi.org/10.1002/14651858.CD007847.pub2

19. Margolese RG, Cecchini RS, Julian TB, Ganz PA, Costantino JP, Vallow LA, Albain KS, Whitworth PW, Cianfrocca ME, Brufsky AM, Gross HM, Soori GS, Hopkins JO, Fehrenbacher L, Sturtz K, Wozniak TF, Seay TE, Mamounas EP, Wolmark N (2016) Anastrozole versus tamoxifen in postmenopausal women with ductal carcinoma in situ undergoing lumpectomy plus radiotherapy (NSABP B-35): a randomised, double-blind, phase 3 clinical trial. Lancet (London, England) 387(10021):849–856. https://doi.org/10.1016/s0140-6736(15)01168-x

20. (EBCTCG)† EBCTCG (2015) Aromatase inhibitors versus tamoxifen in early breast cancer: patient-level meta-analysis of the randomised trials. Lancet 386(10001):1341–1352

21. Burstein HJ, Lacchetti C, Anderson H, Buchholz TA, Davidson NE, Gelmon KE, Giordano SH, Hudis CA, Solky AJ, Stearns V, Winer EP, Griggs JJ (2016) Adjuvant endocrine therapy for women with hormone receptor–positive breast cancer: American Society of Clinical Oncology clinical practice guideline update on ovarian suppression. J Clin Oncol 34(14):1689–1701. https://doi.org/10.1200/jco.2015.65.9573

22. Pagani O, Regan MM, Walley BA, Fleming GF, Colleoni M, Lang I, Gomez HL, Tondini C, Burstein HJ, Perez EA, Ciruelos E, Stearns V, Bonnefoi HR, Martino S, Geyer CE Jr, Pinotti G, Puglisi F, Crivellari D, Ruhstaller T, Winer EP, Rabaglio-Poretti M, Maibach R, Ruepp B, Giobbie-Hurder A, Price KN, Bernhard J, Luo W, Ribi K, Viale G, Coates AS, Gelber RD, Goldhirsch A, Francis PA (2014) Adjuvant exemestane with ovarian suppression in premenopausal breast cancer. N Engl J Med 371(2):107–118. https://doi.org/10.1056/NEJMoa1404037

23. Francis PA, Regan MM, Fleming GF, Lang I, Ciruelos E, Bellet M, Bonnefoi HR, Climent MA, Da Prada GA, Burstein HJ, Martino S, Davidson NE, Geyer CE Jr, Walley BA, Coleman R, Kerbrat P, Buchholz S, Ingle JN, Winer EP, Rabaglio-Poretti M, Maibach R, Ruepp B, Giobbie-Hurder A, Price KN, Colleoni M, Viale G, Coates AS, Goldhirsch A, Gelber RD (2015) Adjuvant ovarian suppression in premenopausal breast cancer. N Engl J Med 372(5):436–446. https://doi.org/10.1056/NEJMoa1412379

24. Regan MM, Francis PA, Pagani O, Fleming GF, Walley BA, Viale G, Colleoni M, Lang I, Gomez HL, Tondini C, Pinotti G, Price KN, Coates AS, Goldhirsch A, Gelber RD (2016) Absolute benefit of adjuvant endocrine therapies for premenopausal women with hormone receptor-positive, human epidermal growth factor receptor 2-negative early breast cancer: TEXT and SOFT trials. J Clin Oncol 34(19):2221–2231. https://doi.org/10.1200/jco.2015.64.3171

25. Cuzick J, Sestak I, Baum M, Buzdar A, Howell A, Dowsett M, Forbes JF (2010) Effect of anastrozole and tamoxifen as adjuvant treatment for early-stage breast cancer: 10-year analysis of the ATAC trial. Lancet Oncol 11(12):1135–1141. https://doi.org/10.1016/S1470-2045(10)70257-6

26. Mouridsen H, Giobbie-Hurder A, Goldhirsch A, Thurlimann B, Paridaens R, Smith I, Mauriac L, Forbes J, Price KN, Regan MM, Gelber RD, Coates AS (2009) Letrozole therapy alone or in sequence with tamoxifen in women with breast cancer. N Engl J Med 361(8):766–776. https://doi.org/10.1056/NEJMoa0810818

27. Regan MM, Neven P, Giobbie-Hurder A, Goldhirsch A, Ejlertsen B, Mauriac L, Forbes JF, Smith I, Lang I, Wardley A, Rabaglio M, Price KN, Gelber RD, Coates AS, Thurlimann B (2011) Assessment of letrozole and tamoxifen alone and in sequence for postmenopausal women with steroid hormone receptor-positive breast cancer: the BIG 1-98 randomised clinical trial at 8.1 years median follow-up. Lancet Oncol 12(12):1101–1108. https://doi.org/10.1016/s1470-2045(11)70270-4

28. van de Velde CJ, Rea D, Seynaeve C, Putter H, Hasenburg A, Vannetzel JM, Paridaens R, Markopoulos C, Hozumi Y, Hille ET, Kieback DG, Asmar L, Smeets J, Nortier JW, Hadji P, Bartlett JM, Jones SE (2011) Adjuvant tamoxifen and exemestane in early breast cancer (TEAM): a randomised phase 3 trial. Lancet (London, England) 377(9762):321–331. https://doi.org/10.1016/s0140-6736(10)62312-4

29. Early Breast Cancer Trialists' Collaborative Group (2015) Aromatase inhibitors versus tamoxifen in early breast cancer: patient-level meta-analysis of the randomised trials. Lancet (London, England) 386(10001):1341–1352. https://doi.org/10.1016/s0140-6736(15)61074-1

30. Davies C, Pan H, Godwin J, Gray R, Arriagada R, Raina V, Abraham M, Alencar VHM, Badran A, Bonfill X, Bradbury J, Clarke M, Collins R, Davis SR, Delmestri A, Forbes JF, Haddad P, Hou M-F, Inbar M, Khaled H, Kielanowska J, Kwan W-H, Mathew BS, Mittra I, Müller B, Nicolucci A, Peralta O, Pernas F, Petruzelka L, Pienkowski T, Radhika R, Rajan B, Rubach MT, Tort S, Urrútia G, Valentini M, Wang Y, Peto R (2013) Long-term effects of continuing adjuvant tamoxifen to 10 years versus stopping at 5 years after diagnosis of oestrogen receptor-positive breast cancer: ATLAS, a randomised trial. Lancet 381(9869):805–816. https://doi.org/10.1016/S0140-6736(12)61963-1

31. Goss PE, Ingle JN, Martino S, Robert NJ, Muss HB, Piccart MJ, Castiglione M, Tu D, Shepherd LE, Pritchard KI, Livingston RB, Davidson NE, Norton L, Perez EA, Abrams JS, Therasse P, Palmer MJ, Pater JL (2003) A randomized trial of letrozole in postmenopausal women after five years of tamoxifen therapy for early-stage breast cancer. N Engl J Med 349(19):1793–1802. https://doi.org/10.1056/NEJMoa032312

32. Jin H, Tu D, Zhao N, Shepherd LE, Goss PE (2012) Longer-term outcomes of letrozole versus placebo after 5 years of tamoxifen in the NCIC CTG MA.17 trial: analyses adjusting for treatment crossover. J Clin Oncol 30(7):718–721. https://doi.org/10.1200/jco.2010.34.4010

33. Goss PE, Ingle JN, Martino S, Robert NJ, Muss HB, Piccart MJ, Castiglione M, Tu D, Shepherd LE, Pritchard KI, Livingston RB, Davidson NE, Norton L, Perez EA, Abrams JS, Cameron DA, Palmer MJ, Pater JL (2005) Randomized trial of letrozole following tamoxifen as extended adjuvant therapy in receptor-positive breast cancer: updated findings from NCIC CTG MA.17. J Natl Cancer Inst 97(17):1262–1271. https://doi.org/10.1093/jnci/dji250

34. Mamounas EP, Jeong JH, Wickerham DL, Smith RE, Ganz PA, Land SR, Eisen A, Fehrenbacher L, Farrar WB, Atkins JN, Pajon ER, Vogel VG, Kroener JF, Hutchins LF, Robidoux A, Hoehn JL, Ingle JN, Geyer CE Jr, Costantino JP, Wolmark N (2008) Benefit from exemestane as extended adjuvant therapy after 5 years of adjuvant tamoxifen: intention-to-treat analysis of the National Surgical Adjuvant Breast and Bowel Project B-33 trial. J Clin Oncol 26(12):1965–1971. https://doi.org/10.1200/jco.2007.14.0228

35. Pan H, Gray R, Braybrooke J, Davies C, Taylor C, McGale P, Peto R, Pritchard KI, Bergh J, Dowsett M, Hayes DF (2017) 20-year risks of breast-cancer recurrence after stopping endocrine therapy at 5 years. N Engl J Med 377(19):1836–1846. https://doi.org/10.1056/NEJMoa1701830

36. Smith I (2014) Preoperative endocrine therapy for operable breast cancer. In: Harris JR, Lippman ME, Morrow M, Kent Osborne C (eds) Diseases of the breast: Fifth edition. Wolters Kluwer Health Adis (ESP).
37. Chiba A, Hoskin T, Heins C, Hunt K, Habermann E, Boughey J (2017) Trends in neoadjuvant endocrine therapy use and impact on rates of breast conservation in hormone receptor-positive breast cancer: a National Cancer Data Base Study. Ann Surg Oncol 24:418
38. Gray RG, Rea D, Handley K, Bowden SJ, Perry P, Earl HM, Poole CJ, Bates T, Chetiyawardana S, Dewar JA, Fernando IN, Grieve R, Nicoll J, Rayter Z, Robinson A, Salman A, Yarnold J, Bathers S, Marshall A, Lee M, Group obotaC (2013) aTTom: long-term effects of continuing adjuvant tamoxifen to 10 years versus stopping at 5 years in 6,953 women with early breast cancer. J Clin Oncol 31(18_suppl):5. https://doi.org/10.1200/jco.2013.31.18_suppl.5
39. Davies C, Pan H, Godwin J, Gray R, Arriagada R, Raina V, Abraham M, Medeiros Alencar VH, Badran A, Bonfill X, Bradbury J, Clarke M, Collins R, Davis SR, Delmestri A, Forbes JF, Haddad P, Hou MF, Inbar M, Khaled H, Kielanowska J, Kwan WH, Mathew BS, Mittra I, Muller B, Nicolucci A, Peralta O, Pernas F, Petruzelka L, Pienkowski T, Radhika R, Rajan B, Rubach MT, Tort S, Urrutia G, Valentini M, Wang Y, Peto R (2013) Long-term effects of continuing adjuvant tamoxifen to 10 years versus stopping at 5 years after diagnosis of oestrogen receptor-positive breast cancer: ATLAS, a randomised trial. Lancet (London, England) 381(9869):805–816. https://doi.org/10.1016/s0140-6736(12)61963-1
40. Rea D, Gray R, Bowden S, Handley K, Earl H, Poole C, Bates T, Dewar J, Raytor Z, Lee M (2013) Overall and subgroup findings of the aTTom trial: a randomised comparison of continuing adjuvant tamoxifen to 10 years compared to stopping after 5 years in 6953 women with ER positive or ER untested early breast cancer. . The European Cancer Congress, 2013 (2013) Scientific Programme – Proffered Papers. Eur J Cancer 49(Supplement 2):S298–S449 Abstract 1860
41. Tjan-Heijnen VCG, van Hellemond IEG, Peer PGM, Swinkels ACP, Smorenburg CH, van der Sangen MJC, Kroep JR, De Graaf H, Honkoop AH, Erdkamp FLG, van den Berkmortel F, de Boer M, de Roos WK, Linn SC, Imholz ALT, Seynaeve CM (2017) Extended adjuvant aromatase inhibition after sequential endocrine therapy (DATA): a randomised, phase 3 trial. Lancet Oncol 18(11):1502–1511. https://doi.org/10.1016/s1470-2045(17)30600-9
42. Blok EJ, Kroep JR, Meershoek-Klein Kranenbarg E, Duijm-de Carpentier M, Putter H, van den Bosch J, Maartense E, van Leeuwen-Stok AE, Liefers GJ, Nortier JWR, Rutgers EJT, van de Velde CJH (2018) Optimal duration of extended adjuvant endocrine therapy for early breast cancer; results of the IDEAL trial (BOOG 2006-05). J Natl Cancer Inst 110(1):40. https://doi.org/10.1093/jnci/djx134
43. Mamounas E, Bandos H, Lembersky B, Geyer C, Fehrenbacher L, Graham M, Chia S, Brufsky A, Hennessy B, Soori G, Dakil S, Seay T, Wade J, McCarron E, Paik S, Swain S, Wickerham D, Wolmark N (2017) Abstract S1–05: a randomized, double-blinded, placebo-controlled clinical trial of extended adjuvant endocrine therapy (tx) with letrozole (L) in postmenopausal women with hormone-receptor (+) breast cancer (BC) who have completed previous adjuvant tx with an aromatase inhibitor (AI): results from NRG oncology/NSABP B-42. Cancer Res 77(4 Supplement):S1-05-S01-05. https://doi.org/10.1158/1538-7445.sabcs16-s1-05
44. Goss PE, Ingle JN, Pritchard KI, Robert NJ, Muss H, Gralow J, Gelmon K, Whelan T, Strasser-Weippl K, Rubin S, Sturtz K, Wolff AC, Winer E, Hudis C, Stopeck A, Beck JT, Kaur JS, Whelan K, Tu D, Parulekar WR (2016) Extending aromatase-inhibitor adjuvant therapy to 10 years. N Engl J Med 375(3):209–219. https://doi.org/10.1056/NEJMoa1604700
45. Jakesz R, Greil R, Gnant M, Schmid M, Kwasny W, Kubista E, Mlineritsch B, Tausch C, Stierer M, Hofbauer F, Renner K, Dadak C, Rucklinger E, Samonigg H (2007) Extended adjuvant therapy with anastrozole among postmenopausal breast cancer patients: results from the randomized Austrian Breast and Colorectal Cancer Study Group trial 6a. J Natl Cancer Inst 99(24):1845–1853. https://doi.org/10.1093/jnci/djm246
46. Goldvaser H, Barnes TA, Seruga B, Cescon DW, Ocana A, Ribnikar D, Amir E (2018) Toxicity of extended adjuvant therapy with aromatase inhibitors in early breast cancer: a systematic review and meta-analysis. J Natl Cancer Inst 110(1):31. https://doi.org/10.1093/jnci/djx141

47. Bliss JM, Kilburn LS, Coleman RE, Forbes JF, Coates AS, Jones SE, Jassem J, Delozier T, Andersen J, Paridaens R, van de Velde CJ, Lonning PE, Morden J, Reise J, Cisar L, Menschik T, Coombes RC (2012) Disease-related outcomes with long-term follow-up: an updated analysis of the intergroup exemestane study. J Clin Oncol 30(7):709–717. https://doi.org/10.1200/jco.2010.33.7899

48. Jakesz R, Jonat W, Gnant M, Mittlboeck M, Greil R, Tausch C, Hilfrich J, Kwasny W, Menzel C, Samonigg H, Seifert M, Gademann G, Kaufmann M, Wolfgang J (2005) Switching of postmenopausal women with endocrine-responsive early breast cancer to anastrozole after 2 years' adjuvant tamoxifen: combined results of ABCSG trial 8 and ARNO 95 trial. Lancet (London, England) 366(9484):455–462. https://doi.org/10.1016/s0140-6736(05)67059-6

49. Kaufmann M, Jonat W, Hilfrich J, Eidtmann H, Gademann G, Zuna I, von Minckwitz G (2007) Improved overall survival in postmenopausal women with early breast cancer after anastrozole initiated after treatment with tamoxifen compared with continued tamoxifen: the ARNO 95 study. J Clin Oncol 25(19):2664–2670. https://doi.org/10.1200/jco.2006.08.8054

50. Dubsky PC, Jakesz R, Mlineritsch B, Postlberger S, Samonigg H, Kwasny W, Tausch C, Stoger H, Haider K, Fitzal F, Singer CF, Stierer M, Sevelda P, Luschin-Ebengreuth G, Taucher S, Rudas M, Bartsch R, Steger GG, Greil R, Filipcic L, Gnant M (2012) Tamoxifen and anastrozole as a sequencing strategy: a randomized controlled trial in postmenopausal patients with endocrine-responsive early breast cancer from the Austrian Breast and Colorectal Cancer Study Group. J Clin Oncol 30(7):722–728. https://doi.org/10.1200/jco.2011.36.8993

51. Boccardo F, Guglielmini P, Bordonaro R, Fini A, Massidda B, Porpiglia M, Roagna R, Serra P, Orzalesi L, Ucci G, Rubagotti A (2013) Switching to anastrozole versus continued tamoxifen treatment of early breast cancer: long term results of the Italian tamoxifen anastrozole trial. Eur J Cancer (Oxford, England: 1990) 49(7):1546–1554. https://doi.org/10.1016/j.ejca.2012.12.025

52. Coombes RC, Kilburn LS, Snowdon CF, Paridaens R, Coleman RE, Jones SE, Jassem J, Van de Velde CJ, Delozier T, Alvarez I, Del Mastro L, Ortmann O, Diedrich K, Coates AS, Bajetta E, Holmberg SB, Dodwell D, Mickiewicz E, Andersen J, Lonning PE, Cocconi G, Forbes J, Castiglione M, Stuart N, Stewart A, Fallowfield LJ, Bertelli G, Hall E, Bogle RG, Carpentieri M, Colajori E, Subar M, Ireland E, Bliss JM (2007) Survival and safety of exemestane versus tamoxifen after 2-3 years' tamoxifen treatment (intergroup exemestane study): a randomised controlled trial. Lancet (London, England) 369(9561):559–570. https://doi.org/10.1016/s0140-6736(07)60200-1

53. Jonat W, Gnant M, Boccardo F, Kaufmann M, Rubagotti A, Zuna I, Greenwood M, Jakesz R (2006) Effectiveness of switching from adjuvant tamoxifen to anastrozole in postmenopausal women with hormone-sensitive early-stage breast cancer: a meta-analysis. Lancet Oncol 7(12):991–996. https://doi.org/10.1016/s1470-2045(06)70948-2

54. Reinert T, Ramalho S, Gonçalves R, Barrios C, Graudenz M, Bines J et al (2016) Multidisciplinary approach to neoadjuvant endocrine therapy in breast cancer: a comprehensive review. Rev Bras Ginecol Obstet 38(12):615–622

55. Peto R, Davies C, Godwin J et al (2012) Comparisons between different polychemotherapy regimens for early breast cancer: meta-analyses of long-term outcomes among 100.000 women in 123 randomised trials. Lancet 379(9814):432–444

56. Lee B, Liedke P, Barrios C et al (2012) Breast cancer in Brazil: present status and future goals. Lancet Oncol 13:e95–e102

57. Reinert T, Gonçalves R, Ellis M (2018) Current status of neoadjuvant endocrine therapy in early stage breast cancer. Curr Treat Options in Oncol 19(5):23

58. Ellis M, Suman V, Hoog J et al (2011) Randomized phase II neoadjuvant comparison between letrozole, anastrozole, and exemestane for postmenopausal women with estrogen receptor–rich stage 2 to 3 breast cancer: clinical and biomarker outcomes and predictive value of the baseline PAM50-based intrinsic subtype—ACOSOG Z1031. J Clin Oncol 29(17):2342–2349

59. DIxon J, Renshhaw L, Mackaskill EJ et al (2009) Increase in response rate by prolonged treatment with neoadjuvant letrozole. Breast Cancer Res Treat 113(1):145–151

60. Carpenter R, Doughty J, Cordiner C et al (2014) Optimum duration of neoadjuvant letrozole to permit breast conserving surgery. Breast Cancer Res Treat 144(3):569–576
61. Smith IE, Dowsett M, Ebbs SR, Dixon JM, Skene A, Blohmer JU, Ashley SE, Francis S, Boeddinghaus I, Walsh G (2005) Neoadjuvant treatment of postmenopausal breast cancer with anastrozole, tamoxifen, or both in combination: the immediate preoperative anastrozole, tamoxifen, or combined with tamoxifen (IMPACT) multicenter double-blind randomized trial. J Clin Oncol 23(22):5108–5116. https://doi.org/10.1200/JCO.2005.04.005
62. Eiermann W, Paepke S, Appfelstaedt J et al (2001) Preoperative treatment of postmenopasusal breast cancer patients with letrozole: a randomized double-blind multicenter study. Ann Oncol 12:1527–1532
63. Cataliotti L, Buzdar A, Noguchi S, Bines J et al (2006) Comparison of anastrozole versus tamoxifen as preoperative therapy in postmenopausal women with hormone receptor-positive breast cancer the pre-operative "Arimidex" compared to tamoxifen (PROACT) trial. Cancer 106(10):2095–2103
64. Masuda N, Sagara Y, Kinoshita T et al (2012) Neoadjuvant anastrozole versus tamoxifen in patients receiving goserelin for premenopausal breast cancer (STAGE): a double-blind, randomised phase 3 trial. Lancet Oncol 13(4):345–352
65. Semiglazov V (2005) Neoadjuvant endocrine therapy: exemestane vs tamoxifen in postmenopausal ER+ breast cancer patients (T1-4, N1-2, M0). J Clin Oncol 23(11s):Abstract 530
66. Lerebours F, Bourgier C, Alran S et al (2012) Abstract PD07-04: a randomized phase II neoadjuvant trial evaluating anastrozole and fulvestrant efficiency for post-menopausal ER-positive, HER2-negative breast cancer patients: first results of the UNICANCER CARMINA 02 French trial. Cancer Res 72(24 Suppl):Abstract nr PD07-04
67. Semiglazov V, Semiglazov V, Dashyan G et al (2007) Phase 2 randomized trial of primary endocrine therapy versus chemotherapy in postmenopausal patients with estrogen receptor-positive breast cancer. Cancer 110:244–254
68. Alba E, Calvo L, Albanell L et al (2012) Chemotherapy and hormonetherapy as neoadjuvant treatment in luminal breast cancer patients: results from the GEICAM/2006-03, a multicenter, randomized, phase II study. Ann Oncol 23(12):3069–3074
69. Palmieri C, Cleator S, Kliburn L et al (2014) NEOCENT: a randomised feasibility and translational study comparing neoadjuvant endocrine therapy with chemotherapy in ER-rich postmenopausal primary breast cancer. Breast Cancer Res Treat 148(3):581–590
70. Cottu P et al (2017) LBA9 – letrozole and palbociclib versus 3rd generation chemotherapy as neoadjuvant treatment of luminal breast cancer. Results of the UNICANCER-NeoPAL study. Ann Oncol 28(Suppl 5):Abstr LBA9
71. Ellis MJ, Tao Y, Luo J, A'Hern R, Evans DB, Bhatnagar AS, Chaudri Ross HA, von Kameke A, Miller WR, Smith I, Eiermann W, Dowsett M (2008) Outcome prediction for estrogen receptor-positive breast cancer based on postneoadjuvant endocrine therapy tumor characteristics. J Natl Cancer Inst 100(19):1380–1388. https://doi.org/10.1093/jnci/djn309
72. Cardoso F, Costa A, Senkus E et al (2016) 3rd ESO–ESMO international consensus guidelines for advanced breast cancer (ABC 3). Ann Oncol 28:16–33
73. Barrios CHFJ, Jonat W et al (2012) The sequential use of endocrine treatment for advanced breast cancer: where are we? Ann Oncol 23:1378–1386
74. Finn R, Martin M, Rugo H et al (2016) PALOMA-2: primary results from a phase III trial of palbociclib (P) with letrozole (L) compared with letrozole alone in postmenopausal women with ER+/HER2– advanced breast cancer (ABC). J Clin Oncol 34(suppl):abstr 507
75. Hortobagyi G, Stemmer S, Burris H et al (2016) Ribociclib as first-line therapy for HR-positive, advanced breast cancer. N Engl J Med 375:1738–1748
76. Goetz M, Toi M, Campone M, Sohn J et al (2017) MONARCH 3: abemaciclib as initial therapy for advanced breast cancer. J Clin Oncol 35:3638–3646
77. Tripathy D et al (2017) First-line ribociclib vs placebo with goserelin and tamoxifen or a nonsteroidal aromatase inhibitor in premenopausal women with hormone receptor-positive, HER2-negative advanced breast cancer: results from the randomized phase III MONALEESA-7 trial. In: SABCS proceedings

78. Finn R, Martin M, Rugo H, Jones S, Im S, Gelmon K et al (2016) Palbociclib and letrozole in advanced breast cancer. N Engl J Med 375(20):1926–1936
79. Finn RS, Crown JP, Lang I et al (2015) The cyclin-dependent kinase 4/6 inhibitor palbociclib in combination with letrozole versus letrozole alone as first-line treatment of oestrogen receptor-positive, HER2-negative, advanced breast cancer (PALOMA-1/TRIO-18): a randomised phase 2 stud. Lancet Oncol 16:25–35
80. Hortobagyi G, Stemmer S, Burris H, Yap Y, Sonke G, Paluch-Shimon S et al (2018) Updated results from MONALEESA-2, a phase 3 trial of first-line ribociclib + letrozole in hormone receptor-positive (HR+), HER2-negative (HER2−), advanced breast cancer (ABC). J Clin Oncol 29:1541–1547
81. Goetz M, Toi M, Klise S, Frenzel M, Bourayou N, Di Leo A et al (2015) MONARCH 3: a randomized phase III study of anastrozole or letrozole plus abemaciclib, a CDK4/6 inhibitor, or placebo in firstline treatment of women with HR+, HER2locoregionally recurrent or metastatic breast cancer (MBC). J Clin Oncol 33:abstract TPS624
82. Wolff A (2017) CDK4 and CDK6 inhibition in breast cancer - a new standard. N Engl J Med 375(20):1993–1994
83. Ellis M (2004) Overcoming endocrine therapy resistance by signal transduction inhibition. Oncologist 9(suppl 3):20–26. https://doi.org/10.1634/theoncologist.9-suppl_3-20
84. Baselga J, Campone M, Piccart M, Burris HA 3rd, Rugo HS, Sahmoud T, Noguchi S, Gnant M, Pritchard KI, Lebrun F, Beck JT, Ito Y, Yardley D, Deleu I, Perez A, Bachelot T, Vittori L, Xu Z, Mukhopadhyay P, Lebwohl D, Hortobagyi GN (2012) Everolimus in postmenopausal hormone-receptor-positive advanced breast cancer. N Engl J Med 366(6):520–529. https://doi.org/10.1056/NEJMoa1109653
85. Yardley D, Noguchi S, Pritchard K et al (2013) Everolimus plus exemestane in postmenopausal patients with HR(+) breast cancer: BOLERO-2 final progression-free survival analysis. Adv Ther 30(10):870–884
86. Turner NCRJ, André F et al (2015) Palbociclib in hormone-receptor positive advanced breast cancer. N Engl J Med 373:1672–1673
87. Sledge G, Toi M, Neven P et al (2017) MONARCH 2: abemaciclib in combination with fulvestrant in women with HR+/HER2- advanced breast cancer who had progressed while receiving endocrine therapy. J Clin Oncol 35(25):2875–2884
88. Di Leo A, Jerusalem G, Petruzelka L et al (2014) Final overall survival: fulvestrant 500mg vs 250mg in the randomized CONFIRM trial. J Nat Cancer Inst 106(1):337
89. Turner NC, Ro J, Andre F, Loi S, Verma S, Iwata H, Harbeck N, Loibl S, Huang Bartlett C, Zhang K, Giorgetti C, Randolph S, Koehler M, Cristofanilli M, Group PS (2015) Palbociclib in hormone-receptor-positive advanced breast cancer. N Engl J Med 373(3):209–219. https://doi.org/10.1056/NEJMoa1505270
90. Chavarri-Guerra YHM, Szymonifka J, Cigler T, Liedke P, Partridge A et al (2014) Drug withdrawal in women with progressive metastatic breast cancer while on aromatase inhibitor therapy. Br J Cancer 111(11):2046–2050
91. Buchanan RBBR, Durrant KR et al (1986) A randomized comparison of tamoxifen with surgical oophorectomy in premenopausal patients with advanced breast cancer. J Clin Oncol 4:1326–1330
92. Boccardo FRA, Perrotta A et al (1994) Ovarian ablation versus goserelin with or without tamoxifen in pre-perimenopausal patients with advanced breast cancer: results of a multicentric Italian study. Ann Oncol 5:337–342
93. Klijn JGBR, Boccardo F et al (2001) Combined tamoxifen and luteinizing hormone-releasing hormone (LHRH) agonist versus LHRH agonist alone in premenopausal advanced breast cancer: a meta-analysis of four randomized trials. J Clin Oncol 19:343–353
94. Klijn JGBL, Mauriac L et al (2000) Combined treatment with buserelin and tamoxifen in premenopausal metastatic breast cancer: a randomized study. J Natl Cancer Inst 92:903–911
95. Park IHRJ, Lee KS et al (2010) Phase II parallel group study showing comparable efficacy between premenopausal metastatic breast cancer patients treated with letrozole plus goserelin

and postmenopausal patients treated with letrozole alone as first-line hormone therapy. J Clin Oncol 28:2705–2711

96. Carlson RWTR, Schurman CM, Rivera E, Chung CT, Phan SP et al (2010) Phase II trial of anastrozole plus goserelin in the treatment of hormone receptor–positive, metastatic carcinoma of the breast in premenopausal women. J Clin Oncol 28:3917–3921

97. Ellis MJ, Ding L, Shen D, Luo J, Suman VJ, Wallis JW, Van Tine BA, Hoog J, Goiffon RJ, Goldstein TC, Ng S, Lin L, Crowder R, Snider J, Ballman K, Weber J, Chen K, Koboldt DC, Kandoth C, Schierding WS, McMichael JF, Miller CA, Lu C, Harris CC, McLellan MD, Wendl MC, DeSchryver K, Allred DC, Esserman L, Unzeitig G, Margenthaler J, Babiera GV, Marcom PK, Guenther JM, Leitch M, Hunt K, Olson J, Tao Y, Maher CA, Fulton LL, Fulton RS, Harrison M, Oberkfell B, Du F, Demeter R, Vickery TL, Elhammali A, Piwnica-Worms H, McDonald S, Watson M, Dooling DJ, Ota D, Chang LW, Bose R, Ley TJ, Piwnica-Worms D, Stuart JM, Wilson RK, Mardis ER (2012) Whole-genome analysis informs breast cancer response to aromatase inhibition. Nature 486(7403):353–360. https://doi.org/10.1038/nature11143

98. Ellis MJ, Perou CM (2013) The genomic landscape of breast cancer as a therapeutic roadmap. Cancer Discov 3(1):27–34

99. Miller C, Gindin Y, Lu C et al (2016) Aromatase inhibition remodels the clonal architecture of estrogen-receptor-positive breast cancers. Nat Commun 7:12498

Structural Insights into Estrogen Receptors and Antiestrogen Therapies

Ian Mitchelle S. de Vera, Udayanga S. Wanninayake, and Thomas P. Burris

Abstract The differential impact of distinct antiestrogens (AEs) is the result of varying structural perturbations they confer to estrogen receptors (ERs) when these small-molecule synthetic compounds compete with endogenous hormones, such as 17β-estradiol. These structural changes translate to altered ability of ERs to conscript cofactors and consequently alter the transcription of their target genes. AEs, depending on the mechanism of action, are classified as either selective estrogen receptor modulators (SERMs), which display tamoxifen-like partial agonism, or as selective estrogen receptor downregulators (SERDs) that confer structurally induced posttranslational modifications (PTMs) that destine these receptors for proteosomal degradation. The conformational plasticity of the ER helix 12 (H12) and how its dynamics and conformational sampling is altered by different AEs are crucial to cofactor recruitment and selectivity, translating to varying degrees of receptor modulation and downstream functional effects. Dissecting these conformational state fluctuations within the context of variable cofactor profiles in different tissues, PTM induction, and emergence of hormonal treatment-related resistance mutations in ERs could lead to improved design of novel therapeutic molecules for breast cancer.

Keywords Nuclear receptor · Estrogen · Tamoxifen · Breast cancer · SERM · Raloxifene

I. M. S. de Vera · U. S. Wanninayake
Department of Pharmacology & Physiology, Saint Louis University School of Medicine, St. Louis, MO, USA

T. P. Burris (✉)
Center for Clinical Pharmacology, Washington University School of Medicine and St. Louis College of Pharmacy, St. Louis, MO, USA
e-mail: burristhomas@wustl.edu

© Springer Nature Switzerland AG 2019
X. Zhang (ed.), *Estrogen Receptor and Breast Cancer*, Cancer Drug Discovery and Development, https://doi.org/10.1007/978-3-319-99350-8_10

241

1 Introduction

Estrogen receptors (ERs) are ligand-dependent transcription factors regulated by the main circulating estrogen hormone, 17β-estradiol (E2), which is normally produced by the ovaries or via alternative metabolic pathway starting with precursor hormones, such as testosterone [1]. Associated metabolites of E2, estriol and estrone, are also estrogen agonists but generally weaker than E2, and some have been found to have tissue-specific roles (Fig. 1a) [2]. These receptors regulate the function of the female reproductive system, control bone density maintenance, and have protective roles on the central nervous and cardiovascular systems. The effect of E2 on target tissues and organs is mediated by two distinct receptors, ERα (NR3A1) and ERβ (NR3A2), which are encoded by distinct genes [3, 4]. ERs have been implicated in pathological conditions ranging from breast and uterine cancers to cardiovascular and bone disease [5, 6]. Small synthetic molecules, such as

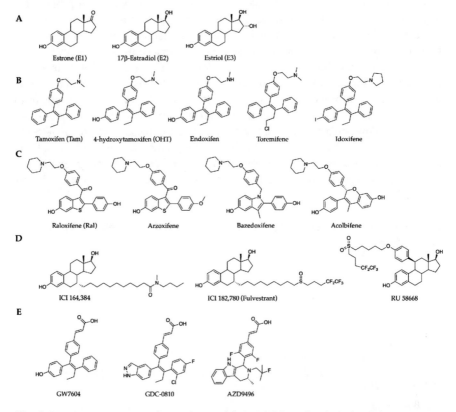

Fig. 1 Estrogen receptor agonists and antagonists. (**a**) Most abundant circulating estrogens, estrone, 17β-estradiol, and estriol. (**b**) Tamoxifen, its active metabolite, 4-hydroxytamoxifen, and SERMs derived from tamoxifen. (**c**) SERM antiestrogens with a steroid-like backbone and a tertiary amine side chain. (**d**) Pure antiestrogens with long side chains attached to a steroid-like scaffold. (**e**) SERDs with steroid-like scaffolds and an acrylic acid functional group

antiestrogen steroid or steroid mimics that are designed to block ERs, are used to treat breast cancer (Fig. 1b–e). Several antiestrogens demonstrate tissue-specific activity, such as selective estrogen receptor modulators (SERMs), tamoxifen and raloxifene (Fig. 1b, c).

Structural studies have illuminated ligand-binding induced conformational reorganization of ER ligand-binding domain (LBD) that leads to stabilization of the ER dimer, thereby promoting interaction with coregulator proteins [7, 8]. Since coregulator proteins have cell-specific expression, estrogens have distinct cellular effects. In general, ERα is the principal receptor mediating E2 signaling in the mammary gland, skeletal muscle, uterus, adipose tissue, and pituitary gland, while ERβ plays a less dominant role in these tissues. In contrast, ERβ is found to be dominant in the central nervous and cardiovascular systems, as well as in the lung, ovary, and prostate gland [9–11]. Understanding the structural properties of ER and the molecular mechanisms underlying ligand-dependent conformational changes has led to the development of more selective ER ligands for more effective antiestrogen therapy. Antiestrogens, in a simplistic binary conformational description (i.e., active vs. inactive receptor), are thought to occupy the ligand-binding pocket, thereby blocking E2 access and locking ER into inactive conformations not conducive to coactivator recruitment. However, current evidence suggests an antagonist-specific continuum of conformational states in ERs that allow exposure of unique surfaces for coregulator recruitment [12, 13]. Furthermore the cell type-specific profiles of coregulators also dictate the transcriptional activities of ERs bound to antagonists [14].

Detailed ER domain structural analysis has proven critical to our understanding of receptor function [15]. X-ray crystallography studies provide structural snapshots that have revealed mechanisms of E2-ER interaction thereby providing invaluable clues to future drug design targeting the estrogen receptor. This chapter will focus on how the structural perturbations in estrogen receptors induced as a result of interaction with agonists and antagonists, posttranslational modifications (PTMs), and endocrine treatment-induced resistance mutations affect cofactor recruitment, transcription of target genes, and antiestrogenicity.

2 Structural Organization of ERs

2.1 Architecture and Sequence Homology of ER Subtypes

Similar to other transcription factors in the nuclear hormone receptor (NHR) family, ERs have distinct domains with structural and functional roles (Fig. 2) [16]. ERα and ERβ are encoded by distinct genes with varying expression levels in different tissues. Full-length ERα is a 66-kDa protein containing 595 amino acids [17], whereas ERβ is slightly smaller at 60 kDa, spanning 530 amino acids [18].

Typically, there are six functional regions [A–E (and in some receptors such as ERα, an F region as well)] in NHRs with significant level of sequence homology.

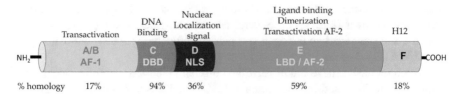

Fig. 2 Schematic of the ER architecture and details of the structural regions. A/B domain at the N-terminus contains activation function-1 (AF-1), the central C region is the DNA-binding domain (DBD), the hinge D contains the nuclear localization signal (NLS), region E is the ligand-binding domain and overlaps with the AF-2, and finally, domain F is the C-terminus of the AF-2 and contains the conformationally flexible helix 12 (H12). Percent homology of ERβ with respect to ERα are reported

Transcriptional activation is facilitated by two activation functions (AF) within the ERs, namely, the constitutively active AF-1 at the NH$_2$ terminus (A/B region, the least conserved between the ERs) and the ligand-dependent AF-2 at the COOH-terminal region (E region) that overlaps with the ligand-binding domain (LBD). The two ER subtypes share an overall sequence identity of 47%, which is primarily driven by high sequence identity in the central DNA-binding domain (DBD; C domain) and ligand-binding domain (LBD; E domain) with 94% and 59% identity between the receptor isotypes, respectively. Region D is considered a flexible hinge that also contains the nuclear localization signal (36% identity) [19]. The highly conserved DBD is responsible for DNA binding and recognition, while the LBD located at the COOH-terminal region is the site for small-molecule ligand binding. Both subtypes show high affinity for E2, which consequently stimulate transcription of an ER responsive gene containing an estrogen-responsive element (ERE) [20].

2.2 ER Ligand-Binding Domain Structure and the Helix 12 Conformational Switch

Like the LBDs of all NHRs, the ER LBDs form three-layered antiparallel α-helical folds [21]. ERα LBD has 12 helices, where the central core is formed by helices H5/H6, H9, and H10 sandwiched between helical layers, L1 (H1–4 and H7) and L2 (H8 and H11), which creates a ligand-binding pocket associated with helices H3, H6, H8, H11, H12, and the hairpin S1/S2 [22]. The dynamically mobile H12 and small two-stranded antiparallel β-sheet flank the major triple layer scaffold [21, 22]. ERβ closely resembles ERα as both have an unstructured F region. However, the ERβ COOH terminus has only an extremely short extended F region. While the F domain of ERα appears to have a role on transcriptional activity modulation, dimerization, receptor stabilization, and coactivator recruitment, the analogous role in ERβ remains unclear [23–25].

The LBDs of ERα and ERβ display considerable structural similarities, with the ligand-binding pocket of ERβ differing only at two residue positions with respect to ERα. Amino acid residues outside the binding cleft influence the size and shape of the respective ER pockets, which explains the subtype-selective binding of certain ligands, as exemplified by the ERβ-specific agonist, diarylpropionitrile [26]. Subtype-selective agonists and antagonists are invaluable for dissecting the biological effects specific to ERα and ERβ, which could corroborate findings from ER-knockout animal models.

Dimerization is crucial to ER function as amino acid substitutions that interfere with dimer formation abrogate receptor transcriptional activity [27]. The dimerization domain of ERα is created predominantly by helix 11, with some contribution from the DBD, amino terminal ends, and residues from H8 and loop H9/H10 of each monomer [28]. The ERα dimer binds ligands via hydrogen bond interactions and hydrophobic contacts with nonpolar ligands in a hydrophobic groove formed by helices, H3, H4, H5, and H12 [29]. Charged residues, namely, E353, R394, H524 and E260, R301, H430 in human ERα and Rat ERβ, respectively, stabilize the binding of agonist and antagonist by interacting with the hydroxyl groups of the estrogenic steroidal backbone.

The ligand-dependent transcriptional activation function-2 (AF-2) of ER is a conformationally dynamic region of the LBD that contains the conformational switch, helix 12 (H12). Depending on the class of ligand bound to ER, H12 is oriented differently with respect to the rest of the LBD (Fig. 3). Binding of an agonist, 17β-estradiol (E2), positions H12 over the ligand-binding cavity to generate a competent AF-2 interaction surface for coactivator docking, which is essential for transcriptional activation (Fig. 3a, b). Specifically, this opens up a new surface

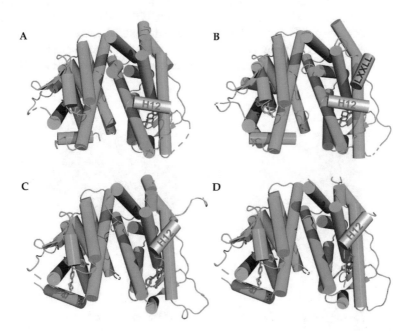

Fig. 3 ERα bound to agonists or antagonists with or without coactivator peptide. (**a**) ERα LBD bound to estradiol (E2) (PDB ID 1ERE). (**b**) ERα LBD bound to E2 and SRC-2 NR box 3 (PDB ID 1GWR). (**c**) ERα LBD bound to 4-hydroxytamoxifen (4-OHT) antagonist (PDB ID 3ERT). (**d**) ERα LBD bound to SERM antagonist, raloxifene (PDB ID 1ERR)

consisting of D538, L539, E542, and M543 to facilitate the interaction with a coactivator [22, 30, 31]. In this H12 conformation, the AF2 surface is conducive to recruitment of helical segments with LXXLL motif, where L and X are leucine and any residue, respectively—a motif found in many coactivators including the p160 steroid receptor coactivators (SRC) [30, 32]. In addition, the 17-OH group in E2 interacts with H524, which is forced to form an H-bond with the peptidic carbonyl group of E419 in loop 6–7. This facilitates the salt bridge formation between E339 from H3 and E419 from H7 to form a salt bridge network with K531 from H11 that favors the agonist orientation of H12 (Fig. 4a) [22].

In contrast, binding of an antagonist, such as 4-hydroxytamoxifen (4-OHT), disrupts the formation of the salt bridge network (Fig. 4b), thereby conferring increased conformational plasticity to H12 and ability to adopt a conformation that occludes the AF-2 groove, which physically blocks coactivator binding (Fig. 3c, d). This physical occlusion is made possible by an internal sequence in H12 that mimics an LXXLL motif, which enables a part of H12 to bind the coactivator groove [30]. A more compelling alternative explanation is that H12 contains an extended corepressor box sequence that binds the AF-1 surface, thereby preventing or hampering corepressor interaction [33, 34]. The latter explains why deletion of H12 confers strong enhancement of ER interaction with corepressors, such as NCoR and SMRT [35, 36]. Even though the importance of NR corepressors to ER signaling remains unclear, studies show that both agonist- and antagonist-bound ERs are capable of recruiting other proteins that repress ER activity [37]. Molecular dynamics (MD) simulation of 4-hydroxytamoxifen (4-OHT)-bound ERα demonstrates structural flexibility of H12, which fluctuates from an initial antagonist position to structurally distinct continuum of H12 positions between an agonist and antagonist conformation, explaining the mixed agonist-antagonist effects of 4-OHT [38].

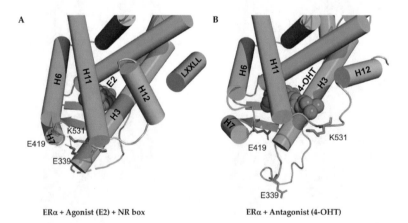

ERα + Agonist (E2) + NR box   ERα + Antagonist (4-OHT)

Fig. 4 (a) ERα LBD bound to E2 and SRC-2 NR box 3 reveals two salt bridges: K531-E419 and K531-E339 (PDB ID 1GWR). (b) When bound to the 4-OHT antagonist (PDB ID 3ERT), the salt bridges are disrupted

2.3 ER DNA-Binding Domain Structure and Response Element Recognition

The centrally positioned DNA-binding domains of the ERs are highly conserved and interact with identical DNA sequences. Crystal structures of ERα DBD with or without DNA reveal a topology characterized by two zinc finger-like motifs consisting of four cysteine residues that each coordinate with Zn^{2+} in a tetrahedral geometry (Fig. 5) [39–42]. Amino acid residues in the D box contribute to ER dimerization and discriminate half site spacing, while residues in the P box are involved in estrogen response element (ERE) recognition. Specifically, P box residues E203, G204, and A207 determine DNA-binding specificity and sequence discrimination and are critical to ERE binding. EREs, which are located at various positions from the transcription start site and/or within a gene locus, are variations of the palindromic sequence, 5′-GGTCAnnnTGACC-3′, where n is any nucleotide acting as a spacer [43, 44].

Gene expression modulated by the binding of E2-complexed ER (E2-ER) to EREs relies on a signaling pathway described as "ERE-dependent" [45–49]. Meanwhile, regulation of target gene expression that is mediated by transcription factor interaction with E2-ER, such as activation protein (AP) 1 and stimulatory

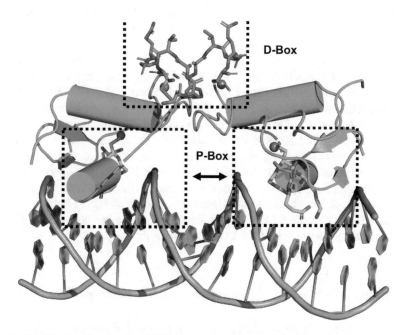

Fig. 5 The DNA-binding domain (DBD) of estrogen receptor α (ERα) dimerbound to the consensus sequence of the estrogen response element (ERE), GGTCAnnnTGACC, where n are nonspecific bases acting as spacer (PDB ID 1HCQ). The first zinc-finger module called P box determine DNA-binding specificity, while the second zinc module termed D box is involved in half-site spacing discrimination

protein (SP) 1 bound to associated regulatory elements on DNA, is classified as "ERE-independent" and employs a signaling pathway mechanism that remains unclear [45, 46, 49, 50]. ER could interact with transcription factors directly or indirectly through coregulatory proteins using interaction surfaces that include the DBD, while transcription control is conferred by combined effects transmitted through the NH_2 and COOH termini.

2.4   The Intrinsically Disordered ER NH_2 Terminus

The amino terminus (domain A/B in Fig. 2) encompasses the AF-1 region and is highly variable among members of the nuclear hormone receptor family [51]. In yeast and chicken cells, ERα AF-1 functions independently of the AF-2 in a ligand- and promoter-independent manner, but decoupling of AF-1 from AF-2 in mammalian cells resulted in a dysfunctional AF-1 in terms of influencing transcription [52–55]. Therefore, ERα AF-1 function depends on three factors, namely, cell type, ligand agonism, and structural integrity of the LBD. This is supported by further studies that demonstrate full activity of ER only when AF-1 and AF-2 are functionally integrated [54, 56–58].

Due to the intrinsically disordered nature of the ER AF-1, the underlying biochemical and structural mechanism of AF-1 action remains elusive. Interestingly, this disordered nature leads to the formation of a large ensemble of rapidly and reversibly interconverting conformational states [51, 59–61]. Inter-domain allosteric cooperativity, protein interaction, and posttranslational modifications (i.e., phosphorylation) control these conformational changes. For instance, interaction of the TATA box-binding protein upon interacting with the NH_2 terminus of ERα induces formation of an ordered structure [61]. Meanwhile, the S118 phosphorylation of ERα complexed with either E2 or tamoxifen via growth factor signaling led to Pin1 recruitment, which isomerizes the S118-P199 bond from cis to trans and promotes a conformational change that favors ligand-independent and agonist-inducible ERα activity [62]. Protein interactions with ERα are important for inducing conformational changes that stabilize interaction with coregulatory proteins, which translates to effective transcription [51]. In contrast, ERβ NH_2 terminus is devoid of AF-1 [48, 58, 63–65], does not interact with the COOH terminus [58], and impairs the ERβ-ERE interactions [66].

3   Structure-Activity Relationships in Antiestrogen Therapy

3.1   Selective ER Modulators and Selective ER Downregulators

Selective ER modulators (SERMs) such as tamoxifen, raloxifene, and analogues (Fig. 1b, c) are ER ligands that display gene- and/or tissue-specific agonist/antagonist activity. The first clinically approved SERM, tamoxifen, is the standard therapeutic regimen for all stages of breast cancer and has benefitted 70% of women with ERα-positive breast cancer [67, 68]. Aside from the antagonist effects of tamoxifen that inhibit breast cancer proliferation, the drug has desirable agonist effects on bone and lipid profiles [69–72]. However, tamoxifen and its active metabolite, 4-hydroxytamoxifen (OHT) has an estrogenic effect in the uterus of mice and rat models, which translates to higher risk of endometrial cancer development during the course of treatment [73, 74]. Moreover, the emergence of tamoxifen resistance without loss of ERα expression has been observed in primary tumors in majority of metastatic cancer patients [75, 76], although remissions are observed after tamoxifen withdrawal or altered treatment regimen, suggesting ongoing ER signaling activity in some tamoxifen-resistant tumors [77, 78].

To hamper the unwanted side effects while concomitantly improving the efficacy of tamoxifen, synthetic analogues (Fig. 1b) were designed, such as the halogenic/pyrrolidino derivatives, toremifene and idoxifene, and the secondary amine variant of 4-OHT, endoxifen [67]. Unfortunately, these tamoxifen analogues did not demonstrate improved efficacy or prevent drug resistance [67, 77, 79]. The benzothiophene SERM derivative, raloxifene (Fig. 1c), retained 76% of tamoxifen efficacy while reducing endometrial cancer incidence but is ineffective against tamoxifen-resistant breast cancer cells [67, 77, 80]. Meanwhile, the raloxifene analogue, arzoxifene, failed to be on par with tamoxifen efficacy for metastatic breast cancer in a phase III clinical trial [81] despite being more potent than tamoxifen and 4-OHT on inhibiting human mammary carcinoma cell proliferation [82, 83]. Relative to tamoxifen and raloxifene, a structural analogue bazedoxifene is more effective than other SERMs at inhibiting gene expression in MCF-7 cells and hampering the growth of tamoxifen-resistant xenograft [84].

Steroidal compounds with long side chains, such as ICI 164,384, ICI 182,780 (fulvestrant), and RU 58668 (Fig. 1d), were developed to minimize partial agonist activity. These drugs were initially referred to as pure antiestrogens (AEs) due to their lack of partial agonist effects in breast and endometrial cell lines [85–88] but were later designated as selective ER downregulators (SERDs) as they promote ERα degradation via the ubiquitin-proteasome pathway in ERα-positive breast cancer cells [89–92]. The pure AE character of fulvestrant did not confer an advantage over tamoxifen against advanced or metastatic breast cancer [79, 93], which could be attributed to its poor pharmacokinetic properties. This limitation is circumvented by doubling the intramuscular injection dosage to 500 mg, which increased patient survival rate [94–96]. In comparison, certain SERM derivatives of tamoxifen, such as GW7604, GDC-0810, and AZD9496, demonstrate SERD ability to induce ERα degradation with similar efficacy as fulvestrant but with improved oral bioavailability [78, 97–99].

In aggregate, antiestrogens demonstrate varying SERD activity, ranging from drugs that lack ERα downregulating capacity, such as tamoxifen, to SERM analogues with disparate levels of ERα reduction ability (e.g., raloxifene, bazedoxifene, GDC-0810, and GW7604). The strongest SERD activity is associated with pure AEs with long side chains, such as ICI 164,384, fulvestrant, and RU 58668.

3.2 Molecular Rationale of Antiestrogen Effects

AEs bind to ERα LBD akin to estradiol—with bulky side chains attached at steroid core positions 7α or 11β conferring antiestrogenicity by positioning these substituents between H3 and H11 of the binding cavity. Presence of bulky functional groups of different length and size results in structural rearrangements that can cause varying levels of steric hindrance to the positioning of H12 over the ligand-binding pocket.

Tamoxifen, raloxifene, and synthetic SERM analogues (Fig. 1b, c) contain alkylaminoethoxy side chains with varying tertiary amine groups. The dimethylamino group of tamoxifen or the piperidyl group of raloxifene sterically hinders the positioning of H12 to the coactivator-binding site. In an unobstructed state, H12 will dock to the coactivator groove via its hydrophobic residues, L540, M543, and L544, in a manner similar to the LXXLL motif in coactivators [22, 30, 100]. Synthetic analogues and ER mutants were made to validate this structural observation. For instance, a raloxifene derivative with a nitrogen-to-carbon replacement of a crucial compound side chain abrogated the drug's antagonist activity [101]. Furthermore, substitution of the crucial D351 residue to glutamic acid altered the effect of raloxifene from a pure antagonist to a tamoxifen-like antagonist in HepG2 cells. A hydrogen bond binds the tertiary amine of raloxifene to D351 in ERα LBD; the mutation to E351 altered this crucial interaction [22, 102]. In transfected MDA-MB-231 cells, a similar mutation D351G abolished tamoxifen-induced expression of TGFA—an estrogen target gene [103]. In addition, a D351A substitution rendered ERα inactive on a reporter gene in tamoxifen-induced HepG2 cells [102], corroborating the importance of D351 in mediating the partial agonist activity of SERMs.

Relative to SERMs, pure AEs such as fulvestrant and ICI 164,384 (Fig. 1d) have longer side chains. A crystal structure of the latter with rat ERβ shows position 7α protruding out of the ligand-binding cleft reminiscent of SERM side chains but bends at carbon 5 by 90°, thereby positioning the rest of the chain onto the coactivator-binding surface [104]. Side chains L261, M264, I265, and L286 in the coactivator-binding surface of rat ERβ form hydrophobic contacts with the terminal n-butyl group of ICI 164,384, which displaces H12 from the same position in crystal structures of 4-OHT and raloxifene-bound ERα (Fig. 3c, d). The long side chain sterically clashes with H12 residues L540 and M543 in the agonist conformation and with L536 and L540 when H12 is positioned in the coactivator-binding surface. Substitution of the aforementioned residues to alanine increased the pure AE-induced ERα transcriptional activity [105–108].

In contrast to ICI 164,384, fulvestrant antiestrogenicity is not affected by D351 mutations, but introduction of tertiary amine functional group in analogues ZK-253 and ZK-703 improved growth inhibition ability toward mouse xenografts from tamoxifen-resistant and estrogen-sensitive breast cancer cell lines [109]. However, these studies did not address whether direct interaction with pure AEs is crucial for enhanced activity.

Aside from amine functional groups, the effect of chain length was also investigated. To reveal optimal chain length for pure antiestrogenicity, derivatives of ICI 164,384 with variable side chain lengths were synthesized. Side chain lengths consisting of 15–19 atoms display optimal antiestrogenicity, while shorter side chains (13–14 carbon atoms) show agonist or SERM-like activity in reporter assays in HepG2 cells transiently transfected with ERα. These results suggest that longer chains are necessary for pure AEs to reach the coactivator-binding surface. Moreover, hydrophobicity and presence of terminal pentafluoropentyl group are crucial factors for pure AE activity, as supported by a study that shows higher potency and efficacy of fulvestrant relative to ICI 164,384 for growth inhibition in *in cellula* and in vivo human breast cancer models [88].

Partial or full SERD activity has been observed upon changing the shorter side chains of SERM analogues. For instance, the derivative bazedoxifene differs from raloxifene by having a larger heterocyclic amine ring (Fig. 1c) conferring enhanced steric clash with H12. Furthermore, GW5638 (Etacstil), the prodrug of the active metabolite GW7604 (Fig. 1e), is a tamoxifen derivative where the dimethyl-aminoethyl group is substituted with an acrylic acid side chain. In its protonated state, the carboxylate group in GW5638 form hydrogen bonds with the peptidic backbone of H12 and E351, inducing a conformation of H12 where the side chain of hydrophobic residues L536, L539, L540, and M543 are pointing toward the aqueous environment, which effectively increases the hydrophobic surface area of H12 relative to 4-OHT-bound ERα while concomitantly maintaining interaction in the coactivator-binding surface [110]. Therefore, pure antiestrogenicity positively correlates with hydrophobic surface area of H12 and is independent of H12 positioning in crystal structures. However, the effect of these structural perturbations on protein-protein interactions and overall ERα stability is not yet clear.

3.3 Effect of AE Binding on Cofactor Recruitment and Gene Transcription

The AF1 and AF2 activation functions at the N- and C-termini, respectively, are utilized by ERs to conscript a large number of cofactors in the presence of agonists. Such cofactors include chromatin remodeling complexes, histone acetyltransferases (HAT), methyltransferases (HMTs) and deacetylases (HDACs), and transcriptional machinery components [111]. The altered recruitment of cofactors to ERα is conformationally induced by AEs that modify the protein surface available for interaction [84]. HATs such as SRC1–3 (NCOA1–3) and CMP/p300 and HMTs including CARM1 and PRMT1 are some of the coactivators that interact directly with the AF2 of E2-ERα or perturb it allosterically [112, 113]. Tamoxifen, but not raloxifene, selectively recruit SRC-1 to promoter genes in Ishikawa and ECC-1 cell lines. Repression of SRC-1 in Ishikawa cells abrogates the partial agonist activity of tamoxifen on target genes [14]. In contrast, when SRC-1 is overexpressed in MCF-7 cells, the behavior of tamoxifen switches from agonist to antagonist suggesting that difference of SRC-1 expression level in breast and uterine cells explains the tissue-specific tamoxifen effects on transcription [14]. Analogously, SRC-2 and p300 overexpression in HeLa cells transfected with ERα amplified the partial agonist activity of tamoxifen but only have moderate and negligible effects in the presence of raloxifene and fulvestrant, respectively [36]. These results suggest that presence of coactivators may contribute to cell- and gene-specific partial agonist activity of SERMs. In addition, 11% of breast tumors show increased SRC-3 expression and is associated with unfavorable prognosis and tumor phenotype, which is explained by the impact of SRC-3 on the cell cycle regulation of both ERα+ and ERα⁻ tumors [114].

The activity and ligand-independent AF-1 function of ERα is linked to the partial agonist activity of tamoxifen and, to some degree, of raloxifene in a cell- and promoter-specific manner [56, 115, 116]. Case in point is the agonist effect of tamoxifen in HEC1 cells that is dependent on the AF1 of ERα [65]. In addition, Zwart and coworkers swapped the AF1 domain of ERα with that of ERβ and consequently abolished tamoxifen-induced transcriptional activity in U2OS cells, showing that the AF1 region is crucial to the partial agonist activity of tamoxifen. This result is corroborated by studies that show the ability of ERα, but not of ERβ, to conscript SRC-1 via the AF1 region [117, 118].

ERα recruits corepressors NCOR1 and NCOR2 (SMRT) in the presence of tamoxifen in MCF-7 cells resulting in the repression of estrogen target genes. Increase of ER target gene expression is observed in the same cells in the presence of tamoxifen after siRNA knockdown of the aforementioned corepressors. Analogously, recruitment of corepressors is absent on genes upregulated by tamoxifen in Ishikawa cells [14, 119, 120]. Moreover, SMRT2 overexpression in HepG2 cells inhibits partial agonist activity of tamoxifen [121]. In comparison to SERMs, ERα bound to fulvestrant is more efficient than raloxifene or tamoxifen at recruiting NCOR1 C-terminal fragment in ChIP experiments in HeLa cells [36]. However, the difference in corepressor recruitment mechanism between SERMs and SERDs remains elusive. It only became possible for raloxifene-bound ERα to co-crystallize with a corepressor NR sequence after H12 deletion, where the peptide occupies the AF2 surface subtended by H3 and H5, and with the raloxifene side chain packed against the peptide N-terminus. Further studies are needed to confirm whether the differential H12 conformation between SERM- and SERD-bound ERα increases corepressor recruitment in the presence of SERDs.

3.4 Impact of ERα Posttranslational Modifications to Pure Antiestrogenicity

Cofactor recruitment is likely modulated by ER posttranslational modifications (PTMs). Mass spectrometry has become an invaluable tool for the identification of acetylation, methylation, and phosphorylation sites in ERα. A study shows that phosphorylation of S104, S106, and S118 in the AF1 region and of S305 in the AF2 may be linked with tamoxifen resistance [122]. Presence of pure AEs induce the phosphorylation of the same serine residues on the AF-1 region, but the link of these PTMs to SERD transcriptional downregulation remains unclear [123, 124]. MCF-7 breast cancer cells with dephosphorylated Y537 displayed increased sensitization to SERMs and fulvestrant [125]. Sensitization of breast cancer cells to AEs may also be induced by other PTMs on ERα, such as acetylation, SUMOylation, ubiquitination, and methylation [122, 126].

SERDs induce the degradation of ERα in breast and uterine cancer cell lines. Presence of 4-OHT increases ERα expression [92, 106, 127], with some level of decrease in the presence of endoxifen, raloxifene, and bazedoxifene and substantial decrease in the presence of pure AE, such as fulvestrant [84]. Moreover, ERα ubiquitination is doubled in the presence of fulvestrant [92].

ERα turnover differs in the presence of AEs and E2. For instance, α-amanitin transcriptional inhibition prevents E2-induced degradation of ERα, but not by fulvestrant [128]. Similarly, partial inhibition of ERα degradation by E2 but not by pure AEs is afforded by cycloheximide or kinase inhibitor treatment [129, 130]. In spite of the aforementioned differences in degradation mechanisms between E2 and SERDs, the Neddylation pathway seems to be important for both E2- and pure AE-induced turnover [131].

Overexpression of ERα to saturate the degradation process has no effect on the capacity of SERDs to act as AEs in MCF-7 cells [132]. Moreover, the steady-state level of ERα unexpectedly increased in the presence of fulvestrant in HepG2 cells, but this ligand still functioned as an inverse agonist while tamoxifen has partial agonist activity [106, 127] suggesting an alternative mechanism to afford enhanced efficacy of pure AEs for inhibiting ERα activity in HepG2 cells. SUMOylation of ERα is strongly induced by pure AEs in MCF-7 breast cancer cells, HEK293 and HepG2 cells, and abolishing SUMOylation attenuates transcription in the presence of pure AEs, with no effect on the corresponding activity induced by E2 or tamoxifen, suggesting that SUMOylation contributes to pure antiestrogenicity [127]. Interestingly, SUMOylation activity peaked at 15–19 carbon atom chain length and decreased when chain length is >22, which correlates with inverse agonist activity in HepG2 cells and with the ability of the AE side chain to dock at the coactivator-binding cleft. Furthermore, the SERM raloxifene also induce SUMOylation to a lesser extent, which positively correlates with its ability to suppress basal transcription activity in HepG2 cells [127]. Possibly, differential SUMOylation could explain the varying SERM effects in different tissues.

3.5   Effect of ER Mutations on AE Action

Emergence of endocrine treatment resistance remains a challenging issue in treatment of patients with ER+ breast cancers. After developing resistance, majority of tumors still express ERα, suggesting the role of ERα in tumor growth. Coactivator overexpression inducing estrogen-dependent transcription is a potential mechanism of desensitization, as is the signaling pathway activation that controls the activity of ERα and/or its associated coactivators [133]. A recent review has highlighted the role of ERα mutations as an additional hormonal treatment resistance mechanism [134], as initially hinted by a constitutively active ERα Y537N mutant isolated from metastatic breast cancer cells [135]. Majority of hormone therapy-resistant tumors contain gain-of-function mutations, such as E380Q, L536Q/R, Y537S/C/N, and D538G that result in ERα activity that is ligand-independent [136–138]. These mutants show higher levels of S118 phosphorylation, enhanced recruitment of SRC1-3, increased ligand-independent tumor growth, and/or S118 phosphorylation [138–140].

Crystal structures of ERα mutants Y537S and D438G in the apo state adopt an agonist-like conformation [138–141]. As a result, affinity of binding of E2 and 4-OHT to said mutants is tenfold weaker relative to wild-type ERα, and higher doses of 4-OHT and fulvestrant are required to affect levels of activity inhibition in mutant ERα similar to wild type. This could lead to clinical resistance to AE therapy when required concentrations for activity suppression of ER mutants are not reached [136, 138, 140]. Furthermore, the structural changes relative to wild type in 4-OHT-bound ERα mutant LBDs may result in different effects on ER target genes at saturation [139].

4 Epilogue

ERα and ERβ have similar structures but display distinct as well as overlapping regulatory potentials in cells in a tissue-specific manner. Antiestrogens have diverse conformations and structures that modulate AF-1 and/or AF-2 activity that translate to varying levels of antiestrogenicity in breast cancer cells. The conformational dynamics of AE binding to ERs has several downstream consequences on posttranslational modifications and ER degradation mechanisms and needs to be explored further. Hormone therapy resistance is caused by the emergence of ER mutants that need to be characterized for their individual responses to various clinically available AEs, which will guide the design of future drugs for breast cancer.

References

1. Gruber CJ, Tschugguel W, Schneeberger C, Huber JC (2002) Production and actions of estrogens. N Engl J Med 346(5):340–352. https://doi.org/10.1056/NEJMra000471
2. Gruber DM, Huber JC (1999) Conjugated estrogens--the natural SERMs. Gynecol Endocrinol 13(Suppl 6):9–12
3. Green S, Walter P, Kumar V, Krust A, Bornert JM, Argos P, Chambon P (1986) Human oestrogen receptor cDNA: sequence, expression and homology to v-erb-A. Nature 320(6058):134–139. https://doi.org/10.1038/320134a0

4. Leygue E, Dotzlaw H, Lu B, Glor C, Watson PH, Murphy LC (1998) Estrogen receptor beta: mine is longer than yours? J Clin Endocrinol Metab 83(10):3754–3755. https://doi.org/10.1210/jcem.83.10.5187-1

5. Deroo BJ, Korach KS (2006) Estrogen receptors and human disease. J Clin Invest 116(3):561–570. https://doi.org/10.1172/JCI27987

6. Nilsson S, Makela S, Treuter E, Tujague M, Thomsen J, Andersson G, Enmark E, Pettersson K, Warner M, Gustafsson JA (2001) Mechanisms of estrogen action. Physiol Rev 81(4):1535–1565. https://doi.org/10.1152/physrev.2001.81.4.1535

7. Bai Y, Giguere V (2003) Isoform-selective interactions between estrogen receptors and steroid receptor coactivators promoted by estradiol and ErbB-2 signaling in living cells. Mol Endocrinol 17(4):589–599. https://doi.org/10.1210/me.2002-0351

8. Mak HY, Hoare S, Henttu PM, Parker MG (1999) Molecular determinants of the estrogen receptor-coactivator interface. Mol Cell Biol 19(5):3895–3903

9. Harris HA (2007) Estrogen receptor-beta: recent lessons from in vivo studies. Mol Endocrinol 21(1):1–13. https://doi.org/10.1210/me.2005-0459

10. Hewitt SC, Winuthayanon W, Korach KS (2016) What's new in estrogen receptor action in the female reproductive tract. J Mol Endocrinol 56(2):R55–R71. https://doi.org/10.1530/JME-15-0254

11. Hamilton KJ, Arao Y, Korach KS (2014) Estrogen hormone physiology: reproductive findings from estrogen receptor mutant mice. Reprod Biol 14(1):3–8. https://doi.org/10.1016/j.repbio.2013.12.002

12. Heldring N, Nilsson M, Buehrer B, Treuter E, Gustafsson JA (2004) Identification of tamoxifen-induced coregulator interaction surfaces within the ligand-binding domain of estrogen receptors. Mol Cell Biol 24(8):3445–3459

13. Paige LA, Christensen DJ, Gron H, Norris JD, Gottlin EB, Padilla KM, Chang CY, Ballas LM, Hamilton PT, McDonnell DP, Fowlkes DM (1999) Estrogen receptor (ER) modulators each induce distinct conformational changes in ER alpha and ER beta. Proc Natl Acad Sci U S A 96(7):3999–4004

14. Shang Y, Brown M (2002) Molecular determinants for the tissue specificity of SERMs. Science 295(5564):2465–2468. https://doi.org/10.1126/science.1068537

15. Pike AC (2006) Lessons learnt from structural studies of the oestrogen receptor. Best Pract Res Clin Endocrinol Metab 20(1):1–14. https://doi.org/10.1016/j.beem.2005.09.002

16. Kumar V, Green S, Stack G, Berry M, Jin JR, Chambon P (1987) Functional domains of the human estrogen receptor. Cell 51(6):941–951

17. Ponglikitmongkol M, Green S, Chambon P (1988) Genomic organization of the human oestrogen receptor gene. EMBO J 7(11):3385–3388

18. Ogawa S, Inoue S, Watanabe T, Hiroi H, Orimo A, Hosoi T, Ouchi Y, Muramatsu M (1998) The complete primary structure of human estrogen receptor beta (hER beta) and its heterodimerization with ER alpha in vivo and in vitro. Biochem Biophys Res Commun 243(1):122–126. https://doi.org/10.1006/bbrc.1997.7893

19. Muramatsu M, Inoue S (2000) Estrogen receptors: how do they control reproductive and nonreproductive functions? Biochem Biophys Res Commun 270(1):1–10. https://doi.org/10.1006/bbrc.2000.2214

20. Kuiper GG, Carlsson B, Grandien K, Enmark E, Haggblad J, Nilsson S, Gustafsson JA (1997) Comparison of the ligand binding specificity and transcript tissue distribution of estrogen receptors alpha and beta. Endocrinology 138(3):863–870. https://doi.org/10.1210/endo.138.3.4979

21. Pike AC, Brzozowski AM, Hubbard RE (2000) A structural biologist's view of the oestrogen receptor. J Steroid Biochem Mol Biol 74(5):261–268

22. Brzozowski AM, Pike AC, Dauter Z, Hubbard RE, Bonn T, Engstrom O, Ohman L, Greene GL, Gustafsson JA, Carlquist M (1997) Molecular basis of agonism and antagonism in the oestrogen receptor. Nature 389(6652):753–758. https://doi.org/10.1038/39645

23. Arao Y, Hamilton KJ, Coons LA, Korach KS (2013) Estrogen receptor alpha L543A,L544A mutation changes antagonists to agonists, correlating with the ligand binding domain

dimerization associated with DNA binding activity. J Biol Chem 288(29):21105–21116. https://doi.org/10.1074/jbc.M113.463455

24. Koide A, Zhao C, Naganuma M, Abrams J, Deighton-Collins S, Skafar DF, Koide S (2007) Identification of regions within the F domain of the human estrogen receptor alpha that are important for modulating transactivation and protein-protein interactions. Mol Endocrinol 21(4):829–842. https://doi.org/10.1210/me.2006-0203

25. Montano MM, Muller V, Trobaugh A, Katzenellenbogen BS (1995) The carboxy-terminal F domain of the human estrogen receptor: role in the transcriptional activity of the receptor and the effectiveness of antiestrogens as estrogen antagonists. Mol Endocrinol 9(7):814–825. https://doi.org/10.1210/mend.9.7.7476965

26. Meyers MJ, Sun J, Carlson KE, Marriner GA, Katzenellenbogen BS, Katzenellenbogen JA (2001) Estrogen receptor-beta potency-selective ligands: structure-activity relationship studies of diarylpropionitriles and their acetylene and polar analogues. J Med Chem 44(24):4230–4251

27. Lees JA, Fawell SE, White R, Parker MG (1990) A 22-amino-acid peptide restores DNA-binding activity to dimerization-defective mutants of the estrogen receptor. Mol Cell Biol 10(10):5529–5531

28. Tamrazi A, Carlson KE, Daniels JR, Hurth KM, Katzenellenbogen JA (2002) Estrogen receptor dimerization: ligand binding regulates dimer affinity and dimer dissociation rate. Mol Endocrinol 16(12):2706–2719. https://doi.org/10.1210/me.2002-0250

29. Vajdos FF, Hoth LR, Geoghegan KF, Simons SP, LeMotte PK, Danley DE, Ammirati MJ, Pandit J (2007) The 2.0 A crystal structure of the ERalpha ligand-binding domain complexed with lasofoxifene. Protein Sci 16(5):897–905. https://doi.org/10.1110/ps.062729207

30. Shiau AK, Barstad D, Loria PM, Cheng L, Kushner PJ, Agard DA, Greene GL (1998) The structural basis of estrogen receptor/coactivator recognition and the antagonism of this interaction by tamoxifen. Cell 95(7):927–937

31. Warnmark A, Treuter E, Gustafsson JA, Hubbard RE, Brzozowski AM, Pike AC (2002) Interaction of transcriptional intermediary factor 2 nuclear receptor box peptides with the coactivator binding site of estrogen receptor alpha. J Biol Chem 277(24):21862–21868. https://doi.org/10.1074/jbc.M200764200

32. Tetel MJ (2009) Nuclear receptor coactivators: essential players for steroid hormone action in the brain and in behaviour. J Neuroendocrinol 21(4):229–237. https://doi.org/10.1111/j.1365-2826.2009.01827.x

33. Heldring N, Pike A, Andersson S, Matthews J, Cheng G, Hartman J, Tujague M, Strom A, Treuter E, Warner M, Gustafsson JA (2007) Estrogen receptors: how do they signal and what are their targets. Physiol Rev 87(3):905–931. https://doi.org/10.1152/physrev.00026.2006

34. Heldring N, Pawson T, McDonnell D, Treuter E, Gustafsson JA, Pike AC (2007) Structural insights into corepressor recognition by antagonist-bound estrogen receptors. J Biol Chem 282(14):10449–10455. https://doi.org/10.1074/jbc.M611424200

35. Huang HJ, Norris JD, McDonnell DP (2002) Identification of a negative regulatory surface within estrogen receptor alpha provides evidence in support of a role for corepressors in regulating cellular responses to agonists and antagonists. Mol Endocrinol 16(8):1778–1792. https://doi.org/10.1210/me.2002-0089

36. Webb P, Nguyen P, Kushner PJ (2003) Differential SERM effects on corepressor binding dictate ERalpha activity in vivo. J Biol Chem 278(9):6912–6920. https://doi.org/10.1074/jbc.M208501200

37. Dobrzycka KM, Townson SM, Jiang S, Oesterreich S (2003) Estrogen receptor corepressors -- à role in human breast cancer? Endocr Relat Cancer 10(4):517–536

38. Chakraborty S, Levenson AS, Biswas PK (2013) Structural insights into Resveratrol's antagonist and partial agonist actions on estrogen receptor alpha. BMC Struct Biol 13:27. https://doi.org/10.1186/1472-6807-13-27

39. Schwabe JW, Chapman L, Finch JT, Rhodes D (1993) The crystal structure of the estrogen receptor DNA-binding domain bound to DNA: how receptors discriminate between their response elements. Cell 75(3):567–578

40. Schwabe JW, Chapman L, Finch JT, Rhodes D, Neuhaus D (1993) DNA recognition by the oestrogen receptor: from solution to the crystal. Structure 1(3):187–204
41. Schwabe JW, Chapman L, Rhodes D (1995) The oestrogen receptor recognizes an imperfectly palindromic response element through an alternative side-chain conformation. Structure 3(2):201–213
42. Schwabe JW, Neuhaus D, Rhodes D (1990) Solution structure of the DNA-binding domain of the oestrogen receptor. Nature 348(6300):458–461. https://doi.org/10.1038/348458a0
43. Klinge CM (2001) Estrogen receptor interaction with estrogen response elements. Nucleic Acids Res 29(14):2905–2919
44. Lin CY, Vega VB, Thomsen JS, Zhang T, Kong SL, Xie M, Chiu KP, Lipovich L, Barnett DH, Stossi F, Yeo A, George J, Kuznetsov VA, Lee YK, Charn TH, Palanisamy N, Miller LD, Cheung E, Katzenellenbogen BS, Ruan Y, Bourque G, Wei CL, Liu ET (2007) Whole-genome cartography of estrogen receptor alpha binding sites. PLoS Genet 3(6):e87. https://doi.org/10.1371/journal.pgen.0030087
45. Bjornstrom L, Sjoberg M (2002) Mutations in the estrogen receptor DNA-binding domain discriminate between the classical mechanism of action and cross-talk with Stat5b and activating protein 1 (AP-1). J Biol Chem 277(50):48479–48483. https://doi.org/10.1074/jbc.C200570200
46. Cheung E, Acevedo ML, Cole PA, Kraus WL (2005) Altered pharmacology and distinct coactivator usage for estrogen receptor-dependent transcription through activating protein-1. Proc Natl Acad Sci U S A 102(3):559–564. https://doi.org/10.1073/pnas.0407113102
47. Hall JM, Couse JF, Korach KS (2001) The multifaceted mechanisms of estradiol and estrogen receptor signaling. J Biol Chem 276(40):36869–36872. https://doi.org/10.1074/jbc.R100029200
48. Huang J, Li X, Hilf R, Bambara RA, Muyan M (2005) Molecular basis of therapeutic strategies for breast cancer. Curr Drug Targets Immune Endocr Metabol Disord 5(4):379–396
49. Safe S (2001) Transcriptional activation of genes by 17 beta-estradiol through estrogen receptor-Sp1 interactions. Vitam Horm 62:231–252
50. Kushner PJ, Agard DA, Greene GL, Scanlan TS, Shiau AK, Uht RM, Webb P (2000) Estrogen receptor pathways to AP-1. J Steroid Biochem Mol Biol 74(5):311–317
51. Kumar R, Thompson EB (2003) Transactivation functions of the N-terminal domains of nuclear hormone receptors: protein folding and coactivator interactions. Mol Endocrinol 17(1):1–10. https://doi.org/10.1210/me.2002-0258
52. Bocquel MT, Kumar V, Stricker C, Chambon P, Gronemeyer H (1989) The contribution of the N- and C-terminal regions of steroid receptors to activation of transcription is both receptor and cell-specific. Nucleic Acids Res 17(7):2581–2595
53. Metzger D, Ali S, Bornert JM, Chambon P (1995) Characterization of the amino-terminal transcriptional activation function of the human estrogen receptor in animal and yeast cells. J Biol Chem 270(16):9535–9542
54. Tasset D, Tora L, Fromental C, Scheer E, Chambon P (1990) Distinct classes of transcriptional activating domains function by different mechanisms. Cell 62(6):1177–1187
55. Tora L, White J, Brou C, Tasset D, Webster N, Scheer E, Chambon P (1989) The human estrogen receptor has two independent nonacidic transcriptional activation functions. Cell 59(3):477–487
56. Benecke A, Chambon P, Gronemeyer H (2000) Synergy between estrogen receptor alpha activation functions AF1 and AF2 mediated by transcription intermediary factor TIF2. EMBO Rep 1(2):151–157. https://doi.org/10.1038/sj.embor.embor609
57. Kraus WL, McInerney EM, Katzenellenbogen BS (1995) Ligand-dependent, transcriptionally productive association of the amino- and carboxyl-terminal regions of a steroid hormone nuclear receptor. Proc Natl Acad Sci U S A 92(26):12314–12318
58. Yi P, Bhagat S, Hilf R, Bambara RA, Muyan M (2002) Differences in the abilities of estrogen receptors to integrate activation functions are critical for subtype-specific transcriptional responses. Mol Endocrinol 16(8):1810–1827. https://doi.org/10.1210/me.2001-0323

59. Kumar R, Litwack G (2009) Structural and functional relationships of the steroid hormone receptors' N-terminal transactivation domain. Steroids 74(12):877–883. https://doi.org/10.1016/j.steroids.2009.07.012

60. Kumar R, Zakharov MN, Khan SH, Miki R, Jang H, Toraldo G, Singh R, Bhasin S, Jasuja R (2011) The dynamic structure of the estrogen receptor. J Amino Acids 2011:812540. https://doi.org/10.4061/2011/812540

61. Warnmark A, Wikstrom A, Wright AP, Gustafsson JA, Hard T (2001) The N-terminal regions of estrogen receptor alpha and beta are unstructured in vitro and show different TBP binding properties. J Biol Chem 276(49):45939–45944. https://doi.org/10.1074/jbc.M107875200

62. Rajbhandari P, Finn G, Solodin NM, Singarapu KK, Sahu SC, Markley JL, Kadunc KJ, Ellison-Zelski SJ, Kariagina A, Haslam SZ, Lu KP, Alarid ET (2012) Regulation of estrogen receptor alpha N-terminus conformation and function by peptidyl prolyl isomerase Pin1. Mol Cell Biol 32(2):445–457. https://doi.org/10.1128/MCB.06073-11

63. Cowley SM, Parker MG (1999) A comparison of transcriptional activation by ER alpha and ER beta. J Steroid Biochem Mol Biol 69(1–6):165–175

64. Delaunay F, Pettersson K, Tujague M, Gustafsson JA (2000) Functional differences between the amino-terminal domains of estrogen receptors alpha and beta. Mol Pharmacol 58(3):584–590

65. McInerney EM, Weis KE, Sun J, Mosselman S, Katzenellenbogen BS (1998) Transcription activation by the human estrogen receptor subtype beta (ER beta) studied with ER beta and ER alpha receptor chimeras. Endocrinology 139(11):4513–4522. https://doi.org/10.1210/endo.139.11.6298

66. Huang J, Li X, Maguire CA, Hilf R, Bambara RA, Muyan M (2005) Binding of estrogen receptor beta to estrogen response element in situ is independent of estradiol and impaired by its amino terminus. Mol Endocrinol 19(11):2696–2712. https://doi.org/10.1210/me.2005-0120

67. Martinkovich S, Shah D, Planey SL, Arnott JA (2014) Selective estrogen receptor modulators: tissue specificity and clinical utility. Clin Interv Aging 9:1437–1452. https://doi.org/10.2147/CIA.S66690

68. Jordan C (2002) Historical perspective on hormonal therapy of advanced breast cancer. Clin Ther 24(Suppl A):A3–A16

69. Love RR, Barden HS, Mazess RB, Epstein S, Chappell RJ (1994) Effect of tamoxifen on lumbar spine bone-mineral density in postmenopausal women after 5 years. Arch Intern Med 154(22):2585–2588. https://doi.org/10.1001/archinte.154.22.2585

70. Love RR, Wiebe DA, Feyzi JM, Newcomb PA, Chappell RJ (1994) Effects of tamoxifen on cardiovascular risk factors in postmenopausal women after 5 years of treatment. J Natl Cancer Inst 86(20):1534–1539

71. Turner RT, Wakley GK, Hannon KS, Bell NH (1988) Tamoxifen inhibits osteoclast-mediated resorption of trabecular bone in ovarian hormone-deficient rats. Endocrinology 122(3):1146–1150. https://doi.org/10.1210/endo-122-3-1146

72. Ward RL, Morgan G, Dalley D, Kelly PJ (1993) Tamoxifen reduces bone turnover and prevents lumbar spine and proximal femoral bone loss in early postmenopausal women. Bone Miner 22(2):87–94

73. Davies P, Syne JS, Nicholson RI (1979) Effects of estradiol and the antiestrogen tamoxifen on steroid hormone receptor concentration and nuclear ribonucleic acid polymerase activities in rat uteri. Endocrinology 105(6):1336–1342. https://doi.org/10.1210/endo-105-6-1336

74. Martin L, Middleton E (1978) Prolonged oestrogenic and mitogenic activity of tamoxifen in the ovariectomized mouse. J Endocrinol 78(1):125–129

75. Jordan VC (2004) Selective estrogen receptor modulation: concept and consequences in cancer. Cancer Cell 5(3):207–213

76. Musgrove EA, Sutherland RL (2009) Biological determinants of endocrine resistance in breast cancer. Nat Rev Cancer 9(9):631–643. https://doi.org/10.1038/nrc2713

77. Ali S, Buluwela L, Coombes RC (2011) Antiestrogens and their therapeutic applications in breast cancer and other diseases. Annu Rev Med 62:217–232. https://doi.org/10.1146/annurev-med-052209-100305

78. McDonnell DP, Wardell SE, Norris JD (2015) Oral selective estrogen receptor downregulators (SERDs), a breakthrough endocrine therapy for breast cancer. J Med Chem 58(12):4883–4887. https://doi.org/10.1021/acs.jmedchem.5b00760

79. Howell A (2006) Pure oestrogen antagonists for the treatment of advanced breast cancer. Endocr Relat Cancer 13(3):689–706. https://doi.org/10.1677/erc.1.00846

80. Vogel VG, Costantino JP, Wickerham DL, Cronin WM, Cecchini RS, Atkins JN, Bevers TB, Fehrenbacher L, Pajon ER, Wade JL 3rd, Robidoux A, Margolese RG, James J, Runowicz CD, Ganz PA, Reis SE, McCaskill-Stevens W, Ford LG, Jordan VC, Wolmark N, National Surgical Adjuvant B, Bowel P (2010) Update of the National Surgical Adjuvant Breast and Bowel Project study of tamoxifen and raloxifene (STAR) P-2 trial: preventing breast cancer. Cancer Prev Res (Phila) 3(6):696–706. https://doi.org/10.1158/1940-6207.CAPR-10-0076

81. Deshmane V, Krishnamurthy S, Melemed AS, Peterson P, Buzdar AU (2007) Phase III double-blind trial of arzoxifene compared with tamoxifen for locally advanced or metastatic breast cancer. J Clin Oncol 25(31):4967–4973. https://doi.org/10.1200/JCO.2006.09.5992

82. Palkowitz AD, Glasebrook AL, Thrasher KJ, Hauser KL, Short LL, Phillips DL, Muehl BS, Sato M, Shetler PK, Cullinan GJ, Pell TR, Bryant HU (1997) Discovery and synthesis of [6-hydroxy-3-[4-[2-(1-piperidinyl)ethoxy]phenoxy]-2-(4-hydroxyphenyl)]b enzo[b] thiophene: a novel, highly potent, selective estrogen receptor modulator. J Med Chem 40(10):1407–1416. https://doi.org/10.1021/jm970167b

83. Suh N, Glasebrook AL, Palkowitz AD, Bryant HU, Burris LL, Starling JJ, Pearce HL, Williams C, Peer C, Wang Y, Sporn MB (2001) Arzoxifene, a new selective estrogen receptor modulator for chemoprevention of experimental breast cancer. Cancer Res 61(23):8412–8415

84. Wardell SE, Nelson ER, Chao CA, McDonnell DP (2013) Bazedoxifene exhibits antiestrogenic activity in animal models of tamoxifen-resistant breast cancer: implications for treatment of advanced disease. Clin Cancer Res 19(9):2420–2431. https://doi.org/10.1158/1078-0432. CCR-12-3771

85. Barsalou A, Gao W, Anghel SI, Carriere J, Mader S (1998) Estrogen response elements can mediate agonist activity of anti-estrogens in human endometrial Ishikawa cells. J Biol Chem 273(27):17138–17146

86. Bowler J, Lilley TJ, Pittam JD, Wakeling AE (1989) Novel steroidal pure antiestrogens. Steroids 54(1):71–99

87. Van de Velde P, Nique F, Bouchoux F, Bremaud J, Hameau MC, Lucas D, Moratille C, Viet S, Philibert D, Teutsch G (1994) RU 58,668, a new pure antiestrogen inducing a regression of human mammary carcinoma implanted in nude mice. J Steroid Biochem Mol Biol 48(2–3):187–196

88. Wakeling AE, Dukes M, Bowler J (1991) A potent specific pure antiestrogen with clinical potential. Cancer Res 51(15):3867–3873

89. Dauvois S, Danielian PS, White R, Parker MG (1992) Antiestrogen ICI 164,384 reduces cellular estrogen receptor content by increasing its turnover. Proc Natl Acad Sci U S A 89(9):4037–4041

90. El Khissiin A, Leclercq G (1999) Implication of proteasome in estrogen receptor degradation. FEBS Lett 448(1):160–166

91. Gibson MK, Nemmers LA, Beckman WC Jr, Davis VL, Curtis SW, Korach KS (1991) The mechanism of ICI 164,384 antiestrogenicity involves rapid loss of estrogen receptor in uterine tissue. Endocrinology 129(4):2000–2010. https://doi.org/10.1210/endo-129-4-2000

92. Wijayaratne AL, McDonnell DP (2001) The human estrogen receptor-alpha is a ubiquitinated protein whose stability is affected differentially by agonists, antagonists, and selective estrogen receptor modulators. J Biol Chem 276(38):35684–35692. https://doi.org/10.1074/jbc.M101097200

93. Howell A, Robertson JF, Abram P, Lichinitser MR, Elledge R, Bajetta E, Watanabe T, Morris C, Webster A, Dimery I, Osborne CK (2004) Comparison of fulvestrant versus tamoxifen for the treatment of advanced breast cancer in postmenopausal women previously untreated with endocrine therapy: a multinational, double-blind, randomized trial. J Clin Oncol 22(9):1605–1613. https://doi.org/10.1200/JCO.2004.02.112

94. Di Leo A, Jerusalem G, Petruzelka L, Torres R, Bondarenko IN, Khasanov R, Verhoeven D, Pedrini JL, Smirnova I, Lichinitser MR, Pendergrass K, Garnett S, Lindemann JP, Sapunar F, Martin M (2010) Results of the CONFIRM phase III trial comparing fulvestrant 250 mg with fulvestrant 500 mg in postmenopausal women with estrogen receptor-positive advanced breast cancer. J Clin Oncol 28(30):4594–4600. https://doi.org/10.1200/JCO.2010.28.8415

95. Di Leo A, Jerusalem G, Petruzelka L, Torres R, Bondarenko IN, Khasanov R, Verhoeven D, Pedrini JL, Smirnova I, Lichinitser MR, Pendergrass K, Malorni L, Garnett S, Rukazenkov Y, Martin M (2014) Final overall survival: fulvestrant 500 mg vs 250 mg in the randomized CONFIRM trial. J Natl Cancer Inst 106(1):djt337. https://doi.org/10.1093/jnci/djt337

96. Robertson JF, Lindemann J, Garnett S, Anderson E, Nicholson RI, Kuter I, Gee JM (2014) A good drug made better: the fulvestrant dose-response story. Clin Breast Cancer 14(6): 381–389. https://doi.org/10.1016/j.clbc.2014.06.005

97. Bentrem D, Dardes R, Liu H, MacGregor-Schafer J, Zapf J, Jordan V (2001) Molecular mechanism of action at estrogen receptor alpha of a new clinically relevant antiestrogen (GW7604) related to tamoxifen. Endocrinology 142(2):838–846. https://doi.org/10.1210/endo.142.2.7932

98. Lai A, Kahraman M, Govek S, Nagasawa J, Bonnefous C, Julien J, Douglas K, Sensintaffar J, Lu N, Lee KJ, Aparicio A, Kaufman J, Qian J, Shao G, Prudente R, Moon MJ, Joseph JD, Darimont B, Brigham D, Grillot K, Heyman R, Rix PJ, Hager JH, Smith ND (2015) Identification of GDC-0810 (ARN-810), an orally bioavailable selective estrogen receptor degrader (SERD) that demonstrates robust activity in tamoxifen-resistant breast cancer xenografts. J Med Chem 58(12):4888–4904. https://doi.org/10.1021/acs.jmedchem.5b00054

99. Wijayaratne AL, Nagel SC, Paige LA, Christensen DJ, Norris JD, Fowlkes DM, McDonnell DP (1999) Comparative analyses of mechanistic differences among antiestrogens. Endocrinology 140(12):5828–5840. https://doi.org/10.1210/endo.140.12.7164

100. Pike AC, Brzozowski AM, Hubbard RE, Bonn T, Thorsell AG, Engstrom O, Ljunggren J, Gustafsson JA, Carlquist M (1999) Structure of the ligand-binding domain of oestrogen receptor beta in the presence of a partial agonist and a full antagonist. EMBO J 18(17): 4608–4618. https://doi.org/10.1093/emboj/18.17.4608

101. Grese TA, Cho S, Finley DR, Godfrey AG, Jones CD, Lugar CW 3rd, Martin MJ, Matsumoto K, Pennington LD, Winter MA, Adrian MD, Cole HW, Magee DE, Phillips DL, Rowley ER, Short LL, Glasebrook AL, Bryant HU (1997) Structure-activity relationships of selective estrogen receptor modulators: modifications to the 2-arylbenzothiophene core of raloxifene. J Med Chem 40(2):146–167. https://doi.org/10.1021/jm9606352

102. Dayan G, Lupien M, Auger A, Anghel SI, Rocha W, Croisetiere S, Katzenellenbogen JA, Mader S (2006) Tamoxifen and raloxifene differ in their functional interactions with aspartate 351 of estrogen receptor alpha. Mol Pharmacol 70(2):579–588. https://doi.org/10.1124/mol.105.021931

103. MacGregor Schafer J, Liu H, Bentrem DJ, Zapf JW, Jordan VC (2000) Allosteric silencing of activating function 1 in the 4-hydroxytamoxifen estrogen receptor complex is induced by substituting glycine for aspartate at amino acid 351. Cancer Res 60(18):5097–5105

104. Pike AC, Brzozowski AM, Walton J, Hubbard RE, Thorsell AG, Li YL, Gustafsson JA, Carlquist M (2001) Structural insights into the mode of action of a pure antiestrogen. Structure 9(2):145–153

105. Arao Y, Hamilton KJ, Ray MK, Scott G, Mishina Y, Korach KS (2011) Estrogen receptor alpha AF-2 mutation results in antagonist reversal and reveals tissue selective function of estrogen receptor modulators. Proc Natl Acad Sci U S A 108(36):14986–14991. https://doi.org/10.1073/pnas.1109180108

106. Lupien M, Jeyakumar M, Hebert E, Hilmi K, Cotnoir-White D, Loch C, Auger A, Dayan G, Pinard GA, Wurtz JM, Moras D, Katzenellenbogen J, Mader S (2007) Raloxifene and ICI182,780 increase estrogen receptor-alpha association with a nuclear compartment via overlapping sets of hydrophobic amino acids in activation function 2 helix 12. Mol Endocrinol 21(4):797–816. https://doi.org/10.1210/me.2006-0074

107. Mahfoudi A, Roulet E, Dauvois S, Parker MG, Wahli W (1995) Specific mutations in the estrogen receptor change the properties of antiestrogens to full agonists. Proc Natl Acad Sci U S A 92(10):4206–4210

108. Norris JD, Fan D, Stallcup MR, McDonnell DP (1998) Enhancement of estrogen receptor transcriptional activity by the coactivator GRIP-1 highlights the role of activation function 2 in determining estrogen receptor pharmacology. J Biol Chem 273(12):6679–6688

109. Hoffmann J, Bohlmann R, Heinrich N, Hofmeister H, Kroll J, Kunzer H, Lichtner RB, Nishino Y, Parczyk K, Sauer G, Gieschen H, Ulbrich HF, Schneider MR (2004) Characterization of new estrogen receptor destabilizing compounds: effects on estrogen-sensitive and tamoxifen-resistant breast cancer. J Natl Cancer Inst 96(3):210–218

110. Wu YL, Yang X, Ren Z, McDonnell DP, Norris JD, Willson TM, Greene GL (2005) Structural basis for an unexpected mode of SERM-mediated ER antagonism. Mol Cell 18(4):413–424. https://doi.org/10.1016/j.molcel.2005.04.014

111. Hall JM, McDonnell DP (2005) Coregulators in nuclear estrogen receptor action: from concept to therapeutic targeting. Mol Interv 5(6):343–357. https://doi.org/10.1124/mi.5.6.7

112. Johnson AB, O'Malley BW (2012) Steroid receptor coactivators 1, 2, and 3: critical regulators of nuclear receptor activity and steroid receptor modulator (SRM)-based cancer therapy. Mol Cell Endocrinol 348(2):430–439. https://doi.org/10.1016/j.mce.2011.04.021

113. Smith CL, O'Malley BW (2004) Coregulator function: a key to understanding tissue specificity of selective receptor modulators. Endocr Rev 25(1):45–71. https://doi.org/10.1210/er.2003-0023

114. Burandt E, Jens G, Holst F, Janicke F, Muller V, Quaas A, Choschzick M, Wilczak W, Terracciano L, Simon R, Sauter G, Lebeau A (2013) Prognostic relevance of AIB1 (NCoA3) amplification and overexpression in breast cancer. Breast Cancer Res Treat 137(3):745–753. https://doi.org/10.1007/s10549-013-2406-4

115. Metivier R, Penot G, Flouriot G, Pakdel F (2001) Synergism between ERalpha transactivation function 1 (AF-1) and AF-2 mediated by steroid receptor coactivator protein-1: requirement for the AF-1 alpha-helical core and for a direct interaction between the N- and C-terminal domains. Mol Endocrinol 15(11):1953–1970. https://doi.org/10.1210/mend.15.11.0727

116. Tzukerman MT, Esty A, Santiso-Mere D, Danielian P, Parker MG, Stein RB, Pike JW, McDonnell DP (1994) Human estrogen receptor transactivational capacity is determined by both cellular and promoter context and mediated by two functionally distinct intramolecular regions. Mol Endocrinol 8(1):21–30. https://doi.org/10.1210/mend.8.1.8152428

117. Merot Y, Metivier R, Penot G, Manu D, Saligaut C, Gannon F, Pakdel F, Kah O, Flouriot G (2004) The relative contribution exerted by AF-1 and AF-2 transactivation functions in estrogen receptor alpha transcriptional activity depends upon the differentiation stage of the cell. J Biol Chem 279(25):26184–26191. https://doi.org/10.1074/jbc.M402148200

118. Webb P, Nguyen P, Shinsako J, Anderson C, Feng W, Nguyen MP, Chen D, Huang SM, Subramanian S, McKinerney E, Katzenellenbogen BS, Stallcup MR, Kushner PJ (1998) Estrogen receptor activation function 1 works by binding p160 coactivator proteins. Mol Endocrinol 12(10):1605–1618. https://doi.org/10.1210/mend.12.10.0185

119. Keeton EK, Brown M (2005) Cell cycle progression stimulated by tamoxifen-bound estrogen receptor-alpha and promoter-specific effects in breast cancer cells deficient in N-CoR and SMRT. Mol Endocrinol 19(6):1543–1554. https://doi.org/10.1210/me.2004-0395

120. Lavinsky RM, Jepsen K, Heinzel T, Torchia J, Mullen TM, Schiff R, Del-Rio AL, Ricote M, Ngo S, Gemsch J, Hilsenbeck SG, Osborne CK, Glass CK, Rosenfeld MG, Rose DW (1998) Diverse signaling pathways modulate nuclear receptor recruitment of N-CoR and SMRT complexes. Proc Natl Acad Sci U S A 95(6):2920–2925

121. Smith CL, Nawaz Z, O'Malley BW (1997) Coactivator and corepressor regulation of the agonist/antagonist activity of the mixed antiestrogen, 4-hydroxytamoxifen. Mol Endocrinol 11(6):657–666. https://doi.org/10.1210/mend.11.6.0009

122. Le Romancer M, Poulard C, Cohen P, Sentis S, Renoir JM, Corbo L (2011) Cracking the estrogen receptor's posttranslational code in breast tumors. Endocr Rev 32(5):597–622. https://doi.org/10.1210/er.2010-0016

123. Ali S, Metzger D, Bornert JM, Chambon P (1993) Modulation of transcriptional activation by ligand-dependent phosphorylation of the human oestrogen receptor A/B region. EMBO J 12(3):1153–1160

124. Thomas RS, Sarwar N, Phoenix F, Coombes RC, Ali S (2008) Phosphorylation at serines 104 and 106 by Erk1/2 MAPK is important for estrogen receptor-alpha activity. J Mol Endocrinol 40(4):173–184. https://doi.org/10.1677/JME-07-0165

125. Suresh PS, Ma S, Migliaccio A, Chen G (2014) Protein-tyrosine phosphatase H1 increases breast cancer sensitivity to antiestrogens by dephosphorylating estrogen receptor at Tyr537. Mol Cancer Ther 13(1):230–238. https://doi.org/10.1158/1535-7163.MCT-13-0610

126. Ascenzi P, Bocedi A, Marino M (2006) Structure-function relationship of estrogen receptor alpha and beta: impact on human health. Mol Asp Med 27(4):299–402. https://doi.org/10.1016/j.mam.2006.07.001

127. Hilmi K, Hussein N, Mendoza-Sanchez R, El-Ezzy M, Ismail H, Durette C, Bail M, Rozendaal MJ, Bouvier M, Thibault P, Gleason JL, Mader S (2012) Role of SUMOylation in full antiestrogenicity. Mol Cell Biol 32(19):3823–3837. https://doi.org/10.1128/MCB.00290-12

128. Reid G, Hubner MR, Metivier R, Brand H, Denger S, Manu D, Beaudouin J, Ellenberg J, Gannon F (2003) Cyclic, proteasome-mediated turnover of unliganded and liganded ERalpha on responsive promoters is an integral feature of estrogen signaling. Mol Cell 11(3):695–707

129. Borras M, Laios I, el Khissiin A, Seo HS, Lempereur F, Legros N, Leclercq G (1996) Estrogenic and antiestrogenic regulation of the half-life of covalently labeled estrogen receptor in MCF-7 breast cancer cells. J Steroid Biochem Mol Biol 57(3–4):203–213

130. Marsaud V, Gougelet A, Maillard S, Renoir JM (2003) Various phosphorylation pathways, depending on agonist and antagonist binding to endogenous estrogen receptor alpha (ERalpha), differentially affect ERalpha extractability, proteasome-mediated stability, and transcriptional activity in human breast cancer cells. Mol Endocrinol 17(10):2013–2027. https://doi.org/10.1210/me.2002-0269

131. Fan M, Bigsby RM, Nephew KP (2003) The NEDD8 pathway is required for proteasome-mediated degradation of human estrogen receptor (ER)-alpha and essential for the antiproliferative activity of ICI 182,780 in ERalpha-positive breast cancer cells. Mol Endocrinol 17(3):356–365. https://doi.org/10.1210/me.2002-0323

132. Wardell SE, Marks JR, McDonnell DP (2011) The turnover of estrogen receptor alpha by the selective estrogen receptor degrader (SERD) fulvestrant is a saturable process that is not required for antagonist efficacy. Biochem Pharmacol 82(2):122–130. https://doi.org/10.1016/j.bcp.2011.03.031

133. Nardone A, De Angelis C, Trivedi MV, Osborne CK, Schiff R (2015) The changing role of ER in endocrine resistance. Breast 24(Suppl 2):S60–S66. https://doi.org/10.1016/j.breast.2015.07.015

134. Jeselsohn R, Buchwalter G, De Angelis C, Brown M, Schiff R (2015) ESR1 mutations-a mechanism for acquired endocrine resistance in breast cancer. Nat Rev Clin Oncol 12(10):573–583. https://doi.org/10.1038/nrclinonc.2015.117

135. Zhang QX, Borg A, Wolf DM, Oesterreich S, Fuqua SA (1997) An estrogen receptor mutant with strong hormone-independent activity from a metastatic breast cancer. Cancer Res 57(7):1244–1249

136. Jeselsohn R, Yelensky R, Buchwalter G, Frampton G, Meric-Bernstam F, Gonzalez-Angulo AM, Ferrer-Lozano J, Perez-Fidalgo JA, Cristofanilli M, Gomez H, Arteaga CL, Giltnane J, Balko JM, Cronin MT, Jarosz M, Sun J, Hawryluk M, Lipson D, Otto G, Ross JS, Dvir A, Soussan-Gutman L, Wolf I, Rubinek T, Gilmore L, Schnitt S, Come SE, Pusztai L, Stephens P, Brown M, Miller VA (2014) Emergence of constitutively active estrogen receptor-alpha mutations in pretreated advanced estrogen receptor-positive breast cancer. Clin Cancer Res 20(7):1757–1767. https://doi.org/10.1158/1078-0432.CCR-13-2332

137. Robinson DR, Wu YM, Vats P, Su F, Lonigro RJ, Cao X, Kalyana-Sundaram S, Wang R, Ning Y, Hodges L, Gursky A, Siddiqui J, Tomlins SA, Roychowdhury S, Pienta KJ, Kim SY,

Roberts JS, Rae JM, Van Poznak CH, Hayes DF, Chugh R, Kunju LP, Talpaz M, Schott AF, Chinnaiyan AM (2013) Activating ESR1 mutations in hormone-resistant metastatic breast cancer. Nat Genet 45(12):1446–1451. https://doi.org/10.1038/ng.2823

138. Toy W, Shen Y, Won H, Green B, Sakr RA, Will M, Li Z, Gala K, Fanning S, King TA, Hudis C, Chen D, Taran T, Hortobagyi G, Greene G, Berger M, Baselga J, Chandarlapaty S (2013) ESR1 ligand-binding domain mutations in hormone-resistant breast cancer. Nat Genet 45(12):1439–1445. https://doi.org/10.1038/ng.2822

139. Fanning SW, Mayne CG, Dharmarajan V, Carlson KE, Martin TA, Novick SJ, Toy W, Green B, Panchamukhi S, Katzenellenbogen BS, Tajkhorshid E, Griffin PR, Shen Y, Chandarlapaty S, Katzenellenbogen JA, Greene GL (2016) Estrogen receptor alpha somatic mutations Y537S and D538G confer breast cancer endocrine resistance by stabilizing the activating function-2 binding conformation. elife 5. https://doi.org/10.7554/eLife.12792

140. Merenbakh-Lamin K, Ben-Baruch N, Yeheskel A, Dvir A, Soussan-Gutman L, Jeselsohn R, Yelensky R, Brown M, Miller VA, Sarid D, Rizel S, Klein B, Rubinek T, Wolf I (2013) D538G mutation in estrogen receptor-alpha: a novel mechanism for acquired endocrine resistance in breast cancer. Cancer Res 73(23):6856–6864. https://doi.org/10.1158/0008-5472.CAN-13-1197

141. Nettles KW, Bruning JB, Gil G, Nowak J, Sharma SK, Hahm JB, Kulp K, Hochberg RB, Zhou H, Katzenellenbogen JA, Katzenellenbogen BS, Kim Y, Joachmiak A, Greene GL (2008) NFkappaB selectivity of estrogen receptor ligands revealed by comparative crystallographic analyses. Nat Chem Biol 4(4):241–247. https://doi.org/10.1038/nchembio.76

Molecular Mechanisms of Endocrine Resistance

Xiaoyong Fu, Carmine De Angelis, Jamunarani Veeraraghavan, C. Kent Osborne, and Rachel Schiff

Abstract Estrogen receptor-positive (ER+) breast cancer is the most common subtype of breast cancer. Endocrine therapy targeting the ER pathway is effective, yet endocrine resistance is prevalent and remains a clinical challenge. The mechanisms underlying endocrine resistance are multifaceted and are likely to continue evolving over time in response to various endocrine regimens. The expression of ER in most endocrine-resistant tumors underscores ER's continuing role, although altered, often via crosstalk with hyperactive growth factor receptor and intracellular kinase signaling pathways. These interactions can alter ER's sensitivity to various endocrine agents and lead to the activation of distinct transcriptional programs that provide proliferation and survival signaling to escape endocrine therapy. Additional molecular determi-

Xiaoyong Fu is a co-corresponding author for this chapter.

X. Fu
Lester & Sue Smith Breast Center, Baylor College of Medicine, Houston, TX, USA

Dan L. Duncan Comprehensive Cancer Center, Baylor College of Medicine, Houston, TX, USA

Department of Molecular and Cellular Biology, Baylor College of Medicine, Houston, TX, USA
e-mail: xiaoyonf@bcm.edu

C. De Angelis · J. Veeraraghavan
Lester & Sue Smith Breast Center, Baylor College of Medicine, Houston, TX, USA

Dan L. Duncan Comprehensive Cancer Center, Baylor College of Medicine, Houston, TX, USA

C. K. Osborne · R. Schiff (✉)
Lester & Sue Smith Breast Center, Baylor College of Medicine, Houston, TX, USA

Dan L. Duncan Comprehensive Cancer Center, Baylor College of Medicine, Houston, TX, USA

Department of Molecular and Cellular Biology, Baylor College of Medicine, Houston, TX, USA

Department of Medicine, Baylor College of Medicine, Houston, TX, USA
e-mail: rschiff@bcm.edu

© Springer Nature Switzerland AG 2019
X. Zhang (ed.), *Estrogen Receptor and Breast Cancer*, Cancer Drug Discovery and Development, https://doi.org/10.1007/978-3-319-99350-8_11

nants inflicting ER transcriptional reprogramming to promote endocrine resistance include alterations of ER coregulators and pioneer factors, and genetic aberrations of ER itself. Recent advances in our understanding of the mechanisms of endocrine resistance, mostly provided by large-scale sequencing studies, further establish the roles of epigenetic alterations, the DNA damage response, the tumor microenvironment, and the immune response in promoting the endocrine-resistant ER+ disease. Progress has been made in translating several of these findings into effective new targeted therapies, such as inhibitors targeting the key signaling node mTOR and the cyclin-dependent kinases CDK4 and CDK6. However, considerable challenges remain in (1) developing new tailored treatment strategies with enhanced efficacy and reduced toxicity, (2) improving the patient selection approaches for these new treatments, and (3) advancing our understanding of how to harness the recent developments in immunotherapy to support other therapeutic strategies to prevent or overcome endocrine resistance and disease progression. It is our hope that continuing translational research will unveil more converging targets and pathways associated with altered ER transcriptional reprogramming, which can be therapeutically exploited to prevent and/or reverse endocrine resistance.

Keywords Estrogen receptor · Endocrine resistance · Growth factor receptor · Crosstalk · Genetic aberrations · Transcriptional reprogramming · Tumor microenvironment

1 Introduction

Breast cancer is a heterogeneous disease with varying clinical, histopathological, and molecular subtypes. Early breast cancer classification was mainly based on the presence of estrogen receptor (ER), progesterone receptor (PR), and HER2 (also known as ERBB2) [1], most commonly assessed by immunohistochemistry (IHC). Recent gene expression profiling reveals several intrinsic breast cancer subtypes: luminal A, luminal B, HER2-enriched, basal-like, and normal-like breast cancer [2, 3], while additional subtypes have been further characterized such as those within the most diversified basal-like subtype [4–6]. Approximately 75% of breast cancers express ER, mainly constituting the luminal subtypes of so-called ER-positive (+) breast cancer [7]. They include the more differentiated, indolent, and endocrine-sensitive luminal A subtype and the more aggressive and relatively less endocrine-sensitive luminal B subtype [2, 3]. ER and its ligand estrogen play a fundamental role in normal mammary gland development and in the etiology and progression of ER+ breast cancer [8]. Accordingly, endocrine therapies, which target the ER pathway, are the mainstay of standard care for patients with ER+ breast cancer in both the early and the advanced stages.

ER is predominantly a nuclear protein that functions as a ligand-dependent transcription factor. ER shares a common structural and functional organization with other members of the nuclear receptor superfamily [9]. Estrogen binding to ER induces its dimerization and enhances its nuclear localization. The formation of an

ER-ligand complex along with its coregulators leads to direct ER binding at a specific DNA sequence called the estrogen response element (ERE) [10] and to the recruitment of additional coregulators and epigenetic modulators (e.g., p300/CBP) to control the classical (i.e., estrogen-dependent) transcriptional program and promote breast cancer cell proliferation and survival [11, 12]. In addition, ER, especially when activated by high growth factor or cellular kinase signaling, can engage in a nonclassical genomic transcriptional program via interaction with DNA at sites such as the AP-1 binding motif through a tethering mechanism [13, 14]. In contrast to the ER genomic activity via ER binding to chromatin, ER can also transduce rapid signaling via its extranuclear non-genomic function, which involves its interaction with various tyrosine kinase receptors (e.g., growth factor receptors) and other signaling molecules (e.g., SRC) to promote cell proliferation and survival [15–18 and references therein].

Three primary modalities of endocrine therapies are used to block the oncogenic ER signaling in breast cancer, including selective estrogen receptor modulators (SERMs, e.g., tamoxifen) that complex with ER and inhibit estrogen binding, estrogen synthesis inhibitors [e.g., aromatase inhibitors (AIs)] that deprive the receptor of its ligand, and selective estrogen receptor downregulators (SERDs, e.g., fulvestrant) that directly degrade ER protein, which results in a more complete inhibition of the ER pathway.

While endocrine therapy is the most effective treatment for ER+ breast cancer, its effectiveness is limited by substantial rates of de novo (intrinsic) resistance and acquired resistance, the latter developed during or after treatment [19, 20]. Tamoxifen has represented the most successful targeted treatment for ER+ breast cancer for more than four decades [21]. However, ~50% of patients with metastatic disease do not respond to first-line tamoxifen treatment, and almost all patients, including those who initially responded, eventually relapse [22]. In addition, about 25% of patients with early primary disease who received tamoxifen as an adjuvant therapy will present with or eventually develop endocrine resistance [23]. In the past two decades, AIs have been shown to be superior to tamoxifen in both the adjuvant and the metastatic settings [24, 25]. However, either intrinsic or acquired resistance to AIs also commonly occurs [26]. Recent studies have shown that fulvestrant, one of the SERDs, has dose-dependent and superior efficacy over AIs in prolonging progression-free survival (PFS) in patients with locally advanced or metastatic breast cancer [27, 28], although resistance still occurs. Orally active SERDs with improved pharmacokinetics have recently been developed [29, 30], but their clinical efficacy and utility are still under investigation [31].

In the past several decades, numerous efforts have been made to understand the mechanisms of endocrine resistance and to identify novel therapeutic strategies to prevent and overcome it. In this chapter, we provide a review of current knowledge and key recent findings on the molecular mechanisms of endocrine resistance. We mainly focus on the mechanisms involving altered cellular signaling cascades converging on altered ER transcriptional reprogramming in endocrine resistance. We also cover the emerging roles of genetic, epigenetic, and tumor microenvironmental alterations in altering ER activity and/or endocrine sensitivity. With respect to different mechanisms, clinical implications and challenges are also briefly discussed. Of note, given the intra-tumoral heterogeneity, plasticity, and response to a variety of antitumor therapies, one particular mechanism may be predominant in some tumors, while in others different mechanisms of endocrine resistance may operate simultaneously during the course of ER+ disease progression and metastasis [32].

2 Crosstalk Between ER and Receptor Tyrosine and Cellular Kinases

Loss of ER expression, which could account for endocrine resistance, has been observed in 15–20% of patients with metastatic breast cancer [33]. However, in most endocrine-resistant cases, ER continues to be expressed and active, which enables response to sequential multiple lines of endocrine treatments in the advanced metastatic setting [34, 35]. Bidirectional crosstalk between ER and growth factor receptors (GFRs), and/or downstream intracellular kinase signaling, especially in the presence of hyperactive GFR signaling, has been well documented and suggested as one of the predominant mechanisms that mediates resistance to various endocrine therapies [36–41]. Such signaling circuits (Fig. 1), which may already preexist or may arise during the course of treatment, either alter ER activity and activate distinct transcriptional programs, also called "ER transcriptional reprogramming," to operate in spite of the presence of endocrine therapy, or bypass ER blockade by providing alternative proliferation and survival signals [40].

2.1 Activation of the HER Family

Preclinical and clinical evidence has revealed extensive mutual interplay between ER and the receptor tyrosine kinase (RTK) HER family as an important contributor to endocrine resistance [38, 42, 43]. About 10% of ER+ breast cancers are ER+/HER2+, and these tumors have been shown to be less responsive to endocrine therapy [44]. Overexpression of HER2 in MCF7 cells and xenograft tumors confers endocrine resistance by activating downstream kinases including the phosphatidylinositol 3-kinase (PI3K) and p42/44 mitogen-activated protein kinase (MAPK) pathways, which in turn activate and/or alter the ER transcriptional activity and its transcriptional programs, via posttranslational modifications (e.g., phosphorylation) of ER itself, its coregulators, or other transcriptional machinery components [40, 45–47]. Increased levels of HER2 and EGFR have been found in acquired tamoxifen-resistant (TamR) preclinical cell and xenograft models [45, 48], and high levels of EGFR are associated with poor distant metastasis-free survival in patients treated with adjuvant tamoxifen [49, 50].

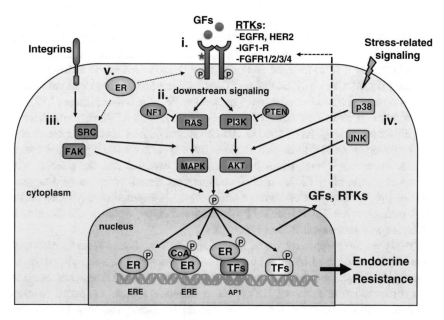

Fig. 1 Crosstalk between ER and multiple receptor tyrosine and intracellular kinases in endocrine resistance. (**i** and **ii**) Hyperactivation of growth factor receptors (GFRs), including the HER2-activating mutations (marked by a blue star), and multiple GFR downstream signaling phosphorylate (p) and activate ER, ER coactivators (CoA), and other transcription factors (TFs) in the nucleus, resulting in altered ER-chromatin interactions including enhanced binding to non-estrogen response elements (ERE) via tethering to other TFs such as AP-1. The altered ER binding and activity, also called "ER transcriptional reprogramming," and activation of other TFs result in an enhancement of the transcriptional induction of growth factors (GFs) and receptor tyrosine kinases (RTKs), which in turn enhance the signaling elicited at the level of GFRs to reinforce the activation of ER. (**iii** and **iv**) Signaling from the tumor microenvironment activates members of the integrin family and the stress-related pathways. These pathways then trigger downstream FAK/SRC and p38/JNK kinase pathways that can further modulate components of the transcriptional machinery, including ER. (**v**) A small fraction of the cellular ER pool associates with RTKs and intracellular SRC kinase to exert its non-genomic function of activating downstream kinase signaling, contributing to endocrine resistance. Alterations in each of these signaling elements can mediate resistance to endocrine therapy by modulating ER activity and by acting as escape pathways to provide alternative proliferation and survival stimuli to resistant breast cancer cells

Notably, signaling of the ER pathway can also activate or inhibit HER pathways by direct and indirect mechanisms [41]. ER can induce the expression of various HER ligands such as amphiregulin and transforming growth factor-α (TGFα), as well as other GFRs/ligands such as insulin-like growth factor receptor (IGF1R) and its ligand IGF1 [51–53], or activate these pathways via its non-genomic membrane activity [51, 54]. On the other hand, ER signaling can also transcriptionally or post-transcriptionally, via activating microRNAs, inhibit the expression of key GFRs such as EGFR and HER2 [55, 56]. As such, endocrine therapy, by blocking ER genomic activity, can relieve this repression, resulting in increased expression of EGFR/HER2 and activation of downstream signaling [20], which in turn can further promote endocrine resistance. In addition, it has been shown in ER+ breast cancer cells that the ER degrader fulvestrant can induce expression of HER3, HER4, and ligands of the epidermal growth factor (EGF) family that activate the HER signaling, which may lead to reduced and ultimately limited therapeutic efficacy of fulvestrant [57, 58]. Clinically, adding an EGFR inhibitor (gefitinib) to tamoxifen or an AI demonstrated a modest advantage in treating ER+ metastatic disease [59, 60]. The addition of an EGFR/HER2 inhibitor (lapatinib) to an AI (letrozole) conferred a significant advantage in PFS in the HER2+ subset of ER+ metastatic breast cancer; however, in the HER2-negative subset, there was no overall significant benefit [61]. A more recent analysis of this trial further revealed that the patients with tumors expressing low ER levels received the most benefit from the dual-targeted therapies [62]. Perhaps those tumors with lower ER expression rely more on the HER pathway when ER is blocked by endocrine therapy, which is consistent with the findings of preclinical studies [46, 63, 64].

Finally, in the recent few years, activating HER2 recurrent somatic mutations have been reported in ~1.6% of primary ER+/HER2-negative (non-amplified) breast cancer [65]. These mutations, largely clustering in the tyrosine kinase and extracellular dimerization domains of HER2, are enriched in lobular vs. ductal invasive carcinomas [66, 67], as well as in the metastatic disease [68–70]. Importantly, recently completed and ongoing clinical trials indicate that many patients with tumors harboring these HER2 mutations are sensitive to the irreversible pan-HER tyrosine kinase inhibitor neratinib [66, 68], especially when combined with fulvestrant [71]. These data strongly indicate the causal role of these HER2 mutations in breast cancer endocrine resistance and metastasis and also demonstrate their predictive and therapeutic value in endocrine-resistant and metastatic ER+ breast cancer.

2.2 Activation of IGF Pathway

IGF1R and insulin receptor (InsR) are both receptor tyrosine kinases (RTKs) that have been shown to drive the signaling that promotes cancer cell growth, proliferation, and migration [72]. Similar to the HER family, the binding of ligands to IGF1R and InsR leads to the downstream signaling activation of PI3K/AKT and RAS/RAF/MAPK pathways [73]. Preclinical studies have shown that IGF1R and InsR modulate ER function and/or endocrine sensitivity at least partly by ER phosphorylation and activation, and gene expression signatures of IGF pathway activation were associated with poor prognosis of patients with ER+ breast cancer [74–77]. Reciprocally, ER can induce the gene expression of IGF1 and IGF1R under estrogen stimulation and can also initiate a non-genomic effect on IGF1R signaling activation by binding to IGF1R in the cytoplasm and cell membrane upon estrogen or IGF1 treatment [51, 78, 79]. The expression of IGF1/IGF1R is reduced upon SERM (e.g., tamoxifen) treatment and remains suppressed when resistance occurs, as shown in preclinical models [45, 80]. In contrast, increased IGF1R expression and signaling have been shown in long-term estrogen-deprived (LTED) cells, possibly due to the hypersensitivity to estrogen [81, 74].

Early preclinical studies demonstrated the efficacy of an anti-IGF1R monoclonal antibody in enhancing endocrine therapy [82]. However, trials with such antibodies targeting IGF1R plus endocrine therapy in ER+ metastatic breast cancer have not shown any advantage over endocrine therapy alone [72 and references therein]. A potential reason for this lack of benefit may be related to the preclinical findings that breast cancer cells that are resistant to tamoxifen are refractory to IGF1R antibody treatment due to low expression levels of IGF1R while remaining sensitive to IGF1R tyrosine kinase inhibitor [80]. On the other hand, preclinical data support the use of SERDs, not tamoxifen, in suppressing LTED cell growth by reducing ER-dependent IGF1R expression and signaling [81], rationalizing the combination of anti-IGF1R therapy to treat ER+ breast cancers that relapse on or after a previous AI. Further, growing evidence indicates that InsR plays an important role in overcoming the inhibitory effect of anti-IGF1R monotherapy either by forming hybrids with the IGF1R or by providing alternative proliferation and survival signaling [83, 84]. The efficacy of dual IGF1R/InsR tyrosine kinase inhibitors has been shown in preclinical endocrine-resistant models [85, 74]. However, the clinical efficacy of these dual inhibitors in combination with endocrine therapy in treating hormone-refractory breast cancer largely remains to be defined.

2.3   Activation of FGFR Signaling

Fibroblast growth factors (FGFs) and their receptors (FGFRs) play essential roles in cell proliferation, survival, differentiation, migration, and apoptosis during embryonic development and adult tissue homeostasis and also in human cancers [86, 87]. Recent clinical sequencing studies revealed breast cancer as the second most commonly affected cancer type with FGFR aberrations (18%) [88], with *FGFR1* amplification (8%) being the most frequent genomic aberration in breast cancer, particularly in the ER+/HER2-negative subtype with shorter overall survival [89]. Preclinical studies confirmed that high FGFR signaling, via *FGFR1* amplification/ overexpression, or high FGFR2/FGF7 signaling contributes to tamoxifen resistance by activating the downstream MAPK and PI3K/mTOR pathways [90, 91]. High-frequency *FGFR1* amplification was observed in the luminal B subtype of breast cancer, and high expression levels of FGFR1/FGFR4 were associated with poor clinical outcome including shorter distant metastasis-free survival (DMFS) and PFS in patients treated with tamoxifen [90, 92]. In addition, *FGFR1* amplification has been identified in clinical samples of invasive lobular carcinoma (ILC) [93], which is mainly ER+/HER2-negative with inferior long-term outcome compared to stage-matched invasive ductal carcinoma (IDC) [67]. This is in line with the preclinical findings that high FGFR1 signaling is required for de novo tamoxifen resistance in one of the ILC cell models (MDA-MB-134VI), where ER drives a unique transcriptional program [94]. Using ER+/*FGFR1*-amplified preclinical cell and patient-derived xenograft (PDX) models, a recent study further uncovered an unexpected role of FGFR1, by its association with ER in nuclei, in maintaining ligand-independent ER activity and mediating resistance to estrogen deprivation in ER+ breast cancer [95], suggesting the complexity of FGFR signaling underlying the molecular mechanisms of endocrine resistance.

Multiple preclinical studies support FGFR1 as a promising therapeutic target to treat endocrine-resistant breast cancer [96, 90]. A phase II trial assessing the efficacy of an FGFR kinase inhibitor (dovitinib, a multi-targeted RTK inhibitor of FGFR1/3) combined with fulvestrant in ER+/HER2-negative advanced breast cancer showed promising clinical activity in the subgroup of patients with *FGFR*-amplified tumors [97]. More data from ongoing or future trials are awaited, including the use of pan or more selective FGFR inhibitors in advanced ER+ breast cancer [98, 99]. Future investigations are needed to elucidate the oncogenic potential and evolving roles of FGFR genomic aberrations in breast cancer endocrine resistance and to explore rational combinations with endocrine and possible other targeted therapies to enhance efficacy or reduce resistance to treatment [100]. In addition, it is also important to develop clinical methods, such as circulating tumor DNA screening [101], to identify tumors with *FGFR* aberrations.

2.4 Intracellular Signaling Cascades

The crosstalk between ER and GFR signaling is mainly manifested by downstream cascades of intracellular signaling that lead to endocrine resistance and disease progression. These intracellular signaling cascades can form a signaling network with extensive intertwined crosstalk that confers an adaptive mechanism to targeted therapies, a phenomenon that has to be considered in the development of new treatment strategies [102, 103].

2.4.1 PI3K/AKT/mTOR

PI3K is a central signaling node mediating various signals transmitted from GFRs and other receptors, such as G-protein-coupled receptors (GPCRs), down to the kinase cascade comprised of AKT and mammalian target of rapamycin (mTOR) [104, 105]. Molecular analysis delineates PI3K as the most frequently altered pathway in 70% of breast cancer, including recurrent mutations and/or amplification of the gene encoding the PI3K catalytic subunit p110α (*PIK3CA*) [106–108]. *PIK3CA* is the most frequently mutated gene in the PI3K pathway in breast cancer, most commonly in luminal ER+ tumors [109]. Oncogenic mutations of *PIK3CA*, paradoxically, are associated with better outcome in ER+ breast cancer patients treated with endocrine therapy [106, 110], possibly due to the low downstream mTOR signaling in these tumors. In contrast, PI3K pathway activation signatures, derived from ER+ tumors at both transcriptomic and proteomic levels, have been shown to correlate with lower ER levels and activity and with the more aggressive and less endocrine-sensitive luminal B subtype [111].

Preclinical models have shown that PI3K pathway activation including PTEN downregulation in ER+/HER2-negative breast cancer cells confers endocrine resistance [112–114]. PI3K pathway inhibitors can restore the expression levels of ER and its regulated genes, by a mechanism that has recently been linked to the epigenetic regulation of ER-dependent transcription [115], resulting in enhanced endocrine sensitivity in preclinical ER+ cell models [111, 116]. In the ER+ MCF7 breast cancer cells, overexpression of constitutively active AKT1 induced resistance to an estrogen deprivation treatment, which was overcome by addition of an AKT inhibitor [117]. Currently, dozens of small-molecule inhibitors targeting multiple components of the PI3K pathway, such as PI3K, AKT, and mTOR, have been developed and tested in preclinical models and/or clinical trials for ER+ breast cancer [105, 118–121]. Several trials have demonstrated the efficacy of mTOR and PI3K inhibitors in overcoming or delaying endocrine resistance in ER+/HER2-negative metastatic breast cancer patients [122–126]. Nevertheless, the efficacy of these targeted therapies is commonly restrained by the extensive feedback regulation throughout the intracellular signaling cascades, including the ER pathway, as has been demonstrated in both preclinical and clinical studies [115, 127–130]. For example, AKT phosphorylates the FOXO family of transcription factors and prevents their nuclear localization and activation [131]. Thus, PI3K/AKT inhibitors can relieve FOXO-dependent negative feedback to induce transcription of key signaling molecules (e.g., HER3, IGF1R, and FGFR2), at least partly in cooperation with ER, leading to reduced efficacy of these inhibitors in hormone-refractory tumors [132, 133]. Overall, while combinatorial therapy co-targeting the ER and PI3K pathways may be potent for a subset of ER+/HER2-negative breast cancer [134], the substantial side effects commonly observed with this strategy call for additional development of more selective inhibitors along these pathways.

2.4.2 RAS/RAF/MEK/ERK

The MAPK cascades are evolutionarily conserved central signaling pathways that control a wide variety of cellular processes in response to various extracellular stimuli that operate via various receptors [135]. The ERK1/2 cascade, also known as the p42/44 MAPK, is the first MAPK pathway elucidated [136] and is considered a prototype of these kinase cascades. Upon activation by various receptors at the plasma membrane, a cascade of events involving multiple kinases eventually activates ERK1/2 [136], which in turn activates its downstream signaling including additional kinases and a variety of transcription factors, such as AP-1 and ER, localized either in the cytoplasm, nucleus, or other cellular organelles [137]. Bidirectional crosstalk between the ERK1/2 pathway and ER has been suggested to play a role in endocrine resistance [46, 138]. It has been reported that activation of ERK1/2 by overexpression of RTKs or its upstream kinases in endocrine-sensitive MCF7 cells results in downregulation of ER mRNA and protein levels [139].

Importantly, however, hyperactive ERK1/2, via phosphorylation of serine 118 in the ligand-independent activation function 1 (AF1) domain of ER, can enhance ER activity in the presence of endocrine therapy, resulting in reduced endocrine sensitivity [140]. Loss of the *NF1* gene that encodes a negative regulator of RAS can also activate ERK1/2, conferring tamoxifen resistance in ER+ breast cancer cells [141, 142]. In addition, preclinical studies have also shown that endocrine resistance is associated with elevated ERK1/2 phosphorylation and MAPK signaling activation [143, 144]. Conversely, MAPK signaling can be activated by estrogen-bound ER via both its non-genomic and genomic activities [145]. Interestingly, since a large number of substrates of MAPK cascades are localized primarily in the nucleus, the nuclear function of ERK1/2 has been linked to gene regulation partly via engaging in chromatin remodeling [146, 147]. For example, ERK2 and another less studied member of the MAPK cascade, ERK5, which has previously been shown to promote endocrine resistance [148], can be activated by estrogen-dependent ER signaling and function as coregulators of ER-dependent gene transcription to promote cell proliferation and invasiveness [149, 150]. However, the definite role of ERK nuclear signaling in promoting endocrine resistance remains to be clarified.

ER expression can be restored in some ER-negative tumor cells or upregulated in low ER-expressing tumors by MAPK inhibitors, leading to recovered endocrine sensitivity [151]. However, both preclinical and clinical studies so far do not support a therapeutic benefit of MAPK inhibitors in combination with endocrine therapy for treating hormone-refractory breast cancer [152, 153]. Whether better biomarkers are needed to select appropriate patients to receive MAPK-targeted therapy is an open question.

2.4.3   SRC/FAK Signaling

SRC is an intracellular tyrosine kinase that plays a key role in transducing signals emanating from cell surface integrin and growth factor receptors, resulting in altered cell-matrix contacts and cell migration [154]. Of note, studies have shown the critical role of a few integrins, especially integrins β1 and β4, in endocrine sensitivity and resistance [155–157]. SRC activity is tightly linked to the focal adhesion kinase (FAK), another cytoplasmic non-RTK that is often deregulated in malignancy to promote cell proliferation, survival, and motility [158]. The crosstalk between ER and SRC/FAK signaling has been shown in estrogen- or growth factor-treated endocrine-sensitive breast cancer cells, where activated SRC/FAK forms a complex with ER and mediates ER extranuclear signaling to promote cell proliferation as well as cytoskeletal remodeling that leads to enhanced cell migration and invasion [159, 160]. It has also been shown that elevated levels of activated SRC promote adhesion-independent FAK phosphorylation in MCF7-TamR cells, resulting in increased cellular motility and invasion [161, 162]. High levels of activated SRC have been found in metastases of ER+ tumors [163], and its cytoplasmic localization was associated with reduced survival in ER+ breast cancer patients treated with endocrine therapy [164]. Somatic mutations in another SRC family kinase, LYN, have been reported in clinical ER+ tumors that progressed under AI treatment, and in preclinical models, these mutations lead to increased kinase activity and reduced response to fulvestrant [165]. Emerging evidence also indicates the role of FAK signaling in maintenance of the cancer stem cells (CSCs) that contribute to tamoxifen resistance [166].

Preclinical studies demonstrated the therapeutic potential of SRC inhibition in either preventing endocrine resistance or resensitizing resistant cells to endocrine therapy [167, 168]. However, a pan-SRC inhibitor recently tested in clinical trials in advanced ER+ breast cancer has shown mixed success, possibly due to the lack of biomarkers for selection of patients most likely to benefit from this therapy [169, 170]. Small-molecule FAK inhibitors have so far not been tested in patients with ER+ endocrine-resistant tumors, though their antitumor activity has been shown in other cancer types [171]. Further mechanistic studies using appropriate preclinical models to examine the interactions between SRC/FAK-targeted therapies and sequentially applied antiestrogen agents would provide a rationale and strategy to develop future clinical trials.

2.4.4 p38, JNK/AP-1, and NFκB Signaling

Preclinical and clinical studies have shown that intrinsic and acquired endocrine resistance is associated with activation of two important stress-related signaling pathways, JNK/AP-1 and p38 [39, 172, 173], which can also be activated by phosphorylation under hyperactive GFR signaling. In the TCGA dataset, frequent mutations in *MAP3K1* and *MAP2K4* (8% and 4%, respectively), the two upstream kinases of the stress-related kinases p38 and JNK1, as well as ERK1/2, have been found to be enriched in luminal/ER+ primary breast tumors [109]. These mutations are predicted to be inactivating, but their functional relationship with response to endocrine therapy is not clear. It has been shown that JNK and p38 kinases directly regulate a wide range of transcription factors. Activated JNK and p38 can phosphorylate and activate ER and/or its coactivators such as SRC3, thus altering ER activity and sensitivity to endocrine agents [20, 174]. One of the best-known transcription factors regulated by JNK is c-Jun [175], a key component of the transcription factor AP-1 complex [176]. Preclinical studies employing genetic strategies have suggested that inhibition of AP-1 alters ER activity and circumvents endocrine resistance [177]. Conversely, overexpression of the AP-1 component c-Jun can modulate ER-chromatin binding and activity, resulting in reduced sensitivity to tamoxifen in ER+ breast cancer cells [178].

Another key transcription factor downstream of stress-related and other signaling elicited largely by inflammatory cytokines and various extracellular stresses is NFκB [179]. Activation of NFκB induces expression of stress-related genes in inflammatory and immune responses and drives breast cancer aggressiveness and resistance to endocrine therapy [180, 181]. Numerous studies have shown that the activation profiles of ER and NFκB are inversely correlated in breast cancer

[182–184] and that the activated NFκB pathway is associated with hormone independence and resistance to endocrine therapy [185–187]. It has been shown that estrogen-stimulated ER prevents NFκB-DNA binding [188] or directly competes with NFκB for binding to transcriptional coactivators [189, 190]. As such, attenuated ER activation, due to endocrine therapy, releases NFκB from the ER-mediated inhibition, leading to NFκB-driven hormone-independent tumor progression. Conversely, NFκB activation, via activation of PKC/AKT signaling, inactivates FOXO3a, leading to decreased ER transcription [191].

Additional studies, however, demonstrated that ER and NFκB can stabilize each other's interaction with their respective response elements [192–194]. Further, ER can be tethered to chromatin-bound NFκB and its transcriptional complex to activate cyclin D1 gene transcription [195]. Preclinical data suggest that NFκB inhibition restores endocrine sensitivity [196, 197]. However, the clinical efficacy of NFκB-targeted therapy (e.g., bortezomib, a proteasome inhibitor) in treating endocrine-resistant breast cancer is not satisfactory [198]. Finally, preclinical studies also suggest the role of autophagy, which is initiated in response to stress or nutrient deprivation and which interplays with the NF-kB signaling pathway [199], in acquired endocrine resistance [200]. Inhibition of autophagy can potentiate resensitization of previously endocrine-resistant breast cancer cells [201]. Due to the complexity of these stress-related pathways that often interact with tumor microenvironment (see below), further basic and mechanistic research is needed to facilitate their clinical application.

2.5   CDK4/6/RB and the Cell Cycle Pathway

Cell cycle deregulation leads to uncontrolled cell proliferation, which is one of the hallmarks of cancer [202]. In response to mitogenic/oncogenic signaling, intracellular signaling cascades activate cyclin D1-dependent kinase (CDK) 4/6 complexes [203], which subsequently phosphorylate the tumor suppressor RB leading to its inactivation. As a consequence, CDK4/6 complexes reduce RB capacity to sequester the E2F transcription factors, thus promoting cell cycle progression from G1 into S phase [204]. ER+ tumors are dependent on estrogen signaling for proliferation and survival, which is antagonized by endocrine therapy targeting the ER pathway leading to cell cycle arrest and reduced tumor cell viability [205]. Preclinical studies and clinical evidence support a strong relationship between ER signaling and CDK4/6/RB pathway activity [206, 207]. A higher frequency of *CDK4* copy number gain is found in luminal B compared to luminal A subtype [109]. ER signaling activates the cyclin D1 gene (*CCND1*) promoter [208], and overexpression of cyclin D1 reverses the growth-inhibitory effects of antiestrogens [209]. High levels of cyclin D1 are associated with the luminal B subtype and with poor prognosis [109, 210]. In fact, *CCND1* amplification is common in breast cancer, occurring in 29% of luminal A, 58% of luminal B, and 38% of the HER2-enriched molecular subtypes [109].

In addition, cyclin D1 binds to ER and enhances ligand-independent ER activity, which can further explain its role in promoting endocrine resistance [211]. Likewise, deregulation of the negative cell cycle regulators p21 and p27 is also associated with poor response to endocrine therapy [212, 213]. In ER+ breast cancer, an RB-loss gene signature has been shown to be correlated with poor disease outcome, especially in patients treated with tamoxifen [214]. Similarly, an ER-dependent E2F activation gene signature has been associated with a reduced response to AIs [215].

In the preclinical setting, the selective CDK4/6 inhibitor palbociclib was preferentially effective in inhibiting the cell proliferation of ER+ cancer cells, including those resistant to endocrine therapies [216]. Three different CDK4/6 inhibitors, palbociclib, ribociclib, and abemaciclib, have recently been approved by the FDA for the treatment of ER+ breast cancer in the advanced or metastatic setting, and their full clinical roles and utilities are still currently being explored in various clinical trials [217]. The prolongation of progression-free survival by these agents in combination with AIs or fulvestrant is striking in ER+ metastatic disease but resistance ultimately occurs [218, 219]. While the overall survival data from these studies are pending, further preclinical and clinical investigations are needed for the development of predictive biomarkers for CDK4/6 inhibitors, as well as for the identification of potential drivers of resistance to anti-CDK4/6 therapy and strategies to overcome such resistance.

3 Additional Factors in Altering ER Activity and Transcriptional Programming

As mentioned earlier, most endocrine-resistant tumors still continuously express ER [33]. Further, ER+-resistant tumors are often still responsive to alternative subsequent lines of endocrine therapy [34], suggesting a continued, albeit altered, role and activity of ER. This altered ER activity may result in changes in ER sensitivity to various endocrine agents, such as hypersensitivity to low estrogen ligand, ligand-independent activity, or increased agonistic activity in the presence of SERMs [220]. Further, altered ER activity can also lead to transcriptional reprogramming by massively altering the gene expression profiles of cancer cells to activate a more aggressive and pro-metastatic program [13, 63, 221]. Here we will briefly discuss other major molecular determinants responsible for altered ER activity, including transcriptional coregulators, pioneer factors, and genomic aberrations of ER itself (Fig. 2). Of note, as discussed above, hyperactive GFRs and cellular signaling, via their bidirectional crosstalk with ER signaling, can also alter each of these other determinants and thus ER activity. A more comprehensive review of these key molecular determinants in regulating ER activity and endocrine sensitivity is discussed in chapters "Estrogen Receptor-Mediated Gene Transcription and Cistrome"; "Structural Studies with Coactivators for the Estrogen Receptor"; "The Estrogen-Regulated Transcriptome: Rapid, Robust, Extensive, and Transient"; and "Estrogen Receptor Regulation of MicroRNAs in Breast Cancer" of this book.

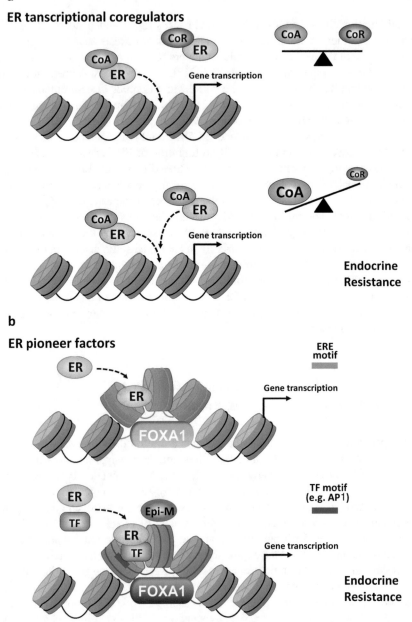

Fig. 2 Additional molecular determinants altering ER activity and transcriptional programming in endocrine resistance. (**a**) Changes in the balance of ER coregulators (CoA, coactivator; CoR, corepressor) occurring due to increased levels and/or activity of CoA (e.g., SRC3) and decreased levels and activity of CoR (N-CoR, SMRT), either by genetic aberrations or in the presence of hyper GFR signaling, result in altered ER sensitivity to various endocrine agents, enhanced or reprogrammed ER-chromatin binding, and altered transcriptional programs, conferring endocrine resistance. (**b**) Augmentation of the ER pioneer factor FOXA1, via gene amplification, active mutations, and/or

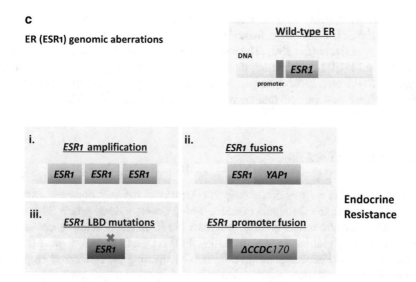

Fig. 2 (continued) overexpression, facilitates a distinct chromatin binding of ER and other tran-scription factors (TFs) and together with other epigenetic modulators (Epi-M) alters ER-chromatin interactions (e.g., tethering to AP-1) and transcriptional programs. (c) *ESR1* genetic aberrations, including (i) *ESR1* gene amplification, (ii) *ESR1* fusions with other oncogenes (e.g., *YAP1*) and *ESR1* promoter hijacking fusion to drive other oncogenes (e.g., *ΔCCDC170*), and (iii) ligand-binding domain (LBD) mutations, resulting in increased ER expression level; hyper transcriptional activity by the fusion protein or increased signaling from the oncogene fused to ER; and constitu-tively active/ligand-independent ER protein, respectively. Overall, these genetic aberrations can lead to altered activity of ER or other oncogenes and their associated transcriptional programs to promote endocrine resistance and aggressive phenotypes

3.1 *Transcriptional Coregulators*

Regulation of gene expression by ER requires positive and negative transcriptional coregulators, termed nuclear receptor coactivators (NCOAs) and nuclear receptor corepressors (NCORs), respectively [222]. These coregulator complexes often impose enzymatic activities such as acetylation or deacetylation on the chromatin to regulate local transcriptional initiation and elongation [223]. Expression levels and posttranslational modifications (e.g., phosphorylation, by GFR signaling) of these coregulators may directly control the equilibrium between agonist and antagonist activity of SERMs such as tamoxifen or the ligand-independent activity of ER [38, 41] (Fig. 2a). As such, overexpression or increased phosphorylation of NCOA3 (also known as AIB1/SRC3) is associated with preclinical resistance to tamoxifen [40], and poor prognosis in patients with tumors harboring high levels of HER fam-ily members [36, 224, 225]. In contrast, reduced expression of NCORs correlates with preclinical and clinical resistance to tamoxifen [226–228]. Of note, about 10% of primary ER+ tumors have been found to harbor either *NCOA2* or *NCOA3* genetic aberrations (amplification and mutations) [67, 229]. Further, the mutations or deletion of *NCOR1* have been found in 6% and 8% of primary and metastatic ER+ tumors, respectively [67, 230]. The role of additional new ER coactivators such as RUNX2 and MED1 in activating distinct ER transcriptional programs (e.g., target genes of *SOX9* and *ERBB2*, respectively) has recently been identified in ER+ or ER+/HER2+ breast cancers that are resistant to tamoxifen [231, 232].

3.2   Pioneer Factors

Pioneer factors are a group of transcription factors that have a unique and important role in unmasking the chromatin domains during developmental processes to facilitate lineage-specific transcriptional programs [233]. In ER+ breast cancer, several luminal-defining pioneer factors, including FOXA1 and GATA3, impose cancer-associated luminal gene expression programs by opening the condensed chromatin and facilitating the binding and function of lineage-specific transcription factors such as ER [234–236]. Previous genome-wide profiling of protein-chromatin binding (cistrome) revealed the process of "ER transcriptional reprogramming," in which pioneer factors such as FOXA1 coordinate with ER in altering genome-wide DNA binding on gene regulatory elements to induce a distinct gene transcriptional profile associated with more aggressive phenotypes (Fig. 2b) [13, 235, 237]. Further, FOXA1 has been shown to engage in such ER reprogramming both in preclinical cell models and in clinical ER+ tumors with poor outcome [115, 221, 238, 239]. In preclinical endocrine-resistant cell models, it has been shown that FOXA1 augmentation, via gene amplification and/or overexpression, elicits gene signatures and proteomic profiles associated with ligand-independent ER activation and the induction of multiple oncogenic signaling pathways, leading to endocrine-resistant, aggressive, and metastasis-related phenotypes [237]. Recent clinical studies suggest that *FOXA1* aberrations, which occur in ~10% of primary ER+ tumors (e.g., amplification) [240], are further enriched in ER+ metastases [67, 241–243], suggesting a potential driver role of FOXA1 in endocrine-resistant and metastatic disease. Interestingly, potentially activating *FOXA1* mutations are more frequent in invasive lobular carcinoma (ILC) than invasive ductal carcinoma (IDC), where GATA3 mutations are more prevalent, suggesting a differential role of these ER pioneer factors in ILC vs. IDC [67]. Nevertheless, future studies are needed to understand the precise impact of *FOXA1* aberrations as well as its interplay with ER in endocrine resistance, which may guide the development of FOXA1-targeting therapeutic strategies.

3.3   Genomic Alterations of ESR1

Recent whole genome sequencing and targeted next-generation sequencing have revealed various genomic aberrations at the ER gene *ESR1*, including gene amplification, rearrangements, and missense mutations (Fig. 2c). *ESR1* amplification, while remaining controversial, has been shown to occur in about 2% of primary breast cancers [109] and, as has recently been reported, in 21% of relapsed tumors after AI treatment [244], suggesting that *ESR1* amplification might play a role in endocrine resistance. Several rare recurrent *ESR1* gene fusions have also been reported recently [245 and references therein]. All of these fusions use the ER promoter to direct the transcription of the fused genes that mostly lose the ER ligand-binding domain (LBD) and the ligand-dependent activation function 2 (AF2), resulting in ligand-independent tumor growth and resistance to endocrine therapy. The *YAP1-ESR1* gene fusion identified in a patient-derived xenograft (PDX) model generated from a metastatic ER+ tumor gave rise to ligand-independent tumor growth and complete resistance to fulvestrant [246]. In addition, a recent report reveals that the ER promoter can be hijacked to express a truncated form (Δ) of CCDC170 involved in alternative survival pathways that can promote endocrine resistance [247].

The recent discovery of recurrent *ESR1* mutations mostly within the region of the ER LBD in endocrine-resistant metastatic ER+ breast cancer sheds new light on a common mechanism of clinical endocrine resistance, especially to AIs [246, 248–252]. These missense mutations are found in >20% of patients who received endocrine therapies and mainly occur in "hotspots" of the LBD, where Y537 and D538 are the most mutated residues [246, 248–252]. Functional and mechanistic studies demonstrated that the mutations confer a constitutive ligand-independent agonistic conformation to the ER LBD, resulting in enhanced recruitment of NCOAs [250, 252] and ligand-independent and altered ER transcriptional activity that leads to tumor growth and enhanced migratory properties [250, 253]. Breast cancers harboring these mutations also display relative resistance to tamoxifen and fulvestrant, which could be overcome with high doses of these antiestrogens or potentially with new oral SERDs [70, 246, 248, 250–252]. A recent study demonstrated that the allele-specific (i.e., Y537 vs. D538) neomorphic properties linked to these mutations promote a metastatic phenotype, in addition to supporting estrogen-independent growth [254]. The fact that enriched and recurrent *ESR1* mutations were found in relapsed vs. primary tumors after endocrine treatments, especially with AIs, highly suggests the clonal selection of either preexisting very rare mutant clones or the later acquisition of mutations under the pressure of endocrine therapy, as new and major mechanisms of resistance [255]. Clinically, it will be important to manage the emergence and frequency of ER-LBD mutations by developing sensitive assays such as liquid biopsies [256], as well as by exploring new treatment strategies (e.g., developing new-generation SERMs/SERDs [257]) to treat endocrine-resistant tumors by preventing and eradicating the emergence of *ESR1*-mutated subpopulations.

4 Epigenetic Alterations in Endocrine Resistance

Epigenetic alterations, such as DNA methylation, histone modifications, and alteration of micro (mi)-RNA expression, influence often inheritable gene expression without changing the DNA sequence [258]. As mentioned, these can lead to global changes in transcriptional programs to activate alternative survival pathways or directly impact ER levels and activity. As such, DNA methylation and histone deacetylation of the ER promoter itself can repress ER expression, leading to loss of ER and, as a result, to global changes in transcriptional program and to endocrine resistance [259]. Further, genome-wide profiles of DNA methylation of endocrine-resistant cells revealed the role of methylated estrogen-regulated enhancers in predicting response to endocrine therapy [260]. In addition, studies of chromatin landscape mapping have demonstrated genome-wide epigenetic reprogramming that results in global changes in transcriptional networks in breast cancer endocrine resistance [261, 262]. These studies led to the identification of key genes/pathways, beyond the ER pathway, regulated by chromatin reprogramming as potential targets to treat endocrine-resistant tumors [261, 262]. Compared to genetic alterations, epigenetic modifications, even stemming from genetic aberrations, are often enzymatically reversible, thus offering desirable therapeutic targets for cancer treatment. For example, preclinical studies and a phase II clinical trial showed efficacy of histone deacetylase (HDAC) inhibitors in treating TamR cells [263] and patients who had progressed on tamoxifen therapy [264].

Epigenetic modifications are also involved in the formation, maintenance, and function of breast cancer stemlike cells (CSCs), which have been proposed to play a role in endocrine resistance [265] and to be enriched after neoadjuvant AI treatment [266]. Likewise, tamoxifen, but not estrogen, can increase mammosphere-forming capacity of ER+ cells in vitro, partly due to the induction of the stem cell transcription factors Nanog and Sox2 [267]. In PDX tumors with acquired tamoxifen resistance, targeting JAG1-NOTCH4-dependent CSC activity overcomes resistance [268]. The polycomb repressive complex (PRC), which represses gene expression through histone modifications and chromatin condensation, regulates breast CSCs [269]. Of interest, resistance to AI and tamoxifen has been associated with the role of histone methyltransferase EZH2, a main component of the PRC, in repressing the apoptotic and antagonistic signaling of antiestrogens [270, 271]. Epigenetic regulation also alters miRNA expression profiles of breast CSCs. A cluster of miRNAs associated with endocrine resistance has recently been identified, including upregulation of those involved in modulating ER levels, activation of the epithelial-mesenchymal transition (EMT) process, and endocrine-resistant phenotypes [272–274].

In spite of the emerging body of evidence supporting epigenetic deregulation in the acquisition of endocrine resistance, many basic questions remain to be answered. Before translational applications can be rationally deployed, a better understanding of how the interplay between ER and its coregulators and epigenetic modifiers evolves in endocrine resistance is needed. Finally, genetic mutations of epigenetic regulators, including writers, readers, and erasers of epigenetic markers identified in ER+ breast tumors [109, 243], further illustrate the complexity of possible co-dependence of genetic and epigenetic regulatory events in the course of endocrine-resistant disease progression [275].

5 Emerging Mechanisms of Endocrine Resistance and Clinical Implications

5.1 DNA Damage Response Pathway

Defects in the DNA damage response and repair (DDR) machinery, as recently reviewed [276], create a permissive state for accumulation of mutations and unchecked cell proliferation and are associated with resistance to DNA-damaging agents. Over the course of breast cancer management, DNA-damaging chemotherapy or radiation is often used sequentially or simultaneously with endocrine therapy in ER+ disease [277]. Despite the conflicting data as to whether hormones are carcinogenic or cancer-protective [278] and regarding a potential link between tamoxifen and DNA damage [279], recent studies suggest that crosstalk between the DDR machinery and hormone signaling pathways influences both disease progression and therapeutic response [280]. In vitro studies describe hormone signals as direct regulators of DNA repair pathways, and a number of DDR factors serve as steroid receptor regulators, often forming feed-forward loops [280]. For instance, activated ER induces miR-18a/miR-106a to reduce the expression of the DNA damage response kinase ATM and its activity in cell cycle checkpoint control, allowing the cell cycle to proceed [281]. As such, in addition to the DNA damage that may be caused by SERMs, such as tamoxifen [282], DDR signaling can be activated as a result of inhibition of estrogen-induced ER signaling. Conversely, the nuclear DDR enzyme poly(ADP-ribose) polymerase 1 (PARP1) can bind to and PARylate ER to enhance ER-DNA binding and transcriptional activity [283]. Interestingly, a recent study showed that defects in a subset of mismatch repair pathway (MMR) components, unleashing the cell cycle checkpoint control, confer endocrine resistance [284]. Importantly, the CDK4 hyperactivity due to the loss of cell cycle checkpoint inhibitory control sensitizes these MMR-deficient ER+ tumors to the CDK4/6 inhibitor palbociclib [284]. Accumulating data from clinical tumor sequencing and functional studies may provide a deeper understanding of how deregulation of the DDR signaling impacts endocrine resistance and may help to facilitate the identification of potential biomarkers and new targets.

5.2 Tumor Microenvironment and Immune Response

Multiple layers of evidence suggest that both tumor progression and response to therapy are modulated by the tumor microenvironment, comprised of fibroblasts, lymph and blood vessels, and immune cells, as well as the extracellular matrix (ECM) [285]. The interaction between stromal cells and tumor cells has been shown to modulate ER-dependent and ER-independent proliferation of luminal breast cancer cells [286]. Indeed, gene expression analysis identified distinct stromal signatures that are strongly associated with clinical outcome of multiple breast cancer subtypes including ER+ tumors [287]. Overexpression of an ECM gene cluster (e.g., *TIMP3*, *FN1*, and *LOX*) in primary ER+ breast cancer correlates with resistance to adjuvant tamoxifen therapy and poor DMFS [288]. Cancer-associated fibroblast (CAF)-derived soluble factors such as fibronectin can modulate resistance to tamoxifen in epithelial cells via interaction with and activation of β1 integrin [289]. Further, more recent studies using PDX and other experimental models revealed the role of CAF-derived circulating extracellular vesicles (also known as exosomes) in conferring endocrine resistance via activation of ER-independent oxidative phosphorylation in CSCs to enhance their propagation [290, 291].

Many studies also support a specific role of the immune system as a regulator of breast cancer development and progression. Considerable evidence supports the notion that inflammation, a hallmark of cancer, is an important tumor microenvironmental factor mediating various breast cancer risk factors (e.g., pregnancy and obesity) and promoting the development of a more aggressive disease that fails to respond to therapies, including endocrine therapy [292 and references therein]. Increased pro-inflammatory cytokines, such as IL1β and TNFα, are released from macrophages and other innate immune cells, inducing invasiveness and metastasis of ER+ breast cancer cells [292]. In addition, a recent preclinical study has shown that in endocrine-resistant cell models with augmented FOXA1 levels, the ER transcriptional reprogramming induces several pro-tumorigenic inflammatory cytokines, such as IL8, which enhance endocrine-resistant and invasive phenotypes [237]. Conversely, it has also been shown that cytokine-induced IKKβ signaling leads to ER phosphorylation at S305 in the hinge domain, resulting in ligand-independent ER activation and endocrine resistance [293]. Clinical gene expression studies have further linked immune-related genes to endocrine resistance in ER+ tumors treated with adjuvant tamoxifen [294] or with neoadjuvant AI [295].

Additionally, tumor-associated macrophage (TAM)-derived ECM factors can also lead to endocrine resistance by directly suppressing ER expression via activating MAPK signaling [296]. The TAMs comprise up to 50% of the breast tumor mass, with their increased infiltration positively correlated with angiogenesis and with poor prognosis and low survival rates [297]. Although one study found an inverse correlation between the macrophage content and ER expression in breast cancer [298], other studies have suggested that TAMs can regulate proliferation and invasiveness of ER+ tumors, partially via directly producing estrogen and activating the NFκB/JNK pathways [299, 300]. TAMs also include the alternative M2 macrophages that upon activation can provide a favorable microenvironment by suppressing antitumor immunity and promoting tumor development and progression [301]. Accumulating evidence implicates estrogen as a potential mediator of immunosuppression through modulation of pro-tumorigenic responses, independent of its direct activity on tumor cells [302 and references therein]. For example, estrogen signaling has been shown to have a dramatic effect on enhancing cytokine-induced expansion of myeloid-derived suppressor cells, resulting in accelerated tumor growth due to blunted antitumor immunity [303]. As such, endocrine therapy is expected to counteract the effect of estrogen on pro-immunosuppression, thus favoring antitumor immunity. However, decreased cellular immunity has been reported in breast cancer patients with endocrine-resistant disease, manifested by clinical symptoms of immunodeficiency such as frequent infections of the respiratory or urinary tract [304], suggesting the complexity and evolving role of immunity during the course of endocrine resistance. Therefore, further research on the crosstalk between ER signaling and the tumor microenvironment and immune system is needed before clinical deployment can be considered for current immune-modulating therapies, such as immune checkpoint inhibitors against PD-1 and PD-L1, in combination with either endocrine therapy or other targeted therapies for endocrine-resistant tumors to achieve overall better outcomes [305].

6 Conclusions

ER-targeted endocrine therapy, the oldest and one of the most successful targeted therapies implemented in the past four decades, has greatly improved the quality of life and survival of millions of women with breast cancer worldwide. However, the battle to defeat endocrine resistance is still challenging and demands additional mechanistic and clinical investigations of the causes and molecular mechanisms of resistance before new and more effective therapeutic strategies can be further developed. One facet of the complexity of endocrine resistance is the diverse bidirectional crosstalk and feedback loops between ER signaling and alternative survival pathways such as GFR signaling that evolve during the course of treatment. The recent advent of large-scale sequencing studies based on multi-OMICS approaches further unveils the complexities of advanced ER+ breast cancer, including the intratumoral heterogeneity and interactions with the tumor microenvironment and the immune system, in the context of tumor response and resistance to endocrine and other targeted therapies. Such studies have also been generating new insights and potential new perspectives in improving the management of ER+ disease. With the increase of new therapeutic agents being tested in clinical trials to treat endocrine-resistant and advanced ER+ breast cancer, and those that have successfully moved into clinical practice such as the CDK4/6 inhibitors, future investigations need to focus on the identification of biomarkers that can predict and monitor the efficacy of these new regimens to improve patient outcome. Finally, acquisition of clinical specimens (e.g., liquid and metastatic tissue biopsies) and development of new preclinical resistant cell and PDX models are of critical importance to further our exploration and translation of new mechanisms and findings into clinical practice. Given the complexity and the inter- and intra-tumoral heterogeneity of the endocrine-resistant disease, especially in the advanced setting, it is the hope that these future studies will help underscore more converging pathways and targets associated with altered ER transcriptional programming, improve our capabilities to stratify patients using a more tailored approach, and facilitate harnessing the new developments in immunotherapy to prevent and overcome endocrine resistance.

Acknowledgments The authors would like to acknowledge funding from the NIH: SPORE Grants P50 CA058183 and CA186784 (to RS and CKO); Cancer Center Grant P30 CA125123; Breast Cancer Research Foundation BCRF-17-143 (to RS and CKO); and the DoD Breakthrough Award FL2 W81XWH-14-1-0326 (to XF) to support several of our research projects, the concepts and findings from which have been included in this chapter.

References

1. Parise CA, Bauer KR, Brown MM, Caggiano V (2009) Breast cancer subtypes as defined by the estrogen receptor (ER), progesterone receptor (PR), and the human epidermal growth factor receptor 2 (HER2) among women with invasive breast cancer in California, 1999-2004. Breast J 15(6):593–602. https://doi.org/10.1111/j.1524-4741.2009.00822.x
2. Perou CM, Sorlie T, Eisen MB, van de Rijn M, Jeffrey SS, Rees CA, Pollack JR, Ross DT, Johnsen H, Akslen LA, Fluge O, Pergamenschikov A, Williams C, Zhu SX, Lonning PE, Borresen-Dale AL, Brown PO, Botstein D (2000) Molecular portraits of human breast tumours. Nature 406(6797):747–752. https://doi.org/10.1038/35021093
3. Sorlie T, Perou CM, Tibshirani R, Aas T, Geisler S, Johnsen H, Hastie T, Eisen MB, van de Rijn M, Jeffrey SS, Thorsen T, Quist H, Matese JC, Brown PO, Botstein D, Lonning PE, Borresen-Dale AL (2001) Gene expression patterns of breast carcinomas distinguish tumor subclasses with clinical implications. Proc Natl Acad Sci U S A 98(19):10869–10874. https://doi.org/10.1073/pnas.191367098
4. Lehmann BD, Bauer JA, Chen X, Sanders ME, Chakravarthy AB, Shyr Y, Pietenpol JA (2011) Identification of human triple-negative breast cancer subtypes and preclinical models for selection of targeted therapies. J Clin Invest 121(7):2750–2767. https://doi.org/10.1172/JCI45014
5. Kreike B, van Kouwenhove M, Horlings H, Weigelt B, Peterse H, Bartelink H, van de Vijver MJ (2007) Gene expression profiling and histopathological characterization of triple-negative/basal-like breast carcinomas. Breast Cancer Res 9(5):R65. https://doi.org/10.1186/bcr1771
6. Shah SP, Roth A, Goya R, Oloumi A, Ha G, Zhao Y, Turashvili G, Ding J, Tse K, Haffari G, Bashashati A, Prentice LM, Khattra J, Burleigh A, Yap D, Bernard V, McPherson A, Shumansky K, Crisan A, Giuliany R, Heravi-Moussavi A, Rosner J, Lai D, Birol I, Varhol R, Tam A, Dhalla N, Zeng T, Ma K, Chan SK, Griffith M, Moradian A, Cheng SW, Morin GB, Watson P, Gelmon K, Chia S, Chin SF, Curtis C, Rueda OM, Pharoah PD, Damaraju S, Mackey J, Hoon K, Harkins T, Tadigotla V, Sigaroudinia M, Gascard P, Tlsty T, Costello JF, Meyer IM, Eaves CJ, Wasserman WW, Jones S, Huntsman D, Hirst M, Caldas C, Marra MA, Aparicio S (2012) The clonal and mutational evolution spectrum of primary triple-negative breast cancers. Nature 486(7403):395–399. https://doi.org/10.1038/nature10933
7. Clark GM, Osborne CK, McGuire WL (1984) Correlations between estrogen receptor, progesterone receptor, and patient characteristics in human breast cancer. J Clin Oncol 2(10):1102–1109. https://doi.org/10.1200/JCO.1984.2.10.1102
8. Huang B, Warner M, Gustafsson JA (2015) Estrogen receptors in breast carcinogenesis and endocrine therapy. Mol Cell Endocrinol 418(Pt 3):240–244. https://doi.org/10.1016/j.mce.2014.11.015
9. Olefsky JM (2001) Nuclear receptor minireview series. J Biol Chem 276(40):36863–36864. https://doi.org/10.1074/jbc.R100047200
10. Klinge CM (2001) Estrogen receptor interaction with estrogen response elements. Nucleic Acids Res 29(14):2905–2919
11. Osborne CK, Schiff R, Fuqua SA, Shou J (2001) Estrogen receptor: current understanding of its activation and modulation. Clin Cancer Res 7(12 Suppl):4338s–4342s discussion 4411s–4412s

12. McKenna NJ, Lanz RB, O'Malley BW (1999) Nuclear receptor coregulators: cellular and molecular biology. Endocr Rev 20(3):321–344. https://doi.org/10.1210/edrv.20.3.0366

13. Lupien M, Meyer CA, Bailey ST, Eeckhoute J, Cook J, Westerling T, Zhang X, Carroll JS, Rhodes DR, Liu XS, Brown M (2010) Growth factor stimulation induces a distinct ER(alpha) cistrome underlying breast cancer endocrine resistance. Genes Dev 24(19):2219–2227. https://doi.org/10.1101/gad.1944810

14. Biddie SC, John S, Sabo PJ, Thurman RE, Johnson TA, Schiltz RL, Miranda TB, Sung MH, Trump S, Lightman SL, Vinson C, Stamatoyannopoulos JA, Hager GL (2011) Transcription factor AP1 potentiates chromatin accessibility and glucocorticoid receptor binding. Mol Cell 43(1):145–155. https://doi.org/10.1016/j.molcel.2011.06.016

15. Nemere I, Pietras RJ, Blackmore PF (2003) Membrane receptors for steroid hormones: signal transduction and physiological significance. J Cell Biochem 88(3):438–445. https://doi.org/10.1002/jcb.10409

16. Levin ER (2012) Elusive extranuclear estrogen receptors in breast cancer. Clin Cancer Res 18(1):6–8. https://doi.org/10.1158/1078-0432.CCR-11-2547

17. Boonyaratanakornkit V, Hamilton N, Marquez-Garban DC, Pateetin P, McGowan EM, Pietras RJ (2018) Extranuclear signaling by sex steroid receptors and clinical implications in breast cancer. Mol Cell Endocrinol 466:51–72. https://doi.org/10.1016/j.mce.2017.11.010

18. Levin ER (2018) Membrane estrogen receptors signal to determine transcription factor function. Steroids 132:1–4. https://doi.org/10.1016/j.steroids.2017.10.014

19. Clarke R, Tyson JJ, Dixon JM (2015) Endocrine resistance in breast cancer--an overview and update. Mol Cell Endocrinol 418(Pt 3):220–234. https://doi.org/10.1016/j.mce.2015.09.035

20. Osborne CK, Schiff R (2011) Mechanisms of endocrine resistance in breast cancer. Annu Rev Med 62:233–247. https://doi.org/10.1146/annurev-med-070909-182917

21. Osborne CK (1998) Tamoxifen in the treatment of breast cancer. N Engl J Med 339(22):1609–1618. https://doi.org/10.1056/NEJM199811263392207

22. Ring A, Dowsett M (2004) Mechanisms of tamoxifen resistance. Endocr Relat Cancer 11(4):643–658. https://doi.org/10.1677/erc.1.00776

23. Early Breast Cancer Trialists' Collaborative Group (2005) Effects of chemotherapy and hormonal therapy for early breast cancer on recurrence and 15-year survival: an overview of the randomised trials. Lancet 365(9472):1687–1717. https://doi.org/10.1016/S0140-6736(05)66544-0

24. Early Breast Cancer Trialists' Collaborative Group (2015) Aromatase inhibitors versus tamoxifen in early breast cancer: patient-level meta-analysis of the randomised trials. Lancet 386(10001):1341–1352. https://doi.org/10.1016/S0140-6736(15)61074-1

25. Rugo HS, Rumble RB, Macrae E, Barton DL, Connolly HK, Dickler MN, Fallowfield L, Fowble B, Ingle JN, Jahanzeb M, Johnston SR, Korde LA, Khatcheressian JL, Mehta RS, Muss HB, Burstein HJ (2016) Endocrine therapy for hormone receptor-positive metastatic breast cancer: American Society of Clinical Oncology guideline. J Clin Oncol 34(25):3069–3103. https://doi.org/10.1200/JCO.2016.67.1487

26. Brodie A, Sabnis G (2011) Adaptive changes result in activation of alternate signaling pathways and acquisition of resistance to aromatase inhibitors. Clin Cancer Res 17(13):4208–4213. https://doi.org/10.1158/1078-0432.CCR-10-2920

27. Robertson JF, Lindemann J, Garnett S, Anderson E, Nicholson RI, Kuter I, Gee JM (2014) A good drug made better: the fulvestrant dose-response story. Clin Breast Cancer 14(6):381–389. https://doi.org/10.1016/j.clbc.2014.06.005

28. Robertson JFR, Bondarenko IM, Trishkina E, Dvorkin M, Panasci L, Manikhas A, Shparyk Y, Cardona-Huerta S, Cheung KL, Philco-Salas MJ, Ruiz-Borrego M, Shao Z, Noguchi S, Rowbottom J, Stuart M, Grinsted LM, Fazal M, Ellis MJ (2016) Fulvestrant 500 mg versus anastrozole 1 mg for hormone receptor-positive advanced breast cancer (FALCON): an international, randomised, double-blind, phase 3 trial. Lancet 388(10063):2997–3005. https://doi.org/10.1016/S0140-6736(16)32389-3

29. Wardell SE, Nelson ER, Chao CA, Alley HM, McDonnell DP (2015) Evaluation of the pharmacological activities of RAD1901, a selective estrogen receptor degrader. Endocr Relat Cancer 22(5):713–724. https://doi.org/10.1530/ERC-15-0287
30. McDonnell DP, Wardell SE, Norris JD (2015) Oral selective estrogen receptor downregulators (SERDs), a breakthrough endocrine therapy for breast cancer. J Med Chem 58(12):4883–4887. https://doi.org/10.1021/acs.jmedchem.5b00760
31. Huang D, Yang F, Wang Y, Guan X (2017) Mechanisms of resistance to selective estrogen receptor down-regulator in metastatic breast cancer. Biochim Biophys Acta 1868(1):148–156. https://doi.org/10.1016/j.bbcan.2017.03.008
32. Zardavas D, Irrthum A, Swanton C, Piccart M (2015) Clinical management of breast cancer heterogeneity. Nat Rev Clin Oncol 12(7):381–394. https://doi.org/10.1038/nrclinonc.2015.73
33. Hoefnagel LD, Moelans CB, Meijer SL, van Slooten HJ, Wesseling P, Wesseling J, Westenend PJ, Bart J, Seldenrijk CA, Nagtegaal ID, Oudejans J, van der Valk P, van Gils CH, van der Wall E, van Diest PJ (2012) Prognostic value of estrogen receptor alpha and progesterone receptor conversion in distant breast cancer metastases. Cancer 118(20):4929–4935. https://doi.org/10.1002/cncr.27518
34. Dodwell D, Wardley A, Johnston S (2006) Postmenopausal advanced breast cancer: options for therapy after tamoxifen and aromatase inhibitors. Breast 15(5):584–594. https://doi.org/10.1016/j.breast.2006.01.007
35. Robertson JF, Osborne CK, Howell A, Jones SE, Mauriac L, Ellis M, Kleeberg UR, Come SE, Vergote I, Gertler S, Buzdar A, Webster A, Morris C (2003) Fulvestrant versus anastrozole for the treatment of advanced breast carcinoma in postmenopausal women: a prospective combined analysis of two multicenter trials. Cancer 98(2):229–238. https://doi.org/10.1002/cncr.11468
36. Schiff R, Massarweh S, Shou J, Osborne CK (2003) Breast cancer endocrine resistance: how growth factor signaling and estrogen receptor coregulators modulate response. Clin Cancer Res 9(1 Pt 2):447S–454S
37. Spears M, Bartlett J (2009) The potential role of estrogen receptors and the SRC family as targets for the treatment of breast cancer. Expert Opin Ther Targets 13(6):665–674. https://doi.org/10.1517/14728220902911509
38. Arpino G, Wiechmann L, Osborne CK, Schiff R (2008) Crosstalk between the estrogen receptor and the HER tyrosine kinase receptor family: molecular mechanism and clinical implications for endocrine therapy resistance. Endocr Rev 29(2):217–233. https://doi.org/10.1210/er.2006-0045
39. Gutierrez MC, Detre S, Johnston S, Mohsin SK, Shou J, Allred DC, Schiff R, Osborne CK, Dowsett M (2005) Molecular changes in tamoxifen-resistant breast cancer: relationship between estrogen receptor, HER-2, and p38 mitogen-activated protein kinase. J Clin Oncol 23(11):2469–2476. https://doi.org/10.1200/JCO.2005.01.172
40. Shou J, Massarweh S, Osborne CK, Wakeling AE, Ali S, Weiss H, Schiff R (2004) Mechanisms of tamoxifen resistance: increased estrogen receptor-HER2/neu cross-talk in ER/HER2-positive breast cancer. J Natl Cancer Inst 96(12):926–935
41. Osborne CK, Shou J, Massarweh S, Schiff R (2005) Crosstalk between estrogen receptor and growth factor receptor pathways as a cause for endocrine therapy resistance in breast cancer. Clin Cancer Res 11(2 Pt 2):865s–870s
42. Giuliano M, Trivedi MV, Schiff R (2013) Bidirectional crosstalk between the estrogen receptor and human epidermal growth factor receptor 2 signaling pathways in breast cancer: molecular basis and clinical implications. Breast Care 8(4):256–262. https://doi.org/10.1159/000354253
43. Schettini F, Buono G, Cardalesi C, Desideri I, De Placido S, Del Mastro L (2016) Hormone receptor/human epidermal growth factor receptor 2-positive breast cancer: where we are now and where we are going. Cancer Treat Rev 46:20–26. https://doi.org/10.1016/j.ctrv.2016.03.012
44. De Laurentiis M, Arpino G, Massarelli E, Ruggiero A, Carlomagno C, Ciardiello F, Tortora G, D'Agostino D, Caputo F, Cancello G, Montagna E, Malorni L, Zinno L, Lauria R, Bianco

AR, De Placido S (2005) A meta-analysis on the interaction between HER-2 expression and response to endocrine treatment in advanced breast cancer. Clin Cancer Res 11(13):4741–4748. https://doi.org/10.1158/1078-0432.CCR-04-2569

45. Massarweh S, Osborne CK, Creighton CJ, Qin L, Tsimelzon A, Huang S, Weiss H, Rimawi M, Schiff R (2008) Tamoxifen resistance in breast tumors is driven by growth factor receptor signaling with repression of classic estrogen receptor genomic function. Cancer Res 68(3):826–833. https://doi.org/10.1158/0008-5472.CAN-07-2707

46. Massarweh S, Osborne CK, Jiang S, Wakeling AE, Rimawi M, Mohsin SK, Hilsenbeck S, Schiff R (2006) Mechanisms of tumor regression and resistance to estrogen deprivation and fulvestrant in a model of estrogen receptor-positive, HER-2/neu-positive breast cancer. Cancer Res 66(16):8266–8273. https://doi.org/10.1158/0008-5472.CAN-05-4045

47. Font de Mora J, Brown M (2000) AIB1 is a conduit for kinase-mediated growth factor signaling to the estrogen receptor. Mol Cell Biol 20(14):5041–5047

48. Britton DJ, Hutcheson IR, Knowlden JM, Barrow D, Giles M, McClelland RA, Gee JM, Nicholson RI (2006) Bidirectional cross talk between ERalpha and EGFR signalling pathways regulates tamoxifen-resistant growth. Breast Cancer Res Treat 96(2):131–146. https://doi.org/10.1007/s10549-005-9070-2

49. Dihge L, Bendahl PO, Grabau D, Isola J, Lovgren K, Ryden L, Ferno M (2008) Epidermal growth factor receptor (EGFR) and the estrogen receptor modulator amplified in breast cancer (AIB1) for predicting clinical outcome after adjuvant tamoxifen in breast cancer. Breast Cancer Res Treat 109(2):255–262. https://doi.org/10.1007/s10549-007-9645-1

50. Foley J, Nickerson NK, Nam S, Allen KT, Gilmore JL, Nephew KP, Riese DJ 2nd (2010) EGFR signaling in breast cancer: bad to the bone. Semin Cell Dev Biol 21(9):951–960. https://doi.org/10.1016/j.semcdb.2010.08.009

51. Fagan DH, Yee D (2008) Crosstalk between IGF1R and estrogen receptor signaling in breast cancer. J Mammary Gland Biol Neoplasia 13(4):423–429. https://doi.org/10.1007/s10911-008-9098-0

52. El-Ashry D, Chrysogelos SA, Lippman ME, Kern FG (1996) Estrogen induction of TGF-alpha is mediated by an estrogen response element composed of two imperfect palindromes. J Steroid Biochem Mol Biol 59(3–4):261–269

53. Wang X, Masri S, Phung S, Chen S (2008) The role of amphiregulin in exemestane-resistant breast cancer cells: evidence of an autocrine loop. Cancer Res 68(7):2259–2265. https://doi.org/10.1158/0008-5472.CAN-07-5544

54. Fan P, Agboke FA, Cunliffe HE, Ramos P, Jordan VC (2014) A molecular model for the mechanism of acquired tamoxifen resistance in breast cancer. Eur J Cancer 50(16):2866–2876. https://doi.org/10.1016/j.ejca.2014.08.011

55. Wilson MA, Chrysogelos SA (2002) Identification and characterization of a negative regulatory element within the epidermal growth factor receptor gene first intron in hormone-dependent breast cancer cells. J Cell Biochem 85(3):601–614. https://doi.org/10.1002/jcb.10168

56. Bailey ST, Westerling T, Brown M (2015) Loss of estrogen-regulated microRNA expression increases HER2 signaling and is prognostic of poor outcome in luminal breast cancer. Cancer Res 75(2):436–445. https://doi.org/10.1158/0008-5472.CAN-14-1041

57. Hutcheson IR, Goddard L, Barrow D, McClelland RA, Francies HE, Knowlden JM, Nicholson RI, Gee JM (2011) Fulvestrant-induced expression of ErbB3 and ErbB4 receptors sensitizes oestrogen receptor-positive breast cancer cells to heregulin beta1. Breast Cancer Res 13(2):R29. https://doi.org/10.1186/bcr2848

58. Zhang X, Diaz MR, Yee D (2013) Fulvestrant regulates epidermal growth factor (EGF) family ligands to activate EGF receptor (EGFR) signaling in breast cancer cells. Breast Cancer Res Treat 139(2):351–360. https://doi.org/10.1007/s10549-013-2541-y

59. Osborne CK, Neven P, Dirix LY, Mackey JR, Robert J, Underhill C, Schiff R, Gutierrez C, Migliaccio I, Anagnostou VK, Rimm DL, Magill P, Sellers M (2011) Gefitinib or placebo in combination with tamoxifen in patients with hormone receptor-positive metastatic

breast cancer: a randomized phase II study. Clin Cancer Res 17(5):1147–1159. https://doi.
org/10.1158/1078-0432.CCR-10-1869

60. Cristofanilli M, Valero V, Mangalik A, Royce M, Rabinowitz I, Arena FP, Kroener JF, Curcio
E, Watkins C, Bacus S, Cora EM, Anderson E, Magill PJ (2010) Phase II, randomized trial to
compare anastrozole combined with gefitinib or placebo in postmenopausal women with hormone receptor-positive metastatic breast cancer. Clin Cancer Res 16(6):1904–1914. https://
doi.org/10.1158/1078-0432.CCR-09-2282

61. Johnston S, Pippen J Jr, Pivot X, Lichinitser M, Sadeghi S, Dieras V, Gomez HL, Romieu G,
Manikhas A, Kennedy MJ, Press MF, Maltzman J, Florance A, O'Rourke L, Oliva C, Stein S,
Pegram M (2009) Lapatinib combined with letrozole versus letrozole and placebo as first-line
therapy for postmenopausal hormone receptor-positive metastatic breast cancer. J Clin Oncol
27(33):5538–5546. https://doi.org/10.1200/JCO.2009.23.3734

62. Finn RS, Press MF, Dering J, O'Rourke L, Florance A, Ellis C, Martin AM, Johnston S
(2014) Quantitative ER and PgR assessment as predictors of benefit from lapatinib in postmenopausal women with hormone receptor-positive, HER2-negative metastatic breast cancer. Clin Cancer Res 20(3):736–743. https://doi.org/10.1158/1078-0432.CCR-13-1260

63. Creighton CJ, Massarweh S, Huang S, Tsimelzon A, Hilsenbeck SG, Osborne CK, Shou
J, Malorni L, Schiff R (2008) Development of resistance to targeted therapies transforms
the clinically associated molecular profile subtype of breast tumor xenografts. Cancer Res
68(18):7493–7501. https://doi.org/10.1158/0008-5472.CAN-08-1404

64. Morrison G, Fu X, Shea M, Nanda S, Giuliano M, Wang T, Klinowska T, Osborne CK,
Rimawi MF, Schiff R (2014) Therapeutic potential of the dual EGFR/HER2 inhibitor
AZD8931 in circumventing endocrine resistance. Breast Cancer Res Treat 144(2):263–272.
https://doi.org/10.1007/s10549-014-2878-x

65. Bose R, Kavuri SM, Searleman AC, Shen W, Shen D, Koboldt DC, Monsey J, Goel N,
Aronson AB, Li S, Ma CX, Ding L, Mardis ER, Ellis MJ (2013) Activating HER2 mutations
in HER2 gene amplification negative breast cancer. Cancer Discov 3(2):224–237. https://doi.
org/10.1158/2159-8290.CD-12-0349

66. Ma CX, Bose R, Gao F, Freedman RA, Telli ML, Kimmick G, Winer E, Naughton M,
Goetz MP, Russell C, Tripathy D, Cobleigh M, Forero A, Pluard TJ, Anders C, Niravath
PA, Thomas S, Anderson J, Bumb C, Banks KC, Lanman RB, Bryce R, Lalani AS, Pfeifer
J, Hayes DF, Pegram M, Blackwell K, Bedard PL, Al-Kateb H, Ellis MJC (2017) Neratinib
efficacy and circulating tumor DNA detection of HER2 mutations in HER2 nonamplified
metastatic breast cancer. Clin Cancer Res 23(19):5687–5695. https://doi.org/10.1158/1078-
0432.CCR-17-0900

67. Ciriello G, Gatza ML, Beck AH, Wilkerson MD, Rhie SK, Pastore A, Zhang H, McLellan M,
Yau C, Kandoth C, Bowlby R, Shen H, Hayat S, Fieldhouse R, Lester SC, Tse GM, Factor
RE, Collins LC, Allison KH, Chen YY, Jensen K, Johnson NB, Oesterreich S, Mills GB,
Cherniack AD, Robertson G, Benz C, Sander C, Laird PW, Hoadley KA, King TA, Network
TR, Perou CM (2015) Comprehensive molecular portraits of invasive lobular breast cancer.
Cell 163(2):506–519. https://doi.org/10.1016/j.cell.2015.09.033

68. Hyman DM, Piha-Paul SA, Won H, Rodon J, Saura C, Shapiro GI, Juric D, Quinn DI,
Moreno V, Doger B, Mayer IA, Boni V, Calvo E, Loi S, Lockhart AC, Erinjeri JP, Scaltriti M,
Ulaner GA, Patel J, Tang J, Beer H, Selcuklu SD, Hanrahan AJ, Bouvier N, Melcer M, Murali
R, Schram AM, Smyth LM, Jhaveri K, Li BT, Drilon A, Harding JJ, Iyer G, Taylor BS,
Berger MF, Cutler RE Jr, Xu F, Butturini A, Eli LD, Mann G, Farrell C, Lalani AS, Bryce RP,
Arteaga CL, Meric-Bernstam F, Baselga J, Solit DB (2018) HER kinase inhibition in patients
with HER2- and HER3-mutant cancers. Nature 554(7691):189–194. https://doi.org/10.1038/
nature25475

69. Nayar U, Cohen O, Kapstad C, Waks A, Wander SA, Painter C, Freeman S, Ram P, Persky N,
Marini L, Helvie K, Oliver N, Ma CX, Winer EP, Lin NU, Wagle N (2018) Acquired HER2
mutations in ER+ metastatic breast cancer confer resistance to ER-directed therapies. In:
Proceedings of the American Association for Cancer Research Annual Meeting 2018. Cancer
Res 78(13 Suppl):Abstract nr 4952

70. Toy W, Weir H, Razavi P, Lawson M, Goeppert AU, Mazzola AM, Smith A, Wilson J, Morrow C, Wong WL, De Stanchina E, Carlson KE, Martin TS, Uddin S, Li Z, Fanning S, Katzenellenbogen JA, Greene G, Baselga J, Chandarlapaty S (2017) Activating ESR1 mutations differentially affect the efficacy of ER antagonists. Cancer Discov 7(3):277–287. https://doi.org/10.1158/2159-8290.CD-15-1523

71. Hyman DP-PS, Saura C, Arteaga C, Mayer I, Shapiro G, Loi S, Lalani A, Xu F, Cutler R, Butturini A, Bryce R, Meric-Bernstam F, Baselga J, Solit D (2017) Neratinib + fulvestrant in ERBB2-mutant, HER2–non-amplified, estrogen receptor (ER)-positive, metastatic breast cancer (MBC): preliminary analysis from the phase II SUMMIT trial. In: Proceedings of the 2016 San Antonio Breast Cancer Symposium. Cancer Res 77(4 Suppl):Abstract nr PD2-08

72. Yang Y, Yee D (2012) Targeting insulin and insulin-like growth factor signaling in breast cancer. J Mammary Gland Biol Neoplasia 17(3–4):251–261. https://doi.org/10.1007/s10911-012-9268-y

73. Christopoulos PF, Msaouel P, Koutsilieris M (2015) The role of the insulin-like growth factor-1 system in breast cancer. Mol Cancer 14:43. https://doi.org/10.1186/s12943-015-0291-7

74. Fox EM, Miller TW, Balko JM, Kuba MG, Sanchez V, Smith RA, Liu S, Gonzalez-Angulo AM, Mills GB, Ye F, Shyr Y, Manning HC, Buck E, Arteaga CL (2011) A kinome-wide screen identifies the insulin/IGF-I receptor pathway as a mechanism of escape from hormone dependence in breast cancer. Cancer Res 71(21):6773–6784. https://doi.org/10.1158/0008-5472.CAN-11-1295

75. Becker MA, Ibrahim YH, Cui X, Lee AV, Yee D (2011) The IGF pathway regulates ERalpha through a S6K1-dependent mechanism in breast cancer cells. Mol Endocrinol 25(3):516–528. https://doi.org/10.1210/me.2010-0373

76. Creighton CJ, Casa A, Lazard Z, Huang S, Tsimelzon A, Hilsenbeck SG, Osborne CK, Lee AV (2008) Insulin-like growth factor-I activates gene transcription programs strongly associated with poor breast cancer prognosis. J Clin Oncol 26(25):4078–4085. https://doi.org/10.1200/JCO.2007.13.4429

77. Farabaugh SM, Boone DN, Lee AV (2015) Role of IGF1R in breast cancer subtypes, stemness, and lineage differentiation. Front Endocrinol 6:59. https://doi.org/10.3389/fendo.2015.00059

78. Sisci D, Surmacz E (2007) Crosstalk between IGF signaling and steroid hormone receptors in breast cancer. Curr Pharm Des 13(7):705–717

79. Song RX, Chen Y, Zhang Z, Bao Y, Yue W, Wang JP, Fan P, Santen RJ (2010) Estrogen utilization of IGF-1-R and EGF-R to signal in breast cancer cells. J Steroid Biochem Mol Biol 118(4–5):219–230. https://doi.org/10.1016/j.jsbmb.2009.09.018

80. Fagan DH, Uselman RR, Sachdev D, Yee D (2012) Acquired resistance to tamoxifen is associated with loss of the type I insulin-like growth factor receptor: implications for breast cancer treatment. Cancer Res 72(13):3372–3380. https://doi.org/10.1158/0008-5472.CAN-12-0684

81. Martin LA, Pancholi S, Chan CM, Farmer I, Kimberley C, Dowsett M, Johnston SR (2005) The anti-oestrogen ICI 182,780, but not tamoxifen, inhibits the growth of MCF-7 breast cancer cells refractory to long-term oestrogen deprivation through down-regulation of oestrogen receptor and IGF signalling. Endocr Relat Cancer 12(4):1017–1036. https://doi.org/10.1677/erc.1.00905

82. Sachdev D, Li SL, Hartell JS, Fujita-Yamaguchi Y, Miller JS, Yee D (2003) A chimeric humanized single-chain antibody against the type I insulin-like growth factor (IGF) receptor renders breast cancer cells refractory to the mitogenic effects of IGF-I. Cancer Res 63(3):627–635

83. Singh P, Alex JM, Bast F (2014) Insulin receptor (IR) and insulin-like growth factor receptor 1 (IGF-1R) signaling systems: novel treatment strategies for cancer. Med Oncol 31(1):805. https://doi.org/10.1007/s12032-013-0805-3

84. Chen J, Nagle AM, Wang YF, Boone DN, Lee AV (2018) Controlled dimerization of insulin-like growth factor-1 and insulin receptors reveal shared and distinct activities of holo and hybrid receptors. J Biol Chem. https://doi.org/10.1074/jbc.M117.789503

85. Chakraborty A, Hatzis C, DiGiovanna MP (2017) Co-targeting the HER and IGF/insulin receptor axis in breast cancer, with triple targeting with endocrine therapy for hormone-sensitive disease. Breast Cancer Res Treat 163(1):37–50. https://doi.org/10.1007/s10549-017-4169-9

86. Fearon AE, Gould CR, Grose RP (2013) FGFR signalling in women's cancers. Int J Biochem Cell Biol 45(12):2832–2842. https://doi.org/10.1016/j.biocel.2013.09.017

87. Haugsten EM, Wiedlocha A, Olsnes S, Wesche J (2010) Roles of fibroblast growth factor receptors in carcinogenesis. Mol Cancer Res 8(11):1439–1452. https://doi.org/10.1158/1541-7786.MCR-10-0168

88. Helsten T, Elkin S, Arthur E, Tomson BN, Carter J, Kurzrock R (2016) The FGFR landscape in cancer: analysis of 4,853 tumors by next-generation sequencing. Clin Cancer Res 22(1):259–267. https://doi.org/10.1158/1078-0432.CCR-14-3212

89. Elbauomy Elsheikh S, Green AR, Lambros MB, Turner NC, Grainge MJ, Powe D, Ellis IO, Reis-Filho JS (2007) FGFR1 amplification in breast carcinomas: a chromogenic in situ hybridisation analysis. Breast Cancer Res 9(2):R23. https://doi.org/10.1186/bcr1665

90. Turner N, Pearson A, Sharpe R, Lambros M, Geyer F, Lopez-Garcia MA, Natrajan R, Marchio C, Iorns E, Mackay A, Gillett C, Grigoriadis A, Tutt A, Reis-Filho JS, Ashworth A (2010) FGFR1 amplification drives endocrine therapy resistance and is a therapeutic target in breast cancer. Cancer Res 70(5):2085–2094. https://doi.org/10.1158/0008-5472.CAN-09-3746

91. Turczyk L, Kitowska K, Mieszkowska M, Mieczkowski K, Czaplinska D, Piasecka D, Kordek R, Skladanowski AC, Potemski P, Romanska HM, Sadej R (2017) FGFR2-driven signaling counteracts tamoxifen effect on ERalpha-positive breast cancer cells. Neoplasia 19(10):791–804. https://doi.org/10.1016/j.neo.2017.07.006

92. Meijer D, Sieuwerts AM, Look MP, van Agthoven T, Foekens JA, Dorssers LC (2008) Fibroblast growth factor receptor 4 predicts failure on tamoxifen therapy in patients with recurrent breast cancer. Endocr Relat Cancer 15(1):101–111. https://doi.org/10.1677/ERC-07-0080

93. Brunello E, Brunelli M, Bogina G, Calio A, Manfrin E, Nottegar A, Vergine M, Molino A, Bria E, Massari F, Tortora G, Cingarlini S, Pedron S, Chilosi M, Zamboni G, Miller K, Martignoni G, Bonetti F (2012) FGFR-1 amplification in metastatic lymph-nodal and haematogenous lobular breast carcinoma. J Exp Clin Cancer Res 31:103. https://doi.org/10.1186/1756-9966-31-103

94. Sikora MJ, Cooper KL, Bahreini A, Luthra S, Wang G, Chandran UR, Davidson NE, Dabbs DJ, Welm AL, Oesterreich S (2014) Invasive lobular carcinoma cell lines are characterized by unique estrogen-mediated gene expression patterns and altered tamoxifen response. Cancer Res 74(5):1463–1474. https://doi.org/10.1158/0008-5472.CAN-13-2779

95. Formisano L, Stauffer KM, Young CD, Bhola NE, Guerrero-Zotano AL, Jansen VM, Estrada MM, Hutchinson KE, Giltnane JM, Schwarz LJ, Lu Y, Balko JM, Deas O, Cairo S, Judde JG, Mayer IA, Sanders M, Dugger TC, Bianco R, Stricker T, Arteaga CL (2017) Association of FGFR1 with ERalpha maintains ligand-independent ER transcription and mediates resistance to estrogen deprivation in ER(+) breast cancer. Clin Cancer Res 23(20):6138–6150. https://doi.org/10.1158/1078-0432.CCR-17-1232

96. Andre F, Bachelot T, Campone M, Dalenc F, Perez-Garcia JM, Hurvitz SA, Turner N, Rugo H, Smith JW, Deudon S, Shi M, Zhang Y, Kay A, Porta DG, Yovine A, Baselga J (2013) Targeting FGFR with dovitinib (TKI258): preclinical and clinical data in breast cancer. Clin Cancer Res 19(13):3693–3702. https://doi.org/10.1158/1078-0432.CCR-13-0190

97. Musolino A, Campone M, Neven P, Denduluri N, Barrios CH, Cortes J, Blackwell K, Soliman H, Kahan Z, Bonnefoi H, Squires M, Zhang Y, Deudon S, Shi MM, Andre F (2017) Phase II, randomized, placebo-controlled study of dovitinib in combination with fulvestrant in postmenopausal patients with HR(+), HER2(−) breast cancer that had progressed during or after prior endocrine therapy. Breast Cancer Res 19(1):18. https://doi.org/10.1186/s13058-017-0807-8

98. Papadopoulos KP, El-Rayes BF, Tolcher AW, Patnaik A, Rasco DW, Harvey RD, LoRusso PM, Sachdev JC, Abbadessa G, Savage RE, Hall T, Schwartz B, Wang Y, Kazakin J, Shaib WL (2017) A phase 1 study of ARQ 087, an oral pan-FGFR inhibitor in patients with advanced solid tumours. Br J Cancer 117(11):1592–1599. https://doi.org/10.1038/bjc.2017.330

99. Soria JC, DeBraud F, Bahleda R, Adamo B, Andre F, Dienstmann R, Delmonte A, Cereda R, Isaacson J, Litten J, Allen A, Dubois F, Saba C, Robert R, D'Incalci M, Zucchetti M, Camboni MG, Tabernero J (2014) Phase I/IIa study evaluating the safety, efficacy, pharmacokinetics, and pharmacodynamics of lucitanib in advanced solid tumors. Ann Oncol 25(11):2244–2251. https://doi.org/10.1093/annonc/mdu390

100. Babina IS, Turner NC (2017) Advances and challenges in targeting FGFR signalling in cancer. Nat Rev Cancer 17(5):318–332. https://doi.org/10.1038/nrc.2017.8

101. Pearson A, Smyth E, Babina IS, Herrera-Abreu MT, Tarazona N, Peckitt C, Kilgour E, Smith NR, Geh C, Rooney C, Cutts R, Campbell J, Ning J, Fenwick K, Swain A, Brown G, Chua S, Thomas A, Johnston SRD, Ajaz M, Sumpter K, Gillbanks A, Watkins D, Chau I, Popat S, Cunningham D, Turner NC (2016) High-level clonal FGFR amplification and response to FGFR inhibition in a translational clinical trial. Cancer Discov 6(8):838–851. https://doi.org/10.1158/2159-8290.CD-15-1246

102. Cortes J, Im SA, Holgado E, Perez-Garcia JM, Schmid P, Chavez-MacGregor M (2017) The next era of treatment for hormone receptor-positive, HER2-negative advanced breast cancer: triplet combination-based endocrine therapies. Cancer Treat Rev 61:53–60. https://doi.org/10.1016/j.ctrv.2017.09.011

103. Turner NC, Neven P, Loibl S, Andre F (2017) Advances in the treatment of advanced oestrogen-receptor-positive breast cancer. Lancet 389(10087):2403–2414. https://doi.org/10.1016/S0140-6736(16)32419-9

104. Mills GB, Kohn E, Lu Y, Eder A, Fang X, Wang H, Bast RC, Gray J, Jaffe R, Hortobagyi G (2003) Linking molecular diagnostics to molecular therapeutics: targeting the PI3K pathway in breast cancer. Semin Oncol 30(5 Suppl 16):93–104

105. Hennessy BT, Smith DL, Ram PT, Lu Y, Mills GB (2005) Exploiting the PI3K/AKT pathway for cancer drug discovery. Nat Rev Drug Discov 4(12):988–1004. https://doi.org/10.1038/nrd1902

106. Stemke-Hale K, Gonzalez-Angulo AM, Lluch A, Neve RM, Kuo WL, Davies M, Carey M, Hu Z, Guan Y, Sahin A, Symmans WF, Pusztai L, Nolden LK, Horlings H, Berns K, Hung MC, van de Vijver MJ, Valero V, Gray JW, Bernards R, Mills GB, Hennessy BT (2008) An integrative genomic and proteomic analysis of PIK3CA, PTEN, and AKT mutations in breast cancer. Cancer Res 68(15):6084–6091. https://doi.org/10.1158/0008-5472.CAN-07-6854

107. Ellis MJ, Lin L, Crowder R, Tao Y, Hoog J, Snider J, Davies S, DeSchryver K, Evans DB, Steinseifer J, Bandaru R, Liu W, Gardner H, Semiglazov V, Watson M, Hunt K, Olson J, Baselga J (2010) Phosphatidyl-inositol-3-kinase alpha catalytic subunit mutation and response to neoadjuvant endocrine therapy for estrogen receptor positive breast cancer. Breast Cancer Res Treat 119(2):379–390. https://doi.org/10.1007/s10549-009-0575-y

108. Campbell IG, Russell SE, Choong DY, Montgomery KG, Ciavarella ML, Hooi CS, Cristiano BE, Pearson RB, Phillips WA (2004) Mutation of the PIK3CA gene in ovarian and breast cancer. Cancer Res 64(21):7678–7681. https://doi.org/10.1158/0008-5472.CAN-04-2933

109. Cancer Genome Atlas Network (2012) Comprehensive molecular portraits of human breast tumours. Nature 490(7418):61–70. https://doi.org/10.1038/nature11412

110. Loi S, Haibe-Kains B, Majjaj S, Lallemand F, Durbecq V, Larsimont D, Gonzalez-Angulo AM, Pusztai L, Symmans WF, Bardelli A, Ellis P, Tutt AN, Gillett CE, Hennessy BT, Mills GB, Phillips WA, Piccart MJ, Speed TP, McArthur GA, Sotiriou C (2010) PIK3CA mutations associated with gene signature of low mTORC1 signaling and better outcomes in estrogen receptor-positive breast cancer. Proc Natl Acad Sci U S A 107(22):10208–10213. https://doi.org/10.1073/pnas.0907011107

111. Creighton CJ, Fu X, Hennessy BT, Casa AJ, Zhang Y, Gonzalez-Angulo AM, Lluch A, Gray JW, Brown PH, Hilsenbeck SG, Osborne CK, Mills GB, Lee AV, Schiff R (2010) Proteomic and transcriptomic profiling reveals a link between the PI3K pathway and lower estrogen-receptor (ER) levels and activity in ER+ breast cancer. Breast Cancer Res 12(3):R40. https://doi.org/10.1186/bcr2594

112. Miller TW, Perez-Torres M, Narasanna A, Guix M, Stal O, Perez-Tenorio G, Gonzalez-Angulo AM, Hennessy BT, Mills GB, Kennedy JP, Lindsley CW, Arteaga CL (2009) Loss of phosphatase and tensin homologue deleted on chromosome 10 engages ErbB3 and insulin-like growth factor-I receptor signaling to promote antiestrogen resistance in breast cancer. Cancer Res 69(10):4192–4201. https://doi.org/10.1158/0008-5472.CAN-09-0042

113. Miller TW, Hennessy BT, Gonzalez-Angulo AM, Fox EM, Mills GB, Chen H, Higham C, Garcia-Echeverria C, Shyr Y, Arteaga CL (2010) Hyperactivation of phosphatidylinositol-3 kinase promotes escape from hormone dependence in estrogen receptor-positive human breast cancer. J Clin Invest 120(7):2406–2413. https://doi.org/10.1172/JCI41680

114. Fu X, Creighton CJ, Biswal NC, Kumar V, Shea M, Herrera S, Contreras A, Gutierrez C, Wang T, Nanda S, Giuliano M, Morrison G, Nardone A, Karlin KL, Westbrook TF, Heiser LM, Anur P, Spellman P, Guichard SM, Smith PD, Davies BR, Klinowska T, Lee AV, Mills GB, Rimawi MF, Hilsenbeck SG, Gray JW, Joshi A, Osborne CK, Schiff R (2014) Overcoming endocrine resistance due to reduced PTEN levels in estrogen receptor-positive breast cancer by co-targeting mammalian target of rapamycin, protein kinase B, or mitogen-activated protein kinase kinase. Breast Cancer Res 16(5):430. https://doi.org/10.1186/s13058-014-0430-x

115. Toska E, Osmanbeyoglu HU, Castel P, Chan C, Hendrickson RC, Elkabets M, Dickler MN, Scaltriti M, Leslie CS, Armstrong SA, Baselga J (2017) PI3K pathway regulates ER-dependent transcription in breast cancer through the epigenetic regulator KMT2D. Science 355(6331):1324–1330. https://doi.org/10.1126/science.aah6893

116. Bosch A, Li Z, Bergamaschi A, Ellis H, Toska E, Prat A, Tao JJ, Spratt DE, Viola-Villegas NT, Castel P, Minuesa G, Morse N, Rodon J, Ibrahim Y, Cortes J, Perez-Garcia J, Galvan P, Grueso J, Guzman M, Katzenellenbogen JA, Kharas M, Lewis JS, Dickler M, Serra V, Rosen N, Chandarlapaty S, Scaltriti M, Baselga J (2015) PI3K inhibition results in enhanced estrogen receptor function and dependence in hormone receptor-positive breast cancer. Sci Transl Med 7(283):283ra251. https://doi.org/10.1126/scitranslmed.aaa4442

117. Vilquin P, Villedieu M, Grisard E, Ben Larbi S, Ghayad SE, Heudel PE, Bachelot T, Corbo L, Treilleux I, Vendrell JA, Cohen PA (2013) Molecular characterization of anastrozole resistance in breast cancer: pivotal role of the Akt/mTOR pathway in the emergence of de novo or acquired resistance and importance of combining the allosteric Akt inhibitor MK-2206 with an aromatase inhibitor. Int J Cancer 133(7):1589–1602. https://doi.org/10.1002/ijc.28182

118. Schettini F, Buono G, Trivedi MV, De Placido S, Arpino G, Giuliano M (2017) PI3K/mTOR inhibitors in the treatment of luminal breast cancer. Why, when and to whom? Breast Care 12(5):290–294. https://doi.org/10.1159/000481657

119. Ciruelos Gil EM (2014) Targeting the PI3K/AKT/mTOR pathway in estrogen receptor-positive breast cancer. Cancer Treat Rev 40(7):862–871. https://doi.org/10.1016/j.ctrv.2014.03.004

120. Zardavas D, Fumagalli D, Loi S (2012) Phosphatidylinositol 3-kinase/AKT/mammalian target of rapamycin pathway inhibition: a breakthrough in the management of luminal (ER+/HER2-) breast cancers? Curr Opin Oncol 24(6):623–634. https://doi.org/10.1097/CCO.0b013e328358a2b5

121. Agarwal R, Carey M, Hennessy B, Mills GB (2010) PI3K pathway-directed therapeutic strategies in cancer. Curr Opin Investig Drugs 11(6):615–628

122. Baselga J, Campone M, Piccart M, Burris HA 3rd, Rugo HS, Sahmoud T, Noguchi S, Gnant M, Pritchard KI, Lebrun F, Beck JT, Ito Y, Yardley D, Deleu I, Perez A, Bachelot T, Vittori L, Xu Z, Mukhopadhyay P, Lebwohl D, Hortobagyi GN (2012) Everolimus in postmenopausal hormone-receptor-positive advanced breast cancer. N Engl J Med 366(6):520–529. https://doi.org/10.1056/NEJMoa1109653

123. Bachelot T, Bourgier C, Cropet C, Ray-Coquard I, Ferrero JM, Freyer G, Abadie-Lacourtoisie S, Eymard JC, Debled M, Spaeth D, Legouffe E, Allouache D, El Kouri C, Pujade-Lauraine E (2012) Randomized phase II trial of everolimus in combination with tamoxifen in patients with hormone receptor-positive, human epidermal growth factor receptor 2-negative metastatic breast cancer with prior exposure to aromatase inhibitors: a GINECO study. J Clin Oncol 30(22):2718–2724. https://doi.org/10.1200/JCO.2011.39.0708

124. Zhang X, Li XR, Zhang J (2013) Current status and future perspectives of PI3K and mTOR inhibitor as anticancer drugs in breast cancer. Curr Cancer Drug Targets 13(2):175–187

125. Baselga JDS, Cortés H et al (2018) Phase III study of taselisib (GDC-0032) + fulvestrant (FULV) v FULV in patients (pts) with estrogen receptor (ER)-positive, PIK3CA-mutant (MUT), locally advanced or metastatic breast cancer (MBC): primary analysis from SANDPIPER. In: Proceedings of the 2018 ASCO Annual Meeting. J Clin Oncol suppl:abstr LBA1006

126. Dickler MN, Saura C, Richards D, Krop I, Cervantes A, Bedard PL, Patel MR, Pusztai L, Oliveira M, Cardenas AK, Cui N, Wilson TR, Stout TJ, Wei MC, Hsu JY, Baselga J (2018) Phase II study of taselisib (GDC0032) in combination with fulvestrant in patients with HER2-negative, hormone receptor-positive advanced breast cancer. Clin Cancer Res. https://doi.org/10.1158/1078-0432.CCR-18-0613

127. Courtois-Cox S, Genther Williams SM, Reczek EE, Johnson BW, McGillicuddy LT, Johannessen CM, Hollstein PE, MacCollin M, Cichowski K (2006) A negative feedback signaling network underlies oncogene-induced senescence. Cancer Cell 10(6):459–472. https://doi.org/10.1016/j.ccr.2006.10.003

128. Gluck S (2017) Consequences of the convergence of multiple alternate pathways on the estrogen receptor in the treatment of metastatic breast cancer. Clin Breast Cancer 17(2):79–90. https://doi.org/10.1016/j.clbc.2016.08.004

129. O'Reilly KE, Rojo F, She QB, Solit D, Mills GB, Smith D, Lane H, Hofmann F, Hicklin DJ, Ludwig DL, Baselga J, Rosen N (2006) mTOR inhibition induces upstream receptor tyrosine kinase signaling and activates Akt. Cancer Res 66(3):1500–1508. https://doi.org/10.1158/0008-5472.CAN-05-2925

130. Fu X, Osborne CK, Schiff R (2013) Biology and therapeutic potential of PI3K signaling in ER+/HER2-negative breast cancer. Breast 22(Suppl 2):S12–S18. https://doi.org/10.1016/j.breast.2013.08.001

131. Huang H, Tindall DJ (2007) Dynamic FoxO transcription factors. J Cell Sci 120(Pt 15):2479–2487. https://doi.org/10.1242/jcs.001222

132. Chandarlapaty S, Sawai A, Scaltriti M, Rodrik-Outmezguine V, Grbovic-Huezo O, Serra V, Majumder PK, Baselga J, Rosen N (2011) AKT inhibition relieves feedback suppression of receptor tyrosine kinase expression and activity. Cancer Cell 19(1):58–71. https://doi.org/10.1016/j.ccr.2010.10.031

133. Chakrabarty A, Sanchez V, Kuba MG, Rinehart C, Arteaga CL (2012) Feedback upregulation of HER3 (ErbB3) expression and activity attenuates antitumor effect of PI3K inhibitors. Proc Natl Acad Sci U S A 109(8):2718–2723. https://doi.org/10.1073/pnas.1018001108

134. Loi S, Michiels S, Baselga J, Bartlett JM, Singhal SK, Sabine VS, Sims AH, Sahmoud T, Dixon JM, Piccart MJ, Sotiriou C (2013) PIK3CA genotype and a PIK3CA mutation-related gene signature and response to everolimus and letrozole in estrogen receptor positive breast cancer. PLoS One 8(1):e53292. https://doi.org/10.1371/journal.pone.0053292

135. Raman M, Chen W, Cobb MH (2007) Differential regulation and properties of MAPKs. Oncogene 26(22):3100–3112. https://doi.org/10.1038/sj.onc.1210392

136. Seger R, Krebs EG (1995) The MAPK signaling cascade. FASEB J 9(9):726–735

137. Yao Z, Seger R (2009) The ERK signaling cascade--views from different subcellular compartments. Biofactors 35(5):407–416. https://doi.org/10.1002/biof.52

138. Thomas RS, Sarwar N, Phoenix F, Coombes RC, Ali S (2008) Phosphorylation at serines 104 and 106 by Erk1/2 MAPK is important for estrogen receptor-alpha activity. J Mol Endocrinol 40(4):173–184. https://doi.org/10.1677/JME-07-0165

139. Creighton CJ, Hilger AM, Murthy S, Rae JM, Chinnaiyan AM, El-Ashry D (2006) Activation of mitogen-activated protein kinase in estrogen receptor alpha-positive breast cancer cells in vitro induces an in vivo molecular phenotype of estrogen receptor alpha-negative human breast tumors. Cancer Res 66(7):3903–3911. https://doi.org/10.1158/0008-5472.CAN-05-4363

140. Kato S, Endoh H, Masuhiro Y, Kitamoto T, Uchiyama S, Sasaki H, Masushige S, Gotoh Y, Nishida E, Kawashima H, Metzger D, Chambon P (1995) Activation of the estrogen receptor through phosphorylation by mitogen-activated protein kinase. Science 270(5241):1491–1494

141. Mendes-Pereira AM, Sims D, Dexter T, Fenwick K, Assiotis I, Kozarewa I, Mitsopoulos C, Hakas J, Zvelebil M, Lord CJ, Ashworth A (2012) Genome-wide functional screen identifies a compendium of genes affecting sensitivity to tamoxifen. Proc Natl Acad Sci U S A 109(8):2730–2735. https://doi.org/10.1073/pnas.1018872108

142. Wallace MD, Pfefferle AD, Shen L, McNairn AJ, Cerami EG, Fallon BL, Rinaldi VD, Southard TL, Perou CM, Schimenti JC (2012) Comparative oncogenomics implicates the neurofibromin 1 gene (NF1) as a breast cancer driver. Genetics 192(2):385–396. https://doi.org/10.1534/genetics.112.142802

143. Martin LA, Farmer I, Johnston SR, Ali S, Dowsett M (2005) Elevated ERK1/ERK2/estrogen receptor cross-talk enhances estrogen-mediated signaling during long-term estrogen deprivation. Endocr Relat Cancer 12(Suppl 1):S75–S84. https://doi.org/10.1677/erc.1.01023

144. Stires H, Heckler MM, Fu X, Li Z, Grasso CS, Quist MJ, Lewis JA, Klimach U, Zwart A, Mahajan A, Gyorffy B, Cavalli LR, Riggins RB (2017) Integrated molecular analysis of tamoxifen-resistant invasive lobular breast cancer cells identifies MAPK and GRM/mGluR signaling as therapeutic vulnerabilities. Mol Cell Endocrinol. https://doi.org/10.1016/j.mce.2017.09.024

145. Marino M, Galluzzo P, Ascenzi P (2006) Estrogen signaling multiple pathways to impact gene transcription. Curr Genomics 7(8):497–508

146. Zhong SP, Ma WY, Dong Z (2000) ERKs and p38 kinases mediate ultraviolet B-induced phosphorylation of histone H3 at serine 10. J Biol Chem 275(28):20980–20984. https://doi.org/10.1074/jbc.M909934199

147. Rao PS, Satelli A, Zhang S, Srivastava SK, Srivenugopal KS, Rao US (2009) RNF2 is the target for phosphorylation by the p38 MAPK and ERK signaling pathways. Proteomics 9(10):2776–2787. https://doi.org/10.1002/pmic.200800847

148. Antoon JW, Martin EC, Lai R, Salvo VA, Tang Y, Nitzchke AM, Elliott S, Nam SY, Xiong W, Rhodes LV, Collins-Burow B, David O, Wang G, Shan B, Beckman BS, Nephew KP, Burow ME (2013) MEK5/ERK5 signaling suppresses estrogen receptor expression and promotes hormone-independent tumorigenesis. PLoS One 8(8):e69291. https://doi.org/10.1371/journal.pone.0069291

149. Madak-Erdogan Z, Lupien M, Stossi F, Brown M, Katzenellenbogen BS (2011) Genomic collaboration of estrogen receptor alpha and extracellular signal-regulated kinase 2 in regulating gene and proliferation programs. Mol Cell Biol 31(1):226–236. https://doi.org/10.1128/MCB.00821-10

150. Madak-Erdogan Z, Ventrella R, Petry L, Katzenellenbogen BS (2014) Novel roles for ERK5 and cofilin as critical mediators linking ERalpha-driven transcription, actin reorganization, and invasiveness in breast cancer. Mol Cancer Res 12(5):714–727. https://doi.org/10.1158/1541-7786.MCR-13-0588

151. Bayliss J, Hilger A, Vishnu P, Diehl K, El-Ashry D (2007) Reversal of the estrogen receptor negative phenotype in breast cancer and restoration of antiestrogen response. Clin Cancer Res 13(23):7029–7036. https://doi.org/10.1158/1078-0432.CCR-07-0587

152. Polo ML, Arnoni MV, Riggio M, Wargon V, Lanari C, Novaro V (2010) Responsiveness to PI3K and MEK inhibitors in breast cancer. Use of a 3D culture system to study pathways related to hormone independence in mice. PLoS One 5(5):e10786. https://doi.org/10.1371/journal.pone.0010786

153. Zaman K, Winterhalder R, Mamot C, Hasler-Strub U, Rochlitz C, Mueller A, Berset C, Wiliders H, Perey L, Rudolf CB, Hawle H, Rondeau S, Neven P (2015) Fulvestrant with or without selumetinib, a MEK 1/2 inhibitor, in breast cancer progressing after aromatase inhibitor therapy: a multicentre randomised placebo-controlled double-blind phase II trial, SAKK 21/08. Eur J Cancer 51(10):1212–1220. https://doi.org/10.1016/j.ejca.2015.03.016

154. Playford MP, Schaller MD (2004) The interplay between Src and integrins in normal and tumor biology. Oncogene 23(48):7928–7946. https://doi.org/10.1038/sj.onc.1208080

155. Pontiggia O, Sampayo R, Raffo D, Motter A, Xu R, Bissell MJ, Joffe EB, Simian M (2012) The tumor microenvironment modulates tamoxifen resistance in breast cancer: a role for soluble stromal factors and fibronectin through beta1 integrin. Breast Cancer Res Treat 133(2):459–471. https://doi.org/10.1007/s10549-011-1766-x

156. Bon G, Folgiero V, Bossi G, Felicioni L, Marchetti A, Sacchi A, Falcioni R (2006) Loss of beta4 integrin subunit reduces the tumorigenicity of MCF7 mammary cells and causes apoptosis upon hormone deprivation. Clin Cancer Res 12(11 Pt 1):3280–3287. https://doi.org/10.1158/1078-0432.CCR-05-2223

157. Nistico P, Di Modugno F, Spada S, Bissell MJ (2014) β1 and β4 integrins: from breast development to clinical practice. Breast Cancer Res 16(5):459

158. Schlaepfer DD, Mitra SK, Ilic D (2004) Control of motile and invasive cell phenotypes by focal adhesion kinase. Biochim Biophys Acta 1692(2–3):77–102. https://doi.org/10.1016/j.bbamcr.2004.04.008

159. Frei A, MacDonald G, Lund I, Gustafsson JA, Hynes NE, Nalvarte I (2016) Memo interacts with c-Src to control estrogen receptor alpha sub-cellular localization. Oncotarget 7(35):56170–56182. https://doi.org/10.18632/oncotarget.10856

160. Chakravarty D, Nair SS, Santhamma B, Nair BC, Wang L, Bandyopadhyay A, Agyin JK, Brann D, Sun LZ, Yeh IT, Lee FY, Tekmal RR, Kumar R, Vadlamudi RK (2010) Extranuclear functions of ER impact invasive migration and metastasis by breast cancer cells. Cancer Res 70(10):4092–4101. https://doi.org/10.1158/0008-5472.CAN-09-3834

161. Hiscox S, Morgan L, Green TP, Barrow D, Gee J, Nicholson RI (2006) Elevated Src activity promotes cellular invasion and motility in tamoxifen resistant breast cancer cells. Breast Cancer Res Treat 97(3):263–274. https://doi.org/10.1007/s10549-005-9120-9

162. Hiscox S, Jordan NJ, Morgan L, Green TP, Nicholson RI (2007) Src kinase promotes adhesion-independent activation of FAK and enhances cellular migration in tamoxifen-resistant breast cancer cells. Clin Exp Metastasis 24(3):157–167. https://doi.org/10.1007/s10585-007-9065-y

163. Planas-Silva MD, Bruggeman RD, Grenko RT, Stanley Smith J (2006) Role of c-Src and focal adhesion kinase in progression and metastasis of estrogen receptor-positive breast cancer. Biochem Biophys Res Commun 341(1):73–81. https://doi.org/10.1016/j.bbrc.2005.12.164

164. Morgan L, Gee J, Pumford S, Farrow L, Finlay P, Robertson J, Ellis I, Kawakatsu H, Nicholson R, Hiscox S (2009) Elevated Src kinase activity attenuates tamoxifen response in vitro and is associated with poor prognosis clinically. Cancer Biol Ther 8(16):1550–1558

165. Schwarz LJ, Fox EM, Balko JM, Garrett JT, Kuba MG, Estrada MV, Gonzalez-Angulo AM, Mills GB, Red-Brewer M, Mayer IA, Abramson V, Rizzo M, Kelley MC, Meszoely IM, Arteaga CL (2014) LYN-activating mutations mediate antiestrogen resistance in estrogen receptor-positive breast cancer. J Clin Invest 124(12):5490–5502. https://doi.org/10.1172/JCI72573

166. Ojo D, Wei F, Liu Y, Wang E, Zhang H, Lin X, Wong N, Bane A, Tang D (2015) Factors promoting tamoxifen resistance in breast cancer via stimulating breast cancer stem cell expansion. Curr Med Chem 22(19):2360–2374

167. Hiscox S, Jordan NJ, Smith C, James M, Morgan L, Taylor KM, Green TP, Nicholson RI (2009) Dual targeting of Src and ER prevents acquired antihormone resistance in breast cancer cells. Breast Cancer Res Treat 115(1):57–67. https://doi.org/10.1007/s10549-008-0058-6

168. Guest SK, Ribas R, Pancholi S, Nikitorowicz-Buniak J, Simigdala N, Dowsett M, Johnston SR, Martin LA (2016) Src is a potential therapeutic target in endocrine-resistant breast cancer exhibiting low estrogen receptor-mediated transactivation. PLoS One 11(6):e0157397. https://doi.org/10.1371/journal.pone.0157397

169. Mayer EL, Baurain JF, Sparano J, Strauss L, Campone M, Fumoleau P, Rugo H, Awada A, Sy O, Llombart-Cussac A (2011) A phase 2 trial of dasatinib in patients with advanced HER2-positive and/or hormone receptor-positive breast cancer. Clin Cancer Res 17(21):6897–6904. https://doi.org/10.1158/1078-0432.CCR-11-0070

170. Herold CI, Chadaram V, Peterson BL, Marcom PK, Hopkins J, Kimmick GG, Favaro J, Hamilton E, Welch RA, Bacus S, Blackwell KL (2011) Phase II trial of dasatinib in patients

with metastatic breast cancer using real-time pharmacodynamic tissue biomarkers of Src inhibition to escalate dosing. Clin Cancer Res 17(18):6061–6070. https://doi.org/ 10.1158/1078-0432.CCR-11-1071

171. Kang Y, Hu W, Ivan C, Dalton HJ, Miyake T, Pecot CV, Zand B, Liu T, Huang J, Jennings NB, Rupaimoole R, Taylor M, Pradeep S, Wu SY, Lu C, Wen Y, Huang J, Liu J, Sood AK (2013) Role of focal adhesion kinase in regulating YB-1-mediated paclitaxel resistance in ovarian cancer. J Natl Cancer Inst 105(19):1485–1495. https://doi.org/10.1093/jnci/djt210

172. Johnston SR, Lu B, Scott GK, Kushner PJ, Smith IE, Dowsett M, Benz CC (1999) Increased activator protein-1 DNA binding and c-Jun NH2-terminal kinase activity in human breast tumors with acquired tamoxifen resistance. Clin Cancer Res 5(2):251–256

173. Schiff R, Reddy P, Ahotupa M, Coronado-Heinsohn E, Grim M, Hilsenbeck SG, Lawrence R, Deneke S, Herrera R, Chamness GC, Fuqua SA, Brown PH, Osborne CK (2000) Oxidative stress and AP-1 activity in tamoxifen-resistant breast tumors in vivo. J Natl Cancer Inst 92(23):1926–1934

174. Wu RC, Qin J, Yi P, Wong J, Tsai SY, Tsai MJ, O'Malley BW (2004) Selective phosphorylations of the SRC-3/AIB1 coactivator integrate genomic responses to multiple cellular signaling pathways. Mol Cell 15(6):937–949. https://doi.org/10.1016/j.molcel.2004.08.019

175. Hibi M, Lin A, Smeal T, Minden A, Karin M (1993) Identification of an oncoprotein- and UV-responsive protein kinase that binds and potentiates the c-Jun activation domain. Genes Dev 7(11):2135–2148

176. Shaulian E (2010) AP-1--the Jun proteins: oncogenes or tumor suppressors in disguise? Cell Signal 22(6):894–899. https://doi.org/10.1016/j.cellsig.2009.12.008

177. Malorni L, Giuliano M, Migliaccio I, Wang T, Creighton CJ, Lupien M, Fu X, Hilsenbeck SG, Healy N, De Angelis C, Mazumdar A, Trivedi MV, Massarweh S, Gutierrez C, De Placido S, Jeselsohn R, Brown M, Brown PH, Osborne CK, Schiff R (2016) Blockade of AP-1 potentiates endocrine therapy and overcomes resistance. Mol Cancer Res 14(5):470–481. https:// doi.org/10.1158/1541-7786.MCR-15-0423

178. He H, Sinha I, Fan R, Haldosen LA, Yan F, Zhao C, Dahlman-Wright K (2018) c-Jun/AP-1 overexpression reprograms ERalpha signaling related to tamoxifen response in ERalpha-positive breast cancer. Oncogene. https://doi.org/10.1038/s41388-018-0165-8

179. Chen LF, Greene WC (2004) Shaping the nuclear action of NF-kappaB. Nat Rev Mol Cell Biol 5(5):392–401. https://doi.org/10.1038/nrm1368

180. Karin M, Cao Y, Greten FR, Li ZW (2002) NF-kappaB in cancer: from innocent bystander to major culprit. Nat Rev Cancer 2(4):301–310. https://doi.org/10.1038/nrc780

181. Bennett L, Quinn J, McCall P, Mallon EA, Horgan PG, McMillan DC, Paul A, Edwards J (2017) High IKKalpha expression is associated with reduced time to recurrence and cancer specific survival in oestrogen receptor (ER)-positive breast cancer. Int J Cancer 140(7):1633–1644. https://doi.org/10.1002/ijc.30578

182. Van Laere SJ, Van der Auwera I, Van den Eynden GG, van Dam P, Van Marck EA, Vermeulen PB, Dirix LY (2007) NF-kappaB activation in inflammatory breast cancer is associated with oestrogen receptor downregulation, secondary to EGFR and/or ErbB2 overexpression and MAPK hyperactivation. Br J Cancer 97(5):659–669. https://doi.org/10.1038/sj.bjc.6603906

183. Van Laere SJ, Van der Auwera I, Van den Eynden GG, Elst HJ, Weyler J, Harris AL, van Dam P, Van Marck EA, Vermeulen PB, Dirix LY (2006) Nuclear factor-kappaB signature of inflammatory breast cancer by cDNA microarray validated by quantitative real-time reverse transcription-PCR, immunohistochemistry, and nuclear factor-kappaB DNA-binding. Clin Cancer Res 12(11 Pt 1):3249–3256. https://doi.org/10.1158/1078-0432.CCR-05-2800

184. Ghisletti S, Meda C, Maggi A, Vegeto E (2005) 17beta-estradiol inhibits inflammatory gene expression by controlling NF-kappaB intracellular localization. Mol Cell Biol 25(8):2957–2968. https://doi.org/10.1128/MCB.25.8.2957-2968.2005

185. Jones RL, Rojo F, A'Hern R, Villena N, Salter J, Corominas JM, Servitja S, Smith IE, Rovira A, Reis-Filho JS, Dowsett M, Albanell J (2011) Nuclear NF-kappaB/p65 expression and response to neoadjuvant chemotherapy in breast cancer. J Clin Pathol 64(2):130–135. https:// doi.org/10.1136/jcp.2010.082966

186. Montagut C, Tusquets I, Ferrer B, Corominas JM, Bellosillo B, Campas C, Suarez M, Fabregat X, Campo E, Gascon P, Serrano S, Fernandez PL, Rovira A, Albanell J (2006) Activation of nuclear factor-kappa B is linked to resistance to neoadjuvant chemotherapy in breast cancer patients. Endocr Relat Cancer 13(2):607–616. https://doi.org/10.1677/erc.1.01171

187. Zhou Y, Eppenberger-Castori S, Marx C, Yau C, Scott GK, Eppenberger U, Benz CC (2005) Activation of nuclear factor-kappaB (NFkappaB) identifies a high-risk subset of hormone-dependent breast cancers. Int J Biochem Cell Biol 37(5):1130–1144. https://doi.org/10.1016/j.biocel.2004.09.006

188. Paimela T, Ryhanen T, Mannermaa E, Ojala J, Kalesnykas G, Salminen A, Kaarniranta K (2007) The effect of 17beta-estradiol on IL-6 secretion and NF-kappaB DNA-binding activity in human retinal pigment epithelial cells. Immunol Lett 110(2):139–144. https://doi.org/10.1016/j.imlet.2007.04.008

189. Nettles KW, Gil G, Nowak J, Metivier R, Sharma VB, Greene GL (2008) CBP is a dosage-dependent regulator of nuclear factor-kappaB suppression by the estrogen receptor. Mol Endocrinol 22(2):263–272. https://doi.org/10.1210/me.2007-0324

190. Frasor J, El-Shennawy L, Stender JD, Kastrati I (2015) NFkappaB affects estrogen receptor expression and activity in breast cancer through multiple mechanisms. Mol Cell Endocrinol 418(Pt 3):235–239. https://doi.org/10.1016/j.mce.2014.09.013

191. Belguise K, Sonenshein GE (2007) PKCtheta promotes c-Rel-driven mammary tumorigenesis in mice and humans by repressing estrogen receptor alpha synthesis. J Clin Invest 117(12):4009–4021. https://doi.org/10.1172/JCI32424

192. Frasor J, Weaver A, Pradhan M, Dai Y, Miller LD, Lin CY, Stanculescu A (2009) Positive cross-talk between estrogen receptor and NF-kappaB in breast cancer. Cancer Res 69(23):8918–8925. https://doi.org/10.1158/0008-5472.CAN-09-2608

193. Frasor J, Weaver AE, Pradhan M, Mehta K (2008) Synergistic up-regulation of prostaglandin E synthase expression in breast cancer cells by 17beta-estradiol and proinflammatory cytokines. Endocrinology 149(12):6272–6279. https://doi.org/10.1210/en.2008-0352

194. Pradhan M, Bembinster LA, Baumgarten SC, Frasor J (2010) Proinflammatory cytokines enhance estrogen-dependent expression of the multidrug transporter gene ABCG2 through estrogen receptor and NF{kappa}B cooperativity at adjacent response elements. J Biol Chem 285(41):31100–31106. https://doi.org/10.1074/jbc.M110.155309

195. Rubio MF, Werbajh S, Cafferata EG, Quaglino A, Colo GP, Nojek IM, Kordon EC, Nahmod VE, Costas MA (2006) TNF-alpha enhances estrogen-induced cell proliferation of estrogen-dependent breast tumor cells through a complex containing nuclear factor-kappa B. Oncogene 25(9):1367–1377. https://doi.org/10.1038/sj.onc.1209176

196. Riggins RB, Zwart A, Nehra R, Clarke R (2005) The nuclear factor kappa B inhibitor parthenolide restores ICI 182,780 (faslodex; fulvestrant)-induced apoptosis in antiestrogen-resistant breast cancer cells. Mol Cancer Ther 4(1):33–41

197. deGraffenried LA, Chandrasekar B, Friedrichs WE, Donzis E, Silva J, Hidalgo M, Freeman JW, Weiss GR (2004) NF-kappa B inhibition markedly enhances sensitivity of resistant breast cancer tumor cells to tamoxifen. Ann Oncol 15(6):885–890

198. Trinh XB, Sas L, Van Laere SJ, Prove A, Deleu I, Rasschaert M, Van de Velde H, Vinken P, Vermeulen PB, Van Dam PA, Wojtasik A, De Mesmaeker P, Tjalma WA, Dirix LY (2012) A phase II study of the combination of endocrine treatment and bortezomib in patients with endocrine-resistant metastatic breast cancer. Oncol Rep 27(3):657–663. https://doi.org/10.3892/or.2011.1562

199. Trocoli A, Djavaheri-Mergny M (2011) The complex interplay between autophagy and NF-kappaB signaling pathways in cancer cells. Am J Cancer Res 1(5):629–649

200. Cook KL, Shajahan AN, Clarke R (2011) Autophagy and endocrine resistance in breast cancer. Expert Rev Anticancer Ther 11(8):1283–1294. https://doi.org/10.1586/era.11.111

201. Yu X, Luo A, Liu Y, Wang S, Li Y, Shi W, Liu Z, Qu X (2015) MiR-214 increases the sensitivity of breast cancer cells to tamoxifen and fulvestrant through inhibition of autophagy. Mol Cancer 14:208. https://doi.org/10.1186/s12943-015-0480-4

202. Hanahan D, Weinberg RA (2000) The hallmarks of cancer. Cell 100(1):57–70
203. Colleoni B, Paternot S, Pita JM, Bisteau X, Coulonval K, Davis RJ, Raspe E, Roger PP (2017) JNKs function as CDK4-activating kinases by phosphorylating CDK4 and p21. Oncogene 36(30):4349–4361. https://doi.org/10.1038/onc.2017.7
204. Thangavel C, Dean JL, Ertel A, Knudsen KE, Aldaz CM, Witkiewicz AK, Clarke R, Knudsen ES (2011) Therapeutically activating RB: reestablishing cell cycle control in endocrine therapy-resistant breast cancer. Endocr Relat Cancer 18(3):333–345. https://doi.org/10.1530/ERC-10-0262
205. Musgrove EA, Sutherland RL (2009) Biological determinants of endocrine resistance in breast cancer. Nat Rev Cancer 9(9):631–643. https://doi.org/10.1038/nrc2713
206. Butt AJ, McNeil CM, Musgrove EA, Sutherland RL (2005) Downstream targets of growth factor and oestrogen signalling and endocrine resistance: the potential roles of c-Myc, cyclin D1 and cyclin E. Endocr Relat Cancer 12(Suppl 1):S47–S59. https://doi.org/10.1677/erc.1.00993
207. Shah AN, Cristofanilli M (2017) The growing role of CDK4/6 inhibitors in treating hormone receptor-positive advanced breast cancer. Curr Treat Options in Oncol 18(1):6. https://doi.org/10.1007/s11864-017-0443-7
208. Eeckhoute J, Carroll JS, Geistlinger TR, Torres-Arzayus MI, Brown M (2006) A cell-type-specific transcriptional network required for estrogen regulation of cyclin D1 and cell cycle progression in breast cancer. Genes Dev 20(18):2513–2526. https://doi.org/10.1101/gad.1446006
209. Wilcken NR, Prall OW, Musgrove EA, Sutherland RL (1997) Inducible overexpression of cyclin D1 in breast cancer cells reverses the growth-inhibitory effects of antiestrogens. Clin Cancer Res 3(6):849–854
210. Kenny FS, Hui R, Musgrove EA, Gee JM, Blamey RW, Nicholson RI, Sutherland RL, Robertson JF (1999) Overexpression of cyclin D1 messenger RNA predicts for poor prognosis in estrogen receptor-positive breast cancer. Clin Cancer Res 5(8):2069–2076
211. Zwijsen RM, Buckle RS, Hijmans EM, Loomans CJ, Bernards R (1998) Ligand-independent recruitment of steroid receptor coactivators to estrogen receptor by cyclin D1. Genes Dev 12(22):3488–3498
212. Chu IM, Hengst L, Slingerland JM (2008) The Cdk inhibitor p27 in human cancer: prognostic potential and relevance to anticancer therapy. Nat Rev Cancer 8(4):253–267. https://doi.org/10.1038/nrc2347
213. Perez-Tenorio G, Berglund F, Esguerra Merca A, Nordenskjold B, Rutqvist LE, Skoog L, Stal O (2006) Cytoplasmic p21WAF1/CIP1 correlates with Akt activation and poor response to tamoxifen in breast cancer. Int J Oncol 28(5):1031–1042
214. Ertel A, Dean JL, Rui H, Liu C, Witkiewicz AK, Knudsen KE, Knudsen ES (2010) RB-pathway disruption in breast cancer: differential association with disease subtypes, disease-specific prognosis and therapeutic response. Cell Cycle 9(20):4153–4163. https://doi.org/10.4161/cc.9.20.13454
215. Miller TW, Balko JM, Fox EM, Ghazoui Z, Dunbier A, Anderson H, Dowsett M, Jiang A, Smith RA, Maira SM, Manning HC, Gonzalez-Angulo AM, Mills GB, Higham C, Chanthaphaychith S, Kuba MG, Miller WR, Shyr Y, Arteaga CL (2011) ERalpha-dependent E2F transcription can mediate resistance to estrogen deprivation in human breast cancer. Cancer Discov 1(4):338–351. https://doi.org/10.1158/2159-8290.CD-11-0101
216. Finn RS, Dering J, Conklin D, Kalous O, Cohen DJ, Desai AJ, Ginther C, Atefi M, Chen I, Fowst C, Los G, Slamon DJ (2009) PD 0332991, a selective cyclin D kinase 4/6 inhibitor, preferentially inhibits proliferation of luminal estrogen receptor-positive human breast cancer cell lines in vitro. Breast Cancer Res 11(5):R77. https://doi.org/10.1186/bcr2419
217. Cruz M, Reinert T, Cristofanilli M (2017) Emerging innovative therapeutic approaches leveraging cyclin-dependent kinase inhibitors to treat advanced breast cancer. Clin Pharmacol Ther. https://doi.org/10.1002/cpt.965

218. Garrido-Castro AC, Goel S (2017) CDK4/6 inhibition in breast cancer: mechanisms of response and treatment failure. Curr Breast Cancer Rep 9(1):26–33. https://doi.org/10.1007/s12609-017-0232-0

219. Liu M, Liu H, Chen J (2018) Mechanisms of the CDK4/6 inhibitor palbociclib (PD 0332991) and its future application in cancer treatment (review). Oncol Rep 39(3):901–911. https://doi.org/10.3892/or.2018.6221

220. Nardone A, De Angelis C, Trivedi MV, Osborne CK, Schiff R (2015) The changing role of ER in endocrine resistance. Breast 24(Suppl 2):S60–S66. https://doi.org/10.1016/j.breast.2015.07.015

221. Ross-Innes CS, Stark R, Teschendorff AE, Holmes KA, Ali HR, Dunning MJ, Brown GD, Gojis O, Ellis IO, Green AR, Ali S, Chin SF, Palmieri C, Caldas C, Carroll JS (2012) Differential oestrogen receptor binding is associated with clinical outcome in breast cancer. Nature 481(7381):389–393. https://doi.org/10.1038/nature10730

222. Feng Q, O'Malley BW (2014) Nuclear receptor modulation--role of coregulators in selective estrogen receptor modulator (SERM) actions. Steroids 90:39–43. https://doi.org/10.1016/j.steroids.2014.06.008

223. Lonard DM, O'Malley BW (2007) Nuclear receptor coregulators: judges, juries, and executioners of cellular regulation. Mol Cell 27(5):691–700. https://doi.org/10.1016/j.molcel.2007.08.012

224. Osborne CK, Bardou V, Hopp TA, Chamness GC, Hilsenbeck SG, Fuqua SA, Wong J, Allred DC, Clark GM, Schiff R (2003) Role of the estrogen receptor coactivator AIB1 (SRC-3) and HER-2/neu in tamoxifen resistance in breast cancer. J Natl Cancer Inst 95(5):353–361

225. Kirkegaard T, McGlynn LM, Campbell FM, Muller S, Tovey SM, Dunne B, Nielsen KV, Cooke TG, Bartlett JM (2007) Amplified in breast cancer 1 in human epidermal growth factor receptor - positive tumors of tamoxifen-treated breast cancer patients. Clin Cancer Res 13(5):1405–1411. https://doi.org/10.1158/1078-0432.CCR-06-1933

226. Keeton EK, Brown M (2005) Cell cycle progression stimulated by tamoxifen-bound estrogen receptor-alpha and promoter-specific effects in breast cancer cells deficient in N-CoR and SMRT. Mol Endocrinol 19(6):1543–1554. https://doi.org/10.1210/me.2004-0395

227. Lavinsky RM, Jepsen K, Heinzel T, Torchia J, Mullen TM, Schiff R, Del-Rio AL, Ricote M, Ngo S, Gemsch J, Hilsenbeck SG, Osborne CK, Glass CK, Rosenfeld MG, Rose DW (1998) Diverse signaling pathways modulate nuclear receptor recruitment of N-CoR and SMRT complexes. Proc Natl Acad Sci U S A 95(6):2920–2925

228. Tabarestani S, Ghaderian SM, Rezvani H, Mirfakhraie R (2014) Expression profiling of breast cancer patients treated with tamoxifen: prognostic or predictive significance. Med Oncol 31(4):896. https://doi.org/10.1007/s12032-014-0896-5

229. Xu J, Wu RC, O'Malley BW (2009) Normal and cancer-related functions of the p160 steroid receptor co-activator (SRC) family. Nat Rev Cancer 9(9):615–630. https://doi.org/10.1038/nrc2695

230. Gao J, Aksoy BA, Dogrusoz U, Dresdner G, Gross B, Sumer SO, Sun Y, Jacobsen A, Sinha R, Larsson E, Cerami E, Sander C, Schultz N (2013) Integrative analysis of complex cancer genomics and clinical profiles using the cBioPortal. Sci Signal 6(269):pl1. https://doi.org/10.1126/scisignal.2004088

231. Jeselsohn R, Cornwell M, Pun M, Buchwalter G, Nguyen M, Bango C, Huang Y, Kuang Y, Paweletz C, Fu X, Nardone A, De Angelis C, Detre S, Dodson A, Mohammed H, Carroll JS, Bowden M, Rao P, Long HW, Li F, Dowsett M, Schiff R, Brown M (2017) Embryonic transcription factor SOX9 drives breast cancer endocrine resistance. Proc Natl Acad Sci U S A 114(22):E4482–E4491. https://doi.org/10.1073/pnas.1620993114

232. Cui J, Germer K, Wu T, Wang J, Luo J, Wang SC, Wang Q, Zhang X (2012) Cross-talk between HER2 and MED1 regulates tamoxifen resistance of human breast cancer cells. Cancer Res 72(21):5625–5634. https://doi.org/10.1158/0008-5472.CAN-12-1305

233. Cirillo LA, Zaret KS (1999) An early developmental transcription factor complex that is more stable on nucleosome core particles than on free DNA. Mol Cell 4(6):961–969

234. Carroll JS, Meyer CA, Song J, Li W, Geistlinger TR, Eeckhoute J, Brodsky AS, Keeton EK, Fertuck KC, Hall GF, Wang Q, Bekiranov S, Sementchenko V, Fox EA, Silver PA, Gingeras TR, Liu XS, Brown M (2006) Genome-wide analysis of estrogen receptor binding sites. Nat Genet 38(11):1289–1297. https://doi.org/10.1038/ng1901

235. Carroll JS, Liu XS, Brodsky AS, Li W, Meyer CA, Szary AJ, Eeckhoute J, Shao W, Hestermann EV, Geistlinger TR, Fox EA, Silver PA, Brown M (2005) Chromosome-wide mapping of estrogen receptor binding reveals long-range regulation requiring the forkhead protein FoxA1. Cell 122(1):33–43. https://doi.org/10.1016/j.cell.2005.05.008

236. Eeckhoute J, Keeton EK, Lupien M, Krum SA, Carroll JS, Brown M (2007) Positive cross-regulatory loop ties GATA-3 to estrogen receptor alpha expression in breast cancer. Cancer Res 67(13):6477–6483. https://doi.org/10.1158/0008-5472.CAN-07-0746

237. Fu X, Jeselsohn R, Pereira R, Hollingsworth EF, Creighton CJ, Li F, Shea M, Nardone A, De Angelis C, Heiser LM, Anur P, Wang N, Grasso CS, Spellman PT, Griffith OL, Tsimelzon A, Gutierrez C, Huang S, Edwards DP, Trivedi MV, Rimawi MF, Lopez-Terrada D, Hilsenbeck SG, Gray JW, Brown M, Osborne CK, Schiff R (2016) FOXA1 overexpression mediates endocrine resistance by altering the ER transcriptome and IL-8 expression in ER-positive breast cancer. Proc Natl Acad Sci U S A 113(43):E6600–E6609. https://doi.org/10.1073/pnas.1612835113

238. Hurtado A, Holmes KA, Ross-Innes CS, Schmidt D, Carroll JS (2011) FOXA1 is a key determinant of estrogen receptor function and endocrine response. Nat Genet 43(1):27–33. https://doi.org/10.1038/ng.730

239. Wright TM, Wardell SE, Jasper JS, Stice JP, Safi R, Nelson ER, McDonnell DP (2014) Delineation of a FOXA1/ERalpha/AGR2 regulatory loop that is dysregulated in endocrine therapy-resistant breast cancer. Mol Cancer Res 12(12):1829–1839. https://doi.org/10.1158/1541-7786.MCR-14-0195

240. Rheinbay E, Parasuraman P, Grimsby J, Tiao G, Engreitz JM, Kim J, Lawrence MS, Taylor-Weiner A, Rodriguez-Cuevas S, Rosenberg M, Hess J, Stewart C, Maruvka YE, Stojanov P, Cortes ML, Seepo S, Cibulskis C, Tracy A, Pugh TJ, Lee J, Zheng Z, Ellisen LW, Iafrate AJ, Boehm JS, Gabriel SB, Meyerson M, Golub TR, Baselga J, Hidalgo-Miranda A, Shioda T, Bernards A, Lander ES, Getz G (2017) Recurrent and functional regulatory mutations in breast cancer. Nature 547(7661):55–60. https://doi.org/10.1038/nature22992

241. Lefebvre C, Bachelot T, Filleron T, Pedrero M, Campone M, Soria JC, Massard C, Levy C, Arnedos M, Lacroix-Triki M, Garrabey J, Boursin Y, Deloger M, Fu Y, Commo F, Scott V, Lacroix L, Dieci MV, Kamal M, Dieras V, Goncalves A, Ferrerro JM, Romieu G, Vanlemmens L, Mouret Reynier MA, Thery JC, Le Du F, Guiu S, Dalenc F, Clapisson G, Bonnefoi H, Jimenez M, Le Tourneau C, Andre F (2016) Mutational profile of metastatic breast cancers: a retrospective analysis. PLoS Med 13(12):e1002201. https://doi.org/10.1371/journal.pmed.1002201

242. Cohen O, Kim D, Oh C, Waks A, Oliver N, Helvie K, Marini L, Rotem A, Lloyd M, Stover D, Adalsteinsson V, Freeman S, Ha G, Cibulskis C, Anderka K, Tamayo P, Johannessen C, Krop I, Garraway L, Winer E, Lin N, Wagle N (2017) Whole exome and transcriptome sequencing of resistant ER+ metastatic breast cancer. In: Proceedings of the 2016 San Antonio Breast Cancer Symposium. Cancer Res 77(4 Suppl):Abstract nr S1-01

243. Zehir A, Benayed R, Shah RH, Syed A, Middha S, Kim HR, Srinivasan P, Gao J, Chakravarty D, Devlin SM, Hellmann MD, Barron DA, Schram AM, Hameed M, Dogan S, Ross DS, Hechtman JF, DeLair DF, Yao J, Mandelker DL, Cheng DT, Chandramohan R, Mohanty AS, Ptashkin RN, Jayakumaran G, Prasad M, Syed MH, Rema AB, Liu ZY, Nafa K, Borsu L, Sadowska J, Casanova J, Bacares R, Kiecka IJ, Razumova A, Son JB, Stewart L, Baldi T, Mullaney KA, Al-Ahmadie H, Vakiani E, Abeshouse AA, Penson AV, Jonsson P, Camacho N, Chang MT, Won HH, Gross BE, Kundra R, Heins ZJ, Chen HW, Phillips S, Zhang H, Wang J, Ochoa A, Wills J, Eubank M, Thomas SB, Gardos SM, Reales DN, Galle J, Durany R, Cambria R, Abida W, Cercek A, Feldman DR, Gounder MM, Hakimi AA, Harding JJ, Iyer G, Janjigian YY, Jordan EJ, Kelly CM, Lowery MA, Morris LGT, Omuro AM, Raj

N, Razavi P, Shoushtari AN, Shukla N, Soumerai TE, Varghese AM, Yaeger R, Coleman J, Bochner B, Riely GJ, Saltz LB, Scher HI, Sabbatini PJ, Robson ME, Klimstra DS, Taylor BS, Baselga J, Schultz N, Hyman DM, Arcila ME, Solit DB, Ladanyi M, Berger MF (2017) Mutational landscape of metastatic cancer revealed from prospective clinical sequencing of 10,000 patients. Nat Med 23(6):703–713. https://doi.org/10.1038/nm.4333

244. Magnani L, Frige G, Gadaleta RM, Corleone G, Fabris S, Kempe MH, Vershure PJ, Barozzi I, Vircillo V, Hong SP, Perone Y, Saini M, Trumpp A, Viale G, Neri A, Ali S, Colleoni MA, Pruneri G, Minucci S (2017) Acquired CYP19A1 amplification is an early specific mechanism of aromatase inhibitor resistance in ERalpha metastatic breast cancer. Nat Genet 49(3):444–450. https://doi.org/10.1038/ng.3773

245. Veeraraghavan J, Ma J, Hu Y, Wang XS (2016) Recurrent and pathological gene fusions in breast cancer: current advances in genomic discovery and clinical implications. Breast Cancer Res Treat 158(2):219–232. https://doi.org/10.1007/s10549-016-3876-y

246. Li S, Shen D, Shao J, Crowder R, Liu W, Prat A, He X, Liu S, Hoog J, Lu C, Ding L, Griffith OL, Miller C, Larson D, Fulton RS, Harrison M, Mooney T, McMichael JF, Luo J, Tao Y, Goncalves R, Schlosberg C, Hiken JF, Saied L, Sanchez C, Giuntoli T, Bumb C, Cooper C, Kitchens RT, Lin A, Phommaly C, Davies SR, Zhang J, Kavuri MS, McEachern D, Dong YY, Ma C, Pluard T, Naughton M, Bose R, Suresh R, McDowell R, Michel L, Aft R, Gillanders W, DeSchryver K, Wilson RK, Wang S, Mills GB, Gonzalez-Angulo A, Edwards JR, Maher C, Perou CM, Mardis ER, Ellis MJ (2013) Endocrine-therapy-resistant ESR1 variants revealed by genomic characterization of breast-cancer-derived xenografts. Cell Rep 4(6):1116–1130. https://doi.org/10.1016/j.celrep.2013.08.022

247. Veeraraghavan J, Tan Y, Cao XX, Kim JA, Wang X, Chamness GC, Maiti SN, Cooper LJ, Edwards DP, Contreras A, Hilsenbeck SG, Chang EC, Schiff R, Wang XS (2014) Recurrent ESR1-CCDC170 rearrangements in an aggressive subset of oestrogen receptor-positive breast cancers. Nat Commun 5:4577. https://doi.org/10.1038/ncomms5577

248. Jeselsohn R, Yelensky R, Buchwalter G, Frampton G, Meric-Bernstam F, Gonzalez-Angulo AM, Ferrer-Lozano J, Perez-Fidalgo JA, Cristofanilli M, Gomez H, Arteaga CL, Giltnane J, Balko JM, Cronin MT, Jarosz M, Sun J, Hawryluk M, Lipson D, Otto G, Ross JS, Dvir A, Soussan-Gutman L, Wolf I, Rubinek T, Gilmore L, Schnitt S, Come SE, Pusztai L, Stephens P, Brown M, Miller VA (2014) Emergence of constitutively active estrogen receptor-alpha mutations in pretreated advanced estrogen receptor-positive breast cancer. Clin Cancer Res 20(7):1757–1767. https://doi.org/10.1158/1078-0432.CCR-13-2332

249. Jia S, Miedel MT, Ngo M, Hessenius R, Chen N, Wang P, Bahreini A, Li Z, Ding Z, Shun TY, Zuckerman DM, Taylor DL, Puhalla SL, Lee AV, Oesterreich S, Stern AM (2018) Clinically observed estrogen receptor alpha mutations within the ligand-binding domain confer distinguishable phenotypes. Oncology 94(3):176–189. https://doi.org/10.1159/000485510

250. Merenbakh-Lamin K, Ben-Baruch N, Yeheskel A, Dvir A, Soussan-Gutman L, Jeselsohn R, Yelensky R, Brown M, Miller VA, Sarid D, Rizel S, Klein B, Rubinek T, Wolf I (2013) D538G mutation in estrogen receptor-alpha: a novel mechanism for acquired endocrine resistance in breast cancer. Cancer Res 73(23):6856–6864. https://doi.org/10.1158/0008-5472.CAN-13-1197

251. Robinson DR, Wu YM, Vats P, Su F, Lonigro RJ, Cao X, Kalyana-Sundaram S, Wang R, Ning Y, Hodges L, Gursky A, Siddiqui J, Tomlins SA, Roychowdhury S, Pienta KJ, Kim SY, Roberts JS, Rae JM, Van Poznak CH, Hayes DF, Chugh R, Kunju LP, Talpaz M, Schott AF, Chinnaiyan AM (2013) Activating ESR1 mutations in hormone-resistant metastatic breast cancer. Nat Genet 45(12):1446–1451. https://doi.org/10.1038/ng.2823

252. Toy W, Shen Y, Won H, Green B, Sakr RA, Will M, Li Z, Gala K, Fanning S, King TA, Hudis C, Chen D, Taran T, Hortobagyi G, Greene G, Berger M, Baselga J, Chandarlapaty S (2013) ESR1 ligand-binding domain mutations in hormone-resistant breast cancer. Nat Genet 45(12):1439–1445. https://doi.org/10.1038/ng.2822

253. Katzenellenbogen JA, Mayne CG, Katzenellenbogen BS, Greene GL, Chandarlapaty S (2018) Structural underpinnings of oestrogen receptor mutations in endocrine therapy resistance. Nat Rev Cancer. https://doi.org/10.1038/s41568-018-0001-z

254. Jeselsohn R, Bergholz JS, Pun M, Cornwell M, Liu W, Nardone A, Xiao T, Li W, Qiu X, Buchwalter G, Feiglin A, Abell-Hart K, Fei T, Rao P, Long H, Kwiatkowski N, Zhang T, Gray N, Melchers D, Houtman R, Liu XS, Cohen O, Wagle N, Winer EP, Zhao J, Brown M (2018) Allele-specific chromatin recruitment and therapeutic vulnerabilities of ESR1 activating mutations. Cancer Cell 33(2):173–186 e175. https://doi.org/10.1016/j.ccell.2018.01.004

255. Jeselsohn R, Buchwalter G, De Angelis C, Brown M, Schiff R (2015) ESR1 mutations-a mechanism for acquired endocrine resistance in breast cancer. Nat Rev Clin Oncol 12(10):573–583. https://doi.org/10.1038/nrclinonc.2015.117

256. Diaz LA Jr, Bardelli A (2014) Liquid biopsies: genotyping circulating tumor DNA. J Clin Oncol 32(6):579–586. https://doi.org/10.1200/JCO.2012.45.2011

257. Pinkerton JV, Thomas S (2014) Use of SERMs for treatment in postmenopausal women. J Steroid Biochem Mol Biol 142:142–154. https://doi.org/10.1016/j.jsbmb.2013.12.011

258. Maruyama R, Choudhury S, Kowalczyk A, Bessarabova M, Beresford-Smith B, Conway T, Kaspi A, Wu Z, Nikolskaya T, Merino VF, Lo PK, Liu XS, Nikolsky Y, Sukumar S, Haviv I, Polyak K (2011) Epigenetic regulation of cell type-specific expression patterns in the human mammary epithelium. PLoS Genet 7(4):e1001369. https://doi.org/10.1371/journal.pgen.1001369

259. Lustberg MB, Ramaswamy B (2011) Epigenetic therapy in breast cancer. Curr Breast Cancer Rep 3(1):34–43. https://doi.org/10.1007/s12609-010-0034-0

260. Stone A, Zotenko E, Locke WJ, Korbie D, Millar EK, Pidsley R, Stirzaker C, Graham P, Trau M, Musgrove EA, Nicholson RI, Gee JM, Clark SJ (2015) DNA methylation of oestrogen-regulated enhancers defines endocrine sensitivity in breast cancer. Nat Commun 6:7758. https://doi.org/10.1038/ncomms8758

261. Magnani L, Stoeck A, Zhang X, Lanczky A, Mirabella AC, Wang TL, Gyorffy B, Lupien M (2013) Genome-wide reprogramming of the chromatin landscape underlies endocrine therapy resistance in breast cancer. Proc Natl Acad Sci U S A 110(16):E1490–E1499. https://doi.org/10.1073/pnas.1219992110

262. Nguyen VT, Barozzi I, Faronato M, Lombardo Y, Steel JH, Patel N, Darbre P, Castellano L, Gyorffy B, Woodley L, Meira A, Patten DK, Vircillo V, Periyasamy M, Ali S, Frige G, Minucci S, Coombes RC, Magnani L (2015) Differential epigenetic reprogramming in response to specific endocrine therapies promotes cholesterol biosynthesis and cellular invasion. Nat Commun 6:10044. https://doi.org/10.1038/ncomms10044

263. Raha P, Thomas S, Thurn KT, Park J, Munster PN (2015) Combined histone deacetylase inhibition and tamoxifen induces apoptosis in tamoxifen-resistant breast cancer models, by reversing Bcl-2 overexpression. Breast Cancer Res 17:26. https://doi.org/10.1186/s13058-015-0533-z

264. Munster PN, Thurn KT, Thomas S, Raha P, Lacevic M, Miller A, Melisko M, Ismail-Khan R, Rugo H, Moasser M, Minton SE (2011) A phase II study of the histone deacetylase inhibitor vorinostat combined with tamoxifen for the treatment of patients with hormone therapy-resistant breast cancer. Br J Cancer 104(12):1828–1835. https://doi.org/10.1038/bjc.2011.156

265. Dontu G, El-Ashry D, Wicha MS (2004) Breast cancer, stem/progenitor cells and the estrogen receptor. Trends Endocrinol Metab 15(5):193–197. https://doi.org/10.1016/j.tem.2004.05.011

266. Creighton CJ, Li X, Landis M, Dixon JM, Neumeister VM, Sjolund A, Rimm DL, Wong H, Rodriguez A, Herschkowitz JI, Fan C, Zhang X, He X, Pavlick A, Gutierrez MC, Renshaw L, Larionov AA, Faratian D, Hilsenbeck SG, Perou CM, Lewis MT, Rosen JM, Chang JC (2009) Residual breast cancers after conventional therapy display mesenchymal as well as tumor-initiating features. Proc Natl Acad Sci U S A 106(33):13820–13825. https://doi.org/10.1073/pnas.0905718106

267. Ao A, Morrison BJ, Wang H, Lopez JA, Reynolds BA, Lu J (2011) Response of estrogen receptor-positive breast cancer tumorspheres to antiestrogen treatments. PLoS One 6(4):e18810. https://doi.org/10.1371/journal.pone.0018810

268. Simoes BM, O'Brien CS, Eyre R, Silva A, Yu L, Sarmiento-Castro A, Alferez DG, Spence K, Santiago-Gomez A, Chemi F, Acar A, Gandhi A, Howell A, Brennan K, Ryden L, Catalano

S, Ando S, Gee J, Ucar A, Sims AH, Marangoni E, Farnie G, Landberg G, Howell SJ, Clarke RB (2015) Anti-estrogen resistance in human breast tumors is driven by JAG1-NOTCH4-dependent cancer stem cell activity. Cell Rep 12(12):1968–1977. https://doi.org/10.1016/j.celrep.2015.08.050

269. van Vlerken LE, Kiefer CM, Morehouse C, Li Y, Groves C, Wilson SD, Yao Y, Hollingsworth RE, Hurt EM (2013) EZH2 is required for breast and pancreatic cancer stem cell maintenance and can be used as a functional cancer stem cell reporter. Stem Cells Transl Med 2(1):43–52. https://doi.org/10.5966/sctm.2012-0036

270. Pathiraja TN, Nayak SR, Xi Y, Jiang S, Garee JP, Edwards DP, Lee AV, Chen J, Shea MJ, Santen RJ, Gannon F, Kangaspeska S, Jelinek J, Issa JP, Richer JK, Elias A, McIlroy M, Young LS, Davidson NE, Schiff R, Li W, Oesterreich S (2014) Epigenetic reprogramming of HOXC10 in endocrine-resistant breast cancer. Sci Transl Med 6(229):229ra241. https://doi.org/10.1126/scitranslmed.3008326

271. Wu Y, Zhang Z, Cenciarini ME, Proietti CJ, Amasino M, Hong T, Yang M, Liao Y, Chiang HC, Kaklamani VG, Jeselsohn R, Vadlamudi RK, Huang TH, Li R, De Angelis C, Fu X, Elizalde PV, Schiff R, Brown M, Xu K (2018) Tamoxifen resistance in breast cancer is regulated by the EZH2-ERalpha-GREB1 transcriptional axis. Cancer Res 78(3):671–684. https://doi.org/10.1158/0008-5472.CAN-17-1327

272. Muluhngwi P, Klinge CM (2015) Roles for miRNAs in endocrine resistance in breast cancer. Endocr Relat Cancer 22(5):R279–R300. https://doi.org/10.1530/ERC-15-0355

273. Guttilla IK, Phoenix KN, Hong X, Tirnauer JS, Claffey KP, White BA (2012) Prolonged mammosphere culture of MCF-7 cells induces an EMT and repression of the estrogen receptor by microRNAs. Breast Cancer Res Treat 132(1):75–85. https://doi.org/10.1007/s10549-011-1534-y

274. Zhao JJ, Lin J, Yang H, Kong W, He L, Ma X, Coppola D, Cheng JQ (2008) MicroRNA-221/222 negatively regulates estrogen receptor alpha and is associated with tamoxifen resistance in breast cancer. J Biol Chem 283(45):31079–31086. https://doi.org/10.1074/jbc.M806041200

275. Mazor T, Pankov A, Song JS, Costello JF (2016) Intratumoral heterogeneity of the epigenome. Cancer Cell 29(4):440–451. https://doi.org/10.1016/j.ccell.2016.03.009

276. Tian H, Gao Z, Li H, Zhang B, Wang G, Zhang Q, Pei D, Zheng J (2015) DNA damage response--a double-edged sword in cancer prevention and cancer therapy. Cancer Lett 358(1):8–16. https://doi.org/10.1016/j.canlet.2014.12.038

277. Blok EJ, Derks MG, van der Hoeven JJ, van de Velde CJ, Kroep JR (2015) Extended adjuvant endocrine therapy in hormone-receptor positive early breast cancer: current and future evidence. Cancer Treat Rev 41(3):271–276. https://doi.org/10.1016/j.ctrv.2015.02.004

278. Ho SM (2004) Estrogens and anti-estrogens: key mediators of prostate carcinogenesis and new therapeutic candidates. J Cell Biochem 91(3):491–503. https://doi.org/10.1002/jcb.10759

279. de Conti A, Tryndyak V, Churchwell MI, Melnyk S, Latendresse JR, Muskhelishvili L, Beland FA, Pogribny IP (2014) Genotoxic, epigenetic, and transcriptomic effects of tamoxifen in mouse liver. Toxicology 325:12–20. https://doi.org/10.1016/j.tox.2014.08.004

280. Schiewer MJ, Knudsen KE (2016) Linking DNA damage and hormone signaling pathways in cancer. Trends Endocrinol Metab 27(4):216–225. https://doi.org/10.1016/j.tem.2016.02.004

281. Guo X, Yang C, Qian X, Lei T, Li Y, Shen H, Fu L, Xu B (2013) Estrogen receptor alpha regulates ATM expression through miRNAs in breast cancer. Clin Cancer Res 19(18):4994–5002. https://doi.org/10.1158/1078-0432.CCR-12-3700

282. Wozniak K, Kolacinska A, Blasinska-Morawiec M, Morawiec-Bajda A, Morawiec Z, Zadrozny M, Blasiak J (2007) The DNA-damaging potential of tamoxifen in breast cancer and normal cells. Arch Toxicol 81(7):519–527. https://doi.org/10.1007/s00204-007-0188-3

283. Zhang F, Wang Y, Wang L, Luo X, Huang K, Wang C, Du M, Liu F, Luo T, Huang D, Huang K (2013) Poly(ADP-ribose) polymerase 1 is a key regulator of estrogen receptor alpha-dependent gene transcription. J Biol Chem 288(16):11348–11357. https://doi.org/10.1074/jbc.M112.429134

284. Haricharan S, Punturi N, Singh P, Holloway KR, Anurag M, Schmelz J, Schmidt C, Lei JT, Suman V, Hunt K, Olson JA Jr, Hoog J, Li S, Huang S, Edwards DP, Kavuri SM, Bainbridge MN, Ma CX, Ellis MJ (2017) Loss of MutL disrupts CHK2-dependent cell-cycle control through CDK4/6 to promote intrinsic endocrine therapy resistance in primary breast cancer. Cancer Discov 7(10):1168–1183. https://doi.org/10.1158/2159-8290.CD-16-1179

285. Tlsty T (2008) Cancer: whispering sweet somethings. Nature 453(7195):604–605. https://doi.org/10.1038/453604a

286. Haslam SZ, Woodward TL (2003) Host microenvironment in breast cancer development: epithelial-cell-stromal-cell interactions and steroid hormone action in normal and cancerous mammary gland. Breast Cancer Res 5(4):208–215. https://doi.org/10.1186/bcr615

287. Finak G, Bertos N, Pepin F, Sadekova S, Souleimanova M, Zhao H, Chen H, Omeroglu G, Meterissian S, Omeroglu A, Hallett M, Park M (2008) Stromal gene expression predicts clinical outcome in breast cancer. Nat Med 14(5):518–527. https://doi.org/10.1038/nm1764

288. Helleman J, Jansen MP, Ruigrok-Ritstier K, van Staveren IL, Look MP, Meijer-van Gelder ME, Sieuwerts AM, Klijn JG, Sleijfer S, Foekens JA, Berns EM (2008) Association of an extracellular matrix gene cluster with breast cancer prognosis and endocrine therapy response. Clin Cancer Res 14(17):5555–5564. https://doi.org/10.1158/1078-0432.CCR-08-0555

289. Pontiggia O, Rodriguez V, Fabris V, Raffo D, Bumaschny V, Fiszman G, de Kier Joffe EB, Simian M (2009) Establishment of an in vitro estrogen-dependent mouse mammary tumor model: a new tool to understand estrogen responsiveness and development of tamoxifen resistance in the context of stromal-epithelial interactions. Breast Cancer Res Treat 116(2):247–255. https://doi.org/10.1007/s10549-008-0113-3

290. Sansone P, Berishaj M, Rajasekhar VK, Ceccarelli C, Chang Q, Strillacci A, Savini C, Shapiro L, Bowman RL, Mastroleo C, De Carolis S, Daly L, Benito-Martin A, Perna F, Fabbri N, Healey JH, Spisni E, Cricca M, Lyden D, Bonafe M, Bromberg J (2017) Evolution of cancer stem-like cells in endocrine-resistant metastatic breast cancers is mediated by stromal microvesicles. Cancer Res 77(8):1927–1941. https://doi.org/10.1158/0008-5472.CAN-16-2129

291. Sansone P, Savini C, Kurelac I, Chang Q, Amato LB, Strillacci A, Stepanova A, Iommarini L, Mastroleo C, Daly L, Galkin A, Thakur BK, Soplop N, Uryu K, Hoshino A, Norton L, Bonafe M, Cricca M, Gasparre G, Lyden D, Bromberg J (2017) Packaging and transfer of mitochondrial DNA via exosomes regulate escape from dormancy in hormonal therapy-resistant breast cancer. Proc Natl Acad Sci U S A 114(43):E9066–E9075. https://doi.org/10.1073/pnas.1704862114

292. Baumgarten SC, Frasor J (2012) Minireview: inflammation: an instigator of more aggressive estrogen receptor (ER) positive breast cancers. Mol Endocrinol 26(3):360–371. https://doi.org/10.1210/me.2011-1302

293. Stender JD, Nwachukwu JC, Kastrati I, Kim Y, Strid T, Yakir M, Srinivasan S, Nowak J, Izard T, Rangarajan ES, Carlson KE, Katzenellenbogen JA, Yao XQ, Grant BJ, Leong HS, Lin CY, Frasor J, Nettles KW, Glass CK (2017) Structural and molecular mechanisms of cytokine-mediated endocrine resistance in human breast cancer cells. Mol Cell 65(6):1122–1135 e1125. https://doi.org/10.1016/j.molcel.2017.02.008

294. Loi S, Haibe-Kains B, Desmedt C, Wirapati P, Lallemand F, Tutt AM, Gillet C, Ellis P, Ryder K, Reid JF, Daidone MG, Pierotti MA, Berns EM, Jansen MP, Foekens JA, Delorenzi M, Bontempi G, Piccart MJ, Sotiriou C (2008) Predicting prognosis using molecular profiling in estrogen receptor-positive breast cancer treated with tamoxifen. BMC Genomics 9:239. https://doi.org/10.1186/1471-2164-9-239

295. Dunbier AK, Ghazoui Z, Anderson H, Salter J, Nerurkar A, Osin P, A'Hern R, Miller WR, Smith IE, Dowsett M (2013) Molecular profiling of aromatase inhibitor-treated postmenopausal breast tumors identifies immune-related correlates of resistance. Clin Cancer Res 19(10):2775–2786. https://doi.org/10.1158/1078-0432.CCR-12-1000

296. Stossi F, Madak-Erdogan Z, Katzenellenbogen BS (2012) Macrophage-elicited loss of estrogen receptor-alpha in breast cancer cells via involvement of MAPK and c-Jun at the ESR1 genomic locus. Oncogene 31(14):1825–1834. https://doi.org/10.1038/onc.2011.370

297. Leek RD, Lewis CE, Whitehouse R, Greenall M, Clarke J, Harris AL (1996) Association of macrophage infiltration with angiogenesis and prognosis in invasive breast carcinoma. Cancer Res 56(20):4625–4629

298. Steele RJ, Eremin O, Brown M, Hawkins RA (1986) Oestrogen receptor concentration and macrophage infiltration in human breast cancer. Eur J Surg Oncol 12(3):273–276

299. Mor G, Yue W, Santen RJ, Gutierrez L, Eliza M, Berstein LM, Harada N, Wang J, Lysiak J, Diano S, Naftolin F (1998) Macrophages, estrogen and the microenvironment of breast cancer. J Steroid Biochem Mol Biol 67(5–6):403–411

300. Hagemann T, Wilson J, Kulbe H, Li NF, Leinster DA, Charles K, Klemm F, Pukrop T, Binder C, Balkwill FR (2005) Macrophages induce invasiveness of epithelial cancer cells via NF-kappa B and JNK. J Immunol 175(2):1197–1205

301. Chanmee T, Ontong P, Konno K, Itano N (2014) Tumor-associated macrophages as major players in the tumor microenvironment. Cancers 6(3):1670–1690. https://doi.org/10.3390/cancers6031670

302. Rothenberger NJ, Somasundaram A, Stabile LP (2018) The role of the estrogen pathway in the tumor microenvironment. Int J Mol Sci 19(2). https://doi.org/10.3390/ijms19020611

303. Conejo-Garcia JR, Payne KK, Svoronos N (2017) Estrogens drive myeloid-derived suppressor cell accumulation. Oncoscience 4(1–2):5–6. https://doi.org/10.18632/oncoscience.340

304. Zavadova E, Vocka M, Spacek J, Konopasek B, Fucikova T, Petruzelka L (2014) Cellular and humoral immunodeficiency in breast cancer patients resistant to hormone therapy. Neoplasma 61(1):90–98

305. Rugo HS, Vidula N, Ma C (2016) Improving response to hormone therapy in breast cancer: new targets, new therapeutic options. Am Soc Clin Oncol Educ Book 35:e40–e54. https://doi.org/10.14694/EDBK_159198

Estrogen Receptor β and Breast Cancer

Christoforos Thomas and Jan-Åke Gustafsson

Abstract Despite the primary role of estrogen receptor α (ERα) in mediating the effects of estrogen in malignant breast and as therapeutic target, the development of endocrine-resistant and metastatic phenotypes indicates the complexity of the mechanisms that regulate hormone signaling in the disease. The discovery of ERβ and its functional characterization has improved our understanding about the mechanism of estrogen receptor action, the regulation of estrogen signaling in breast tumors, and their response to therapy. The progressive decline of ERβ in pro-invasive lesions and invasive tumors points toward a role as suppressor of both tumorigenesis and progression in breast cancer. The antiproliferative and anti-invasive effects of the receptor and its agonists in preclinical models of breast cancer support these roles and delineate the mechanisms of action. The association of ERβ with clinical outcome proposes the potential use of the receptor as prognostic marker and its agonists in chemoprevention and therapeutic strategies for resistant and metastatic disease.

Keywords Estrogen receptor β · Breast cancer · Estrogen signaling · Breast cancer metastasis · Breast cancer prognosis

1 Introduction

Estrogen is essential for the development and physiological function of mammary gland and is implicated in initiation and progression of breast cancer. It impacts both normal and malignant breast by regulating cell proliferation, differentiation, metabolism, and epithelial-stromal interactions. The effects of the hormone in these conditions are mediated by two estrogen receptor (ER) subtypes. Similar to other members of the nuclear receptor superfamily of transcription factors, ERα and ERβ regulate gene expression in response to ligand binding [1, 2]. Due to distinct ligand-interacting domains, ligands bind to ERα and ERβ with different affinities and

C. Thomas (✉) · J.-Å. Gustafsson
Department of Biology and Biochemistry, Center for Nuclear Receptors and Cell Signaling,
University of Houston, Houston, TX, USA

© Springer Nature Switzerland AG 2019
X. Zhang (ed.), *Estrogen Receptor and Breast Cancer*, Cancer Drug Discovery
and Development, https://doi.org/10.1007/978-3-319-99350-8_12

activate cellular responses with varying potencies. Specificity in ligand binding is associated with differential activation of C- and N-terminal activating function (AF) domains of two ERs. In addition to estrogen, the N-terminal domain differentially regulates the activity of ERα and ERβ through recruitment of various types of regulatory proteins in response to hormone-independent signaling. Thus, due to distinct mechanisms of activation, ERα and ERβ differentially control gene expression and affect major cancer-associated biological processes [1, 3]. Differences in the mechanism of action combined with the ER subtype-specific expression changes account for the differential role of ERs in breast cancer biology and therapy.

Nearly 70% of breast tumors express ERα often at higher levels than the normal gland, linking this ER subtype to oncogenic actions of estrogen and suggesting potential benefit of these tumors from treatment with antiestrogens. Indeed, ERα is an established biological marker that predicts response to endocrine therapies [4]. It also represents a successful therapeutic target because ERα antagonists such as tamoxifen and aromatase inhibitors that cause estrogen deprivation are standard and efficient treatments for ERα-positive breast cancer. In contrast, the clinical importance of ERβ in breast cancer remains unclear. Despite some controversial reports about its expression in breast tumors, most authors agree that ERβ declines during the development and progression of the disease [5]. This observation together with the absence or low expression in many breast cancer cell lines is interpreted as hallmark of tumor suppressor activity [5]. Such role is further supported by studies associating the reintroduction of ERβ in breast cancer cells with decreased proliferation and invasion and inhibition of xenograft tumor growth and metastasis. To elicit these antitumor actions, the receptor alters cell cycle progression, DNA damage response and apoptosis, epithelial to mesenchymal transition (EMT), and tumor-stroma interactions by regulating various signaling pathways including those that are initiated by growth factors and tumor suppressors. In contrast to antitumor activity, a few studies claimed a pro-tumorigenic function of the receptor based on associations with more aggressive clinical phenotypes and increased cell proliferation proposing a bi-faceted role in the disease [6]. Thus, the tumor suppressor role of ERβ is currently disputed, and its clinical importance is under debate. In this chapter, we will provide comprehensive information on the mechanism of ERβ action attempting to shed more light into its relationship with the biology of breast cancer. In addition, we will discuss older studies and recently published preclinical and clinical findings with the aim to provide an up-to-date and unbiased opinion about the role of the receptor in breast cancer prognosis and therapy.

2 Mechanism of ERβ Action

The human *ESR2* gene is located on chromosome 14q23.2, and its coding region consists of eight exons that produce a protein of 530 amino acids [7]. As with other nuclear receptors including ERα, ERβ has a six-domain structure with separate regions for binding ligands, DNA, and various types of regulatory proteins and domains that control ligand-dependent and ligand-independent functions [8, 9] (Fig. 1).

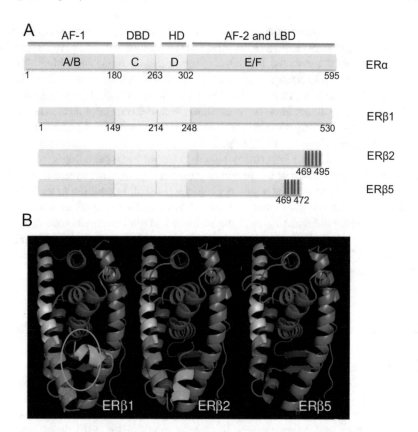

Fig. 1 Schematic illustration of the genomic and functional structure of ERβ. (**a**) Schematic representation of structural and functional domains of estrogen receptors α (ERα) and β (ERβ). The positions of the functional domains are indicated by blue bars on top, the structural domains are highlighted A–F, and the amino acids are shown in black. The regions A/B contain the activation function 1 (AF-1) domain that is responsible for ligand-independent activity and a co-regulatory domain where coactivators and corepressors are recruited. The C and D regions contain the DNA-binding domain (DBD) and hinge domain (HD), respectively. By binding various types of regulatory proteins, the hinge domain regulates conformation, DNA binding, stability, and intracellular localization of the receptor. The region E/F contains the activation function 2 (AF-2) domain that is responsible for hormone-dependent activity and the ligand-binding domain (LBD). This region interacts with co-regulatory proteins and controls receptor dimerization and nuclear translocation. ERβ is modified by alternative splicing that results in truncated proteins. Human ERβ isoforms in breast tumors are formed from alternative splicing of the last coding exon (shown by the striped bars) and are shown below the wild-type receptor. (**b**) Molecular models of ERβ isoforms. Helix 11 has the common region (shown in pink) of each isoform and an isoform-specific region that is labeled in dark red. Helix 12 (green) has a different orientation in ERβ2 compared with that of ERβ1. The helix 12 of ERβ1 is drifted toward the binding pocket (orange oval). Panel (**a**) was reproduced from Thomas and Gustafsson [10] with permission from Elsevier, Copyright (2015). Paned (**b**) was reproduced from Leung et al. [11], Copyright (2006) National Academy of Sciences, USA

Association of estrogen or other agonists with the ligand-binding domain causes swift of its major regulatory element (helix 12) toward a position that allows recruitment of coactivators that are essential for transcription initiation. In contrast, binding of an antagonist promotes a different conformation with a drift of helix 12 away from the rest of the structure that prevents interactions with coactivators [12, 13] (Fig. 2). Upon activation, ERβ forms homodimers or heterodimers with ERα and through the zinc finger-containing DNA-binding domain is recruited to DNA at specific sequences known as estrogen response elements (ERE) (Fig. 2). ERE can vary from canonical palindromic (GGTCAnnnTGACC) to imperfectly palindromic and hemi-palindromic (half sites, GGTCA) and are located at the proximal promoter region, downstream of the transcription start site or at distal regulatory regions [14–16]. In addition to the classical pathway that solely relies on direct ERβ-DNA binding, ERβ triggers transcription by interacting with and regulating other transcription factors. The nonclassical activation occurs either through indirect recruitment (tethering) of ERβ to the motif of its partner transcription factor or association of the receptor and the interacting factor with their cognate response elements (Fig. 2).

2.1 *ERβ Binds DNA as Homodimer or Heterodimer with ERα*

The different modes of ERβ-DNA association are also evident from the analysis of ERβ-binding sites in estrogen-stimulated MCF-7 cells with chromatin immunoprecipitation approaches including ChiP-seq and ChIP-on-chip. The transfected ERβ in these cells binds proximal promoters and regions upstream of the promoters, within the gene and downstream of it. Compared with ERα, ERβ shows a higher tendency to bind sites that surround the transcription start site [14–17]. In addition to proximal regions, enhancers of estrogen-responsive genes in cells expressing both receptors are more likely to have binding sites unique to ERβ than ERα indicating a preference for recruitment of ERβ homodimers to distal regulatory elements [15, 16]. The formation of ERβ homodimers is additionally supported by findings showing less ERα/ERβ shared binding sites in cells expressing both receptors compared with those that express either of them alone [16]. The same observation suggests altered distribution of ERβ-binding sites in the presence of ERα. Indeed, ERα causes a substantial shift of ERβ binding into many new sites that account for 60% of the sites that it occupies when it is expressed alone [16]. In addition to homodimers, ERα/ERβ heterodimer binding impacts the expression of estrogen-responsive genes and may account for the transcriptional repression of ERα in luminal cells [15, 18]. Combination of ChiP-Seq and ChIP-on-chip data with findings from ChiP-qPCR and transcriptome analysis that refers to estrogen-stimulated genes that are differentially regulated by ERβ confirms the versatile nature of ERβ-DNA interaction and identifies a list of primary ERβ target genes [14, 17]. Ontology analysis attests the link between the ERβ-associated genes and regulation of cellular processes (proliferation, survival, apoptosis, metabolism, differentiation, migration, and adhesion) that affect development, progression, and

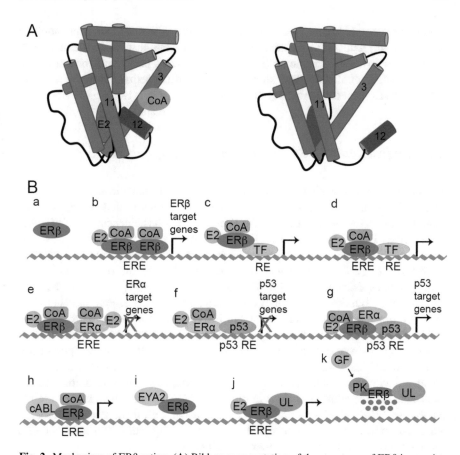

Fig. 2 Mechanism of ERβ action. (**A**) Ribbon representation of the structures of ERβ in agonist- and antagonist-bound conformation. (Left) Estrogen (green) and other agonists cause helix 12 to shift toward helix 3 forming a surface that allows recruitment of coactivators (colored orange). (Right) In an antagonist-bound conformation (antagonist is colored purple), helix 12 is drifted away from helix 3 preventing the interaction of the receptor with coactivators. Helices are shown in blue cylinders. (**B**) Schematic illustration of the mechanism of ERβ action. (a) In the absence of ligand, ERβ does not bind with DNA. (b) Upon estrogen (E2) binding, ERβ forms homodimers, binds DNA at estrogen response elements (ERE), and activates gene expression. (c, d) ERβ can activate gene expression by interacting and activating other transcription factors. This mechanism involves association of ERβ with chromatin through tethering to interacting transcription factor (c) or direct interaction of ERβ and its partner transcription at their cognate response elements (d). (e) ERβ forms heterodimers with and represses the transcriptional activity of ERα. (f) ERα binds to and inhibits the transcriptional activity of p53. (g) By interacting with the ERα-p53 complex, ERβ attenuates the inhibitory effect of ERα on p53. (h) Protein kinases such as cABL activate ERβ in the absence of estrogen. (i) Phosphatases such as EYA2 dephosphorylate and inactivate ERβ. (j) Interaction with ubiquitin ligases and proteasome-dependent degradation combined with new protein synthesis is essential for activation of ERβ in response to estrogen. (k) Upon growth factor stimulation, interaction of ERβ with ubiquitin ligases leads to proteasome-dependent degradation and inactivation. Panel (**a**) of Fig. 1; Reprinted from Thomas C, Gustafsson JA (2015) Estrogen receptor mutations and functional consequences for breast cancer. Trends Endocrinol Metab 26 (9):467–476. Copyright (2015)

therapy response of breast cancer [14, 17]. The enrichment of these gene ontology categories correlates with the inhibitory effect of ERβ on estrogen-induced cell proliferation in studies that analyzed ERβ-DNA binding [14, 15, 19] and strengthens previously published data showing antiproliferative responses of ERβ in ERα-positive breast cancer cells [18, 20, 21].

2.2   Interaction of ERβ with Other Transcription Factors

Sequence analysis reveals the prevalence of imperfectly palindromic ERE or half sites in ERβ-binding sites. In addition to ERE, DNA motifs that belong to other transcription factors are identified in the same DNA regions. Enrichment of FOXA1, AP-1, SP-1, E2F, BACH1, and PAX binding matrices in ERβ-binding sites that contain ERE indicates the importance of other transcription factors in mediating interactions of ERβ with chromatin [22]. Motifs of these and other transcription factors such as GSFC1, NRF1, and ZNF also reside in ERβ-binding sites that lack ERE pointing to indirect ERβ-DNA association that enables gene trans-regulation. Different binding matrices are enriched in ERβ-binding sites when ERα is present including elements of interferon regulatory factor, suggesting regulation of a separate group of estrogen-responsive genes in cells expressing both receptors [16]. In addition to ERα, ERβ-specific agonists promote a distinct ERβ-DNA association compared with estrogen implying that ligand-specific conformations of the receptor determine the selection of chromatin binding [16]. The same ligands increase the number of ERα/ERβ shared binding sites compared with those that are observed when both receptors are co-occupied by estrogen suggesting that ERβ agonists favor a type of ERα/ERβ heterodimer activation [16].

2.3   Ligand-Independent Activation of ERβ

In addition to agonist-dependent activation, ERβ elicits transcriptional responses in the absence of ligand [1, 18, 23]. Membrane and cytoplasmic signaling cascades trigger posttranslation modifications that regulate ERs in a ligand-independent fashion. Such activation of ERα is often associated with estrogen unresponsiveness and antiestrogen resistance [24]. On the other hand, phosphorylation of ERβ at certain serine (Ser-94, Ser-106, Ser-124,) and tyrosine (Tyr-36) residues of AF-1 domain alters the ubiquitination and turnover of the receptor and is coupled with its transcriptional activation and antitumor activity [25]. Proteasome-dependent degradation of ERβ is executed by E3 ubiquitin ligases and their regulatory factors. The aberrant signaling of these proteins in breast tumors is often associated with altered expression and transcriptional activity of ERβ [26, 27]. Molecules that work in concert with E3 ligases to regulate ERβ turnover include members of the MAPK family of kinases. Similar to these kinases, the c-ABL kinase and EYA2 phosphatase regulate through phosphorylation the recruitment of co-regulators (p300, SRC-1, CBP) that enable transcription initiation. While, upon growth factor stimulation, phosphorylation of the transfected receptor in non-breast cancer cells was initially associated with a pro-oncogenic function through recruitment of coactivator SRC-1 [28], phosphorylation of tyrosine-36 (Y-36) mediates the antiproliferative and anti-invasive activity of ERβ in breast cancer cells and xenografts [29, 30]. By interacting with ERβ and exerting opposite actions on tyrosine-36 phosphorylation, EYA2 and c-ABL control the transcriptional activity of the receptor demonstrating how hormone-independent signaling determines the function of the receptor. Given this type of regulation, a high c-ABL/EYA2 expression ratio in some breast cancer cells may explain tumor-repressive effects of the receptor that are observed in the absence of exogenous agonist. In addition to ligand-independent activation, phosphorylation of AF-1 regulates ERβ in response to estrogen binding through interaction with the AF-2 domain. The ERβ agonists 17β-estradiol, DPN, and S-equol that activate the receptor are also known to enhance phosphorylation of ERβ at tyrosine-36 [29, 30].

3   Regulation of ERβ Expression

In contrast to the upregulation of ERα in early luminal tumors, the decline of ERβ expression is observed in atypical hyperplasia and carcinoma in situ and further decrease in invasive lesions [31–34]. The reduced expression of ERβ has been proposed to contribute to breast tumorigenesis. Such anti-tumorigenic role is supported by the observed association between increased expression in breast atypia lobules and decreased risk of developing breast cancer [34]. Similar to human cancer, lower levels of the receptor are detected in mouse mammary tumors compared with normal glands indicating the importance of altered ERβ expression in malignant transformation [35, 36].

3.1   Regulation of ERβ Expression at mRNA Level

Changes in expression of ERβ occur by alterations in protein synthesis and degradation. At the level of transcriptional regulation, increased methylation of ERβ promoter is associated with decreased amounts of the receptor in breast cancer cells and tumors. This association has been experimentally explored by the use of DNA methyltransferase inhibitors that enable re-expression of ERβ [32, 37–39]. Following transcription, the mRNA of ERβ is susceptible to regulation by microRNAs (miRs). As in the case of ERα mRNA that is targeted by various miRs including miR-206, ERβ is regulated by miR-92. miR-92 belongs to a family of miRs that function as oncogenic factors by promoting cell proliferation and repressing apoptosis.

Upregulation of miR-92 in breast cancer cells downregulates ERβ, and its increased expression in primary breast tumors correlates with decreased mRNA and protein levels of the receptor suggesting the miR-dependent regulation of ERβ as one of the mechanisms that account for its silencing in breast cancer [40].

3.2 Regulation of ERβ Expression and Activity at Posttranslational Level

In addition to mRNA, ERβ expression is regulated at posttranslational level. The role of the ubiquitin-proteasome pathway in determining turnover of both ERα and ERβ was emphasized in the initially proposed mechanism. In the absence of ligands, ERs are stable within a complex with heat shock proteins (HSPs), whereas ligand binding causes dissociation from chaperones, poly-ubiquitination, and proteasome-mediated degradation [41–43]. However, this model does not reflect the dynamic fluctuation of the turnover of ERβ in changing cellular conditions. For instance, while poly-ubiquitination of ERβ is observed in both presence and absence of ligand, degradation is largely estrogen-dependent [44]. Furthermore, in early studies, degradation of ERs was associated with decreased transcription of ER target genes [45], whereas the use of proteasome inhibitors suggests that maximal estrogen responses require proteasome processing and new protein synthesis indicating the importance of degradation for receptor transactivation [45]. Other investigations describe the agonist-induced degradation of ERβ as a process to shut off the activity of the receptor when the estrogen response is complete and the amount of the ligand is reduced. Such regulation of protein links the highly dynamic status of the receptor to cellular strategies that adjust protein production to hormone availability and the physiological demand for this signaling [44].

In the absence of ligand, ERs differentially respond to proteasome inhibition with the transcriptional activity of ERα to increase and that of ERβ to remain unaffected. The distinct transcriptional responses of unliganded receptors to proteasome inhibition reflect the differential involvement of AF-1 and AF-2 domains in regulation of protein degradation. The function of AF-1 of ERβ is required for ligand-dependent poly-ubiquitination and degradation. By regulating protein stability, AF-1 affects the nuclear mobility and the association of ERβ with active chromatin templates that is required for transcriptional regulation. Specific amino acids within the AF1 domain (Ser-94, Ser-106) are involved in proteasome-dependent degradation of the receptor. These amino acids are essential for the interaction with specific ubiquitin ligases and control protein stability in response to various stimuli including growth factor signaling. On the other hand, the AF-2 domain seems to protect the unliganded ERβ from proteolysis through reducing its association with the 26S proteasome [44], and this may explain the lack of ERβ response to proteasome inhibition in the absence of estrogen.

3.3 Pathways That Regulate Degradation of ERβ

In addition to estrogen, growth factors such as heregulin-β and downstream effectors (PI3K/AKT) promote poly-ubiquitination and degradation of ERβ by inducing its interaction with the E3 ubiquitin ligase MDM2. In contrast to estrogen, the effect of PI3K/AKT pathway on ERβ stability is associated with reduced receptor-DNA binding and activity and increased proliferation of breast cancer cells suggesting another mechanism that decreases the expression and antitumor activity of the receptor in breast tumors [46]. In addition to MDM2, approaches that combine immunoprecipitation with mass fingerprinting methods have revealed other E3 ubiquitin ligases (CHIP, E6AP), chaperones (HSP-90, HSP-70), transcription factors (EBF1), and regulatory molecules (CBP, MTA1, PES1) as interacting proteins that regulate the stability of ERβ [17, 25, 27, 44, 47]. CHIP, E6AP, and MDM2 regulate ERβ similar to ERα, and EBF1 appears to be more potent in suppressing ERβ. In contrast, PES1 by acting in concert with CHIP elicits opposite effects on the turnover of ERα and ERβ. By enhancing the stability of ERα and targeting ERβ for degradation, PES1 increases breast tumor growth and alters response to tamoxifen treatment [26, 27]. In addition to ER ligands, other compounds including HSP-90 inhibitors (17-DMAG) and phytoestrogens regulate the stability of ERβ and determine its transcriptional activity. Among these are the resveratrol analog and naturally isolated compound Diptoindonesin (Dip G). Dip G increases the protein levels of ERβ and decreases ERα in an ubiquitin-proteasome-dependent manner in the absence and presence of estrogen. The upregulation of ERβ has been observed in a series of transfected breast cancer cell lines and the endogenous receptor in MCF-7 cells. In addition to the fully functional ERβ1, Dip G increases the stability of ERβ2. Dip G acts in common in both isoforms of N-terminus by suppressing its interaction with the E3 ligase CHIP. In accordance with the reverse effect on the stability of ERs, Dip G inhibits the estrogen-induced transcriptional activity of ERα and increases that of ERβ. As a result, the compound reduces the estrogen-induced proliferation of MCF-7 cells and augmented the suppressive effect of tamoxifen. In addition, it potentiates the antiproliferative and anti-invasive activity of ERβ in various breast cancer cell lines [48]. As ERβ levels decline with cancer progression, the effect of this natural product on ERβ stability indicates the potential use of small molecules in therapies targeting ERβ protein. The involvement of multiple proteins and ligands in posttranslational regulation of ERβ underlines the complexity of the mechanisms that lead to decreased levels of the receptor in breast cancer. Genetic aberrations that alter hormone and E3 ligase levels, growth factor signaling, and the activity of other regulatory factors may contribute to malignant transformation and tumor progression through a mechanism that involves, among other alterations, ERβ downregulation.

4 Estrogen Receptor β in Normal Mammary Gland

The mammary gland of hormone receptor-deficient mice before puberty appears normal suggesting that prepubertal development of the organ occurs largely in a hormone-independent manner. In contrast, mature female mice lacking major sources of reproductive hormones show impaired growth of mammary gland, and treatment of hormone-deprived mice with 17β-estradiol, progesterone, and prolactin in conjunction with cortisol and growth hormone (GH) restores normal development. Estrogen signaling is required for ductal elongation during puberty and together with progesterone and/or prolactin promote side branching and alveologenesis in adulthood and pregnancy [49]. The use of ERα-deficient mice and tissue recombination experiments with transplantation of wild-type and ERα knockout glands into wild-type fat pads and vice versa revealed the essential role of epithelial ERα in ductal elongation and side branching [50]. Transplantation experiments using chimeric tissues with wild-type and ERα-deficient epithelial cells suggest involvement of a paracrine mechanism that is employed by estrogen and ERα to drive epithelial cell proliferation and morphogenesis [51]. The mechanism relies on secretion of the paracrine epidermal growth factor receptor (EGFR) ligand amphiregulin (AREG) by a subset of ERα-positive ductal cells that stimulates neighboring cells to proliferate contributing to ductal outgrowth [52].

4.1 ERβ and Cell Proliferation in Normal Gland

In contrast to ERα, the physiological role of ERβ in mammary gland development remains unclear. The analysis of ERβ knockout mice provided with evidence of incomplete differentiation. Despite the development of a normal ductal tree, ERβ-deficient mice fail to generate side branching [53]. This phenotype could be due to lack of ERβ in mammary epithelium and stroma or ovaries. Ovarian dysfunction has been observed in different ERβ knockout mice and could be responsible for a decrease in progesterone synthesis that leads to delayed side branching [54]. Moreover, the detection of cysts together with the expression of proliferation markers in differentiated luminal epithelial cells in aging mice of one ERβ knockout model suggests growth inhibitory activity of the receptor in normal gland [53]. Such activity is consistent with the antiproliferative activity of ERβ in two mammary epithelial cell lines [55–57]. In contrast, treatment of adult virgin female mice with the ERβ agonist diarylpropionitrile (DPN) and WAY increases lateral branching and ductal growth similar to 17β-estradiol suggesting proliferative actions of ERβ in mammary epithelium [58]. However, the effects of these agonists are not fully understood, particularly in tissues that express both ER subtypes. For instance, DPN is reported to elicit antiproliferative effects only when ERβ is highly expressed [59]. Since the expression of ERβ in the mouse mammary gland is not well defined, the proliferative effect of ERβ ligands may be due to activation of ERα in mammary epithelium, ER-subtype-specific regulation of stroma functions including immune response, or altered ovarian function. Thus, comparison of treatments in wild-type and ERβ knockout mice will help to clarify the mechanism of ligand action.

4.2   ERβ and Epithelial Differentiation in Normal Gland

In addition to side branching, ERβ has been suggested to regulate alveologenesis and promote epithelial cell differentiation [53]. The role in alveologenesis is also evident by the estrogen-induced alveolar growth in ERα knockout mice and EGFR-deficient transplants [60]. The contribution of the receptor in differentiation is corroborated by its consistent association with markers of epithelial cell differentiation in mouse mammary tissues and human mammary and breast cancer cell lines. Reduced cell adhesion markers E-cadherin and integrin α2 and the epithelial tight junction protein occludin are expressed in mammary glands of midpregnant and lactating ERβ knockout mice compared with the wild-type mice [53]. Similar to mammary glands, decreased expression of epithelial (CK8, E-cadherin) and upregulation of mesenchymal/basal markers (CK14, vimentin, p63, a-SMA) are observed in p53-deficient breast tumors that are developed in the absence of ERβ. In agreement with the expression of epithelial markers, these tumors either have less well differentiated glands or metaplastic histology and spindle cell morphology compared with the ERβ-proficient tumors [36]. In contrast to contradictory actions on cell proliferation, cell-based studies invariably support the role of ERβ in epithelial differentiation. ERβ and its agonists are linked to epithelial maintenance and decreased invasion in TNBC cells through inhibition of EGFR signaling [23, 30, 61–64]. The inhibitory effect on EGFR in breast cancer cells may imply that a similar mechanism is employed by the receptor to promote differentiation during morphogenesis of the mammary gland where EGFR represents an essential paracrine regulator of estrogen-induced development [51].

5   ERβ Splice Variants

Unlike point mutations in ESR1 gene that occur in a substantial number of ERα-positive metastatic cancers that progressed during hormonal therapy, ESR2 is not part of the list with the significant mutated genes in breast cancer. Instead, several truncated ERβ proteins have been detected in breast tumors [10]. Due to lack of sensitive methods of detection and specific antibodies for immunohistochemical assessment, a few truncated isoforms were analyzed in clinical samples. Some of these proteins result from alternative splicing of the C-terminus. Although this splicing mechanism produces five different isoforms, three of them have been detected in human breast tumors, the fully functional ERβ (ERβ1) and its variants ERβ2 and ERβ5. The last coding exon (exon 8) of ERβ1 has been replaced by exon

9 in ERβ2, and ERβ5 contains part of exon 7 and a different exon 8 [12, 65]. Exons 7 and 8 form a portion of the ligand binding and activation function 2 domains where helix 12 resides providing necessary surfaces for interaction with coactivators that regulate the activity of the receptor in response to ligand. Missing or alteration of these exons in ERβ2 and ERβ5 impairs or prevents association with ligand and results in the lack of or disorientated helix 12 (Fig. 1). Despite that they are incapable of binding ligands, ERβ2 and ERβ5 show higher estrogen-independent transcriptional activity than fully functional ERβ and influence estrogen signaling by forming heterodimers with ERα and ERβ1 resulting in altered ER activity [66]. ERβ2 has been reported to elicit various types of effects in different breast cancer cell models. Upregulation of ERβ2 inhibits the transcriptional activity of ERα in luminal breast cancer cells [67]. This effect is rather due to formation of ERα/ERβ2 heterodimers that promote proteasome-dependent degradation of ERα. On the other hand, inconsistent effects are reported for the same variant in ERα-negative cells. Induction of ERβ2 at lower levels than ERβ1 does not seem to affect cell survival and gene expression in TNBC cells [23, 68, 69]. In contrast, knockdown of endogenous ERβ2 in ERβ-negative TNBC cells inhibits proliferation and invasion by decreasing the stability of hypoxia-inducible factor (HIF-1α) through upregulation of prolyl hydroxylase 3 (PHD3). The inverse correlation between ERβ2 and PHD3 expression is also observed in clinical breast cancer specimens [70, 71]. As with ERβ1, conflicting results have been published regarding the expression of ERβ2 and ERβ5 in human breast tumors. Use of antibodies that specifically recognize these variants in immunohistochemical studies indicates cell type-specific expression in tumors [72]. In addition, their distinct patterns of subcellular localization are associated with prognosis. Their unique expression and mechanism of action suggest involvement in estrogen-mediated biological processes and potential implications in disease outcomes.

6   ERβ, Cell Proliferation, and Survival

While the role of ERα in promoting proliferation of mammary epithelial and breast cancer cells is established, the antiproliferative and pro-apoptotic effects of ERβ have been disputed by a few studies adding to the confusion that still surrounds its clinical importance in breast cancer [6]. The controversy stems from the analysis of genetically engineered mice with functional deletion of ERβ gene by different laboratories. Two independent groups reported defects in ductal side branching in ERβ knockout mice. The authors associated the phenotype with either the lack of the receptor in mammary epithelial cells or the impaired ovarian function that appears in these mice [53, 54]. However, one of these groups reported formation of abnormally large alveoli in lactating ERβ knockout mice and increased proliferation in differentiated epithelial cells and the presence of cysts in aging glands of the same mice [53, 73]. In contrast, the other group did not observe any cystic malformation and increased cell proliferation in the ERβ-deficient glands [54]. Consistent with the increased proliferation of ductal epithelial cells in ERβ knockout mice, independent investigations showed antiproliferative and pro-apoptotic effects of the receptor and its agonists in various mammary epithelial cell lines [55, 57]. Similar to the normal mammary cells, growth-repressive effects are observed following upregulation of the receptor in the majority of human breast cancer cell lines.

6.1   Antiproliferative Effects of ERβ

Most of breast cancer cells express low, almost undetectable by Western blot, levels of ERβ; thereby studying effects on cell proliferation and survival requires cells that are engineered to express ERβ [74]. Inducible and constitutive systems have been used to achieve transient or stable expression of fully functional ERβ and its variant isoforms in both luminal and ERα-negative cells. Expression of ERβ1 at various levels that are often less than ERα in MCF-7 cells is associated with reduced cell growth, inhibition of cell cycle progression, and induction of apoptosis both in the absence and presence of agonists in ERα-positive and ERα-negative cells and tumor xenografts [3, 75–80]. Multiple molecules are linked to tumor-repressive effects of ERβ1 including cell cycle regulators (cyclins E and D, CDC25, CDKs, SKP2) [20, 76, 81], anti-apoptotic proteins (FOXOM1, SURVIVIN, BCL-2) [3], oncogenes (HIF-1) [82], and angiogenesis factors (VEGF, PDGF) [75]. Gene ontology analysis of the top differentially regulated genes in ERβ-expressing cells reveals enrichment in pathways that regulate cell proliferation, apoptosis, and cell cycle progression [14, 18, 77]. Furthermore, upregulation of ERβ represses estrogen-induced cell proliferation and increases the sensitivity to antiestrogens, endoplasmic reticulum (EnR) stress inducers, and DNA-damaging agents [68, 83–86]. The increased sensitivity of ERβ-expressing cells to tamoxifen is associated with downregulation of the HER2/HER3 receptor dimer, its downstream effector AKT, and upregulation of PTEN [85]. The cytotoxic effects in the presence of EnR stress correlate with reduced expression of the pro-survival regulator of the unfolded protein response (UPR) IRE1α and the activity of its target XBP-1 [68, 87]. Finally, in response to chemotherapeutics, ERβ alters components of the DNA damage response (CHK1, BRCA) and p53 pathway (GADD45, p21, PUMA, NOXA) [68, 85–87]. The inhibitory effect of ERβ on estrogen-induced proliferation of ERα-positive cells correlates with repression of estrogen-associated gene expression [14, 18]. This transcriptional effect is mediated by a specific ERβ-chromatin binding that involves a set of primary target genes (HES-1, CDK-6, IRS-1, JAK-2 IGFBP-4, MYC) and transcription factors that control cell proliferation and apoptosis [14, 15, 17]. One of the ERβ-interacting transcription factors in luminal cells is p53. ERα interacts with p53 and induces a repressive heterochromatin conformation that inhibits p53-dependent gene expression. By binding to p53 and reducing the inhibitory interaction with ERα, ERβ stimulates the expression of p53 target genes [80, 84]. In addition to estrogen, ERβ antagonizes proliferative signals of growth factors in ERα-positive cells. Among these factors is heregulin-β that stimulates proliferation in MCF-7 cells by activating the HER2/HER3 pathway and promoting MDM2-depedent degradation of ERβ. The demand for downregulation of ERβ during growth factor-induced cell proliferation is clearly seen in cells with knockdown of MDM2 that do not respond to heregulin-β due to upregulating ERβ [88].

6.2   Contrasting Actions of ERβ on Cell Proliferation

In contrast to cell growth inhibitory effects, increased proliferation was observed in a few cell lines following upregulation of ERβ [6, 89]. The opposite actions on cell proliferation could be explained by differences in the amounts of the transfected receptor. The antiproliferative effect may require certain expression of ERβ that some stably transfected clones lack. In support of this, studies demonstrate that the transfected ERβ in TNBC cells inhibits proliferation only when it further increases by treatment with compounds that inhibit the proteasome pathway [48]. Similar to proteasome inhibitors, the antiproliferative effects in some ERβ-transfected cells are only seen after activation of the receptor with estrogen [77]. Other conditions that account for the loss of antiproliferative effect include the expression of truncated ERβ from plasmids lacking the N-terminus that is essential for activation through interaction with coactivators and DNA binding [29]. In addition, loss of transcription factors such as p53 that cooperates with ERβ on promoters of antiproliferating genes [80, 84], expression of ERα or ERβ isoforms that form inhibitory heterodimers with wild-type ERβ [3, 12, 18], and hyperactive oncogenic signaling that either decreases the stability and activity of the receptor or inhibits pro-apoptotic downstream pathways [27, 29, 47]. Consistent with the antitumor activity of the transfected ERβ, treatment of most of the ERα-positive and TNBC cells with detectable endogenous ERβ with agonists decreases cell proliferation, while downregulation of the receptor in the same cells attenuates the effects of the ligands [29, 30, 68]. In contrast to this trend, one recent investigation reports that ERβ mediates the proliferative effects of estrogens and enhances stem cell activity [90]. It has also been reported that some of the ERβ agonists behave differently when the cells grow in the absence and presence of basement membrane extract that induces growth factor signaling. While under basal conditions agonists inhibit cell growth, the same ligands promote cell proliferation and prevent cell death in the presence of matrigel or EGF- and insulin-containing media that are used in culture of mammary epithelial cells and activate PI3K and MAPK signaling. The role of growth factor signaling in the performance of ligands is further supported by the capacity of PI3K inhibitors to revert the growth stimulatory effects of ERβ agonists in cells that grow in matrigel or with insulin and EGF [58]. The proliferative responses of these compounds in the presence of growth factors may relate to the loss of ERβ expression due to proteasome-dependent degradation that is induced by this oncogenic signaling. In the absence of the receptor, some of the ERβ agonists may lead to activation of highly expressed ERα in luminal cancer cells. Such condition could not be excluded because the protein levels of endogenous ERβ are not often shown or validated by the use of appropriate controls, raising questions about the suggested proliferative phenotypes. Thus, a better characterization of the expression would explain some controversial effects of the receptor and its ligands and determine the optimal expression that is needed for the tumor suppressor activity.

6.3   Effects of ERβ2 on Cell Proliferation

In contrast to the antiproliferative activity of fully functional ERβ1, the role of its variant isoforms on cell survival still remains elusive. mRNA expression of some variants was reported in human breast cancer cells and tissues soon after the cloning of wild-type receptor [91], and the use of antibodies directed against the C-terminus that recognize splice variants suggests the presence of ERβ2 and ERβ5 in human breast tumors [66, 92]. Upregulation of ERβ2 in ERα-positive breast cancer cells was initially associated with inhibition of cell proliferation. Although the antiproliferative activity of ERβ2 was similar to wild-type receptor, gene expression analysis revealed that the two isoforms regulate distinct sets of genes implying the engagement of different mechanism of action [67, 93]. More recently, the endogenous ERβ2 in TNBC cells has been shown to drive proliferation by regulating the HIF-1α pathway [70]. The proliferative activity of ERβ2 is in agreement with its clinical association with worse disease outcome [72].

7   ERβ, Invasion, and Migration

The first evidence linking the receptor to migration and invasion and the mechanisms that regulate metastasis in breast cancer was provided by the analysis of the mammary gland of ERβ knockout mice. The results of this study suggest the involvement of ERβ in differentiation of the mammary epithelial tissue. In particular, increased adhesion of epithelial cells and expression of adhesion molecules (E-cadherin, occludin, integrin α) are observed in mammary glands of wild-type compared with the knockout mice [53]. Similar to ERβ knockout mice, knockdown of the receptor in mouse mammary epithelial cells decreases cell adhesion and the expression of E-cadherin through a mechanism that involves increased lysosomal degradation. The loss of cell adhesion is associated with the failure of ERβ-deficient cells to form polarized acini when they grow in reconstituted base membrane indicating involvement of the receptor in processes that regulate morphogenesis of mammary gland [94]. Since these processes are similar with those that operate and influence initiation and progression of breast cancer, ERβ was assumed to maintain epithelial structure in breast cancer tissues. Effects of ERβ on differentiation of malignant breast are reported in a mouse model with spontaneous p53-deficient tumors. When these tumors are developed in the absence of the receptor, they show less glandular differentiation and more spindle-shaped metaplasia as well as decreased epithelial and increased mesenchymal markers [36]. The association of ERβ with epithelial differentiation and increased cell adhesion has been corroborated in breast cancer cells. Upregulation of ERβ in mesenchymal-like and highly metastatic TNBC cells induces a strong epithelial transformation by increasing the expression of E-cadherin and members of the miR-200 family and suppressing the transcriptional repressor of E-cadherin ZEB. The capacity of ERβ to upregulate E-cadherin is also seen in human breast tumors where a positive correlation between the two proteins is identified. As an inducer of epithelial transformation, ERβ is capable of decreasing migration and the invasiveness of TNBC cells both in vitro and in a xenograft zebrafish invasion model [23]. ERβ impedes EMT and invasion and upregulates E-cadherin by repressing EGFR and its downstream signaling [23, 61]. Similar to breast cancer, ERβ is likely to reinstate epithelial differentiation after ductal elongation in normal gland by inhibiting EGFR and its related paracrine signaling [51]. ERβ represses EGFR signaling by acting on the promoter of EGFR gene and by regulating recycling of the protein [23, 61]. The posttranslational effect is associated with the inhibition of the pro-invasive function of mutant p53 that is expressed in many TNBCs [95]. ERβ inhibits growth factor signaling by interacting with mutant p53 and p63 on promoters of genes (SHARP, ADAMTS-9, Follistatin, CCNG2) that regulate EGFR activity, EMT, and invasion [96]. The anti-invasive activity of ERβ in TNBC cells has been seen in many other studies that implicate additional molecules (androgen receptor) in ERβ function and confirm effects of the receptor on pathways (ZEB1, TGF-β) that regulate E-cadherin and EMT [30, 48, 62–64]. The same studies demonstrate the in vivo anti-metastatic activity of ERβ and the ability of ERβ agonists to decrease the invasiveness of TNBC cells proposing the use of ligands as therapeutic intervention to prevent metastasis. In addition to TNBC cells, a similar anti-migratory activity of ERβ is observed in ERα-positive cells. Upregulation of ERβ in these cells enhances cell adhesion to extracellular matrix by increasing the expression of integrin α1 and β [97]. Thus, the anti-metastatic activity of the receptor is likely to affect breast cancer independent of subtype, growth factor receptor, and ERα status. Depending on the cellular content, ERβ can regulate large gene networks of cell differentiation, adhesion, and migration to ensure epithelial maintenance and control breast cancer metastasis. The ability of the receptor to adjust global anti-metastasis-associated gene expression may relate to its high propensity to bind multiple regulatory elements for various transcription factors and other epigenetic modifiers at enhancer regions [15, 16]. Most of the ERβ target genes that regulate invasion in breast cancer cells are also altered in mammary glands of ERβ knockout mice further validating its role as pro-differentiation factor in breast cancer [53]. In contrast to some ongoing debate on the antiproliferative activity of ERβ, its association with differentiation has not been disputed and is strong enough to define the receptor as tumor suppressor with specific anti-metastatic function. The effects of ERβ on cell adhesion and epithelial maintenance imply involvement of the receptor in initial steps of metastatic process when ductal epithelial cells invade the surrounding tissue but do not exclude specific roles in endothelial transmigration and extravasation as well as colonization in distant sites when tumor cells regain the epithelial phenotype. Such a role is supported by the analysis of prostate cancer tissues showing decline of ERβ during cancer development and re-expression in lymph nodes and bone metastasis [98].

8 Importance of ERβ as a Prognostic Factor in Breast Cancer

8.1 Reduced Expression of ERβ in Breast Tumors

Preclinical, clinical, and epidemiological studies have provided sufficient evidence for the implication of estrogens in etiology of breast cancer. Exposure to estrogens is associated with development of the disease and use of drugs that inhibit estrogen signaling with efficient treatment of ERα-positive tumors [99]. The correlation of ERα with response to endocrine therapy and the ability of its antagonists to reduce the rate of disease recurrence and breast cancer mortality have established the receptor as principal biomarker and primary therapeutic target in breast cancer [1, 100]. Despite the standard application of ERα antagonists in treatment of luminal tumors, one-third of women receiving tamoxifen for 5 years will eventually relapse indicating the complexity of the mechanisms that regulate response to endocrine therapy. It has thus been assumed that a better understanding of the biology of resistant tumors will foster the development of additional prognostic markers and therapeutic targets and improve management of resistant disease. In conjunction with this anticipation, the discovery of ERβ was initially met with great hope that a different ER subtype may complement ERα in prognosis and therapy. However, subsequently published studies failed to define a clear association of the receptor with clinical outcome preventing its routine clinical use. Most authors blame the use of poorly validated antibodies in immunohistochemical studies that vary in sensitivity and specificity as they recognize, among other non-specific epitopes, amino acid sequences that are common to all five known C-terminal splice variants [101]. Two recent studies focused on assessing the specificity of several ERβ antibodies including those that are commonly used to characterize breast cancer cell lines and tissues and evaluate clinical associations. Discrepancies between the two studies in performance of the same antibodies in immunoblotting assays indicate the need for developing more reproducible methods for evaluating ERβ expression in cells. Furthermore, the authors identify two different optimal antibodies for assessing ERβ expression by immunohistochemical means. One study shows expression of ERβ in breast and prostate cancer and consistent with previous findings gradual decline during tumor progression [5]. The other study suggests that ERβ is not expressed in most human tissues including breast cancer [102]. These contrasting results rather sustain the confusion that surrounds the status of the receptor in the disease. Despite the widely use of non-specific reagents, certain investigations performed comprehensive analysis with control cell lines expressing different ERβ isoforms and demonstrated the specificity of a few ERβ antibodies [23, 29, 36, 103]. Using immunoprecipitation or other methods to enrich for nuclear fraction or ERβ protein, they detected low levels of endogenous receptor in MCF-7 cells and a few other cell lines [29, 68, 96]. The decreased expression may account for the poor performance of antibodies in certain assays. The same methodological issue may apply to transfected cells since even efficient expression systems produce levels that are substantially lower compared with the detectable ERα in MCF-7 cells [23]. Differences in the levels of ERβ in transfected clones that were developed and maintained in different laboratories may explain variations in specificity of the same antibodies. Although the low levels of ERβ in breast cancer cells may relate to its tumor suppressor function, it is not yet clear whether this low expression is adequate to elicit some antitumor activity. The reduced expression of ERβ in breast cancer compared with benign tissues has been seen in clinical specimens and is consistent with the decline of the receptor during the development of spontaneous mouse mammary tumors [31–33, 104]. Less than half of these tumors retain ERβ, and within the positive cancers, the receptor is expressed in polarized epithelial cells but not in the poorly differentiated cellular compartment [36]. The presence of ERβ in a subset of cancer cells could imply that it controls tumor growth and progression through inhibition of paracrine factors that trigger proliferation in neighboring cells. These include growth factors that mediate the proliferative effects of ERα during ductal elongation and pro-inflammatory cytokines that stimulate stromal components to initiate oncogenic signals in tumor cells [51].

8.2 Association of ERβ with Clinicopathological Characteristics

The decline of ERβ in ductal hyperplasia and during the transition from carcinoma in situ to invasive cancer points toward a role as suppressor of both development and progression. The anti-tumorigenic role is supported by the analysis of breast tissues from women with atypical hyperplasia that increases the risk of breast cancer. High expression of ERβ in atypia and adjacent normal lobules is associated with decreased risk of developing breast cancer [34]. Despite this association, the prognostic and predictive value of ERβ remains controversial. Initial studies suffered from analysis of small number of samples and use of poorly validated antibodies. Other investigations evaluated only mRNA levels that do not often correlate well with protein expression, and they are not informative for the subcellular localization and the identity of ERβ-positive cells. By analyzing large cohorts with validated antibodies directed to specific regions of the isoforms ERβ1, ERβ2, and ERβ5, more recent studies identify associations between the different variants and clinical outcome. Despite some inconsistency in reported associations, most studies indicate correlation of ERβ1 with favorable prognostic markers (Table 1). Focusing on data from studies that examined large number of tumors (from 123 to 3093) by immunohistochemistry, ERβ1 significantly correlates with ERα in three studies [105–107]. The association with ERα as well as BRCA1 is also observed in a cohort with familial breast carcinomas when ERβ is assessed with an antibody that recognizes all three variants [108]. In support of its association with favorable prognosis, ERβ1 inversely correlates with the expression of HER2, pAKT, loss of PTEN [105, 106, 114], and the basal markers cytokeratin 5/6 and EGFR [106]. In contrast, ERβ1 is associated with Ki-67 in two cohorts of endocrine-treated tumors [110, 111]. In addition to molecular markers, ERβ1 correlates with low histological grade, small tumor size, and negative lymph node status in two studies [106, 109], whereas no association with the above or other known clinicopathological indicators is observed in two other studies [72, 113]. Similar to ERβ1, ERβ2 correlates with ERα positively in three [72, 107, 109] and negatively in one [108] of the four studies that assessed the variant with specific antibodies. ERβ2 also correlates with progesterone receptor, androgen receptor, and BRCA1. Whereas one study reports association of nuclear ERβ2 with low histological grade, another one correlates its cytoplasmic expression with high-grade tumors [72, 109], and two studies do not detect any significant relationship with prognostic factors [107, 108]. Finally, one study identifies association of ERβ5 with moderate Nottingham prognostic index [72].

8.3 Correlation of ERβ with Clinical Outcome

Consistent with the association with favorable prognostic biomarkers, ERβ1 correlates with better clinical outcome in most of the studies (Table 1). Nuclear ERβ1 is reported as independent predictor of both recurrence and mortality particularly in patients with TNBC that receive tamoxifen monotherapy [107]. It is also identified as the second most powerful indicator of favorable prognosis irrespective of ERα status in another study with hormonally treated patients [105]. Consistent, high-nuclear but not cytoplasmic ERβ1 correlates with longer recurrence-free survival in ERα-positive patients that receive adjuvant tamoxifen but not in unselected and TN breast cancers [104]. Similar results are observed in the study with familial breast carcinomas where high-nuclear ERβ1 is associated with longer 15-year survival only in tamoxifen-treated patients [108]. In addition to endocrine therapy, high-nuclear ERβ1 expression correlates with better survival in chemotherapy-treated patients [112, 114]. When mRNA levels of ERβ1 and ERβ2 strongly correlate with protein expression in unselected patients, both mRNA and protein levels of these isoforms are significantly associated with longer disease-free survival [109]. On the

Table 1 Correlation of ERβ with prognostic markers and clinical outcome

Molecular/ clinicopathological markers	Clinical outcome	Number of patients	Treatment	Reference
ERβ1: Positive correlation with ERα	*ERβ1*: Second most powerful indicator of favorable prognosis	181	Adjuvant tamoxifen ± CHT	[105]
ERβ1: Positive correlation with ERα, inverse correlation with HER2, CK5/6, EGFR. Association with low-grade, small size, and negative lymph node	*ERβ1*: No correlation with clinical outcome	3093	No information	[106]
ERβ1: Positive correlation with ERα *ERβ2*: Positive correlation with ERα	*ERβ1*: Association with better survival in tamoxifen-treated TNBCs (independent predictor of recurrence and mortality)	442	Adjuvant: tamoxifen	[107]
ERβ: Positive correlation with ERα and BRAC1 *ERβ2*: Inverse correlation with ERα, positive correlation with PR, AR and BRCA1	*ERβ1*: Association of nuclear ERβ1 with longer 15-year survival only in tamoxifen-treated patients	123	Adjuvant: No treatment, tamoxifen ± CHT	[108]
ERβ1: Correlation with low-grade, small size, negative lymph node *ERβ2*: Positive correlation with ERα, association of cytoplasmic ERβ2 with low histological grade	*ERβ1*: Association with longer disease-free survival *ERβ2*: Association with longer disease-free survival	150	Adjuvant: No treatment, tamoxifen ± CHT	[109]

(continued)

Table 1 (continued)

Molecular/clinicopathological markers	Clinical outcome	Number of patients	Treatment	Reference
ERβ2: Positive correlation with ERα, association of nuclear ERβ2 with low histological grade *ERβ5*: Association with moderate Nottingham prognostic index	*ERβ1*: No association with prognosis *ERβ2*: Association of nuclear ERβ2 with better survival and response to endocrine therapy, cytoplasmic ERβ2, or combined cytoplasmic and nuclear ERβ2 correlates with worse survival, metastasis, recurrence, and breast cancer-specific death *ERβ5*: Association of nuclear ERβ5 moderately with improved survival	757	No treatment, tamoxifen ± Zoladex	[72]
ERβ1: Positive correlation with Ki-67	Not reported	442	Adjuvant: tamoxifen	[110]
ERβ1: Positive correlation with Ki-67	No association	167	Adjuvant: Endocrine ± RT	[111]
No correlation	*ERβ1*: Association of nuclear but not cytoplasmic ERβ1 with longer recurrence-free survival in tamoxifen-treated ERα + patients but not in unselected and TN breast cancers	429	Adjuvant: No treatment, tamoxifen ± Fluoxymesterone	[104]

(continued)

Table 1 (continued)

Molecular/ clinicopathological markers	Clinical outcome	Number of patients	Treatment	Reference
ERβ1: Positive correlation with ERα and AR	*ERβ1*: Association with lower risk of breast cancer, association of nuclear ERβ1 with better survival in chemotherapy-treated but not in endocrine-treated patients	903	Adjuvant: Tamoxifen, AI, CHT, RT, Trastuzumab	[112]
ERβ1: No correlation	*ERβ1*: Association with better survival in node-negative patients that receive hormonal therapy but not chemotherapy Association with higher risk of relapse in nod-positive patients that receive chemotherapy	2170	Adjuvant: Endocrine or CHT	[113]
ERβ1: Inverse correlation with p-AKT and loss of PTEN	*ERβ1*: Association with better overall survival, disease-free survival, distant metastasis-free survival	571	Adjuvant: No treatment, CHT	[114]

AI aromatase inhibitors, *AR* androgen receptor, *CHT* chemotherapy, *PR* progesterone receptor, *RT* radiation therapy

other hand, no significant correlation of ERβ1 with better survival is observed in another cohort with unselected tumors. Instead, nuclear ERβ2 significantly correlates with better survival and response to endocrine therapy and strong nuclear ERβ5 moderately with improved survival [72]. In contrast to nuclear expression, cytoplasmic ERβ2 or combined cytoplasmic and nuclear ERβ2 is linked to worse overall survival, metastasis, recurrence, and breast cancer-specific death [72]. Cytoplasmic ERβ2 expression also correlates with poorer survival in chemotherapy-treated patients [72, 108]. Varying associations are observed in another large study. While ERβ1 does not appear as a significant prognostic factor in unselected tumors, it emerges as significant predictor of better disease-free survival in node-negative patients that received hormonal therapy but not chemotherapy. In contrast, ERβ1 correlates with significantly higher risk of relapse in nod-positive patients that largely receive chemotherapy [113]. Finally, despite the association with good prognostic markers, ERβ1 does not correlate with better survival in the largest study irrespective of ERα status even in tamoxifen-treated patients [106]. These results manifest how molecular heterogeneity, treatment variability, and the complex biology of breast cancer can influence the relationship of the receptor with clinical outcome. Differences in characteristics of patients including varying expression of isoforms among ethnic groups [66], duration and type of treatment (endocrine therapy, chemotherapy) [101], technical issues including variability in antibody specificities, tissue storage and preparation (fixation, antigen retrieval), tissue staining (antibody concentration, chromogen treatment), and evaluation of staining and scoring system could explain contrasting results [5]. Thus, contradictory observations should be interpreted with caution, and further stratification of patients is required to fully determine prognostic and predictive values. Despite the limitations in assessing the clinical importance of ERβ, an overall consideration of the presented data points toward an association of the receptor with favorable prognosis. This is also supported by two recent studies that performed meta-analysis of clinical data. By reviewing data from 20 studies that assessed ERβ isoforms by immunohistochemistry, the first one shows correlation of ERβ1 and ERβ2 with improved disease-free survival and total ERβ and ERβ2 with overall survival. However, when the patients are classified based on clinical subtypes, ERβ is associated with disease-free survival only in ERα-negative but not ERα-positive patients [115]. The second study confirms the significant associations of ERβ1 and ERβ2 but not ERβ5 with improved survival [116].

9   Concluding Remarks

The majority of studies analyzing breast cancer cells expressing ERβ demonstrate antiproliferative and anti-invasive effects. More inconsistent responses are observed with the use of ligands in cells that express endogenous receptor. Some of these studies suffer from poor characterization of cellular levels of the receptor. In cells with inadequate expression of ERβ, the adverse effects of agonists may be due to activation of ERα or ER-independent signaling. A better characterization of breast cancer cell lines will not only indicate the optimal conditions for ligand treatment but more importantly identify cell lines that express enough and functional amount of the receptor. Analysis of these cells after knockout of ERβ and/or treatment with specific agonists would corroborate the tumor suppressor function of the receptor and identify compounds with potential use in clinic for treatment of breast cancer. In addition to ligands, further mechanistic studies are required to delineate the pathways that regulate the expression of the receptor and its variant isoforms. Identification of molecules that cause methylation of the promoter or degradation of the protein will help to understand its reduced expression in cancer. It will also lead to characterization of additional markers with prognostic or therapeutic value. Despite the detection of ERβ in stroma, our understanding of its role in breast cancer entirely relies on evaluation of tumor cellular phenotypes. Given the significant contribution of the immune system and fibroblasts to tumor development and progression, analysis of tumor microenvironment in human tissues and mouse models of breast cancer will help to better understand specific actions of the receptor in the disease. Finally, additional prospective clinical studies with cohorts of hormone refractory tumors will clarify the association of ERβ with mechanisms of endocrine resistance. Implementation of single-cell mRNA assessment and DNA sequencing in primary and metastatic tissues and in serial plasma samples will lead through monitoring genomic and epigenetic changes in real time to more precise evaluation of how ERβ signaling is altered during the progression of the disease and whether these alterations are associated with more aggressive phenotypes and response to therapy.

References

1. Thomas C, Gustafsson JA (2011) The different roles of ER subtypes in cancer biology and therapy. Nat Rev Cancer 11(8):597–608. https://doi.org/10.1038/nrc3093
2. Nilsson S, Makela S, Treuter E, Tujague M, Thomsen J, Andersson G, Enmark E, Pettersson K, Warner M, Gustafsson JA (2001) Mechanisms of estrogen action. Physiol Rev 81(4):1535–1565. https://doi.org/10.1152/physrev.2001.81.4.1535
3. Chang EC, Frasor J, Komm B, Katzenellenbogen BS (2006) Impact of estrogen receptor beta on gene networks regulated by estrogen receptor alpha in breast cancer cells. Endocrinology 147(10):4831–4842. https://doi.org/10.1210/en.2006-0563
4. Harvey JM, Clark GM, Osborne CK, Allred DC (1999) Estrogen receptor status by immunohistochemistry is superior to the ligand-binding assay for predicting response to adjuvant endocrine therapy in breast cancer. J Clin Oncol 17(5):1474–1481. https://doi.org/10.1200/JCO.1999.17.5.1474
5. Nelson AW, Groen AJ, Miller JL, Warren AY, Holmes KA, Tarulli GA, Tilley WD, Katzenellenbogen BS, Hawse JR, Gnanapragasam VJ, Carroll JS (2017) Comprehensive assessment of estrogen receptor beta antibodies in cancer cell line models and tissue reveals critical limitations in reagent specificity. Mol Cell Endocrinol 440:138–150. https://doi.org/10.1016/j.mce.2016.11.016
6. Leygue E, Murphy LC (2013) A bi-faceted role of estrogen receptor beta in breast cancer. Endocr Relat Cancer 20(3):R127–R139. https://doi.org/10.1530/ERC-12-0389
7. Ogawa S, Inoue S, Watanabe T, Orimo A, Hosoi T, Ouchi Y, Muramatsu M (1998) Molecular cloning and characterization of human estrogen receptor betacx: a potential inhibitor of estrogen action in human. Nucleic Acids Res 26(15):3505–3512
8. Katzenellenbogen JA, Katzenellenbogen BS (1996) Nuclear hormone receptors: ligand-activated regulators of transcription and diverse cell responses. Chem Biol 3(7):529–536
9. Green S, Walter P, Greene G, Krust A, Goffin C, Jensen E, Scrace G, Waterfield M, Chambon P (1986) Cloning of the human oestrogen receptor cDNA. J Steroid Biochem 24(1):77–83
10. Thomas C, Gustafsson JA (2015) Estrogen receptor mutations and functional consequences for breast cancer. Trends Endocrinol Metab 26(9):467–476. https://doi.org/10.1016/j.tem.2015.06.007
11. Leung YK, Gao Y, Lau KM, Zhang X, Ho SM (2006) ICI 182,780-regulated gene expression in DU145 prostate cancer cells is mediated by estrogen receptor-beta/NFkappaB crosstalk. Neoplasia 8(4):242–249. https://doi.org/10.1593/neo.05853

12. Leung YK, Mak P, Hassan S, Ho SM (2006) Estrogen receptor (ER)-beta isoforms: a key to understanding ER-beta signaling. Proc Natl Acad Sci U S A 103(35):13162–13167. https://doi.org/10.1073/pnas.0605676103

13. Souza PCT, Textor LC, Melo DC, Nascimento AS, Skaf MS, Polikarpov I (2017) An alternative conformation of ERbeta bound to estradiol reveals H12 in a stable antagonist position. Sci Rep 7(1):3509. https://doi.org/10.1038/s41598-017-03774-x

14. Grober OM, Mutarelli M, Giurato G, Ravo M, Cicatiello L, De Filippo MR, Ferraro L, Nassa G, Papa MF, Paris O, Tarallo R, Luo S, Schroth GP, Benes V, Weisz A (2011) Global analysis of estrogen receptor beta binding to breast cancer cell genome reveals an extensive interplay with estrogen receptor alpha for target gene regulation. BMC Genomics 12:36. https://doi.org/10.1186/1471-2164-12-36

15. Zhao C, Gao H, Liu Y, Papoutsi Z, Jaffrey S, Gustafsson JA, Dahlman-Wright K (2010) Genome-wide mapping of estrogen receptor-beta-binding regions reveals extensive cross-talk with transcription factor activator protein-1. Cancer Res 70(12):5174–5183. https://doi.org/10.1158/0008-5472.CAN-09-4407

16. Charn TH, Liu ET, Chang EC, Lee YK, Katzenellenbogen JA, Katzenellenbogen BS (2010) Genome-wide dynamics of chromatin binding of estrogen receptors alpha and beta: mutual restriction and competitive site selection. Mol Endocrinol 24(1):47–59. https://doi.org/10.1210/me.2009-0252

17. Le TP, Sun M, Luo X, Kraus WL, Greene GL (2013) Mapping ERbeta genomic binding sites reveals unique genomic features and identifies EBF1 as an ERbeta interactor. PLoS One 8(8):e71355. https://doi.org/10.1371/journal.pone.0071355

18. Williams C, Edvardsson K, Lewandowski SA, Strom A, Gustafsson JA (2008) A genome-wide study of the repressive effects of estrogen receptor beta on estrogen receptor alpha signaling in breast cancer cells. Oncogene 27(7):1019–1032. https://doi.org/10.1038/sj.onc.1210712

19. Klionsky DJ, Abdalla FC, Abeliovich H, Abraham RT, Acevedo-Arozena A, Adeli K, Agholme L, Agnello M, Agostinis P, Aguirre-Ghiso JA, Ahn HJ, Ait-Mohamed O, Ait-Si-Ali S, Akematsu T, Akira S, Al-Younes HM, Al-Zeer MA, Albert ML, Albin RL, Alegre-Abarrategui J, Aleo MF, Alirezaei M, Almasan A, Almonte-Becerril M, Amano A, Amaravadi R, Amarnath S, Amer AO, Andrieu-Abadie N, Anantharam V, Ann DK, Anoopkumar-Dukie S, Aoki H, Apostolova N, Arancia G, Aris JP, Asanuma K, Asare NY, Ashida H, Askanas V, Askew DS, Auberger P, Baba M, Backues SK, Baehrecke EH, Bahr BA, Bai XY, Bailly Y, Baiocchi R, Baldini G, Balduini W, Ballabio A, Bamber BA, Bampton ET, Banhegyi G, Bartholomew CR, Bassham DC, Bast RC Jr, Batoko H, Bay BH, Beau I, Bechet DM, Begley TJ, Behl C, Behrends C, Bekri S, Bellaire B, Bendall LJ, Benetti L, Berliocchi L, Bernardi H, Bernassola F, Besteiro S, Bhatia-Kissova I, Bi X, Biard-Piechaczyk M, Blum JS, Boise LH, Bonaldo P, Boone DL, Bornhauser BC, Bortoluci KR, Bossis I, Bost F, Bourquin JP, Boya P, Boyer-Guittaut M, Bozhkov PV, Brady NR, Brancolini C, Brech A, Brenman JE, Brennand A, Bresnick EH, Brest P, Bridges D, Bristol ML, Brookes PS, Brown EJ, Brumell JH, Brunetti-Pierri N, Brunk UT, Bulman DE, Bultman SJ, Bultynck G, Burbulla LF, Bursch W, Butchar JP, Buzgariu W, Bydlowski SP, Cadwell K, Cahova M, Cai D, Cai J, Cai Q, Calabretta B, Calvo-Garrido J, Camougrand N, Campanella M, Campos-Salinas J, Candi E, Cao L, Caplan AB, Carding SR, Cardoso SM, Carew JS, Carlin CR, Carmignac V, Carneiro LA, Carra S, Caruso RA, Casari G, Casas C, Castino R, Cebollero E, Cecconi F, Celli J, Chaachouay H, Chae HJ, Chai CY, Chan DC, Chan EY, Chang RC, Che CM, Chen CC, Chen GC, Chen GQ, Chen M, Chen Q, Chen SS, Chen W, Chen X, Chen YG, Chen Y, Chen YJ, Chen Z, Cheng A, Cheng CH, Cheng Y, Cheong H, Cheong JH, Cherry S, Chess-Williams R, Cheung ZH, Chevet E, Chiang HL, Chiarelli R, Chiba T, Chin LS, Chiou SH, Chisari FV, Cho CH, Cho DH, Choi AM, Choi D, Choi KS, Choi ME, Chouaib S, Choubey D, Choubey V, Chu CT, Chuang TH, Chueh SH, Chun T, Chwae YJ, Chye ML, Ciarcia R, Ciriolo MR, Clague MJ, Clark RS, Clarke PG, Clarke R, Codogno P, Coller HA, Colombo MI, Comincini S, Condello M, Condorelli F, Cookson MR, Coombs GH, Coppens I, Corbalan R, Cossart P, Costelli P, Costes S, Coto-Montes A, Couve E, Coxon FP, Cregg JM, Crespo JL, Cronje MJ,

Cuervo AM, Cullen JJ, Czaja MJ, D'Amelio M, Darfeuille-Michaud A, Davids LM, Davies FE, De Felici M, de Groot JF, de Haan CA, De Martino L, De Milito A, De Tata V, Debnath J, Degterev A, Dehay B, Delbridge LM, Demarchi F, Deng YZ, Dengjel J, Dent P, Denton D, Deretic V, Desai SD, Devenish RJ, Di Gioacchino M, Di Paolo G, Di Pietro C, Diaz-Araya G, Diaz-Laviada I, Diaz-Meco MT, Diaz-Nido J, Dikic I, Dinesh-Kumar SP, Ding WX, Distelhorst CW, Diwan A, Djavaheri-Mergny M, Dokudovskaya S, Dong Z, Dorsey FC, Dosenko V, Dowling JJ, Doxsey S, Dreux M, Drew ME, Duan Q, Duchosal MA, Duff K, Dugail I, Durbeej M, Duszenko M, Edelstein CL, Edinger AL, Egea G, Eichinger L, Eissa NT, Ekmekcioglu S, El-Deiry WS, Elazar Z, Elgendy M, Ellerby LM, Eng KE, Engelbrecht AM, Engelender S, Erenpreisa J, Escalante R, Esclatine A, Eskelinen EL, Espert L, Espina V, Fan H, Fan J, Fan QW, Fan Z, Fang S, Fang Y, Fanto M, Fanzani A, Farkas T, Farre JC, Faure M, Fechheimer M, Feng CG, Feng J, Feng Q, Feng Y, Fesus L, Feuer R, Figueiredo-Pereira ME, Fimia GM, Fingar DC, Finkbeiner S, Finkel T, Finley KD, Fiorito F, Fisher EA, Fisher PB, Flajolet M, Florez-McClure ML, Florio S, Fon EA, Fornai F, Fortunato F, Fotedar R, Fowler DH, Fox HS, Franco R, Frankel LB, Fransen M, Fuentes JM, Fueyo J, Fujii J, Fujisaki K, Fujita E, Fukuda M, Furukawa RH, Gaestel M, Gailly P, Gajewska M, Galliot B, Galy V, Ganesh S, Ganetzky B, Ganley IG, Gao FB, Gao GF, Gao J, Garcia L, Garcia-Manero G, Garcia-Marcos M, Garmyn M, Gartel AL, Gatti E, Gautel M, Gawriluk TR, Gegg ME, Geng J, Germain M, Gestwicki JE, Gewirtz DA, Ghavami S, Ghosh P, Giammarioli AM, Giatromanolaki AN, Gibson SB, Gilkerson RW, Ginger ML, Ginsberg HN, Golab J, Goligorsky MS, Golstein P, Gomez-Manzano C, Goncu E, Gongora C, Gonzalez CD, Gonzalez R, Gonzalez-Estevez C, Gonzalez-Polo RA, Gonzalez-Rey E, Gorbunov NV, Gorski S, Goruppi S, Gottlieb RA, Gozuacik D, Granato GE, Grant GD, Green KN, Gregorc A, Gros F, Grose C, Grunt TW, Gual P, Guan JL, Guan KL, Guichard SM, Gukovskaya AS, Gukovsky I, Gunst J, Gustafsson AB, Halayko AJ, Hale AN, Halonen SK, Hamasaki M, Han F, Han T, Hancock MK, Hansen M, Harada H, Harada M, Hardt SE, Harper JW, Harris AL, Harris J, Harris SD, Hashimoto M, Haspel JA, Hayashi S, Hazelhurst LA, He C, He YW, Hebert MJ, Heidenreich KA, Helfrich MH, Helgason GV, Henske EP, Herman B, Herman PK, Hetz C, Hilfiker S, Hill JA, Hocking LJ, Hofman P, Hofmann TG, Hohfeld J, Holyoake TL, Hong MH, Hood DA, Hotamisligil GS, Houwerzijl EJ, Hoyer-Hansen M, Hu B, Hu CA, Hu HM, Hua Y, Huang C, Huang J, Huang S, Huang WP, Huber TB, Huh WK, Hung TH, Hupp TR, Hur GM, Hurley JB, Hussain SN, Hussey PJ, Hwang JJ, Hwang S, Ichihara A, Ilkhanizadeh S, Inoki K, Into T, Iovane V, Iovanna JL, Ip NY, Isaka Y, Ishida H, Isidoro C, Isobe K, Iwasaki A, Izquierdo M, Izumi Y, Jaakkola PM, Jaattela M, Jackson GR, Jackson WT, Janji B, Jendrach M, Jeon JH, Jeung EB, Jiang H, Jiang JX, Jiang M, Jiang Q, Jiang X, Jimenez A, Jin M, Jin S, Joe CO, Johansen T, Johnson DE, Johnson GV, Jones NL, Joseph B, Joseph SK, Joubert AM, Juhasz G, Juillerat-Jeanneret L, Jung CH, Jung YK, Kaarniranta K, Kaasik A, Kabuta T, Kadowaki M, Kagedal K, Kamada Y, Kaminskyy VO, Kampinga HH, Kanamori H, Kang C, Kang KB, Kang KI, Kang R, Kang YA, Kanki T, Kanneganti TD, Kanno H, Kanthasamy AG, Kanthasamy A, Karantza V, Kaushal GP, Kaushik S, Kawazoe Y, Ke PY, Kehrl JH, Kelekar A, Kerkhoff C, Kessel DH, Khalil H, Kiel JA, Kiger AA, Kihara A, Kim DR, Kim DH, Kim EK, Kim HR, Kim JS, Kim JH, Kim JC, Kim JK, Kim PK, Kim SW, Kim YS, Kim Y, Kimchi A, Kimmelman AC, King JS, Kinsella TJ, Kirkin V, Kirshenbaum LA, Kitamoto K, Kitazato K, Klein L, Klimecki WT, Klucken J, Knecht E, Ko BC, Koch JC, Koga H, Koh JY, Koh YH, Koike M, Komatsu M, Kominami E, Kong HJ, Kong WJ, Korolchuk VI, Kotake Y, Koukourakis MI, Kouri Flores JB, Kovacs AL, Kraft C, Krainc D, Kramer H, Kretz-Remy C, Krichevsky AM, Kroemer G, Kruger R, Krut O, Ktistakis NT, Kuan CY, Kucharczyk R, Kumar A, Kumar R, Kumar S, Kundu M, Kung HJ, Kurz T, Kwon HJ, La Spada AR, Lafont F, Lamark T, Landry J, Lane JD, Lapaquette P, Laporte JF, Laszlo L, Lavandero S, Lavoie JN, Layfield R, Lazo PA, Le W, Le Cam L, Ledbetter DJ, Lee AJ, Lee BW, Lee GM, Lee J, Lee JH, Lee M, Lee MS, Lee SH, Leeuwenburgh C, Legembre P, Legouis R, Lehmann M, Lei HY, Lei QY, Leib DA, Leiro J, Lemasters JJ, Lemoine A, Lesniak MS, Lev D, Levenson VV, Levine B, Levy E, Li F, Li JL, Li L, Li S, Li W, Li XJ, Li YB, Li YP, Liang C, Liang Q, Liao YF, Liberski PP, Lieberman A, Lim HJ, Lim KL, Lim K,

Lin CF, Lin FC, Lin J, Lin JD, Lin K, Lin WW, Lin WC, Lin YL, Linden R, Lingor P, Lippincott-Schwartz J, Lisanti MP, Liton PB, Liu B, Liu CF, Liu K, Liu L, Liu QA, Liu W, Liu YC, Liu Y, Lockshin RA, Lok CN, Lonial S, Loos B, Lopez-Berestein G, Lopez-Otin C, Lossi L, Lotze MT, Low P, Lu B, Lu Z, Luciano F, Lukacs NW, Lund AH, Lynch-Day MA, Ma Y, Macian F, MacKeigan JP, Macleod KF, Madeo F, Maiuri L, Maiuri MC, Malagoli D, Malicdan MC, Malorni W, Man N, Mandelkow EM, Manon S, Manov I, Mao K, Mao X, Mao Z, Marambaud P, Marazziti D, Marcel YL, Marchbank K, Marchetti P, Marciniak SJ, Marcondes M, Mardi M, Marfe G, Marino G, Markaki M, Marten MR, Martin SJ, Martinand-Mari C, Martinet W, Martinez-Vicente M, Masini M, Matarrese P, Matsuo S, Matteoni R, Mayer A, Mazure NM, McConkey DJ, McConnell MJ, McDermott C, McDonald C, McInerney GM, McKenna SL, McLaughlin B, McLean PJ, McMaster CR, McQuibban GA, Meijer AJ, Meisler MH, Melendez A, Melia TJ, Melino G, Mena MA, Menendez JA, Menna-Barreto RF, Menon MB, Menzies FM, Mercer CA, Merighi A, Merry DE, Meschini S, Meyer CG, Meyer TF, Miao CY, Miao JY, Michels PA, Michiels C, Mijaljica D, Milojkovic A, Minucci S, Miracco C, Miranti CK, Mitroulis I, Miyazawa K, Mizushima N, Mograbi B, Mohseni S, Molero X, Mollereau B, Mollinedo F, Momoi T, Monastyrska I, Monick MM, Monteiro MJ, Moore MN, Mora R, Moreau K, Moreira PI, Moriyasu Y, Moscat J, Mostowy S, Mottram JC, Motyl T, Moussa CE, Muller S, Munger K, Munz C, Murphy LO, Murphy ME, Musaro A, Mysorekar I, Nagata E, Nagata K, Nahimana A, Nair U, Nakagawa T, Nakahira K, Nakano H, Nakatogawa H, Nanjundan M, Naqvi NI, Narendra DP, Narita M, Navarro M, Nawrocki ST, Nazarko TY, Nemchenko A, Netea MG, Neufeld TP, Ney PA, Nezis IP, Nguyen HP, Nie D, Nishino I, Nislow C, Nixon RA, Noda T, Noegel AA, Nogalska A, Noguchi S, Notterpek L, Novak I, Nozaki T, Nukina N, Nurnberger T, Nyfeler B, Obara K, Oberley TD, Oddo S, Ogawa M, Ohashi T, Okamoto K, Oleinick NL, Oliver FJ, Olsen LJ, Olsson S, Opota O, Osborne TF, Ostrander GK, Otsu K, Ou JH, Ouimet M, Overholtzer M, Ozpolat B, Paganetti P, Pagnini U, Pallet N, Palmer GE, Palumbo C, Pan T, Panaretakis T, Pandey UB, Papackova Z, Papassideri I, Paris I, Park J, Park OK, Parys JB, Parzych KR, Patschan S, Patterson C, Pattingre S, Pawelek JM, Peng J, Perlmutter DH, Perrotta I, Perry G, Pervaiz S, Peter M, Peters GJ, Petersen M, Petrovski G, Phang JM, Piacentini M, Pierre P, Pierrefite-Carle V, Pierron G, Pinkas-Kramarski R, Piras A, Piri N, Platanias LC, Poggeler S, Poirot M, Poletti A, Pous C, Pozuelo-Rubio M, Praetorius-Ibba M, Prasad A, Prescott M, Priault M, Produit-Zengaffinen N, Progulske-Fox A, Proikas-Cezanne T, Przedborski S, Przyklenk K, Puertollano R, Puyal J, Qian SB, Qin L, Qin ZH, Quaggin SE, Raben N, Rabinowich H, Rabkin SW, Rahman I, Rami A, Ramm G, Randall G, Randow F, Rao VA, Rathmell JC, Ravikumar B, Ray SK, Reed BH, Reed JC, Reggiori F, Regnier-Vigouroux A, Reichert AS, Reiners JJ Jr, Reiter RJ, Ren J, Revuelta JL, Rhodes CJ, Ritis K, Rizzo E, Robbins J, Roberge M, Roca H, Roccheri MC, Rocchi S, Rodemann HP, Rodriguez de Cordoba S, Rohrer B, Roninson IB, Rosen K, Rost-Roszkowska MM, Rouis M, Rouschop KM, Rovetta F, Rubin BP, Rubinsztein DC, Ruckdeschel K, Rucker EB 3rd, Rudich A, Rudolf E, Ruiz-Opazo N, Russo R, Rusten TE, Ryan KM, Ryter SW, Sabatini DM, Sadoshima J, Saha T, Saitoh T, Sakagami H, Sakai Y, Salekdeh GH, Salomoni P, Salvaterra PM, Salvesen G, Salvioli R, Sanchez AM, Sanchez-Alcazar JA, Sanchez-Prieto R, Sandri M, Sankar U, Sansanwal P, Santambrogio L, Saran S, Sarkar S, Sarwal M, Sasakawa C, Sasnauskiene A, Sass M, Sato K, Sato M, Schapira AH, Scharl M, Schatzl HM, Scheper W, Schiaffino S, Schneider C, Schneider ME, Schneider-Stock R, Schoenlein PV, Schorderet DF, Schuller C, Schwartz GK, Scorrano L, Sealy L, Seglen PO, Segura-Aguilar J, Seiliez I, Seleverstov O, Sell C, Seo JB, Separovic D, Setaluri V, Setoguchi T, Settembre C, Shacka JJ, Shanmugam M, Shapiro IM, Shaulian E, Shaw RJ, Shelhamer JH, Shen HM, Shen WC, Sheng ZH, Shi Y, Shibuya K, Shidoji Y, Shieh JJ, Shih CM, Shimada Y, Shimizu S, Shintani T, Shirihai OS, Shore GC, Sibirny AA, Sidhu SB, Sikorska B, Silva-Zacarin EC, Simmons A, Simon AK, Simon HU, Simone C, Simonsen A, Sinclair DA, Singh R, Sinha D, Sinicrope FA, Sirko A, Siu PM, Sivridis E, Skop V, Skulachev VP, Slack RS, Smaili SS, Smith DR, Soengas MS, Soldati T, Song X, Sood AK, Soong TW, Sotgia F, Spector SA, Spies CD, Springer W, Srinivasula SM, Stefanis L, Steffan JS, Stendel R, Stenmark H, Stephanou A, Stern ST,

Sternberg C, Stork B, Stralfors P, Subauste CS, Sui X, Sulzer D, Sun J, Sun SY, Sun ZJ, Sung
JJ, Suzuki K, Suzuki T, Swanson MS, Swanton C, Sweeney ST, Sy LK, Szabadkai G, Tabas
I, Taegtmeyer H, Tafani M, Takacs-Vellai K, Takano Y, Takegawa K, Takemura G, Takeshita
F, Talbot NJ, Tan KS, Tanaka K, Tang D, Tanida I, Tannous BA, Tavernarakis N, Taylor GS,
Taylor GA, Taylor JP, Terada LS, Terman A, Tettamanti G, Thevissen K, Thompson CB,
Thorburn A, Thumm M, Tian F, Tian Y, Tocchini-Valentini G, Tolkovsky AM, Tomino Y,
Tonges L, Tooze SA, Tournier C, Tower J, Towns R, Trajkovic V, Travassos LH, Tsai TF,
Tschan MP, Tsubata T, Tsung A, Turk B, Turner LS, Tyagi SC, Uchiyama Y, Ueno T,
Umekawa M, Umemiya-Shirafuji R, Unni VK, Vaccaro MI, Valente EM, Van den Berghe G,
van der Klei IJ, van Doorn W, van Dyk LF, van Egmond M, van Grunsven LA, Vandenabeele
P, Vandenberghe WP, Vanhorebeek I, Vaquero EC, Velasco G, Vellai T, Vicencio JM, Vierstra
RD, Vila M, Vindis C, Viola G, Viscomi MT, Voitsekhovskaja OV, von Haefen C, Votruba M,
Wada K, Wade-Martins R, Walker CL, Walsh CM, Walter J, Wan XB, Wang A, Wang C,
Wang D, Wang F, Wang G, Wang H, Wang HG, Wang HD, Wang J, Wang K, Wang M, Wang
RC, Wang X, Wang YJ, Wang Y, Wang Z, Wang ZC, Wansink DG, Ward DM, Watada H,
Waters SL, Webster P, Wei L, Weihl CC, Weiss WA, Welford SM, Wen LP, Whitehouse CA,
Whitton JL, Whitworth AJ, Wileman T, Wiley JW, Wilkinson S, Willbold D, Williams RL,
Williamson PR, Wouters BG, Wu C, Wu DC, Wu WK, Wyttenbach A, Xavier RJ, Xi Z, Xia
P, Xiao G, Xie Z, Xu DZ, Xu J, Xu L, Xu X, Yamamoto A, Yamashina S, Yamashita M,
Yan X, Yanagida M, Yang DS, Yang E, Yang JM, Yang SY, Yang W, Yang WY, Yang Z, Yao
MC, Yao TP, Yeganeh B, Yen WL, Yin JJ, Yin XM, Yoo OJ, Yoon G, Yoon SY, Yorimitsu T,
Yoshikawa Y, Yoshimori T, Yoshimoto K, You HJ, Youle RJ, Younes A, Yu L, Yu SW, Yu WH,
Yuan ZM, Yue Z, Yun CH, Yuzaki M, Zabirnyk O, Silva-Zacarin E, Zacks D, Zacksenhaus E,
Zaffaroni N, Zakeri Z, Zeh HJ 3rd, Zeitlin SO, Zhang H, Zhang HL, Zhang J, Zhang JP,
Zhang L, Zhang MY, Zhang XD, Zhao M, Zhao YF, Zhao Y, Zhao ZJ, Zheng X, Zhivotovsky
B, Zhong Q, Zhou CZ, Zhu C, Zhu WG, Zhu XF, Zhu X, Zhu Y, Zoladek T, Zong WX,
Zorzano A, Zschocke J, Zuckerbraun B (2012) Guidelines for the use and interpretation of
assays for monitoring autophagy. Autophagy 8(4):445–544

20. Strom A, Hartman J, Foster JS, Kietz S, Wimalasena J, Gustafsson JA (2004) Estrogen receptor
beta inhibits 17beta-estradiol-stimulated proliferation of the breast cancer cell line T47D. Proc
Natl Acad Sci U S A 101(6):1566–1571. https://doi.org/10.1073/pnas.0308319100

21. Hartman J, Lindberg K, Inzunza J, Wan J, Strom A, Gustafsson J (2006) Estrogen receptor
beta represses breast tumor growth and angiogenesis in vivo. J Clin Oncol 24(18):565s–565s

22. Vivar OI, Zhao X, Saunier EF, Griffin C, Mayba OS, Tagliaferri M, Cohen I, Speed TP,
Leitman DC (2010) Estrogen receptor beta binds to and regulates three distinct classes of
target genes. J Biol Chem 285(29):22059–22066. https://doi.org/10.1074/jbc.M110.114116

23. Thomas C, Rajapaksa G, Nikolos F, Hao R, Katchy A, McCollum CW, Bondesson M, Quinlan
P, Thompson A, Krishnamurthy S, Esteva FJ, Gustafsson JA (2012) ERbeta1 represses basal-
like breast cancer epithelial to mesenchymal transition by destabilizing EGFR. Breast Cancer
Res 14(6):R148. https://doi.org/10.1186/bcr3358

24. Gomez BP, Riggins RB, Shajahan AN, Klimach U, Wang A, Crawford AC, Zhu Y, Zwart A,
Wang M, Clarke R (2007) Human X-box binding protein-1 confers both estrogen independence and antiestrogen resistance in breast cancer cell lines. FASEB J 21(14):4013–4027.
https://doi.org/10.1096/fj.06-7990com

25. Picard N, Charbonneau C, Sanchez M, Licznar A, Busson M, Lazennec G, Tremblay A
(2008) Phosphorylation of activation function-1 regulates proteasome-dependent nuclear
mobility and E6-associated protein ubiquitin ligase recruitment to the estrogen receptor beta.
Mol Endocrinol 22(2):317–330. https://doi.org/10.1210/me.2007-0281

26. Thomas C, Gustafsson JA (2012) Targeting PES1 for restoring the ERalpha/ERbeta ratio in
breast cancer. J Clin Invest 122(8):2771–2773. https://doi.org/10.1172/JCI65133

27. Cheng L, Li J, Han Y, Lin J, Niu C, Zhou Z, Yuan B, Huang K, Jiang K, Zhang H, Ding L,
Xu X, Ye Q (2012) PES1 promotes breast cancer by differentially regulating ERalpha and
ERbeta. J Clin Invest 122(8):2857–2870. https://doi.org/10.1172/JCI62676

28. Tremblay A, Tremblay GB, Labrie F, Giguere V (1999) Ligand-independent recruitment of SRC-1 to estrogen receptor beta through phosphorylation of activation function AF-1. Mol Cell 3(4):513–519

29. Yuan B, Cheng L, Chiang HC, Xu X, Han Y, Su H, Wang L, Zhang B, Lin J, Li X, Xie X, Wang T, Tekmal RR, Curiel TJ, Yuan ZM, Elledge R, Hu Y, Ye Q, Li R (2014) A phosphotyrosine switch determines the antitumor activity of ERbeta. J Clin Invest 124(8):3378–3390. https://doi.org/10.1172/JCI74085

30. Yuan B, Cheng L, Gupta K, Chiang HC, Gupta HB, Sareddy GR, Wang D, Lathrop K, Elledge R, Wang P, McHardy S, Vadlamudi R, Curiel TJ, Hu Y, Ye Q, Li R (2016) Tyrosine phosphorylation regulates ERbeta ubiquitination, protein turnover, and inhibition of breast cancer. Oncotarget 7(27):42585–42597. https://doi.org/10.18632/oncotarget.10018

31. Roger P, Sahla ME, Makela S, Gustafsson JA, Baldet P, Rochefort H (2001) Decreased expression of estrogen receptor beta protein in proliferative preinvasive mammary tumors. Cancer Res 61(6):2537–2541

32. Skliris GP, Munot K, Bell SM, Carder PJ, Lane S, Horgan K, Lansdown MR, Parkes AT, Hanby AM, Markham AF, Speirs V (2003) Reduced expression of oestrogen receptor beta in invasive breast cancer and its re-expression using DNA methyl transferase inhibitors in a cell line model. J Pathol 201(2):213–220. https://doi.org/10.1002/path.1436

33. Huang B, Omoto Y, Iwase H, Yamashita H, Toyama T, Coombes RC, Filipovic A, Warner M, Gustafsson JA (2014) Differential expression of estrogen receptor alpha, beta1, and beta2 in lobular and ductal breast cancer. Proc Natl Acad Sci U S A 111(5):1933–1938. https://doi.org/10.1073/pnas.1323719111

34. Hieken TJ, Carter JM, Hawse JR, Hoskin TL, Bois M, Frost M, Hartmann LC, Radisky DC, Visscher DW, Degnim AC (2015) ERbeta expression and breast cancer risk prediction for women with atypias. Cancer Prev Res (Phila) 8(11):1084–1092. https://doi.org/10.1158/1940-6207.CAPR-15-0198

35. Bardin A, Boulle N, Lazennec G, Vignon F, Pujol P (2004) Loss of ERbeta expression as a common step in estrogen-dependent tumor progression. Endocr Relat Cancer 11(3):537–551

36. Bado I, Nikolos F, Rajapaksa G, Wu W, Castaneda J, Krishnamurthy S, Webb P, Gustafsson JA, Thomas C (2017) Somatic loss of estrogen receptor beta and p53 synergize to induce breast tumorigenesis. Breast Cancer Res 19(1):79. https://doi.org/10.1186/s13058-017-0872-z

37. Swedenborg E, Power KA, Cai W, Pongratz I, Ruegg J (2009) Regulation of estrogen receptor beta activity and implications in health and disease. Cell Mol Life Sci 66(24):3873–3894. https://doi.org/10.1007/s00018-009-0118-z

38. Rody A, Holtrich U, Solbach C, Kourtis K, von Minckwitz G, Engels K, Kissler S, Gatje R, Karn T, Kaufmann M (2005) Methylation of estrogen receptor beta promoter correlates with loss of ER-beta expression in mammary carcinoma and is an early indication marker in premalignant lesions. Endocr Relat Cancer 12(4):903–916. https://doi.org/10.1677/erc.1.01088

39. Zhao C, Lam EW, Sunters A, Enmark E, De Bella MT, Coombes RC, Gustafsson JA, Dahlman-Wright K (2003) Expression of estrogen receptor beta isoforms in normal breast epithelial cells and breast cancer: regulation by methylation. Oncogene 22(48):7600–7606. https://doi.org/10.1038/sj.onc.1207100

40. Al-Nakhle H, Burns PA, Cummings M, Hanby AM, Hughes TA, Satheesha S, Shaaban AM, Smith L, Speirs V (2010) Estrogen receptor {beta}1 expression is regulated by miR-92 in breast cancer. Cancer Res 70(11):4778–4784. https://doi.org/10.1158/0008-5472.CAN-09-4104

41. Tateishi Y, Kawabe Y, Chiba T, Murata S, Ichikawa K, Murayama A, Tanaka K, Baba T, Kato S, Yanagisawa J (2004) Ligand-dependent switching of ubiquitin-proteasome pathways for estrogen receptor. EMBO J 23(24):4813–4823. https://doi.org/10.1038/sj.emboj.7600472

42. Pratt WB, Toft DO (1997) Steroid receptor interactions with heat shock protein and immunophilin chaperones. Endocr Rev 18(3):306–360. https://doi.org/10.1210/edrv.18.3.0303

43. Bagatell R, Khan O, Paine-Murrieta G, Taylor CW, Akinaga S, Whitesell L (2001) Destabilization of steroid receptors by heat shock protein 90-binding drugs: a ligand-independent approach to hormonal therapy of breast cancer. Clin Cancer Res 7(7):2076–2084

44. Tateishi Y, Sonoo R, Sekiya Y, Sunahara N, Kawano M, Wayama M, Hirota R, Kawabe Y, Murayama A, Kato S, Kimura K, Yanagisawa J (2006) Turning off estrogen receptor beta-mediated transcription requires estrogen-dependent receptor proteolysis. Mol Cell Biol 26(21):7966–7976. https://doi.org/10.1128/MCB.00713-06

45. Fan M, Park A, Nephew KP (2005) CHIP (carboxyl terminus of Hsc70-interacting protein) promotes basal and geldanamycin-induced degradation of estrogen receptor-alpha. Mol Endocrinol 19(12):2901–2914. https://doi.org/10.1210/me.2005-0111

46. Alonso L, Gallego E, Gonzalez FJ, Sanchez-Munoz A, Torres E, Pajares BI, Leeflang S, Baha C (2009) Gonadotropin and steroid receptors as prognostic factors in advanced ovarian cancer: a retrospective study. Clin Transl Oncol 11(11):748–752

47. Ohshiro K, Kumar R (2015) MTA1 regulation of ERbeta pathway in salivary gland carcinoma cells. Biochem Biophys Res Commun 464(4):1016–1021. https://doi.org/10.1016/j.bbrc.2015.07.043

48. Zhao Z, Wang L, James T, Jung Y, Kim I, Tan R, Hoffmann FM, Xu W (2015) Reciprocal regulation of ERalpha and ERbeta stability and activity by diptoindonesin G. Chem Biol 22(12):1608–1621. https://doi.org/10.1016/j.chembiol.2015.10.011

49. Sternlicht MD (2006) Key stages in mammary gland development: the cues that regulate ductal branching morphogenesis. Breast Cancer Res 8(1):201. https://doi.org/10.1186/bcr1368

50. Korach KS, Couse JF, Curtis SW, Washburn TF, Lindzey J, Kimbro KS, Eddy EM, Migliaccio S, Snedeker SM, Lubahn DB, Schomberg DW, Smith EP (1996) Estrogen receptor gene disruption: molecular characterization and experimental and clinical phenotypes. Recent Prog Horm Res 51:159–186 discussion 186–158

51. Mallepell S, Krust A, Chambon P, Brisken C (2006) Paracrine signaling through the epithelial estrogen receptor alpha is required for proliferation and morphogenesis in the mammary gland. Proc Natl Acad Sci U S A 103(7):2196–2201. https://doi.org/10.1073/pnas.0510974103

52. Ciarloni L, Mallepell S, Brisken C (2007) Amphiregulin is an essential mediator of estrogen receptor alpha function in mammary gland development. Proc Natl Acad Sci U S A 104(13):5455–5460. https://doi.org/10.1073/pnas.0611647104

53. Forster C, Makela S, Warri A, Kietz S, Becker D, Hultenby K, Warner M, Gustafsson JA (2002) Involvement of estrogen receptor beta in terminal differentiation of mammary gland epithelium. Proc Natl Acad Sci U S A 99(24):15578–15583. https://doi.org/10.1073/pnas.192561299

54. Antal MC, Krust A, Chambon P, Mark M (2008) Sterility and absence of histopathological defects in nonreproductive organs of a mouse ERbeta-null mutant. Proc Natl Acad Sci U S A 105(7):2433–2438. https://doi.org/10.1073/pnas.0712029105

55. Helguero LA, Faulds MH, Gustafsson JA, Haldosen LA (2005) Estrogen receptors alfa (ERalpha) and beta (ERbeta) differentially regulate proliferation and apoptosis of the normal murine mammary epithelial cell line HC11. Oncogene 24(44):6605–6616. https://doi.org/10.1038/sj.onc.1208807

56. Treeck O, Pfeiler G, Mitter D, Lattrich C, Piendl G, Ortmann O (2007) Estrogen receptor {beta}1 exerts antitumoral effects on SK-OV-3 ovarian cancer cells. J Endocrinol 193(3):421–433. https://doi.org/10.1677/JOE-07-0087

57. Treeck O, Lattrich C, Springwald A, Ortmann O (2010) Estrogen receptor beta exerts growth-inhibitory effects on human mammary epithelial cells. Breast Cancer Res Treat 120(3):557–565. https://doi.org/10.1007/s10549-009-0413-2

58. Cotrim CZ, Fabris V, Doria ML, Lindberg K, Gustafsson JA, Amado F, Lanari C, Helguero LA (2013) Estrogen receptor beta growth-inhibitory effects are repressed through activation of MAPK and PI3K signalling in mammary epithelial and breast cancer cells. Oncogene 32(19):2390–2402. https://doi.org/10.1038/onc.2012.261

59. Sotoca AM, van den Berg H, Vervoort J, van der Saag P, Strom A, Gustafsson JA, Rietjens I, Murk AJ (2008) Influence of cellular ERalpha/ERbeta ratio on the ERalpha-agonist induced proliferation of human T47D breast cancer cells. Toxicol Sci 105(2):303–311. https://doi.org/10.1093/toxsci/kfn141

60. Wiesen JF, Young P, Werb Z, Cunha GR (1999) Signaling through the stromal epidermal growth factor receptor is necessary for mammary ductal development. Development 126(2):335–344
61. Samanta S, Sharma VM, Khan A, Mercurio AM (2012) Regulation of IMP3 by EGFR signaling and repression by ERbeta: implications for triple-negative breast cancer. Oncogene 31:4689. https://doi.org/10.1038/onc.2011.620
62. Song W, Tang L, Xu Y, Sun Q, Yang F, Guan X (2017) ERbeta1 inhibits metastasis of androgen receptor-positive triple-negative breast cancer by suppressing ZEB1. J Exp Clin Cancer Res 36(1):75. https://doi.org/10.1186/s13046-017-0545-x
63. Schuler-Toprak S, Haring J, Inwald EC, Moehle C, Ortmann O, Treeck O (2016) Agonists and knockdown of estrogen receptor beta differentially affect invasion of triple-negative breast cancer cells in vitro. BMC Cancer 16(1):951. https://doi.org/10.1186/s12885-016-2973-y
64. Hinsche O, Girgert R, Emons G, Grundker C (2015) Estrogen receptor beta selective agonists reduce invasiveness of triple-negative breast cancer cells. Int J Oncol 46(2):878–884. https://doi.org/10.3892/ijo.2014.2778
65. Vladusic EA, Hornby AE, Guerra-Vladusic FK, Lupu R (1998) Expression of estrogen receptor beta messenger RNA variant in breast cancer. Cancer Res 58(2):210–214
66. Poola I, Fuqua SA, De Witty RL, Abraham J, Marshallack JJ, Liu A (2005) Estrogen receptor alpha-negative breast cancer tissues express significant levels of estrogen-independent transcription factors, ERbeta1 and ERbeta5: potential molecular targets for chemoprevention. Clin Cancer Res 11(20):7579–7585. https://doi.org/10.1158/1078-0432.CCR-05-0728
67. Omoto Y, Eguchi H, Yamamoto-Yamaguchi Y, Hayashi S (2003) Estrogen receptor (ER) beta1 and ERbetacx/beta2 inhibit ERalpha function differently in breast cancer cell line MCF7. Oncogene 22(32):5011–5020. https://doi.org/10.1038/sj.onc.1206787
68. Rajapaksa G, Nikolos F, Bado I, Clarke R, Gustafsson JA, Thomas C (2015) ERbeta decreases breast cancer cell survival by regulating the IRE1/XBP-1 pathway. Oncogene 34(31):4130–4141. https://doi.org/10.1038/onc.2014.343
69. Secreto FJ, Monroe DG, Dutta S, Ingle JN, Spelsberg TC (2007) Estrogen receptor alpha/beta isoforms, but not betacx, modulate unique patterns of gene expression and cell proliferation in Hs578T cells. J Cell Biochem 101(5):1125–1147. https://doi.org/10.1002/jcb.21205
70. Bialesova L, Xu L, Gustafsson JA, Haldosen LA, Zhao C, Dahlman-Wright K (2017) Estrogen receptor beta2 induces proliferation and invasiveness of triple negative breast cancer cells: association with regulation of PHD3 and HIF-1alpha. Oncotarget 8(44):76622–76633. https://doi.org/10.18632/oncotarget.20635
71. Faria M, Karami S, Granados-Principal S, Dey P, Verma A, Choi DS, Elemento O, Bawa-Khalfe T, Chang JC, Strom AM, Gustafsson JA (2018) The ERbeta4 variant induces transformation of the normal breast mammary epithelial cell line MCF-10A; the ERbeta variants ERbeta2 and ERbeta5 increase aggressiveness of TNBC by regulation of hypoxic signaling. Oncotarget 9(15):12201–12211. https://doi.org/10.18632/oncotarget.24134
72. Shaaban AM, Green AR, Karthik S, Alizadeh Y, Hughes TA, Harkins L, Ellis IO, Robertson JF, Paish EC, Saunders PT, Groome NP, Speirs V (2008) Nuclear and cytoplasmic expression of ERbeta1, ERbeta2, and ERbeta5 identifies distinct prognostic outcome for breast cancer patients. Clin Cancer Res 14(16):5228–5235. https://doi.org/10.1158/1078-0432.CCR-07-4528
73. Palmieri C, Cheng GJ, Saji S, Zelada-Hedman M, Warri A, Weihua Z, Van Noorden S, Wahlstrom T, Coombes RC, Warner M, Gustafsson JA (2002) Estrogen receptor beta in breast cancer. Endocr Relat Cancer 9(1):1–13
74. Haldosen LA, Zhao C, Dahlman-Wright K (2014) Estrogen receptor beta in breast cancer. Mol Cell Endocrinol 382(1):665–672. https://doi.org/10.1016/j.mce.2013.08.005
75. Hartman J, Lindberg K, Morani A, Inzunza J, Strom A, Gustafsson JA (2006) Estrogen receptor beta inhibits angiogenesis and growth of T47D breast cancer xenografts. Cancer Res 66(23):11207–11213. https://doi.org/10.1158/0008-5472.CAN-06-0017

76. Paruthiyil S, Parmar H, Kerekatte V, Cunha GR, Firestone GL, Leitman DC (2004) Estrogen receptor beta inhibits human breast cancer cell proliferation and tumor formation by causing a G2 cell cycle arrest. Cancer Res 64(1):423–428

77. Shanle EK, Zhao Z, Hawse J, Wisinski K, Keles S, Yuan M, Xu W (2013) Research resource: global identification of estrogen receptor beta target genes in triple negative breast cancer cells. Mol Endocrinol 27(10):1762–1775. https://doi.org/10.1210/me.2013-1164

78. Lazennec G, Bresson D, Lucas A, Chauveau C, Vignon F (2001) ER beta inhibits proliferation and invasion of breast cancer cells. Endocrinology 142(9):4120–4130. https://doi.org/10.1210/endo.142.9.8395

79. Bivona TG, Hieronymus H, Parker J, Chang K, Taron M, Rosell R, Moonsamy P, Dahlman K, Miller VA, Costa C, Hannon G, Sawyers CL (2011) FAS and NF-kappaB signalling modulate dependence of lung cancers on mutant EGFR. Nature 471(7339):523–526. https://doi.org/10.1038/nature09870

80. Lu W, Katzenellenbogen BS (2017) Estrogen receptor-beta modulation of the ERalpha-p53 loop regulating gene expression, proliferation, and apoptosis in breast cancer. Horm Cancer 8(4):230–242. https://doi.org/10.1007/s12672-017-0298-1

81. Reese JM, Bruinsma ES, Monroe DG, Negron V, Suman VJ, Ingle JN, Goetz MP, Hawse JR (2017) ERbeta inhibits cyclin dependent kinases 1 and 7 in triple negative breast cancer. Oncotarget 8(57):96506–96521. https://doi.org/10.18632/oncotarget.21787

82. Park C, Lee Y (2014) Overexpression of ERbeta is sufficient to inhibit hypoxia-inducible factor-1 transactivation. Biochem Biophys Res Commun 450(1):261–266. https://doi.org/10.1016/j.bbrc.2014.05.107

83. Murphy LC, Peng B, Lewis A, Davie JR, Leygue E, Kemp A, Ung K, Vendetti M, Shiu R (2005) Inducible upregulation of oestrogen receptor-beta1 affects oestrogen and tamoxifen responsiveness in MCF7 human breast cancer cells. J Mol Endocrinol 34(2):553–566. https://doi.org/10.1677/jme.1.01688

84. Bado I, Pham E, Soibam B, Nikolos F, Gustafsson J-Å, Thomas C (2018) ERβ alters the chemosensitivity of luminal breast cancer cells by regulating p53 function. Oncotarget 9(32):22509–22522. https://www.ncbi.nlm.nih.gov/pubmed/29854295

85. Lindberg K, Helguero LA, Omoto Y, Gustafsson JA, Haldosen LA (2011) Estrogen receptor beta represses Akt signaling in breast cancer cells via downregulation of HER2/HER3 and upregulation of PTEN: implications for tamoxifen sensitivity. Breast Cancer Res 13(2):R43. https://doi.org/10.1186/bcr2865

86. Thomas CG, Strom A, Lindberg K, Gustafsson JA (2011) Estrogen receptor beta decreases survival of p53-defective cancer cells after DNA damage by impairing G(2)/M checkpoint signaling. Breast Cancer Res Treat 127(2):417–427. https://doi.org/10.1007/s10549-010-1011-z

87. Rajapaksa G, Thomas C, Gustafsson JA (2016) Estrogen signaling and unfolded protein response in breast cancer. J Steroid Biochem Mol Biol 163:45. https://doi.org/10.1016/j.jsbmb.2016.03.036

88. Sanchez M, Picard N, Sauve K, Tremblay A (2013) Coordinate regulation of estrogen receptor beta degradation by Mdm2 and CREB-binding protein in response to growth signals. Oncogene 32(1):117–126. https://doi.org/10.1038/onc.2012.19

89. Jonsson P, Katchy A, Williams C (2014) Support of a bi-faceted role of estrogen receptor beta (ERbeta) in ERalpha-positive breast cancer cells. Endocr Relat Cancer 21(2):143–160. https://doi.org/10.1530/ERC-13-0444

90. Ma R, Karthik GM, Lovrot J, Haglund F, Rosin G, Katchy A, Zhang X, Viberg L, Frisell J, Williams C, Linder S, Fredriksson I, Hartman J (2017) Estrogen receptor beta as a therapeutic target in breast cancer stem cells. J Natl Cancer Inst 109(3):1–14. https://doi.org/10.1093/jnci/djw236

91. Moore JT, McKee DD, Slentz-Kesler K, Moore LB, Jones SA, Horne EL, Su JL, Kliewer SA, Lehmann JM, Willson TM (1998) Cloning and characterization of human estrogen receptor beta isoforms. Biochem Biophys Res Commun 247(1):75–78. https://doi.org/10.1006/bbrc.1998.8738

92. Green CA, Peter MB, Speirs V, Shaaban AM (2008) The potential role of ER beta isoforms in the clinical management of breast cancer. Histopathology 53(4):374–380. https://doi.org/10.1111/j.1365-2559.2008.02968.x

93. Zhao C, Matthews J, Tujague M, Wan J, Strom A, Toresson G, Lam EW, Cheng G, Gustafsson JA, Dahlman-Wright K (2007) Estrogen receptor beta2 negatively regulates the transactivation of estrogen receptor alpha in human breast cancer cells. Cancer Res 67(8):3955–3962. https://doi.org/10.1158/0008-5472.CAN-06-3505

94. Helguero LA, Lindberg K, Gardmo C, Schwend T, Gustafsson JA, Haldosen LA (2008) Different roles of estrogen receptors alpha and beta in the regulation of E-cadherin protein levels in a mouse mammary epithelial cell line. Cancer Res 68(21):8695–8704. https://doi.org/10.1158/0008-5472.CAN-08-0788

95. Ciriello G, Gatza ML, Beck AH, Wilkerson MD, Rhie SK, Pastore A, Zhang H, McLellan M, Yau C, Kandoth C, Bowlby R, Shen H, Hayat S, Fieldhouse R, Lester SC, Tse GM, Factor RE, Collins LC, Allison KH, Chen YY, Jensen K, Johnson NB, Oesterreich S, Mills GB, Cherniack AD, Robertson G, Benz C, Sander C, Laird PW, Hoadley KA, King TA, Network TR, Perou CM (2015) Comprehensive molecular portraits of invasive lobular breast cancer. Cell 163(2):506–519. https://doi.org/10.1016/j.cell.2015.09.033

96. Bado I, Nikolos F, Rajapaksa G, Gustafsson JA, Thomas C (2016) ERbeta decreases the invasiveness of triple-negative breast cancer cells by regulating mutant p53 oncogenic function. Oncotarget 7(12):13599–13611. https://doi.org/10.18632/oncotarget.7300

97. Lindberg K, Strom A, Lock JG, Gustafsson JA, Haldosen LA, Helguero LA (2010) Expression of estrogen receptor beta increases integrin alpha 1 and integrin beta 1 levels and enhances adhesion of breast cancer cells. J Cell Physiol 222(1):156–167. https://doi.org/10.1002/Jcp.21932

98. Zhu X, Leav I, Leung YK, Wu M, Liu Q, Gao Y, McNeal JE, Ho SM (2004) Dynamic regulation of estrogen receptor-beta expression by DNA methylation during prostate cancer development and metastasis. Am J Pathol 164(6):2003–2012

99. Hankinson SE, Colditz GA, Willett WC (2004) Towards an integrated model for breast cancer etiology: the lifelong interplay of genes, lifestyle, and hormones. Breast Cancer Res 6(5):213–218. https://doi.org/10.1186/bcr921

100. Allred DC, Harvey JM, Berardo M, Clark GM (1998) Prognostic and predictive factors in breast cancer by immunohistochemical analysis. Mod Pathol 11(2):155–168

101. Speirs V, Green AR, Hughes TA, Ellis IO, Saunders PT, Shaaban AM (2008) Clinical importance of estrogen receptor beta isoforms in breast cancer. J Clin Oncol 26(35):5825.; author reply 5825–5826. https://doi.org/10.1200/JCO.2008.19.5909

102. Andersson S, Sundberg M, Pristovsek N, Ibrahim A, Jonsson P, Katona B, Clausson CM, Zieba A, Ramstrom M, Soderberg O, Williams C, Asplund A (2017) Insufficient antibody validation challenges oestrogen receptor beta research. Nat Commun 8:15840. https://doi.org/10.1038/ncomms15840

103. Nikolos F, Thomas C, Rajapaksa G, Bado I, Gustafsson JA (2014) ERbeta regulates NSCLC phenotypes by controlling oncogenic RAS signaling. Mol Cancer Res 12:843. https://doi.org/10.1158/1541-7786.MCR-13-0663

104. Reese JM, Suman VJ, Subramaniam M, Wu X, Negron V, Gingery A, Pitel KS, Shah SS, Cunliffe HE, McCullough AE, Pockaj BA, Couch FJ, Olson JE, Reynolds C, Lingle WL, Spelsberg TC, Goetz MP, Ingle JN, Hawse JR (2014) ERbeta1: characterization, prognosis, and evaluation of treatment strategies in ERalpha-positive and -negative breast cancer. BMC Cancer 14:749. https://doi.org/10.1186/1471-2407-14-749

105. Nakopoulou L, Lazaris AC, Panayotopoulou EG, Giannopoulou I, Givalos N, Markaki S, Keramopoulos A (2004) The favourable prognostic value of oestrogen receptor beta immunohistochemical expression in breast cancer. J Clin Pathol 57(5):523–528

106. Marotti JD, Collins LC, Hu R, Tamimi RM (2010) Estrogen receptor-beta expression in invasive breast cancer in relation to molecular phenotype: results from the Nurses' Health Study. Mod Pathol 23(2):197–204. https://doi.org/10.1038/modpathol.2009.158

107. Honma N, Horii R, Iwase T, Saji S, Younes M, Takubo K, Matsuura M, Ito Y, Akiyama F, Sakamoto G (2008) Clinical importance of estrogen receptor-beta evaluation in breast cancer patients treated with adjuvant tamoxifen therapy. J Clin Oncol 26(22):3727–3734. https://doi.org/10.1200/JCO.2007.14.2968

108. Yan M, Rayoo M, Takano EA, Fox SB (2011) Nuclear and cytoplasmic expressions of ERbeta1 and ERbeta2 are predictive of response to therapy and alters prognosis in familial breast cancers. Breast Cancer Res Treat 126(2):395–405. https://doi.org/10.1007/s10549-010-0941-9

109. Sugiura H, Toyama T, Hara Y, Zhang Z, Kobayashi S, Fujii Y, Iwase H, Yamashita H (2007) Expression of estrogen receptor beta wild-type and its variant ERbetacx/beta2 is correlated with better prognosis in breast cancer. Jpn J Clin Oncol 37(11):820–828. https://doi.org/10.1093/jjco/hym114

110. Honma N, Horii R, Iwase T, Saji S, Younes M, Ito Y, Akiyama F (2015) Ki-67 evaluation at the hottest spot predicts clinical outcome of patients with hormone receptor-positive/HER2-negative breast cancer treated with adjuvant tamoxifen monotherapy. Breast Cancer 22(1):71–78. https://doi.org/10.1007/s12282-013-0455-5

111. O'Neill PA, Davies MP, Shaaban AM, Innes H, Torevell A, Sibson DR, Foster CS (2004) Wild-type oestrogen receptor beta (ERbeta1) mRNA and protein expression in tamoxifen-treated post-menopausal breast cancers. Br J Cancer 91(9):1694–1702. https://doi.org/10.1038/sj.bjc.6602183

112. Elebro K, Borgquist S, Rosendahl AH, Markkula A, Simonsson M, Jirstrom K, Rose C, Ingvar C, Jernstrom H (2017) High estrogen receptor beta expression is prognostic among adjuvant chemotherapy-treated patients-results from a population-based breast cancer cohort. Clin Cancer Res 23(3):766–777. https://doi.org/10.1158/1078-0432.CCR-16-1095

113. Novelli F, Milella M, Melucci E, Di Benedetto A, Sperduti I, Perrone-Donnorso R, Perracchio L, Venturo I, Nistico C, Fabi A, Buglioni S, Natali PG, Mottolese M (2008) A divergent role for estrogen receptor-beta in node-positive and node-negative breast cancer classified according to molecular subtypes: an observational prospective study. Breast Cancer Res 10(5):R74. https://doi.org/10.1186/bcr2139

114. Wang J, Zhang C, Chen K, Tang H, Tang J, Song C, Xie X (2015) ERbeta1 inversely correlates with PTEN/PI3K/AKT pathway and predicts a favorable prognosis in triple-negative breast cancer. Breast Cancer Res Treat 152(2):255–269. https://doi.org/10.1007/s10549-015-3467-3

115. Tan W, Li Q, Chen K, Su F, Song E, Gong C (2016) Estrogen receptor beta as a prognostic factor in breast cancer patients: a systematic review and meta-analysis. Oncotarget 7(9):10373–10385. https://doi.org/10.18632/oncotarget.7219

116. Liu J, Guo H, Mao K, Zhang K, Deng H, Liu Q (2016) Impact of estrogen receptor-beta expression on breast cancer prognosis: a meta-analysis. Breast Cancer Res Treat 156(1):149–162. https://doi.org/10.1007/s10549-016-3721-3

Endocrine Disrupting Chemicals and Breast Cancer: The Saga of Bisphenol A

Nira Ben-Jonathan

Abstract Breast cancer results from time-related complex interactions between internal and external factors. In addition to endogenous estrogens, which play an undisputed role in breast tumorigenesis, exogenous compounds which mimic the actions of estrogen and are referred to as endocrine disruptors (EDCs) or xenoestrogens have strong impacts on breast development during the perinatal period and on carcinogenesis in adults. EDCs include natural compounds such as phytoestrogens and mycoestrogens, as well as numerous man-made chemicals which are widely used by the agriculture, chemical, food, and cosmetic industries, and are included in multiple everyday consumer products. This chapter reviews the evidence on human exposure to the EDCs, their in vitro and in vivo effects on breast cancer, and their proposed mechanisms of action. Emphasis has been placed on bisphenol A (BPA), a prototypical xenoestrogen whose adverse health effects have attracted considerable attention by scientists, industry, regulatory agencies, and the public at large. The disparate positions on health hazards by BPA, which have been undertaken by the chemical and food industries, environmental advocacy groups, health organizations, and regulatory agencies, are reviewed and criticized.

Keywords Estrogen · Estrogen receptors (ER) · Xenoestrogens · Endocrine disruptors (EDC) · Breast cancer risks · Bisphenol A (BPA) · Phytoestrogens · Mycoestrogens · Breast carcinogenesis · Mechanism of action · Health hazards

1 Introduction

Endocrine-disrupting chemicals (EDCs) are defined as exogenous compounds that affect hormone synthesis, secretion, metabolism, and/or actions [1]. EDCs can act either as agonists or as antagonists of receptors of multiple hormones: estrogens (ER), progesterone (PR), androgens (AR), glucocorticoids (GR), mineralocorticoids

N. Ben-Jonathan (✉)
Department of Cancer Biology, University of Cincinnati, Cincinnati, OH, USA
e-mail: Nira.Ben-Jonathan@uc.edu

© Springer Nature Switzerland AG 2019
X. Zhang (ed.), *Estrogen Receptor and Breast Cancer*, Cancer Drug Discovery and Development, https://doi.org/10.1007/978-3-319-99350-8_13

343

(MR), thyroid hormones (TR), G protein-coupled estrogen receptor (GPER), peroxisome proliferator-activated receptor (PPAR), and others. EDCs can also alter the availability of active hormones by affecting hormone synthesis and metabolic enzymes [2].

Xenoestrogens represent a subclass of EDCs which specifically mimic or interfere with actions of estrogens. Xenoestrogens encompass a wide variety of compounds, some of which are naturally made by plants (phytoestrogens) or fungi (mycoestrogens), while others are man-made chemicals. The latter group includes pharmaceuticals, cosmetics, plastic additives, industrial solvents, pesticides, herbicides, and by-products of combustion and industrial manufacturing processes. The times at which exposure to xenoestrogens occurs, i.e., during fetal, neonatal, pubertal, or adult life, are of critical importance in the manifestation of their effects on the development and progression of breast cancer.

This chapter begins with a discussion on the impact of the environment on breast cancer, followed by a short description of the various types of xenoestrogens and their prevalence in the environment. The focus then shifts to bisphenol A (BPA), a prototypical xenoestrogen whose adverse health effects have attracted considerable attention by scientists, industry, regulatory agencies, and the public at large. After appraising the levels of human exposure to BPA, the discussion summarizes in vitro and in vivo data that substantiate its adverse effects on breast cancer. The proposed mechanism(s) of action of BPA through different receptors that activate canonical and noncanonical pathways are then reviewed. Finally, we discuss the disparate positions that have been undertaken by the chemical and food industries, scientific societies, and environmental advocates, on BPA as a risk factor for human health. This is followed by an assessment of the current policies of regulatory agencies in the USA and abroad on banning BPA from consumer products and the shortcoming of other bisphenols which were recently introduced as substitutes for BPA. Figure 1 illustrates the various classes of xenoestrogens which impinge upon breast cancer, with an emphasis on the multiple environmental sources of BPA.

2   Risk Factors of Breast Cancer and Impact of the Environment

Breast cancer is a heterogeneous disease, characterized by considerable diversity among tumors as well as among patients. This heterogeneity must be taken into account upon evaluating the risk of disease occurrence, progression, and therapeutic resistance. The most acceptable determinants of breast cancer risks are gender (female), age (older), and history of the reproductive cycle (early age at menarche, nulliparity, late age at first full-term pregnancy, late age at lactation and short duration, and late menopause). A lifetime cumulative exposure to endogenous estrogens is considered a strong risk factor, although other hormones that affect the development and differentiation of breast epithelial and stromal cells serve as contributing

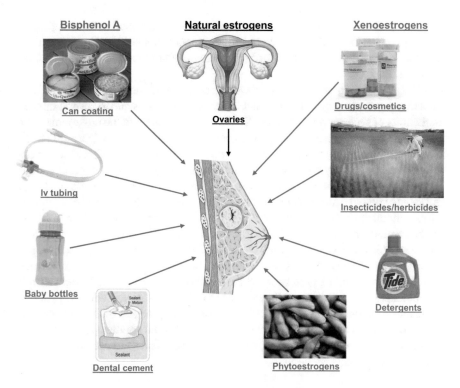

Fig. 1 Various sources of estrogen-like substances that affect breast cancer

factors. Additional risk factors include exogenous estrogens (oral contraceptives and hormone replacement therapy, HRT), radiation exposure, alcohol consumption, obesity, and to a lesser extent higher educational level and socioeconomic status. Notably, only 5–10% of breast cancer cases are hereditary, caused by passing abnormal genes such as BRCA1 and BRCA2 from parent to child. Moreover, all the above risk factors explain only about half of breast cancer cases in the USA, where incidence rates of the disease have been rising slowly for the past two decades [3].

The geographical location has long been recognized as a determinant in the incidence of breast cancer. High incidence rates are found in North America and Northern/Western Europe, intermediate rates are evident in South America and Southern Europe, while low rates are seen in Africa and Asia [4]. As individuals migrate from low- to high-risk geographical areas, the incidence of breast cancer approaches that of the host country within one or two generations, suggesting that most of the differences are due to altered diet and/or environmental exposures.

The role of the environment in breast tumorigenesis has been supported by many epidemiological surveys. For example, a large study has examined the risks of cancer by analyzing data on 44,788 pairs of twins in the Swedish, Danish, and Finnish twin registries [5]. Statistical modeling was used to estimate the relative importance of heritable vs environmental factors in causing many types of cancers. The study found that inherited genetic factors make only a minor contribution to susceptibility to most types of neoplasms, while the environment has a principal role in causing sporadic cancer. More than 60% of breast cancers were found to have an environmental etiology.

Most epidemiological studies, however, do not provide a clear link between human exposure to a specific EDC and breast cancer. This is due to several inherent limitations of such surveys: (a) most EDCs, while prevalent in the environment, are present at very low concentrations, often below conventional analytical methods for their measurement; (b) the length or the timing of exposure to EDCs cannot be easily assessed, especially with respect to the critical "windows of susceptibility" during embryonic life; and (c) EDCs exist in the environment as a mixture, making it difficult to sort out distinct contributions of each compound to adverse health effects.

A comprehensive review [6] compiled information from multiple animal studies on the carcinogenic potential of a variety of chemicals. As many as 216 compounds, which include industrial chemicals, chlorinated solvents, combustion products, pesticides, dyes, pharmaceuticals, and research chemicals, were reported to increase mammary gland tumors in rodents. Of these, 29 are produced in the USA at >1 million pounds/year; 35 are air pollutants, 25 have been associated with occupational exposures of women, and 73 are present in consumer products or as food contaminants. The study concluded that many of these chemicals are mutagenic and cause tumors in multiple organs and species. Such characteristics are considered indicative of carcinogenicity in humans.

3   Natural Xenoestrogens

Xenoestrogens are broadly divided into natural and synthetic compounds. Natural compounds include phytoestrogens, plant-derived compounds whose primary route of exposure is by consumption, and mycoestrogens, products of fungi that are usually present as food contaminants. Most, albeit not all, xenoestrogens are phenolic compounds that structurally resemble 17β-estradiol (E2). Their shared structures include a phenolic ring and a pair of hydroxyl groups, whose position is important for determining their ability to bind ERα and/or ERβ [7]. Table 1 summarizes the sources as well as major exposure pathways for the different classes of xenoestrogens.

3.1   Phytoestrogens

Phytoestrogens include as many as 100 molecules, which are subclassified into 5 groups: flavonoids, isoflavones, stilbens, coumestans, and lignans (Fig. 2). These compounds are found in fruits, vegetables, legumes, teas, and coffees and are mostly

Table 1 Different classes of xenoestrogens, their sources in the environment, and major pathways of human exposure

Class Compounds	Sources	Exposure pathways
Phytoestrogens	Plants	Ingestion
Genestein, resveratrol, daidzein		
Mycoestrogens	Fungi	Ingestion
Zeranol, fusarins		
Pharmaceuticals	Drugs, cosmetics	Skin
DES, HRT, phthalates		
Pesticides and herbicides	Livestock, crops	Skin, inhalation
DDT, atrazine, dieldrin		
Plastics, industrial chemicals	Polycarbonates, epoxy resins	Skin, iv, oral
PCBs, bisphenols		
Food additives	Variety of foods	Ingestion
Propyl gallate, 4-hexyl resorcinol		
Detergents and preservatives	Household goods	Skin
Parabens, alkylphenols		
Combustion by-products	Car exhausts	Inhalation
Dioxin, aromatic hydrocarbons		

Fig. 2 The five classes of phytoestrogens and their proposed mode of action

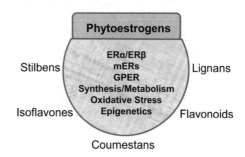

concentrated in the fruit skin and flowers. Four of the most commonly ingested and widely studied phytoestrogens are resveratrol, daidzein, quercetin, and genistein.

The notion on functional associations between phytoestrogens and breast cancer has been based on the observations that high consumption of soy products, which are enriched in phytoestrogens, correlates with low incidence of breast cancer in several Asian countries. However, epidemiological studies have produced inconsistent results, and the role of phytoestrogens in breast chemoprevention remains enigmatic. This uncertainty is due to the multiple modes of actions of phytoestrogens, as well as to their nonlinear, and often antagonistic, dose effects [8]. As compared with E2, phytoestrogens bind only weekly to ERs, except that many have a preferential higher binding affinity to ERβ, whose activation can inhibit the growth-promoting effects of ERα. In general, however, only saturating doses of phytoestrogens exert growth inhibitory effects on breast cancer. In addition to binding to intracellular ERs, some phytoestrogens activate membrane estrogen receptors (mERs) and G protein-coupled receptor, GPER [9]; they can also inhibit local estrogen synthesis, affect metabolic degradation, and can also cause epigenetic changes (Fig. 2).

In vitro and in vivo studies with genistein, daidzein, resveratrol, and quercetin show that they exert their actions by affecting estrogen-metabolizing enzymes, cell cycle progression, cell differentiation, proliferation, apoptosis, and the inflammatory response [7]. Collectively, while there is some evidence supporting a chemoprotective role for phytoestrogens in breast cancer, there are also data showing their adverse effects. Undoubtedly, more research is needed to fully evaluate the estrogenic activities of phytoestrogens and the biological relevance of experimental findings.

3.2 Mycoestrogens

Fusarium is a large family of fungi that reside in soil worldwide. Some *Fusarium* species are economically important because of their harmful impact on crops. *Fusarium* fungi produce two main groups of mycoestrogens: zearalenones and fusarins [10]. The zearalenones act as strong estrogen agonists, with a binding affinity to ER in human cells only ten times lower than that of E2, while the fusarins have a weaker binding affinity, 2.6×10^5 lower than E2 [11]. Zearalenones are present in grains and other plant-derived foods through fungal contamination and in animal products (e.g., meat, eggs, dairy products) through the use of zeranol in livestock to promote growth and improve beef/meat production.

Zeranol, a synthetic derivative of zearalanol, is FDA approved for use as a non-steroidal anabolic growth promoter in beef production in the USA but is banned for this purpose in the European Union. At low concentrations, zeranol accelerated the growth of ER-positive MCF-7 breast cancer cells but did not affect growth of the ER-negative MDA-MB-231 cells [12]. At high concentrations, however, zeranol suppressed growth of both ER-positive and ER-negative cells. Like the typical mode of action of many xenoestrogens, zeranol shows a dose-dependent biphasic effect on ER-positive breast cancer cells: accelerating cell growth at low concentrations but inducing apoptosis at high concentrations. Comparable results were reported for the effects of several fusarelins, whose growth-promoting effects on MCF-7 cells were blocked by the ER antagonist fulvestrant, confirming an action via ERs [11]. Collectively, experimental and epidemiologic data, albeit limited, indicate that mycoestrogens act as endocrine disruptors. Both estrogenic and antiestrogenic effects have been reported, and their actions depend on the dose, hormonal environment, and critical window of developmental exposure.

4 Synthetic Xenoestrogens

Synthetic xenoestrogens encompass a very large class of chemicals which are introduced into the environment by the pharmaceutical, food, cosmetics, agricultural, and chemical industries, as illustrated in Fig. 3.

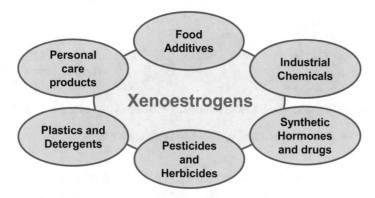

Fig. 3 Man-made chemicals which act as endocrine disruptors

4.1 Pharmaceuticals

Diethylstilbestrol (DES), produced in 1938 as the first potent synthetic estrogen, was prescribed from 1940 to 1971 to several million pregnant women to prevent miscarriage and correct other complications of pregnancy. Astute observations by several physicians in the early 1970s, who noticed increased incidence of a rare vaginal cancer in adolescent women, drew attention to the deleterious effects of DES [13, 14]. In retrospect, there was no good reason for treating pregnant women with DES, except that it was readily available and was considered safe. Like thalidomide, DES had little impact on the treated women themselves, but had a substantial, albeit a delayed, effect on their developing fetuses, demonstrating that drug actions in the fetus cannot be extrapolated from lack of adult responsiveness. During the 1960s–1970s, DES was also used as a growth promoter in 70–80% of poultry and livestock in the USA. Given this widespread practice, the consequences of human exposure to DES via meat consumption cannot be evaluated.

Prenatal exposure to DES caused multiple structural and functional abnormalities in both men and women. A large percentage of daughters of mothers who took DES had benign anomalies of the reproductive tract, with increased incidence of infertility and ectopic pregnancy. The most common cancer was vaginal clear cell adenocarcinoma, affecting 0.1–0.15% of the exposed women. Structural abnormalities in sons included cryptorchidism, malformed urethras, and epididymal cysts, often accompanied by decreased sperm count, increased sperm deformities, and prostatic inflammation. Whereas the congenital malformations caused by thalidomide were recognized at birth, those of DES were more subtle and delayed. Unlike thalidomide, which is not teratogenic in most laboratory animals, DES exerts similar effects in many species, including nonhuman primates [13]. DES-treated fetal or neonatal rodents developed latent tumors of the pituitary, mammary gland, and uterus.

A more recent analysis revealed that daughters of mothers who took DES during pregnancy have a twofold higher risk of breast cancer than those who were not exposed to DES [15]. It was subsequently proposed that DES exposure in utero

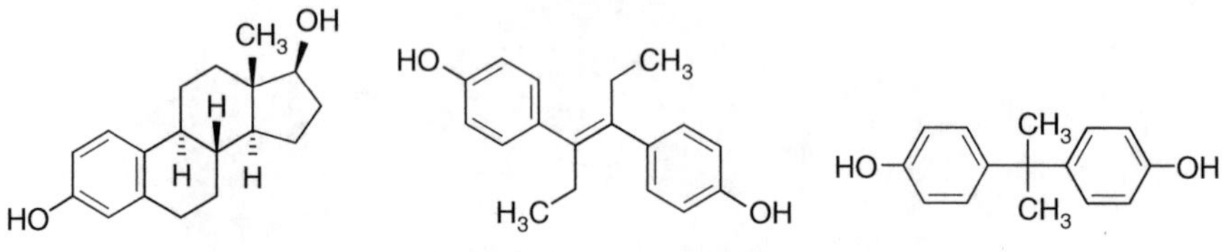

17β-Estradiol (E2)   **Diethylstilbestrol (DES)**   **Bisphenol A (BPA)**

Fig. 4 Chemical structures of estradiol, diethylstilbestrol, and bisphenol A

induces epigenetic alterations such as increased DNA methylation, histone modifications, and microRNA expression. Such alterations often target genes that regulate stem cells and prevent differentiation of their daughter cells. Figure 4 shows the structural similarity of DES and BPA, as compared to the structure of the natural estrogen, 17β-estradiol (E2).

The release of estrogenic-active pharmaceuticals into waterways has been known for some time and has become of increasing concern [16]. Multiple infertility treatment drugs, including HRT and oral contraceptives, are disposed from millions of households into the sewage system. The efficacy of their removal from wastewater varies widely, depending on the chemical structure of each compound and the treatment technologies of the sewage treatment plants. In addition, effluents containing pharmaceuticals from some medical facilities and drug manufacturing plants are released directly into river waters and not collected by a sewer system, becoming a significant contaminant source of hormonally active compounds. A recent study reported on the detection of many pharmaceutical and personal care products at microgram to nanogram per liter concentrations in the great lakes in both surface water and sediments [17].

4.2 Cosmetics

Many personal care products, including facial and body creams, sunscreens, nail polish, hair dyes, and perfumes, contain substances that are intended to increase product stability and preservation or for enhancing absorption through the skin [18]. The main compounds with estrogen-like activity in personal care products are parabens, phthalates, perfluorinated chemicals, triclosan, UV filters, and BPA. Although the concentration of each xenoestrogen in a given product is rather low, they often exist in mixtures. Thus, potential synergism, additivity, or inhibition must be taken into account, since safe doses of a single chemical cannot be predicted as harmless when present in a mixture.

Parabens are low-cost compounds with antimicrobial activity against Gram-positive bacteria, yeast, and molds. They are stable at different pHs and withstand autoclaving [2]. Parabens are widely used in moisturizers, toothpaste, hair/shaving products, toiletries, and food packaging-commodities. Parabens have been measured in breast tumors and were reported to increase the proliferation of MCF-7 cells, to cause DNA damage, and to alter mitochondrial functions [19].

Phthalates are used as plasticizers, lubricants, and solvents in many consumer products, with a yearly global production of over 5 million tons [2]. Phthalates are lipophilic, accounting for their leaching and partitioning properties. In animals, phthalates cause oxidative stress, embryonic developmental problems, reproductive impairments, and neurobehavioral effects. Even at a very low concentration, phthalates induced proliferation of breast cancer cells through the PI3K/AKT signaling pathway.

Two other xenoestrogens used in cosmetics are perfluorinated compounds (PFCs) and triclosan. PFCs are used as surfactants and coating materials in many consumer products. Epidemiological studies, however, yielded inconsistent data with respect to their association with breast cancer [18]. A recent in vitro study, using the estrogen-responsive T47D cells [20], found that although PFCs did not have estrogenic activity per se, they augmented the effects of E2 on cell growth and estrogen-responsive gene expression. The estrogenic effects of triclosan were examined both in vitro and in vivo [21]. Triclosan stimulated the expression of cyclin D1 and p21 in MCF-7 cells, resulting in enhanced cell proliferation, and increased tumor growth in a mouse xenograft model.

4.3   Food Additives

An integrated in silico and in vitro strategy was used to screen dozens of food additives and has identified two compounds, propyl gallate and 4-hexylresorcinol, as having estrogenic activity at the nanomolar range [22]. Propyl gallate is an antioxidant which is widely used in food additives, cosmetics, adhesives, and lubricants. It prevents spoilage by protecting the oils in food products from reacting with hydrogen peroxide and oxygen free radicals. When tested with cells transfected with ERs, propyl gallate was estrogenic in both ERα- and ERβ-expressing cells, being more estrogenic in ERβ-expressing cells [23].

Hexylresorcinol is an organic compound with anesthetic, antiseptic, and anthelmintic properties. In addition to its use as a food additive, hexylresorcinol is included in topical preparations for skin infections, throat lozenges, and antiaging creams. A recent study reported that 4-hexylresorcinol synergized with cisplatin to decrease metastasis and increase survival in a melanoma xenograft model [24], but there are no published records on its activity in breast cancer cells.

4.4   Detergents and Preservatives

Long-chain alkylphenols, primarily nonylphenols and octylphenols, are used in the production of detergents, cleaning products, as antioxidants in some plastics, and in personal care products such as hair dyes. Alkylphenols, especially 4-nonylphenol

(4-NP) and its breakdown products, were detected in house air, sewers, and municipal landfills [25]. 4-NP mimics E2 by acting via both nuclear and cell membrane ERs. In MCF-7 cells, 4-NP altered several genes involved in cell proliferation, while a prenatal exposure of rats to 4-NP affected the development of the mammary gland and caused changes in steroid receptors in other reproductive tissues. Mice exposed to 4-NP had increased risk of mammary cancer.

4.5 Polychlorinated Biphenyls (PCBs)

PCBs are industrialized chemicals used in adhesives, fire retardants, and waxes. Given their lipid solubility and low rate of degradation, PCBs persist and bioaccumulate in the environment, and can pass to humans through the food chain, eventually reaching measurable levels in human tissues, cord blood, and breast milk [26]. The latter suggests that individuals can be exposed to high levels of PCBs during early development, when estrogenic effects may be more detrimental than those affecting adults.

The sex determination process in the red-eared slider turtle has been used as a very sensitive bioassay for establishing the estrogenic activity of PCBs [27]. Like many egg-laying reptiles, the sex of the developing embryo in this species is determined by the incubation temperature. When eggs are incubated at 26.6 °C, all eggs will become male, while at when incubated at 31 °C, all eggs will become female. A 1:1 ratio is found at about 29.2 °C. Because higher temperatures accelerate the conversion of testosterone to estradiol, embryos incubated at a warmer temperature are exposed to more estradiol during the critical period for sex determination and become female. Exploiting the fact that exogenous estrogens can override the temperature effect, it was reported when eggs incubated at all-male or male-biased temperatures were exposed to certain PCBs, more females were generated than expected on the basis of temperature alone [28]. In spite of the clear estrogenic effects of PCBs in reptiles, and some in vitro estrogenic effects in breast cancer cells [29], epidemiological studies on a potential association of PCBs with breast cancer yielded inconsistent results, with some revealing a positive association [30], while others do not [31].

4.6 Polycyclic Aromatic Hydrocarbons (PAH)

PAHs are by-products of combustion, resulting from fossil fuel manufacturing, diesel exhaust, grilled meats, and cigarettes. Inhalation is a major means of PAH exposure, since PAH residues are often associated with suspended particulate matter in the air [25]. The recent stricter emission standards by regulatory agencies in the USA resulted in a significant decrease in PAH release by vehicles, compared to their highest levels in the 1970s. Studies looking at workers exposed regularly to gasoline fumes and vehicular exhaust (major sources of PAHs) found increased risk of breast cancer in premenopausal women, and also of male breast cancer, specifically in men carrying a *BRCA1* or *BRCA2* mutation [25].

Most PAHs are only weakly estrogenic, but they activate the aryl hydrocarbon receptor (AhR), resulting in altered cell signaling, increased DNA mutations, and complex interactions with ER-regulated pathways. AhR is a ligand-activated transcription factor that regulates multiple genes in response to a broad class of environmental chemicals [32]. This receptor was historically characterized for its role in mediating toxicity and adaptive responses to chemicals such as 2,3,7.8,-tetrachlorodibenzo-p-dioxin (TCDD), a prototypical AhR agonist. In addition to its activation by various ligands, AhR is overexpressed, and is constitutively active, in advanced breast cancer, where it has been known to drive progression of the disease.

4.7   Pesticides and Herbicides

DDT (dichloro-diphenyl-trichloroethane), the first widely used synthetic pesticide, is a classic example of the far-reaching endocrine-disruptive effects of pesticides. DDT has been highly effective in eradicating malaria throughout the early 1900s but was subsequently found to have long-term devastating effects on reproductive success in wildlife and adverse health effects in humans [33]. Since the late 1960s, DDT has been banned for agricultural use in most countries, but it is still used for malaria control in few countries, including sub-Saharan Africa [34]. Given its continued use and persistence in the environment, DDT and its main metabolite, DDE, are detectable worldwide. Both animals and humans ingest DDT- and DDE-contaminated foods and retain the chemicals. Significant concentrations of DDT and DDE are found in human fat tissue, breast milk, and placenta, even in geographical locations where it has not been used for decades. The involvement of DDT in breast cancer has been controversial, however, likely because of some inherent flaws of epidemiological surveys, including analysis of contaminant levels at the time of breast cancer diagnosis rather than at the time of exposure to the chemicals during the critical early periods of breast development [35].

Atrazine, heptachlor, dieldrin, and aldrin are among the most widely recognized pesticides and herbicides with respect to their endocrine-disrupting properties [25]. Atrazine is used to control broadleaf weeds in corn and sorghum crops. Over 75 million pounds of atrazine are applied annually in the USA, with elevated levels found during the treatment season in both drinking water and groundwater in agricultural areas. In some rural areas, where use of pesticides is common, serum levels of dieldrin and heptachlor were higher in women with breast cancer than in normal women, raising the concern that they play a role in the genesis of breast cancer [36].

5 BPA and Human Exposure

BPA is a synthetic compound with a $(CH_3)_2C(C_6H_4OH)_2$ formula and a molecular weight of 228. BPA was first synthesized by a Russian chemist in 1891 and was tested in the early 1930s by the British biochemist Edward Dodds as an artificial estrogen. After finding that BPA was much less effective than estradiol, Dodds developed the structurally similar DES, which was then used as a synthetic estrogen in women and animals until it was banned in 1971, as was discussed in Sect. 4. Although BPA has never been utilized as a drug, it has been widely used since 1957 as a constituent of numerous consumer products.

5.1 BPA Production and Environmental Sources

During the 1980s, the world production capacity of BPA was 1 million metric tons, increasing to 7.7 million metric tons in 2015, and is projected to reach 10.6 million metric tons by 2022, making it one of the highest volumes of chemicals produced worldwide. BPA is produced by an acid-catalyzed reaction of phenol and acetone and is composed of two unsaturated phenol rings (see Fig. 4). BPA has good solubility in organic solvents and is poorly soluble in water. Most BPA is used in the manufacture of polycarbonate (60%) and epoxy resins (30%), with the remainder used for the production of polyester resins.

Polycarbonates, which are composed of linked BPA monomers, are made by reacting BPA with phosgene. Polycarbonate material has many desirable commercial qualities such as transparency, moldability, and high impact strength. The carbonate linkages of the polymer are rather stable but can be hydrolyzed at high temperature and at neutral to alkaline pH, resulting in release of small amounts of BPA. Epoxy resins containing BPA diglycidylether (BADGE) have superior adhesive properties. When reacted with a hardener, they become cross-linked and are used in coating and bonding applications. BPA diglycidyl methacrylate (bis-GMA) is a constituent of dental sealants, used to replace tooth structures. Their polymerization (curing) reaction is photo-initiated by UV or visible light. Incompletely polymerized resins may contain 5–10% of free BPA.

Polycarbonate plastic, which is clear and nearly shatterproof, serves as a component of a wide array of consumer products, including baby and water bottles, medical (iv cannulae and eyeglass lenses) and dental (sealants) applications, household electronics (CDs and DVDs), foundry casting, and lining of water pipes. BPA is also used as an antioxidant in plasticizers and as a polymerization inhibitor in PVC. Epoxy resins containing BPA are used to coat the inside of most food and beverage cans. BPA-based resins are also used as susceptors to achieve food browning in some packages for microwave cooking. BPA is also used as a color developer in carbonless copy and thermal receipt papers, as a constituent of some flame retardants, and as a fungicide.

5.2 Discovery of the Endocrine-Disruptive Activity of BPA

The action of BPA as a xenoestrogen was serendipitously discovered in the early 1990s by Stanford University's investigators who identified an estrogen-binding protein in yeast and went on to examine if yeast make the endogenous ligand. After first reporting that yeast produce estradiol, they realized that the estrogenic activity did not come from the yeast, but from the culture media which were prepared with water autoclaved in polycarbonate flasks. As detailed in their seminal 1993 paper [37], using binding to ER as a bioassay, the estrogenic compound was purified by chromatography and identified as BPA. About 2–3 µg/L of BPA were detected in the autoclaved water. They then tested if authentic BPA is estrogenic, using four criteria: (a) binding to ER, (b) proliferation of MCF-7 cells, (c) induction of progesterone receptors, and (d) reversal of estrogenic actions by tamoxifen. BPA satisfied all these criteria as an estrogenic compound, with the lowest effective dose of 10–20 nM.

Intrigued by the finding of BPA in autoclaved water, a Spanish group analyzed liquid from 20 different brands of canned vegetables for BPA content [38]. BPA levels ranged from 0 to 33 µg/can, with the variability attributed to the type of polymer, sterilization procedure, and food variety. They concluded that an alkaline or fatty food favored increased leaching of BPA during heating. In 1996, the same group [39] reported detectable levels of BPA in saliva of patients treated with dental sealants containing bis-GMA. Soon thereafter, our 1997 paper [40] was the first to describe the neuroendocrine effects of BPA. Using rat anterior pituitary cells, we found that BPA stimulated cell proliferation and increased prolactin gene expression and release, albeit at a 1000- to 5000-fold lower potency than estradiol. In spite of its relatively low potency in vitro, BPA unexpectedly had similar efficacy to estradiol in inducing hyperprolactinemia in the estrogen-sensitive Fischer 344 (F344) rats, while Sprague Dawley (SD) rats did not respond to BPA [41, 42]. These data suggested that the responsiveness to BPA in rodents is strain dependence and that BPA may cause adverse effects on the neuroendocrine axis in certain susceptible human subpopulations.

In follow-up studies, we reported that BPA induced growth, differentiation, and c-fos gene expression in the female rat reproductive tract [42] and altered the release of leptin, adiponectin, and interleukin-6 (IL-6) from human adipose explants and adipocyte cell lines [43].

5.3 Human Exposure to BPA

Since the late 1990s, the scientific community has become increasingly concerned with the endocrine-disruptive effects of BPA. As of today, there have been more than 7000 publications with "bisphenol A" in their title. Not surprisingly, the intense research activities ignited considerable public awareness of the adverse effects of

BPA, leading to studies aimed at determining the sources of human exposure to BPA, and its presence in human tissues and body fluids.

A recent review on the global presence and accumulation of BPA [44] suggested that BPA is released into the environment by pre-consumer and postconsumer leaching. Pre-consumer sources include the chemical, plastics, coating, and staining industries, while postconsumer BPA represents discharge from wastewater treatment plants, irrigation pipes, and indirect leaching from plastic, paper, and metal waste in landfills and paper or material recycling companies. Significant levels of BPA have been measured in ambient air, in house dust, as well as in river and drinking water in many countries. As a matter of fact, human exposure to BPA is quite significant, considering that BPA-based polycarbonate and epoxy resins are very common in food and drinking utensils and that BPA leaching is facilitated when food is cooked or sterilized at high temperatures. In addition to ingestion and inhalation, BPA can enter the skin through absorption from several sources, including thermal papers. Table 2 lists the range of BPA concentrations measured in different products, human tissues and body fluids, and ambient environment.

Upon entering the human body, BPA is cleared within few hours through the kidney. Given its lipophilic nature, BPA can be taken up and retained in human fat tissue and breast stroma [45]. Although the amount of circulating free BPA can be reduced by glucuronidation and sulfation, such conjugations are reversible by beta-glucuronidase and arylsulfatase C, respectively [46]. BPA was detected in over 90% of urine samples, collected from thousands of individuals at many geographical locations, and was detected in blood and urine of pregnant women and breast milk [25]. BPA was present in serum and follicular fluid at 1–2 ng/mL, as well as in fetal serum and full-term amniotic fluid, confirming its ability to cross the placenta [47]. These data indicated a significant exposure to BPA during the prenatal period, which must be considered upon evaluating the potential for human exposure to endocrine-disrupting chemicals in early fetuses.

Table 2 BPA levels under various conditions

Type of material	BPA concentration
Canned food	30–50 μg/kg
Canned dairy products	0.5–5 μg/kg
Breast milk	1.5–3 μg/L
Pacifiers	0.3–0.35 μg/product
Children toys	0.15 μg/product
Cosmetics	30 μg/product
Thermal paper	1–3 μg/100 g
Indoor air	0.5–5 ng/m^3
House dust	100–20,000 μg/kg

Modified from various sources

6   In Vitro and In Vivo Studies with BPA

The endocrine-disruptive effects of BPA are widespread and variable and have been documented in animal and human cells derived from both epithelial and mesenchymal origins. Multiple pathophysiological and oncogenic actions of BPA have been reported in a large variety of species, including fish, amphibians, reptiles, birds, rodents, cats, dogs, rabbits, and monkeys. Here we focus only on in vitro and in vivo actions of BPA that impinge upon breast development and tumorigenesis. In addition, only studies that have used environmentally relevant doses of BPA (≤ 100 nM), rather than pharmacological concentrations, are considered.

6.1   Genomic and Non-genomic Effects of BPA on Breast Cells

Several analytical methods have been optimized for evaluating the estrogenicity of xenoestrogens [48]. These include competitive ligand-binding assays, in vitro gene expression analyses, reporter assays, cell proliferation assays (E-screen), and yeast estrogen screen (YES). The endpoint of the E-screen is proliferation of the estrogen-sensitive MCF-7 breast cancer cells, while the YES assay is based on ERα-mediated induction of lacZ, which encodes the enzyme β-galactosidase in yeast.

Many studies with BPA have identified a nonconventional dose-response profile called non-monotonic dose-response (NMDR) relationships [49]. The term "NMDR" defines a curve whose slope changes direction within the range of the tested doses. Non-monotonicity challenges basic concepts in toxicology and risk assessment which posit that the larger the dose of a given substance, the greater is the response. This "linearity" concept has been traditionally applied to therapeutic with pharmaceuticals, as well as for toxicity evaluation. On the other hand, many EDCs, including BPA, exhibit a U- or an inverted U-shape dose-response curve, whereby low doses may either be more effective or act in the opposite direction, than the high doses.

The estrogenicity of low BPA doses have been covered in several reviews [50–52] and will be briefly summarized here. Exposure of normal and malignant human breast cells to low BPA doses altered the expression of hundreds of genes associated with hormone-receptor-mediated processes such as cell proliferation, apoptosis, and carcinogenesis. BPA treatment of cells derived from normal breast tissue of women diagnosed with breast cancer generated a gene-response profile associated with the development of highly aggressive tumors. BPA also activates sets of genes that were distinct from those induced by E2. Pretreatment of MCF-7 and T47D cells with 25–100 nM BPA resulted in increased cell proliferation and reduced apoptosis. In 3D cultures of breast cells, which resemble the structure and functions of breast epithelium in vivo, BPA reduced the number of tubules, increased spherical masses, and caused more deformed acini, indicating an ability to induce neoplastic transformation.

BPA rapidly activated non-genomic signaling by phosphorylating MAPK and Akt in MCF-7 cells within 10 min of exposure. At low doses, BPA also induced rapid influx of calcium in breast cancer cells, which was neither reversed by ICI182780 nor reproduced by E2 or DES, suggesting that classical ERs were not involved.

6.2 Induction of Chemoresistance by Estrogens

As discussed in our review [51], estrogens can activate the PI3K/Akt survival pathway and also increase the expression of anti-apoptotic proteins, serving as the backdrop for their involvement with resistance to chemotherapy. Most studies have linked estrogen-induced chemoresistance to activation of the anti-apoptotic protein Bcl-2. For example, MCF-7 cells grown without estrogens became sensitized to doxorubicin, which was accompanied by decreased Bcl-2 expression, while Bcl-2 reconstitution restored resistance to the drug. Induction of Bcl-2 by estrogen, as well as ERα overexpression in breast cancer cells, caused a significant decrease in taxol-induced apoptosis. A combination of tamoxifen and TRAIL was more effective than each alone in inducing apoptosis in the ERα-negative MDA-MB-231 breast cancer cells and in arresting growth of xenografts. This sensitization was associated with decreased Bcl-2 expression and increased expression of the pro-apoptotic protein Bax.

Additional studies revealed that low doses of E2 (0.01–10 nM) abrogated cisplatin toxicity in breast cancer cells by increasing cell proliferation and by decreasing apoptosis [51]. Protection from anticancer drugs by estrogen occurred in the presence of ERα and ERβ antagonists, in ERα-negative MDA-MB-468 cells, and in T47D cells with ERβ knockdown, indicating independence of classical ERs. E2 increased the expression of Bcl-2 in T47D cells, both in the presence and absence of cisplatin. Given that a potent Bcl-2 inhibitor only partially abrogated protection by E2, other mediators appeared to be involved. In addition to activating anti-apoptotic proteins, estrogen antagonized taxol- and radiation-induced apoptosis by altering JNK activity. Another mechanism by which estrogens increased chemoresistance is by affecting membrane exporters. This was shown by an estrogen-induced increase in cytoplasmic p-glycoprotein in MCF-7 cells, which are resistant to doxorubicin, but not in T47D cells, which are sensitive to the drug.

6.3 Induction of Chemoresistance by BPA

Similar to E2, BPA exhibits multiple interactions with chemotherapeutic agents [53, 54]. Our lab was the first to report that BPA at environmentally relevant doses confers chemoresistance. As summarized in our review [55], we postulated that BPA increases chemoresistance based on the antagonism of chemotherapeutic agents by

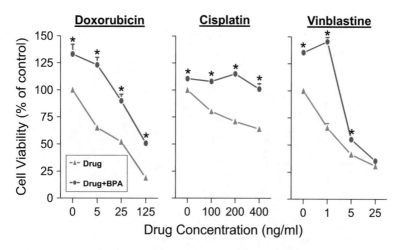

Fig. 5 BPA antagonizes cytotoxicity by doxorubicin, cisplatin, and vinblastine in MDA-MB-468 breast cancer cells treated with the drug alone or pretreated with 1 nM BPA. Cell viability was determined after 4 days (Modified from [54])

estradiol. Notably, BPA antagonized multiple anticancer drugs, often at equimolar potency with estradiol. In fact, BPA antagonized the cytotoxicity of three drugs, doxorubicin, cisplatin, and vinblastine, which induce cell death by different mechanisms (Fig. 5). Doxorubicin causes DNA damage and block transcription by chelating metal ions, generating free radicals, and inhibiting topoisomerase. Cisplatin causes DNA intra-strand cross-linking and inhibits replication, while vinblastine acts by interfering with microtubule dynamics, resulting in mitotic arrest and cell death.

BPA alone, or in combination with doxorubicin or cisplatin, increased Bcl-2 expression. Treatment with a Bcl-2 inhibitor completely blocks the antagonizing effects of BPA, but only partially abrogates those by E2. This suggested that BPA and estrogen protect against drug-induced cytotoxicity by somewhat different mechanisms, i.e., anti-apoptosis vs mitogenesis. This was supported by flow cytometry and BrdU incorporation data showing that BPA alone increased cell survival, while estrogen alone increased cell proliferation. Figure 6 illustrates the proposed mechanisms by which BPA increases resistance to cisplatin by increasing Bcl-2 expression. Although these BPA actions did not appear to be mediated via ERα and ERβ, the receptor involved was not identified. Using colon cancer cells, others reported that BPA can influence chemotherapy outcome [56].

6.4   Perinatal Actions of BPA

As discussed in a recent review [25], even a brief exposure during the perinatal period to environmentally relevant doses of BPA can lead to abnormalities in mammary tissue development, beginning during gestation and lasting into adulthood.

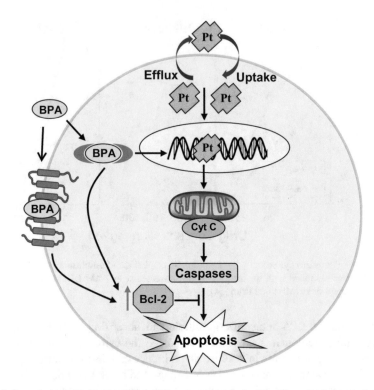

Fig. 6 Proposed mechanism by which BPA antagonizes induction of apoptosis by cisplatin (Pt). Pt enters the nucleus, binds to DNA, causes cell cycle arrest, and induces apoptosis. BPA binds either to cytoplasmic or to membrane ERs and increases Bcl-2 expression which inhibits apoptosis (Modified from [51])

Many of these changes were similar to those observed after prenatal exposure to DES. For example, prenatal exposure of rats to BPA increased the number of pre-cancerous lesions in the mammary glands and increased the animal's susceptibility to mammary tumors formation, following adult exposures to subthreshold doses of carcinogens. In the mouse fetal mammary gland, prenatal exposure to BPA altered the expression of genes involved in extracellular matrix formation, adipogenesis, and lumen formation through ER-dependent and ER-independent pathways. Also, prenatal exposure of mice to BPA resulted in dysregulation of inflammatory cyto-kines in the adult glands, a process that may lead to altered cell growth through inhibition of immune responses that target malignant cells. Similar changes in the mammary glands were observed upon exposure of female rhesus monkeys to envi-ronmentally relevant doses of BPA during gestation [57].

Most of the long-term effects of BPA are dose dependent, with low- and high-dose exposures resulting in a different timing as well as in variable gene expression profiles in the mammary gland. For example, upon chronic exposure of adult mice to BPA, only the low doses decreased the latency of tumor appearance and increased the number of mammary tumors and their rate of metastasis. All doses enhanced mammary cell proliferation, but relatively higher doses counteracted the increased proliferation with parallel increases in programmed cell death [58].

The long-term effects of BPA on the mammary gland are manifested through epigenetic mechanisms. This can lead to changes in gene regulation across the lifetime, as was supported by showing that exposures of rats to low levels of BPA altered the epigenome in mammary tissue, with different profiles seen at weaning and post-puberty [59]. In addition, in utero exposure of mice to BPA was accompanied by altered DNA methylation that preferentially affected ERα-binding genes [60].

Collectively, these data suggested that during gestation and perinatal life, BPA exerts long-lasting effects on multiple cell types within the mammary gland, resulting in structural and functional alterations which ultimately impinge upon the normal functions and the carcinogenic potential of the adult gland.

7   Proposed Mechanisms of Action of BPA

Studies with breast cancer and other cell types have shown that BPA acts, in part, through the same pathways as does estradiol [25, 61]. Yet, the binding affinity of BPA to ERα or ERβ is several orders of magnitude lower than that of E2, while BPA at low nanomolar doses has similar activities to those of E2 [32, 62]. To explain this discordance, several mechanisms of action of BPA have been proposed (Fig. 6): (1) induction of a different conformation of the binding within the LBD of intracellular ERs [63], resulting in the recruitment of a different set of coactivators [64], (2) binding and activation of membrane-associated ERs (mER), (3) activation of GPER, (4) binding to estrogen-related receptors (ERR), and (5) interactions with other steroidal or nonsteroidal receptors. The first mechanism is based on in silico computational models, while significant experimental evidence supports BPA interactions with classical and nonclassical receptors [65]. A summary of the potential mechanisms by which BPA exerts estrogen-like actions is shown in Fig. 7. Below, we also include an evaluation of the properties of bisphenol S (BPS), which has been proposed as a substitute for BPA in multiple consumer products.

7.1   Differential Binding Configuration of Estrogen and BPA to Intracellular ERα/ERβ

ERα and ERβ are the products of different genes, localized to chromosomes 6q25.1 and 14q23–24.1, respectively. Both are ligand-inducible transcription factors composed of several functional domains: (1) N-terminal domain (NTD), (2) DNA-binding domain (DBD), and (3) ligand-binding domain (LBD). Two activation function (AF) domains, AF1 and AF2, located within the NTD and LBD, respectively, are responsible for regulating the transcriptional activity of ERs. As depicted

Fig. 7 Potential mechanisms by which BPA exerts estrogen-like actions. Binding of BPA (double blue hexagon) to either membrane ERs (mERs) or GPER (G protein-coupled estrogen receptor) can activate either genomic or non-genomic pathways. Binding of BPA to cytoplasmic ERs or ERRγ results in genomic alterations

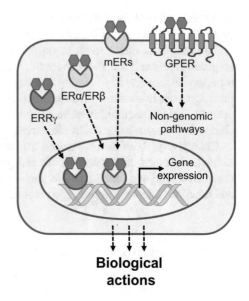

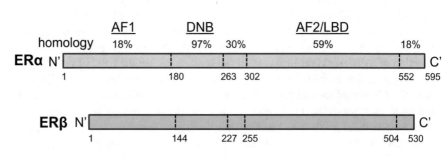

Fig. 8 Comparison of the structures of ERα and ERβ, showing the total amino acids and the percent homology among the different functional domains. *AF1 and AF2* activation functions 1 and 2, *DNB* DNA-binding domain, *LBD* ligand-binding domain

in Fig. 8, ERβ has a high homology to ERα in the DBD (97% amino acid identity) and a lesser homology in the LBD (59% amino acid identity). The NTD of ERβ is shorter than that of ERα, with a poor sequence homology of only ~18%. Despite having similar LBDs, the two ERs have different binding affinities for many xenoestrogens, with BPA having a tenfold higher binding affinity to ERβ than ERα. Also, numerous isoforms of ERα and ERβ have been identified, which likely play unique roles as mediators of the actions of both endogenous estrogens and BPA.

The LBD of ERα is composed of 11 α-helices, folded into three antiparallel layers, forming a globular structure which harbors a hormone-binding site, a homo- or hetero-dimerization interface, and co-regulator (activator and repressor) interaction sites. E2 binds to the ligand-binding cavity through a combination of hydrogen bonds and hydrophobic interactions. Given its structural dissimilarity to E2, BPA interacts differently with the LBD, causing conformational changes that enable the recruitments of different transcriptional coactivators through which BPA exerts its biological actions [66]. For example, the BPA/ERβ complex showed >500-fold greater potency than the BPA/ERα complex for recruiting the coactivator transcriptional mediators/intermediary factor 2 (TIF2). In the presence of ERα, BPA usually mimics E2 and acts as a proliferative agent, while in the presence of ERβ, it often functions as an antagonist.

Collectively, in any given cell, the balance of ERα/ERβ expression ratio, the differential activation by BPA, and the expression levels of ER-regulated targets via coactivators, rather than the relatively weak binding affinity of BPA to the ERs, ultimately determine the overall cell responsiveness to BPA.

7.2   The Role of Membrane ERs

In many cells, a small fraction of cellular ERs are localized within the plasma membrane as ERα and ERβ homodimers or heterodimers [67]. Whereas endothelial cells equally express both ERs at the plasma membrane, breast cancer cells primarily have ERα. Unlike the classical growth factor receptors such as EGFR, mERs have no transmembrane and kinase domains, and are bound to the membrane through palmitoylation, in association with caveolins. Within the caveolae, mERs can form protein complexes with kinases associated with the MAPK, AKT, and other signaling pathways [68].

In contrast to the classical genomic actions that take hours after stimulation with estrogens, low doses of either E2 or BPA can increase cAMP levels within seconds. This rapid action was named "non-genomic," as it is not affected by transcriptional inhibitors such as actinomycin D. The non-genomic estrogen-signaling cascade involves the generation of second messengers such as Ca2+, cAMP, and NO and activation of receptor tyrosine kinases such as EGFR, IGF-1R, and other kinases, such as PI3-kinase, Akt, MAPKs, PKA/PKC, and Src [69].

7.3   Activation of GPER by Estrogens and BPA

All the rapid actions of E2 were initially ascribed to the mERs. However, the cloning of an orphan receptor, named GPR30, in the late 1990s underscored a role for a G protein-coupled receptor (GPCR) as an important mediator of rapid estrogenic actions [70]. Expression of GPER was found in many tissues, including the lung, liver, prostate, ovary, and placenta. Several years later, the putative functions of GPER were identified, based on the induction of protein kinases such as Erk1, Erk2, and c-fos by E2 in breast cancer cell lines expressing GPER, but not in those lacking GPER. The ER antagonists tamoxifen and ICI 182,780 also bind GPER, but unlike their ER-mediated effects, they had agonistic activities for GPER. Highly selective, nonsteroidal GPER agonists and antagonists have also been developed [70].

GPER functions as a typical Gs-coupled heptahelical receptor, which promotes second messenger signaling via both GSα- and Gβγ-dependent activation of plasma membrane-associated matrix metalloproteinases, integrin α5β1, and EGFR. GPER has all the hallmarks associated with plasma membrane action, and agents such as antibodies and peptides that do not cross the plasma membrane block its actions. Using ER-negative breast cancer cell lines, estrogens bind GPER and activate MAP kinase, Erk1/2, and PI3K signaling through transactivation of EGFR and an EGFR-independent activation of adenylyl cyclase. Recent data showed that GPER shuttles between the plasma membrane and intracellular organelles and is translocated to the nucleus via an importin-mediated mechanism, where it affects c-fos and connective tissue growth factor (CTGF) expression [71].

BPA binds to GPER with an IC_{50} of 630 nM, compared with an IC_{50} of 17.8 nM for E2. By activating GPER and its multiple downstream signaling pathways, BPA can alter cellular responses associated with breast carcinogenesis such as cell survival, epithelial-to-mesenchymal transition, migration, invasion of surrounding tissue, and attraction of vascular supply. Changes in the tumor milieu itself, as well as those in the tumor microenvironment, are conducive for tumor cell survival, dissemination, and cancer progression [65].

7.4   Binding of BPA to Estrogen-Related Receptors (ERR)

The ERRs are a subfamily of nuclear receptors whose structure is closely related to those of ERα and ERβ. They were initially thought to share a common biological function with the ERs, but since they do not bind estrogen or endogenous ER ligands, they are considered orphan nuclear receptors. Three ERRs are known: ERRα, ERRβ, and ERRγ [66, 72]. ERRα is primarily present in tissues with high metabolism such as the heart, kidney, GI tract, skeletal muscle, and brown adipose tissue, while expression of ERRβ and ERRγ is more restricted. The ERRs share significant structural homology with the ERs, particularly in the DBD and LBD regions. They are also constitutively active, as their LBD configuration facilitates exposure of AF-2 to binding co-regulators in the absence of ligands [72].

ERRα expression in breast tumors was correlated with expression of the ErbB2 oncogene, an indicator of aggressive tumor behavior and hormonal insensitivity [73]. Although ERRβ expression also showed a direct relationship with Erbβ expression, its potential as a biomarker was unclear. On the other hand, overexpression ERRγ was associated with hormonally responsive ER-positive status, and was correlated with ErbB4, indicating a potential as a biomarker of favorable clinical course and hormonal sensitivity.

BPA operates primarily through to ERRγ, having a K_D of 5.5 nM, which is a more environmentally relevant dose than that needed to activate ERα or ERβ [74]. Triple-negative breast cancer is characterized by the propensity for invasion and metastasis. BPA treatment at nanomolar concentrations significantly increased the expressions of ERRγ, but not that of ERRα or ERRβ, in the triple negative

Fig. 9 Relative expression of various receptors in T47D (estrogen-sensitive) and MDA-MB-468 (triple-negative) breast cancer cells. Data are presented as percent of ERα expression in T47D cells (Modified from [54])

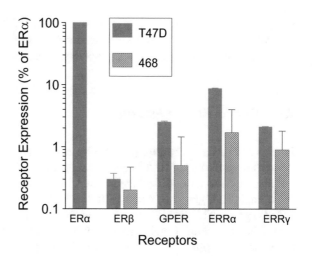

MDA-MB-231 and BT-549 cells [75]. Knockdown of ERRγ attenuated the BPA-induced expression of matrix metalloproteinase-2 (MMP-2) and MMP-9 in these cells, suggesting that BPA, acting via ERRγ, affects cancer cell motility, migration, and invasion. Another study reported that silencing ERRγ significantly abolished BPA-induced proliferation of MCF-7 and SkBr3 cells, while silencing of ERRα was ineffective [76]. In addition, nanomolar doses of BPA upregulated the mRNA and protein levels of ERRγ and triggered its nuclear translocation.

In our studies, we used selective ER antagonists and ruled out the potential involvement of ERα and ERβ in mediating the chemo-protective effects by BPA [54], with the results suggesting that BPA may act via ERRγ. Figure 9 shows the relative expression levels of BPA-responsive receptors in the ER-positive T47D cells and the triple-negative MDA-MB-468 cells. Data are presented as percent of ERα expression in T47D cells. Notably, ERβ expression is similar, but very low, in the two cells lines, being less than 1% that of ERα. ERRα is the most highly expressed of the alternative receptors in both cell lines, nearing 10% of ERα in T47D cells. The expression levels of GPER and ERRγ are similar in T47D cells, with ERRγ being slightly higher than GPER in 468 cells. ERRβ was undetectable in both cell lines.

7.5   Other Molecular Mechanisms

BPA and other EDCs can also affect breast cancer by activating a variety of nuclear receptors, including AR, TR, GR, AhR, pregnane X receptor (hPXR), and PPAR [77, 78], each of which contributes to some degree to breast tumorigenesis. For example, activation of hPXR and upregulation of their target genes by BPA alter the local bioavailability of endogenous androgens and estrogens, providing a pathway for BPA to affect steroid receptor activity without directly binding to these receptors. By activating a variety of nuclear receptors, BPA can also alter hormone synthesis and metabolism by regulating steroid biosynthetic enzymes, cytochrome P450 metabolizing enzymes, conjugation enzymes, and transporters [79].

7.6 BPS, a BPA Substitute

In response to the increasing pressure by concerned scientists and environmental groups to ban the use of BPA in consumer products, the chemical industry began to introduce BPS as a safe substitute for BPA in the mid-2000s. BPS, with the chemical formula of $C_{12}H_{10}O_4S$, consists of two hydroxyphenyl groups connected by a sulfonyl group. The production volume of BPS is between 1000 and 10,000 tons per year. BPS is used as a monomer in synthetic polymers such as polyethersulfone (PES) and polysulfone (PSU), as well as in epoxy resins which are also used for food contact. Figure 10 shows the structural similarities of BPA and BPS and their corresponding polymers. Structural/chemical data showed that PES have excellent thermal, optical, and mechanical properties as plastics.

As depicted in Fig. 11, reports on strong EDC properties of BPS began to appear in 2000, and as of to date, more than 150 publications on its bioactivity have been published. As reviewed in [80], most studies found BPS to be as potent as BPA in terms of estrogenic, antiestrogenic, androgenic, and antiandrogenic activities in vitro and in vivo. BPS also has potencies similar to that of estradiol in membrane-mediated pathways, important for actions such as proliferation, differentiation, and apoptosis. Like BPA, BPS altered organ weights, reproductive endpoints, and enzyme expression. The inevitable conclusion was that BPS is as hormonally active as BPA, with clear endocrine-disrupting effects. Like BPA, BPS has been detected in human blood [81] and urine [82].

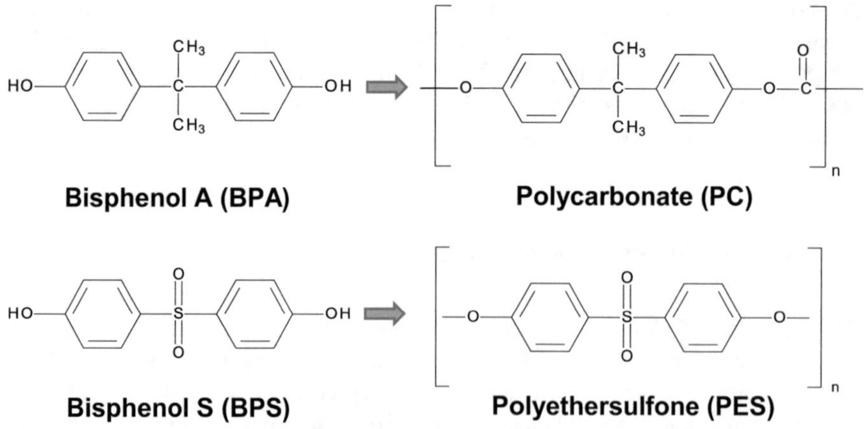

Fig. 10 Structures of bisphenol A (BPA) and bisphenol S (BPS) monomers and their corresponding polymers

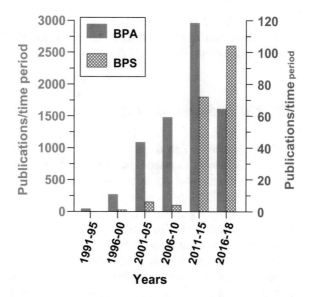

Fig. 11 Number of publications in PubMed on BPA (left axis) and BPS (right axis), per period from 1991 to the beginning of 2018. Note the differences in the range in the Y scales

8   Positions on BPA Undertaken by Various Organizations and Regulatory Agencies

More than any compound in recent memory, BPA has generated highly controversial assessments with respect to the extent of human exposure and adverse health effects. Over the last two decades, several review panels have been convened to evaluate BPA, dozens of million dollars of federal money were spent on studying the pathophysiology of BPA, and several regulatory agencies have debated the hazards of BPA exposure to human health. Thus far, there is no overall consensus whether BPA should be banned from all consumer products. Here we review disparate positions on BPA, undertaken by environmental advocacy groups, the Endocrine Society, the chemical and food industry, health organizations, and regulatory agencies.

8.1   Environmental Advocacy Groups

A number of not-for-profit advocacy groups and organizations have expressed strong opinions about the actions of BPA as an endocrine disruptor. Among these are the following: Consumers Union, the Union of Concerned Scientists, Women's Voices for the Earth, the Conversation Group, and the Environmental Working Group. Almost without exception, their positions indicated that BPA should be banned from all food and beverage containers because of health risks. They have accepted the ample scientific evidence that BPA exposure is linked to increased risk of breast and prostate cancer, early puberty, childhood obesity, autism, and hyperactivity and emphasized that children metabolize BPA more slowly than adults, putting them especially at risk.

8.2   The Endocrine Society

In 2009, alarmed by new discoveries on EDCs, the US Endocrine Society, which represents thousands of research scientists and clinicians, set a precedent for scientific and medical organizations by being the first scientific society to take a public stance on the EDCs. An extensive 2009 publication by the Society was entitled: Endocrine-disrupting chemicals: an Endocrine Society scientific statement" [83]. Another publication, entitled "Endocrine-disrupting chemicals and public health protection: A statement of principles from The Endocrine Society," was published in 2012 [1]. In subsequent years, through their online communication *Endocrine News*, the society continued to review additional scientific evidence, focusing primarily on BPA and its substitute analogs. This resulted in comprehensive statements on what was known and which gaps existed in research on bisphenols. It was emphasized that there is no endocrine system that is immune to EDCs and that the effects of these compounds may be transmitted to future generations. The Society's statement concluded that the evidence for adverse outcomes in multiple physiological systems is strong and mounting. It encouraged the development of partnership with other organizations with scientific and medical expertise to evaluate the effects of EDCs and communicate to other researchers, clinicians, community advocates, and politicians.

8.3   The Chemical Industry

The global BPA market in 2016 was 15.5 billion dollars and was projected to increase to 22.5 billion dollar by 2022. With so much money at stake, it is not surprising that the chemical, food, and cosmetic industries have invested heavily in concerted efforts to provide counterarguments to health hazards by BPA. In 1999, the Bisphenol A Global Industry Group, located in Washington, D.C., initiated a journal named *Bisphenol A*, whose main premise was to establish the safety of BPA. The first issue in October 1999 included ten articles on human safety, migration from plastics, and toxicology. The second issue in April 2000 included eight articles on environmental safety, biodegradation, aquatic toxicity, and safety assessment. Almost all authors came from industry, and their overall conclusions were that there is no significant migration of BPA from polycarbonate plastics, no adverse low-dose effects, no convincing evidence for carcinogenicity, no bioaccumulation in aquatic organisms, and no discernible effects on fetal/neonatal development. The editor indicated that all manuscripts were peer-reviewed, but did not provide listing of editorial board membership or the composition of the pool of reviewers.

8.4 Health Organizations and Regulatory Agencies

Since 1998, several federal health organizations, including the National Institute of Environmental Health Sciences (NIEHS), the Environmental Protection Agency (EPA), and the National Toxicology Program (NTP), have been attempting to develop an integrated, scientific-based assessment on exposure and health hazards of EDCs/BPA. This was initially accomplished by biannual workshops that convened dozens of researchers and government officials to develop criteria for evaluating these compounds. The meetings resulted in several publications in *Environmental Health Perspectives* and other journals.

A 2013 publication entitled "Low-dose effects of bisphenol A" by multiple authors [50] critically evaluated previous assessments of low-dose effects of BPA and examined if these studies have addressed previously identified data gaps. It also examined endpoints across multiple studies and biological targets (cells, animals, and human populations) to identify consistent endpoints affected by BPA exposures. After summarizing hundreds of low-dose studies, the authors concluded that there are sufficient evidence for low-dose effects of BPA on specific endpoints and suggestive evidence for additional endpoints.

8.5 CLARITY-BPA: The Ultimate Effort to Settle the Issue of BPA

Given the overwhelming scientific evidence on the EDC properties of BPA, a relevant question is why it has been so difficult to reach regulatory decisions whether BPA poses hazards to human health. Undoubtedly, replacement of bisphenols is a very costly endeavor to the chemical and polymer industries. Second, among the thousands of published studies, some have used very large doses of bisphenols in vitro or in vivo, providing fodder to contrarians. Third, a legitimate concern has been the lack of standardization among animal studies in terms of routes of administration, pharmacokinetics across species, differences between sexes, sensitive windows of exposure, and specific disease endpoints.

In 2009, a decision was made to form partnership between the NIEHS, FDA, NTP, and more than a dozen academic researchers whose main premise was to formulate and execute a multi-year, multimillion dollar research initiative called CLARITY-BPA. Under the CLARITY-BPA consortium, conducted during 2011–2016, thousands of male and female Sprague Dawley (SD) rats were housed and treated at the National Center for Toxicological Research (NCTR) at Jefferson, Arkansas. Rats were given a daily gavage with vehicle (0.3% carboxymethylcellulose), seven equally spaced BPA doses (0.05, 0.5, 2.5, 25, 250, 2500, 25,000 μg/kg bw/day), or two doses of 17α-ethinylestradiol (EE$_2$; 0.05 and 0.5 μg/kg bw/day) as a reference. The treatments started at early pregnancy, continued during early neonatal life, and lasted up to 2 years of age.

Twelve laboratories across the USA, who submitted competitive grant applications, were selected to cover different endpoints, including behavior, brain development, reproduction, cardiovascular, metabolism, and several cancers. The university-based researchers were provided animals, tissues, and/or serum samples according to their specifications from the NCTR facilities and did the analysis in their own laboratories. In several meetings of all the grantees, results were presented and discussed. Although some interesting data have emerged, others were inconclusive or negative.

A discussion of the entire CLARITY-BPA study is beyond the scope of this chapter. Instead, we appraise few pros and cons of this study. Positive aspects included the uniform animal treatment, the good laboratory practice (GLP) of animal breeding and randomization, the double-blinded data handling, the wide range of BPA doses, the inclusion of EE$_2$ as a reference, the use of both sexes, and the chronic exposure from prenatal to neonatal to old age. On the other hand, several caveats have become apparent, raising concerns as to whether sound conclusions could be made. The first and foremost problem was the selection of SD rats as the animal model, despite previous reports that this strain is significantly less sensitive to BPA than other strains [84, 85] and, therefore, does not truly represent a population with variable sensitivity. Figure 12 shows an example from our own studies showing lack of responsiveness of SD rats to induction of PRL release by either BPA or E2, as compared their significant effects in Fischer 344 (F344) rats. A similar strain differences in the vaginal responses to BPA was also found, leading us to conclude that the choice of a suitable animal model is critically important when seeking to test the estrogenic effects of xenoestrogens.

Other problems have also emerged. The daily oral gavage apparently caused significant stress to the animals, as judged by highly elevated levels of many stress-induced hormones. There was also an inadvertent exposure of some of the

Fig. 12 Induction of hyperprolactinemia in Fischer 344 (F344) but not in Sprague Dawley (SD) rats by estradiol (E2) and bisphenol A (BPA). Ovariectomized rats were implanted with Silastic capsules containing crystalline E2 or BPA for 3 days (Modified from [40])

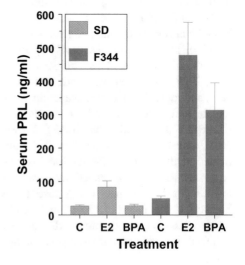

Table 3 The IC50 and relative binding affinity (RBA) of different bisphenols for hERα and hERβ

Compound	hERα		hERβ	
	IC$_{50}$ (nM)	RBA (%)	IC$_{50}$ (nM)	RBA (%)
E2	0.12	100	0.21	100
BPA	840	0.025	400	0.052
BPS	6600	0.001	3500	0.006
BPF	2200	0.005	1500	0.014

Modified from [77]

control rats to high BPA levels, which was discovered late in the study and was only partially corrected. In addition, the mandatory study design did not allow for collection and analysis of certain specific parameters deemed essential for some of the studies. For example, in our studies on the effects of BPA on obesity and metabolism, rats were not provided with high- and low-fat diet as requested. Changes were measured in body weight only, rather than in adipose tissue composition, as should have been done using nuclear magnetic resonance (NMR). Moreover, a single blood sample from each rat was taken at the time of sacrifice, rather than repeated blood sampling for a more appropriate representation of the changing hormonal milieu.

In sum, the CLARITY BPA consortium study likely falls short of providing the ultimate adjudication on the endocrine-disruptive effects of BPA, and additional relevant studies are clearly warranted. The irony is, however, that in addition to BPA and BPS, other bisphenols, including BPF and bisphenol A diglycidyl ether (BADGE), also have EDC properties. This raises the possibility that the vast amount of work invested in characterizing BPA is being erased by its replacement with other bisphenols by the industry. A comparison of the binding affinities of E2 and the various bisphenols to hERα and hERβ is presented in Table 3.

8.6 Legislative Decisions About BPA

In 2012, following the lead of 11 states, the FDA banned BPA from baby bottles and sippy cups nationwide, in fact after the manufacturers of these products had already stopped their use of BPA. Although the change of rules provided some comfort to parents, it has not gone far enough, as has been demanded by the advocacy groups and the Endocrine Society. Meanwhile, several bills for a total ban of BPA have been introduced in the US Congress but have not yet been acted upon. The main problem is that replacements for BPA in plastics and food containers by other chemicals could be just as harmful or even worse. A study by the NTP, which tested 24 replacement chemicals, found that many already in use are structurally and functionally similar to BPA and, just like BPA, may harm the endocrine system.

In parallel with efforts in the USA, the European Food Safety Authority (EFSA) has been leading efforts for a similar ban of BPA from consumer products at Europe.

In 2010, France banned the use of BPA in products that come into direct contact with food for babies and young children. An European Union wide ban followed in 2011. In 2015, France has introduced a new law, banning the use of BPA in all food packaging. China, Canada, and Malaysia are also in the process of legislating a ban on BPA, primarily from products intended for babies and young children.

9 Conclusions and Perspectives

The role of estrogen in breast tumorigenesis is undisputable. Observations that support this argument include the following: (a) a prolonged and uninterrupted exposure to endogenous estrogen is a risk factor for the development of breast cancer, (b) administration of exogenous estrogens to postmenopausal women is associated with increased risk of breast cancer, (c) gonadectomy in premeno-pausal women reduces the risk for developing breast cancer, and (d) pharmaco-logical agents which block estrogen biosynthesis or estrogen receptors serve as effective treatments for breast cancer.

The prevailing notion is that breast cancer results from time-related complex interactions between internal and external factors. Unlike mutagenic or genotoxic chemicals which often act as tumor initiators, xenoestrogens generally act as tumor promoters at many time points during the development of breast cancer. Although some EDCs are more likely to be encountered in an industrial environment, dozens of hormonally active agents have been identified in household dust or air, as well as in food, cosmetics, and other consumer goods. Given that exposures are widespread and breast cancer is common, addressing environmental risk factors has the potential to save thousands of lives each year, even though the relative risks of breast cancer due to xenoestrogens are vastly smaller than those for the BRCA genes.

Many of the effects BPA at low doses mimic estrogen but are not mediated via ERα or ERβ. Therefore, alternative receptors and noncanonical signaling pathways, as characterized by GPER and ERRγ, have been considered. Yet, uncertainty with respect to the exact mechanism of action of BPA still remains. This raises the intriguing possibility that BPA utilizes as yet an unidentified unique receptor. Such prospect is not unprecedented, as exemplified by opioid and cannabinoid receptors which were discovered many years after the bioactivity of their exogenous ligands was recognized. Indeed, there are still hundreds of membrane, cytoplasmic, and nuclear orphan receptors without an identified ligand.

This chapter addresses the growing literature on the connections between important EDCs and the risk of developing breast cancer, based primarily on nonhuman models. Although most experimental paradigms test the effects of each individual chemical, it is important to recognize that these compounds exist in the environment as mixtures which may form various levels of interactions. By interfering with the actions of natural hormones, exposures to EDCs contribute to the development of a wide variety of disease states. Often these effects are most profound when exposures are low-dose and during early development. In humans, ductal development of mammary gland begins between the 12th and the 14th week of gestation, and therefore, exposure to BPA during this time of pregnancy is potentially risky for the fetus.

The issue of human health hazards by EDCs in general and bisphenols in particular is far from being resolved. Although progress has been made in banning some EDCs from products that come in contact with infants, the bans do not encompass the adult population that is constantly exposed to their adverse health effects.

References

1. Zoeller RT, Brown TR, Doan LL, Gore AC, Skakkebaek NE, Soto AM, Woodruff TJ, vom Saal FS (2012) Endocrine-disrupting chemicals and public health protection: a statement of principles from the Endocrine Society. Endocrinology 153(9):4097–4110
2. Giulivo M, Lopez de Alda M, Capri E, Barcelo D (2016) Human exposure to endocrine disrupting compounds: their role in reproductive systems, metabolic syndrome and breast cancer. A review. Environ Res 151:251–264
3. Coyle YM (2004) The effect of environment on breast cancer risk. Breast Cancer Res Treat 84(3):273–288
4. Hortobagyi GN, de la Garza SJ, Pritchard K, Amadori D, Haidinger R, Hudis CA, Khaled H, Liu MC, Martin M, Namer M, O'Shaughnessy JA, Shen ZZ, Albain KS (2005) The global breast cancer burden: variations in epidemiology and survival. Clin Breast Cancer 6(5):391–401
5. Lichtenstein P, Holm NV, Verkasalo PK, Iliadou A, Kaprio J, Koskenvuo M, Pukkala E, Skytthe A, Hemminki K (2000) Environmental and heritable factors in the causation of cancer--analyses of cohorts of twins from Sweden, Denmark, and Finland. N Engl J Med 343(2):78–85
6. Rudel RA, Attfield KR, Schifano JN, Brody JG (2007) Chemicals causing mammary gland tumors in animals signal new directions for epidemiology, chemicals testing, and risk assessment for breast cancer prevention. Cancer 109(12 Suppl):2635–2666
7. Mense SM, Hei TK, Ganju RK, Bhat HK (2008) Phytoestrogens and breast cancer prevention: possible mechanisms of action. Environ Health Perspect 116(4):426–433
8. Bilal I, Chowdhury A, Davidson J, Whitehead S (2014) Phytoestrogens and prevention of breast cancer: the contentious debate. World J Clin Oncol 5(4):705–712
9. Zhao E, Mu Q (2011) Phytoestrogen biological actions on Mammalian reproductive system and cancer growth. Sci Pharm 79(1):1–20
10. Bandera EV, Chandran U, Buckley B, Lin Y, Isukapalli S, Marshall I, King M, Zarbl H (2011) Urinary mycoestrogens, body size and breast development in New Jersey girls. Sci Total Environ 409(24):5221–5227
11. Sondergaard TE, Klitgaard LG, Purup S, Kobayashi H, Giese H, Sorensen JL (2012) Estrogenic effects of fusarielins in human breast cancer cell lines. Toxicol Lett 214(3):259–262
12. Yuri T, Tsukamoto R, Miki K, Uehara N, Matsuoka Y, Tsubura A (2006) Biphasic effects of zeranol on the growth of estrogen receptor-positive human breast carcinoma cells. Oncol Rep 16(6):1307–1312
13. Marselos M, Tomatis L (1992) Diethylstilboestrol: I, pharmacology, toxicology and carcinogenicity in humans. Eur J Cancer 28A(6–7):1182–1189
14. Marselos M, Tomatis L (1992) Diethylstilboestrol: II, pharmacology, toxicology and carcinogenicity in experimental animals. Eur J Cancer 29A(1):149–155
15. Hilakivi-Clarke L (2014) Maternal exposure to diethylstilbestrol during pregnancy and increased breast cancer risk in daughters. Breast Cancer Res 16(2):208
16. Fairbairn DJ, Karpuzcu ME, Arnold WA, Barber BL, Kaufenberg EF, Koskinen WC, Novak PJ, Rice PJ, Swackhamer DL (2016) Sources and transport of contaminants of emerging

concern: a two-year study of occurrence and spatiotemporal variation in a mixed land use watershed. Sci Total Environ 551–552:605–613

17. Blair BD, Crago JP, Hedman CJ, Klaper RD (2013) Pharmaceuticals and personal care products found in the Great Lakes above concentrations of environmental concern. Chemosphere 93(9):2116–2123

18. Nicolopoulou-Stamati P, Hens L, Sasco AJ (2015) Cosmetics as endocrine disruptors: are they a health risk? Rev Endocr Metab Disord 16(4):373–383

19. Charles AK, Darbre PD (2013) Combinations of parabens at concentrations measured in human breast tissue can increase proliferation of MCF-7 human breast cancer cells. J Appl Toxicol 33(5):390–398

20. Sonthithai P, Suriyo T, Thiantanawat A, Watcharasit P, Ruchirawat M, Satayavivad J (2016) Perfluorinated chemicals, PFOS and PFOA, enhance the estrogenic effects of 17beta-estradiol in T47D human breast cancer cells. J Appl Toxicol 36(6):790–801

21. Lee HR, Hwang KA, Nam KH, Kim HC, Choi KC (2014) Progression of breast cancer cells was enhanced by endocrine-disrupting chemicals, triclosan and octylphenol, via an estrogen receptor-dependent signaling pathway in cellular and mouse xenograft models. Chem Res Toxicol 27(5):834–842

22. Amadasi A, Mozzarelli A, Meda C, Maggi A, Cozzini P (2009) Identification of xenoestrogens in food additives by an integrated in silico and in vitro approach. Chem Res Toxicol 22(1):52–63

23. ter Veld MG, Schouten B, Louisse J, van Es DS, van der Saag PT, Rietjens IM, Murk AJ (2006) Estrogenic potency of food-packaging-associated plasticizers and antioxidants as detected in ERalpha and ERbeta reporter gene cell lines. J Agric Food Chem 54(12):4407–4416

24. Lee SW, Kim SG, Park YW, Kweon H, Kim JY, Rotaru H (2013) Cisplatin and 4-hexylresorcinol synergise to decrease metastasis and increase survival rate in an oral mucosal melanoma xenograft model: a preliminary study. Tumour Biol 34(3):1595–1603

25. Gray JM, Rasanayagam S, Engel C, Rizzo J (2017) State of the evidence 2017: an update on the connection between breast cancer and the environment. Environ Health 16(1):94

26. Moysich KB, Menezes RJ, Baker JA, Falkner KL (2002) Environmental exposure to polychlorinated biphenyls and breast cancer risk. Rev Environ Health 17(4):263–277

27. Crews D, Bergeron JM, McLachlan JA (1995) The role of estrogen in turtle sex determination and the effect of PCBs. Environ Health Perspect 103(Suppl 7):73–77

28. Bergeron JM, Crews D, McLachlan JA (1994) PCBs as environmental estrogens: turtle sex determination as a biomarker of environmental contamination. Environ Health Perspect 102(9):780–781

29. Liu S, Li S, Du Y (2010) Polychlorinated biphenyls (PCBs) enhance metastatic properties of breast cancer cells by activating rho-associated kinase (ROCK). PLoS One 5(6):e11272

30. Morgan M, Deoraj A, Felty Q, Roy D (2017) Environmental estrogen-like endocrine disrupting chemicals and breast cancer. Mol Cell Endocrinol 457:89–102

31. Zani C, Ceretti E, Covolo L, Donato F (2017) Do polychlorinated biphenyls cause cancer? A systematic review and meta-analysis of epidemiological studies on risk of cutaneous melanoma and non-Hodgkin lymphoma. Chemosphere 183:97–106

32. Powell JB, Goode GD, Eltom SE (2013) The aryl hydrocarbon receptor: a target for breast cancer therapy. J Cancer Ther 4(7):1177–1186

33. Carson R (1962) Silent Spring. Houghton Mifflin, Boston

34. Gray J, Evans N, Taylor B, Rizzo J, Walker M (2009) State of the evidence: the connection between breast cancer and the environment. Int J Occup Environ Health 15(1):43–78

35. Beard J (2006) DDT and human health. Sci Total Environ 355(1–3):78–89

36. Mathur V, Bhatnagar P, Sharma RG, Acharya V, Sexana R (2002) Breast cancer incidence and exposure to pesticides among women originating from Jaipur. Environ Int 28(5):331–336

37. Krishnan AV, Stathis P, Permuth SF, Tokes L, Feldman D (1993) Bisphenol-A: an estrogenic substance is released from polycarbonate flasks during autoclaving. Endocrinology 132(6):2279–2286

38. Brotons JA, Olea-Serrano MF, Villalobos M, Pedraza V, Olea N (1995) Xenoestrogens released from lacquer coatings in food cans. Environ Health Perspect 103(6):608–612
39. Olea N, Pulgar R, Perez P, Olea-Serrano F, Rivas A, Novillo-Fertrell A, Pedraza V, Soto AM, Sonnenschein C (1996) Estrogenicity of resin-based composites and sealants used in dentistry. Environ Health Perspect 104(3):298–305
40. Steinmetz R, Brown NG, Allen DL, Bigsby RM, Ben-Jonathan N (1997) The environmental estrogen bisphenol A stimulates prolactin release in vitro and in vivo. Endocrinology 138(5):1780–1786
41. Ben-Jonathan N, Steinmetz R (1998) Xenoestrogens: the emerging story of bisphenol A. Trends Endocrinol Metab 9(3):124–128
42. Steinmetz R, Mitchner NA, Grant A, Allen DL, Bigsby RM, Ben-Jonathan N (1998) The xenoestrogen bisphenol A induces growth, differentiation, and c-fos gene expression in the female reproductive tract. Endocrinology 139(6):2741–2747
43. Ben-Jonathan N, Hugo ER, Brandebourg TD (2009) Effects of bisphenol A on adipokine release from human adipose tissue: implications for the metabolic syndrome. Mol Cell Endocrinol 304(1–2):49–54
44. Corrales J, Kristofco LA, Steele WB, Yates BS, Breed CS, Williams ES, Brooks BW (2015) Global assessment of bisphenol A in the environment: review and analysis of its occurrence and bioaccumulation. Dose Response 13(3):1–9
45. Wang L, Xue J, Kannan K (2015) Widespread occurrence and accumulation of bisphenol A diglycidyl ether (BADGE), bisphenol F diglycidyl ether (BFDGE) and their derivatives in human blood and adipose fat. Environ Sci Technol 49(5):3150–3157
46. Ginsberg G, Rice DC (2009) Does rapid metabolism ensure negligible risk from bisphenol A? Environ Health Perspect 117(11):1639–1643
47. Ikezuki Y, Tsutsumi O, Takai Y, Kamei Y, Taketani Y (2002) Determination of bisphenol A concentrations in human biological fluids reveals significant early prenatal exposure. Hum Reprod 17(11):2839–2841
48. Soto AM, Maffini MV, Schaeberle CM, Sonnenschein C (2006) Strengths and weaknesses of in vitro assays for estrogenic and androgenic activity. Best Pract Res Clin Endocrinol Metab 20(1):15–33
49. Vandenberg LN, Colborn T, Hayes TB, Heindel JJ, Jacobs DR Jr, Lee DH, Shioda T, Soto AM, vom Saal FS, Welshons WV, Zoeller RT, Myers JP (2012) Hormones and endocrine-disrupting chemicals: low-dose effects and nonmonotonic dose responses. Endocr Rev 33(3):378–455
50. Vandenberg LN, Ehrlich S, Belcher SM, Ben-Jonathan N, Dolinoy DC, Hugo ER, Hunt PA, Newbold RR, Rubin BS, Saili KS, Soto AM, Wang HS, vom Saal FS (2013) Low dose effects of bisphenol A. Endocr Disruptors 1(1):e1-1–e1-20
51. Idelman G, Jacobson EM, Tuttle TR, Ben-Jonathan N (2011) Lactogens and estrogens in breast cancer chemoresistance. Expert Rev Endocrinol Metab 6(3):411–422
52. Wang Z, Liu H, Liu S (2017) Low-dose bisphenol A exposure: a seemingly instigating carcinogenic effect on breast cancer. Adv Sci (Weinh) 4(2):1600248
53. LaPensee EW, LaPensee CR, Fox S, Schwemberger S, Afton S, Ben-Jonathan N (2010) Bisphenol A and estradiol are equipotent in antagonizing cisplatin-induced cytotoxicity in breast cancer cells. Cancer Lett 290(2):167–173
54. LaPensee EW, Tuttle TR, Fox SR, Ben-Jonathan N (2009) Bisphenol A at low nanomolar doses confers chemoresistance in estrogen receptor-alpha-positive and -negative breast cancer cells. Environ Health Perspect 117(2):175–180
55. LaPensee EW, Ben-Jonathan N (2010) Novel roles of prolactin and estrogens in breast cancer: resistance to chemotherapy. Endocr Relat Cancer 17(2):R91–R107
56. Delgado M, Ribeiro-Varandas E (2015) Bisphenol A at the reference level counteracts doxorubicin transcriptional effects on cancer related genes in HT29 cells. Toxicol In Vitro 29(8):2009–2014
57. Tharp AP, Maffini MV, Hunt PA, VandeVoort CA, Sonnenschein C, Soto AM (2012) Bisphenol A alters the development of the rhesus monkey mammary gland. Proc Natl Acad Sci U S A 109(21):8190–8195

58. Jenkins S, Wang J, Eltoum I, Desmond R, Lamartiniere CA (2011) Chronic oral exposure to bisphenol A results in a nonmonotonic dose response in mammary carcinogenesis and metastasis in MMTV-erbB2 mice. Environ Health Perspect 119(11):1604–1609

59. Dhimolea E, Wadia PR, Murray TJ, Settles ML, Treitman JD, Sonnenschein C, Shioda T, Soto AM (2014) Prenatal exposure to BPA alters the epigenome of the rat mammary gland and increases the propensity to neoplastic development. PLoS One 9(7):e99800

60. Jorgensen EM, Alderman MH III, Taylor HS (2016) Preferential epigenetic programming of estrogen response after in utero xenoestrogen (bisphenol-A) exposure. FASEB J 30(9):3194–3201

61. Fajas L (2003) Adipogenesis: a cross-talk between cell proliferation and cell differentiation. Ann Med 35(2):79–85

62. Feng Y, Jiao Z, Shi J, Li M, Guo Q, Shao B (2016) Effects of bisphenol analogues on steroidogenic gene expression and hormone synthesis in H295R cells. Chemosphere 147:9–19

63. McRobb FM, Kufareva I, Abagyan R (2014) In silico identification and pharmacological evaluation of novel endocrine disrupting chemicals that act via the ligand-binding domain of the estrogen receptor alpha. Toxicol Sci 141(1):188–197

64. Cao H, Wang F, Liang Y, Wang H, Zhang A, Song M (2017) Experimental and computational insights on the recognition mechanism between the estrogen receptor alpha with bisphenol compounds. Arch Toxicol 91(12):3897–3912

65. Castillo SR, Gomez R, Perez SE (2016) Bisphenol A induces migration through a GPER-, FAK-, Src-, and ERK2-dependent pathway in MDA-MB-231 breast cancer cells. Chem Res Toxicol 29(3):285–295

66. Acconcia F, Pallottini V, Marino M (2015) Molecular mechanisms of action of BPA. Dose Response 13(4):1–9

67. Levin ER (2009) Plasma membrane estrogen receptors. Trends Endocrinol Metab 20(10):477–482

68. Song RX, Santen RJ (2006) Membrane initiated estrogen signaling in breast cancer. Biol Reprod 75(1):9–16

69. Albini A, Rosano C, Angelini G, Amaro A, Esposito AI, Maramotti S, Noonan DM, Pfeffer U (2014) Exogenous hormonal regulation in breast cancer cells by phytoestrogens and endocrine disruptors. Curr Med Chem 21(9):1129–1145

70. Barton M, Filardo EJ, Lolait SJ, Thomas P, Maggiolini M, Prossnitz ER (2018) Twenty years of the G protein-coupled estrogen receptor GPER: historical and personal perspectives. J Steroid Biochem Mol Biol 176:4–15

71. Pupo M, Vivacqua A, Perrotta I, Pisano A, Aquila S, Abonante S, Gasperi-Campani A, Pezzi V, Maggiolini M (2013) The nuclear localization signal is required for nuclear GPER translocation and function in breast Cancer-Associated Fibroblasts (CAFs). Mol Cell Endocrinol 376(1–2):23–32

72. Misawa A, Inoue S (2015) Estrogen-related receptors in breast cancer and prostate cancer. Front Endocrinol (Lausanne) 6:83–90

73. Ariazi EA, Clark GM, Mertz JE (2002) Estrogen-related receptor alpha and estrogen-related receptor gamma associate with unfavorable and favorable biomarkers, respectively, in human breast cancer. Cancer Res 62(22):6510–6518

74. Matsushima A, Kakuta Y, Teramoto T, Koshiba T, Liu X, Okada H, Tokunaga T, Kawabata S, Kimura M, Shimohigashi Y (2007) Structural evidence for endocrine disruptor bisphenol A binding to human nuclear receptor ERR gamma. J Biochem 142(4):517–524

75. Zhang XL, Liu N, Weng SF, Wang HS (2016) Bisphenol A increases the migration and invasion of triple-negative breast cancer cells via oestrogen-related receptor gamma. Basic Clin Pharmacol Toxicol 119(4):389–395

76. Song H, Zhang T, Yang P, Li M, Yang Y, Wang Y, Du J, Pan K, Zhang K (2015) Low doses of bisphenol A stimulate the proliferation of breast cancer cells via ERK1/2/ERRgamma signals. Toxicol In Vitro 30(1 Pt B):521–528

77. Molina-Molina JM, Amaya E, Grimaldi M, Saenz JM, Real M, Fernandez MF, Balaguer P, Olea N (2013) In vitro study on the agonistic and antagonistic activities of bisphenol-S and

other bisphenol-A congeners and derivatives via nuclear receptors. Toxicol Appl Pharmacol 272(1):127–136

78. Kitamura S, Suzuki T, Sanoh S, Kohta R, Jinno N, Sugihara K, Yoshihara S, Fujimoto N, Watanabe H, Ohta S (2005) Comparative study of the endocrine-disrupting activity of bisphenol A and 19 related compounds. Toxicol Sci 84(2):249–259

79. Tabb MM, Blumberg B (2006) New modes of action for endocrine-disrupting chemicals. Mol Endocrinol 20(3):475–482

80. Rochester JR, Bolden AL (2015) Bisphenol S and F: a systematic review and comparison of the hormonal activity of bisphenol A substitutes. Environ Health Perspect 123(7):643–650

81. Jin H, Zhu J, Chen Z, Hong Y, Cai Z (2017) Occurrence and partitioning of bisphenol analogues in adults' blood from China. Environ Sci Technol 51(24):14025–14032

82. Liao C, Liu F, Alomirah H, Loi VD, Mohd MA, Moon HB, Nakata H, Kannan K (2012) Bisphenol S in urine from the United States and seven Asian countries: occurrence and human exposures. Environ Sci Technol 46(12):6860–6866

83. Diamanti-Kandarakis E, Bourguignon JP, Giudice LC, Hauser R, Prins GS, Soto AM, Zoeller RT, Gore AC (2009) Endocrine-disrupting chemicals: an Endocrine Society scientific statement. Endocr Rev 30(4):293–342

84. Long X, Steinmetz R, Ben-Jonathan N, Caperell-Grant A, Young PC, Nephew KP, Bigsby RM (2000) Strain differences in vaginal responses to the xenoestrogen bisphenol A. Environ Health Perspect 108(3):243–247

85. Khurana S, Ranmal S, Ben-Jonathan N (2000) Exposure of newborn male and female rats to environmental estrogens: delayed and sustained hyperprolactinemia and alterations in estrogen receptor expression. Endocrinology 141(12):4512–4517

Emerging Therapeutic Approaches to Overcome Breast Cancer Endocrine Resistance

Marissa Leonard, Juan Tan, Yongguang Yang, Mahmoud Charif, Elyse E. Lower, and Xiaoting Zhang

Abstract Antiestrogen therapies have been a staple treatment option for estrogen receptor (ER)-positive breast cancer patients for many decades, but resistance remains a major obstacle for continued successful treatment. In this chapter, we will discuss the preclinical and clinical research advancement in the development of novel strategies to overcome breast cancer endocrine resistance. We will focus on the current successes and emerging future developments in targeting growth signaling pathways (i.e., CDK4/6, PI3K/AKT/mTOR, and IGF-1) and ER cofactors such as SRC family cofactors and Mediator Subunit 1 (MED1) using small molecules, antibodies, and RNA nanotechnology. We will also provide future perspective for other potential novel therapeutic targets such as epigenetic modification, noncoding RNAs, immunotherapy, etc. and the expansion of therapeutic options in endocrine-resistant breast cancers.

Keywords Endocrine resistance · Growth signaling pathways · Transcriptional cofactors · Small-molecule inhibitors · RNA nanotechnology

M. Leonard
Department of Cancer Biology, University of Cincinnati College of Medicine, Cincinnati, OH, USA

Graduate Program in Cancer and Cell Biology, University of Cincinnati College of Medicine, Cincinnati, OH, USA

J. Tan · Y. Yang
Department of Cancer Biology, University of Cincinnati College of Medicine, Cincinnati, OH, USA

M. Charif · E. E. Lower
Division of Hematology and Oncology, Department of Internal Medicine, University of Cincinnati College of Medicine, Cincinnati, OH, USA

X. Zhang (✉)
Department of Cancer Biology, Vontz Center for Molecular Studies, University of Cincinnati College of Medicine, Cincinnati, OH, USA

Graduate Program in Cancer and Cell Biology, University of Cincinnati College of Medicine, Cincinnati, OH, USA
e-mail: zhangxt@ucmail.uc.edu

© Springer Nature Switzerland AG 2019   379
X. Zhang (ed.), *Estrogen Receptor and Breast Cancer*, Cancer Drug Discovery and Development, https://doi.org/10.1007/978-3-319-99350-8_14

1 Introduction

Estrogen receptor (ER) α is expressed in the majority (~75%) of breast cancers and plays crucial roles in driving growth and metastasis of the ER-positive subtype of breast cancer. Since its discovery, a number of approaches have been developed to target ER for the treatment of breast cancer. As described in the previous chapters, antiestrogen therapies including the selective estrogen receptor modulator, tamoxifen, and the estrogen receptor degrader, fulvestrant, as well as estrogen deprivation therapies such as aromatase inhibitors (e.g., letrozole), are the backbone therapies of hormone-dependent breast cancer. However, acquired and de novo resistance to these therapies remain major hurdles in the long-term management of this disease. The preceding chapters have discussed the development and use of antiestrogen therapies in clinics and the molecular mechanisms underlying endocrine resistance. In this chapter, we will focus on the current and emerging approaches being developed and used to overcome endocrine resistance. Most of these approaches are primarily aiming to target the key components of growth signaling pathways or tissue-specific ER transcriptional coactivators that play key roles in mediating endocrine resistance. Specifically, we will discuss examples of novel therapies that are developed to target key signaling pathways (e.g., CDK4/6, PI3K/AKT/mTOR, IGF-1) and used in the treatment of breast cancer and endocrine-resistant breast cancer. In addition, novel regimens or approaches that include RNA nanotechnology are currently being developed to target specific ER transcriptional coactivators (e.g., SRCs, MED1) and will be further described in detail. Some of these have already been approved by the FDA for clinical use alone or in combination with endocrine therapies, while others are still undergoing clinical investigation or are being studied in preclinical settings. Moreover, a future perspective on other potential major targets including additional growth signaling pathways, noncoding RNAs, epigenetic modifiers, and immunotherapies will also be discussed.

2 Combating Endocrine Resistance Through Growth Signaling Pathway Inhibition

Growth factor signaling pathways have long been recognized as key mediators of both de novo and acquired breast cancer resistance to endocrine therapies. Interestingly, the estrogen receptor is able to activate a number of these growth signaling pathways as well because some of the key components of these pathways such as cyclin D and IGF-1 are in fact the direct target genes regulated by ER. Furthermore, these pathways can often activate ER itself through direct phosphorylation of ER or its cofactors to regulate ER-mediated transcription and other functions as described in previous chapters. In recent years, a number of drugs have been developed to target these growth signaling pathways to treat breast cancer and overcome endocrine resistance. Some have recently been approved for clinical use while many of them are still in clinical trials or preclinical development. Here, we will specifically focus on discussing in detail the development, clinical trial status, side effects, and potential future uses of inhibitors of CDK4/6, PI3K/AKT/ mTOR, and IGF-1/IGF-1R pathways in breast cancer.

2.1 CDK4/6 Cell Cycle Signaling

The cell cycle is divided into four phases: G1 (cells decide whether to divide, grow or become dormant), S (DNA synthesis), G2 (preparation for cell division), and M (cell division) [1]. The cyclins and cyclin-dependent kinases (CDKs) are key regulatory machinery of cell cycle progression, while dysregulation of CDKs and cell cycle has been considered to be a hallmark of cancer [2, 3]. Unlike CDK1 and 2 that drive the cell cycle through S and M phases together with cyclins E, A, and B, CDK4 and CDK6 play important roles in controlling the transition from G1 to S phases of the cell cycle by forming holoenzymes with D-type cyclins (D1, D2, and D3). Retinoblastoma protein (pRb) and its family members (RB2, RBL1 (p107)) are primary substrates of CDK4/6. Phosphorylation of pRb by CDK4/6 inactivates pRb and releases the inhibition of the E2F family of transcription factors to allow target genes to be expressed to initiate S phase [4]. Recent studies have also found that tumor suppressor p16^{INK4a} is able to bind and potently inhibit the cyclin D-CDK4 kinase activities. In breast cancer, the cyclin D1 gene is amplified and overexpressed in about 20% and 50% of cases, respectively. Since these alterations often occur in ER+ breast cancer and the ER pathway can also activate the cyclin D-CDK-4/6 pathway to promote tumor growth, inhibition of CDK4/6 has become a highly important strategy for breast cancer therapy [5]. To date, the CDK4/6 inhibitors, in combination with current endocrine therapies, have been approved for the treatment of ER+ advanced breast cancer [6].

There are three major US-approved CDK4/6 inhibitors: palbociclib (PD0332991; Pfizer, New York, USA), abemaciclib (LY2835219; Lilly, Indiana, USA), and ribociclib (LEE011; Novartis, Basel, Switzerland) (Table 1) [7, 8]. All of these orally bioavailable small-molecule inhibitors are highly selective for CDK4/6 with IC$_{50}$ values in the low nanomolar range to specifically compete for binding of ATP to CDK4/6 over other cyclin-dependent kinases [7]. Palbociclib was the first to gain Food and Drug Administration (FDA) and European Commission (EMA) first-line metastatic approval in 2015 for the treatment of HR+, HER2− advanced breast cancers in combination with the aromatase inhibitor letrozole (Novartis Pharmaceuticals, Basel, Switzerland) [7]. In the PALOMA 1 study, which assesses the safety and efficacy of palbociclib plus letrozole in patients with previously untreated ER+, HER2− breast cancer, the median progression-free survival (PFS) significantly doubled with combination therapy versus letrozole alone, 20.2 months versus 10.2 months, respectively ($P = 0.0004$). In the subsequent larger PALOMA 2 study, the median PFS was 24.8 months for palbociclib plus letrozole combination therapy versus 14.5 months in the placebo plus letrozole group. Results of the

Table 1 Overview of the current FDA-approved CDK4/6 inhibitor drugs

Drug	Palbociclib	Ribociclib	Abemaciclib
Chemical structure			
Development status	Approved by FDA and EMA for the treatment of HR+, HER2− ABC in combination with letrozole as first-line treatment, as well as in combination with fulvestrant after disease progression following ET	Approved by FDA and EMA for the treatment of HR+, HER2− MBC in combination with letrozole as first-line therapy	Approved in the USA for the treatment of HR+, HER2− ABC or MBC
Efficacy	PALOMA-2 PFS 24.8 vs 14.5 months PALOMA-3 PFS 9.5 vs 4.6 months	MONALEESA-2 PFS not reached vs 14.7 months	MONARCH-3 PFS not reached vs 14.7 months
Grade 3/4 side effects	Neutropenia: 62–66.5% Fatigue: 1.8–2% Diarrhea: 0–1.4% Possible QTc prolongation	Neutropenia: 59.3% Fatigue: 2.4% Diarrhea: 1.2% QTc prolongation >480 ms: 3.3%	Neutropenia: 21.1% Diarrhea: 9.5% Leukopenia: 7.6%

2016 double-blind phase III PALOMA 3 trial led to the approval of palbociclib in combination with the estrogen receptor downregulator fulvestrant (Faslodex, AstraZeneca) for the treatment of women with HR+, HER2− advanced or metastatic breast cancer (MBC) [7].

Ribociclib received FDA breakthrough therapy designation in 2016 and has been approved by both the FDA and EMA in 2017 after the randomized, double-blind, placebo-controlled phase III trial (MONALEESA 2, NCT01958021). This trial studied combination therapy with letrozole as first-line therapy in HR+, HER2− MBC without prior systemic therapy for advanced disease [7]. A dose-escalation study (NCT01237236) indicated the maximum tolerated dose (MTD) of ribociclib was 900 mg/day and the recommended dose was 600 mg/day on a 21-of-28-d schedule. The MONALEESA 2 study revealed a significantly longer PFS with ribociclib plus letrozole compared to placebo plus letrozole with the median duration of response (DOR) 26.7 months and 18.6 months in the ribociclib arm and placebo arm, respectively. In addition, the average pain reduction was improved in the ribociclib arm (26%) compared to the placebo arm (15%) [9]. The ongoing MONALEESA 3 trial (NCT02422615) examined the effect of ribociclib plus fulvestrant versus placebo plus fulvestrant in men and postmenopausal women with HR+, HER2− breast cancer who received no treatment or only one line of prior endocrine treatment. The MONALEESA 7 trial (NCT02278120) studied the efficacy, safety, and PFS of ribociclib plus either the nonsteroidal aromatase inhibitor (NSAI) or tamoxifen plus goserelin (luteinizing hormone-releasing hormone analog for suppression of sex hormone production) versus placebo plus NSAI or tamoxifen plus goserelin in premenopausal HR+, HER2− advanced breast cancer. The ribociclib investigation pipeline is rich with approximately 30 initiated or ongoing ribociclib trials underway.

Abemaciclib, which received FDA breakthrough therapy designation in 2015, was US approved in 2017 for the treatment of patients with HR+, HER2− advanced or metastatic breast cancer (MBC) after a clinical trial expanded access program (NCT02792725). A phase I study (NCT01394016) on abemaciclib revealed a median PFS of 5.8 months and 8.8 months for all breast cancer patients and HR+ patients, respectively. Further, in the MONARCH 1 trial (NCT02102490), monotherapy of abemaciclib showed an objective response rate (ORR) of 19.7%, clinical benefit rate (CBR) of 42.4%, and median PFS of 6 months. Furthermore, the MONARCH 2 (NCT02107703) study found a median PFS of abemaciclib plus fulvestrant versus fulvestrant treatment alone of 16.4 months and 9.3 months, respectively, while the ORR was 48.1% versus 21.3% in patients who progressed while receiving endocrine therapy. In MONARCH 3 (NCT02246621), anastrozole/letrozole plus abemaciclib versus anastrozole/letrozole plus placebo are examined in postmenopausal HR+, HER2− patients with no prior systemic treatment. Furthermore, in the MONARCH plus trial (NCT02246621), abemaciclib plus anastrozole/letrozole or fulvestrant versus placebo plus anastrozole/letrozole or fulvestrant treatment arms are being compared in postmenopausal HR+, HER2− regionally recurrent or metastatic BC patients.

The most commonly reported adverse effects for CDK/6 inhibitors are neutropenia, leukopenia, fatigue, anemia, thrombocytopenia, arthralgia, diarrhea, nausea, and vomiting [10]. In the palbociclib plus letrozole trial, neutropenia, leukopenia, and fatigue were reported while neutropenia, fatigue, and nausea were found in the combinational trial of palbociclib plus fulvestrant. Likewise, nausea, infection, fatigue, leukopenia, and diarrhea are the most common side effects reported with ribociclib treatment. Although the risk of neutropenic fever is low (1.8%) with palbociclib and ribociclib, hematologic side effects are common, and a rest period of 7 days is recommended during the 1-month cycle. Due to structural differences, abemaciclib-treated patients experience less hematologic toxicity but report more gastrointestinal toxicity and fatigue. Interestingly, de novo and acquired resistance to CDK4/6 inhibitor therapy occurs. Tumors with a loss of Rb function are rendered unresponsive to CDK4/6 inhibitors, and possible additional resistance mechanisms include amplification of cyclin E, activation of CDK2, loss of p27[KIP1] or p21[CIP], etc. Furthermore, there is currently a lack of alternative or better biomarkers identified to predict the treatment response besides ER. Recently, it has been reported that MutL-, ER+ breast tumors are more sensitive to CDK4/6 inhibitor treatment, which partly explains why the inhibition of CDK4/6 is effective in some endocrine therapy-resistant tumors and also suggests a potential new class of biomarkers for CDK4/6-targeted therapies [11].

Because of the success of these completed and ongoing clinical trials, numerous phase II/III/IV studies are now activated and recruiting worldwide. Overall, there are approximately 130 ongoing clinical trials involving CDK4/6 inhibitor treatment alone or in combination with other agents. CDK4/6 inhibitors have been approved for the treatment of ER+ HER2− breast cancer; however, despite positive preclinical data, usage in ER+ HER2+ positive patients remains to be proven. Clinical trials (e.g., NA-PHER2, monarcHER) are underway to investigate the effectiveness of CDK4/6 inhibitors on ER+, HER2+ subtype breast cancer patients with a combination of CDK4/6 inhibitor, endocrine therapy, and anti-HER2 treatment (trastuzumab, pertuzumab). Due to crosstalk between CDK4/6, PI3K, and ER pathways [12], additional triplet combination-based endocrine therapies with CDK4/6 inhibitors and other drugs such as PI3k/mTOR inhibitors are also ongoing. In addition, a recent study showed that CDK4/6 inhibitors cannot only induce cell cycle arrest but also enhance tumor immunogenicity in cell lines, animal models, and patients and combining CDK4/6 inhibitors with immunotherapies appears to also hold promise [13]. Along with these various trial combinations in diverse patient populations and the development of new CDK4/6 inhibitors, we can expect to better understand the biology, clinical applications, and optimal use of the CDK4/6 inhibitors for the treatment of therapy-refractory breast cancers.

2.2 PI3K/AKT/mTOR Pathway

Activation of the PI3K/AKT/mTOR signaling pathway occurs in nearly 70% of breast cancers, and preclinical research indicates that activation of this pathway plays significant roles in these cancers and correlates with high histologic grade and poor clinical prognosis [14]. PI3K and its protein family are activated by a number of growth factor receptor tyrosine kinases and G-protein-coupled receptors to promote cell growth and survival. The PI3K protein family consists of three subtypes of lipid kinase, each of which catalyzes phosphorylation of phosphatidylinositol 4,5-bisphosphate (PIP2) to phosphatidylinositol 3,4,5-triphosphate (PIP3) [15]. Through direct binding mechanisms, PIP3 then activates downstream signaling components such as phosphoinositide-dependent kinase-1 (PDK1) and AKT. Once AKT is activated, it can phosphorylate a number of nuclear and cytoplasmic proteins, including mTOR that is heavily involved in regulation of protein synthesis and cell growth [15]. The PI3K/AKT/mTOR pathway is the most frequently activated and mutated pathway in breast cancers, and crosstalk is also prominent between the PI3K/AKT/mTOR signaling pathway and the ER signaling pathway [16–18]. Activation of the ER pathway can occur through PI3K/AKT/mTOR signaling activity to regulate estrogen-independent ER transcriptional activity and promote cell proliferation even in the absence of estrogen [16, 19]. Significantly, hyperactivation of the PI3K/AKT/mTOR pathway has also been implicated as a key mechanism underlying endocrine resistance in ER+ breast cancers [15, 20–23].

A number of therapeutics, including the highly characterized and FDA-approved mTOR inhibitor everolimus, have been developed to target the PI3K/AKT/mTOR pathway for the treatment of breast cancer (Table 2). Two prominent studies, BOLERO-2 and TAMRAD, have evaluated everolimus in ER+ breast cancer patients with disease progression following aromatase inhibitor (AI) treatment. Briefly, BOLERO-2 was a randomized phase III study of 724 postmenopausal women with HR+/HER2-negative metastatic breast cancer who experienced disease progression after treatment with nonsteroidal aromatase inhibitors letrozole or anastrozole. Findings from this study showed that combination treatment with everolimus and the steroidal aromatase inhibitor, exemestane, significantly prolonged progression-free survival by 4.6 months compared to exemestane alone [23]. The results from these clinical studies provide support for this treatment as a second-line therapy for advanced disease following recurrence during or after adjuvant endocrine therapy [15]. TAMRAD is another clinical investigation of combination therapy using both everolimus and tamoxifen following disease progression post aromatase inhibitor treatment. This randomized phase II study in 111 postmenopausal women with HR+/HER2− AI-resistant metastatic breast cancer demonstrated that concurrent treatment using both everolimus and tamoxifen significantly increased clinical benefit rate (61% versus 42%), delayed time to progression (8.6 versus 4.5 months), and enhanced overall survival rate (70% versus 46%) compared to tamoxifen-only treatment [24]. Combination treatment particularly benefitted patients with secondary endocrine resistance, i.e., patients who had relapsed greater than 6 months following discontinued use of adjuvant aromatase inhibitor treatment [24].

Presently, pan-PI3K inhibitors (e.g., BKM120 [buparlisib], GDC-0941 [pictilisib]), isoform-specific PI3K inhibitors (e.g., BYL719, GDC-0032), and dual PI3K/mTOR inhibitors (e.g., GDC-0980, NVP-BEZ235) are among the many pathway inhibitors that have been developed [25]. Pan-PI3K inhibitors target all PI3K isoforms (i.e., $p110\alpha$, $p110\beta$, $p110\gamma$, $p110\delta$) and the highly potent pan-PI3K inhibitor

Table 2 Examples of PI3K/mTOR/AKT inhibitors and their development status

Class	Compound, manufacturer	Primary target(s), potency (IC$_{50}$, K$_i$)	Clinical status	Common side effects
mTOR inhibitors	Everolimus, Novartis	mTORC1/2, 5–6 nM	FDA approved following phase II NCT017997120 Phase III (BOLERO-2) NCT00863655(+exemestane)	Rash, erythema, stomatitis, nausea
	Ridaforolimus, Merck	mTORC1/2, <1 nM	Phase II, NCT01605396 (+dalotuzumab)	Mouth sores, rash
Pan-PI3K inhibitors	Buparlisib, Novartis	**p110α, 52 nM** p110β, 166 nM p110γ, 262 nM p110δ, 116 nM mTORC1/2, 4610 nM	Phase II NCT02404844 (+tamoxifen) Phase III (BELLE-3): NCT01633060 (+fulvestrant)	Fatigue, anorexia, diarrhea, hyperglycemia, nausea, rash
	Pictilisib, Genentech	**p110α, 3 nM** p110β, 33 nM p110γ, 75 nM **p110δ, 3 nM** mTORC1/2, 580 nM	Phase II, NCT01740336 (+paclitaxel) (FERGI) NCT01437566 (+fulvestrant)	Hyperglycemia, diarrhea, nausea
Isoform-specific PI3K inhibitors	Alpelisib, Novartis	p110α, 5 nM	Phase I NCT02734615 (+LSZ102), NCT01872260 (+letrozole)	Hyperglycemia, rash, nausea, fatigue
	GDC-0032, Genentech	**p110α, <1 nM (0.29)** p110β, 9.1 nM **p110γ, <1 nM (0.12)** p110δ, <1 nM	Phase II (LORELEI) NCT02273973 (+letrozole) Phase III: (SANDPIPER) NCT02340221 + fulvestrant	Hyperglycemia, diarrhea, fatigue, nausea
Dual PI3K/ mTOR inhibitors	Dactolisib (NVP-BEZ235), Genentech	**p110α, 4 nM** p110β, 75 nM p110γ, 7 nM p110δ, 5 nM **mTORC1/ C2, 6 nM**	Phase I: NCT00620594 Phase Ib/II: NCT01495247 (+paclitaxel)	Fatigue, diarrhea, nausea, mucositis
	GDC-0980, Genentech	**p110α, 5 nM** p110β, 27 nM p110γ, 14 nM p110δ, 7 nM **mTORC1/2, 17 K$_i$**	Phase I NCT01254526 (+bevacizumab + paclitaxel) Phase II NCT01437566 (+fulvestrant)	Fatigue, diarrhea, nausea, rash, mucositis, hyperglycemia

(continued)

Table 2 (continued)

Class	Compound, manufacturer	Primary target(s), potency (IC_{50}, K_i)	Clinical status	Common side effects
AKT inhibitors	MK2206, Merck	**AKT1, 8 nM** AKT2, 12 nM AKT3, 65 nM	Phase II NCT01277757 NCT01776008 (+anastrozole, goserelin acetate)	Skin rash, nausea, fatigue, hyperglycemia
	AZD5363, AstraZeneca	**AKT1, 3 nM** AKT2, 7 nM AKT3, 7 nM	Phase II (STAKT) NCT02077569 (PAKT) NCT02423603 (+paclitaxel)	Hyperglycemia, rash, diarrhea

Bold indicates the primary targets of the inhibitors

BKM120 has recently been tested clinically in a series of BELLE (Buparlisib Breast Cancer Clinical Evaluation) trials. Overall, modest benefit was reported in BELLE-2, BELLE-3, and NEOBELLE studies and the BKM120 plus fulvestrant or letrozole study. In addition, a high percentage of patients experienced serious adverse effects that included hyperglycemia and liver damage. Similar toxicities were also found for another pan-PI3K inhibitor GDC-0941 in the FERGI study. Possible solutions to overcome the high toxicity of pan-PI3K inhibitors include new dosing schedules that may be less toxic and/or development of isoform-specific PI3K inhibitors whose safety profiles are more favorable [25]. In a phase Ia study of alpelisib (BLY719), a selective inhibitor of the p110a catalytic subunit of PI3K, the inhibitor demonstrated tolerable safety and promising preliminary activity in ER+/HER2− breast cancer patients with PI3K-altered tumors. A phase Ib clinical trial for ER+ breast cancer patients found the combination of alpelisib with letrozole clinically advantageous in patients with tumors that are PI3K mutant and resistant to adjuvant therapy [26]. Currently, further phase II and III clinical trials are still underway.

Dual PI3K/mTOR inhibitors, like GDC-0980 (apitolisib) and NVP-BEZ235 (dactolisib), potently target both PI3K pathway isoforms and mTORC1/C2 at low nM concentrations, ranging 5–27 nM [15]. Following preclinical studies indicating antitumor activity of apitolisib in mammary tumor orthotopic xenograft mouse models, GDC-0980 recently underwent a phase I clinical study to determine its safety, tolerability, and initial antitumor activity in patients with advanced solid tumors [27]. Findings from this study indicated that GDC-0980 was predominantly well tolerated at doses less than 70 mg/day with antitumor activity [27]. Dual PI3K/ mTOR inhibitor NVP-BEZ235 has also shown potent antitumor activity in preclinical investigation. One study found that this inhibitor disrupted downstream effectors including AKT, S6 ribosomal protein, and 4EBP1 in breast cancer cells. Furthermore, the antiproliferative activity shown by NVP-BEZ235 was greater than the previously described everolimus in a panel of 21 different cancer cell lines. Subsequent clinical studies evaluated the NVP-BEZ235 inhibitor combined with either paclitaxel

(NCT01495247) or trastuzumab (NCT00620594) in hormone receptor-positive, HER-2/neu-driven breast cancer patients; however, results are unavailable.

Furthermore, both catalytic and allosteric AKT inhibitors (e.g., MK2206, AZD5363) are currently undergoing clinical study. Generally, findings from these clinical trials suggest that AKT inhibitors are more antiproliferative than antitumor, with stable disease being the best overall response noted in patients [28]. Yet combination treatment with AKT inhibitors and chemotherapy has induced tumor shrinkage at a tolerable dose [29]. Preclinical analyses found that MK-2206 elicited apoptosis in parental ER+ but not estrogen-deprived cell lines. In those patients that did not respond to MK-2206 alone, fulvestrant was required to induce apoptosis [30]. The same investigators performed a phase I clinical study in patients with ER+/HER2− breast cancer to determine appropriate treatment dose of MK-2206 when administered with either anastrozole, fulvestrant, or both. Results revealed that 31 patients (42%) experienced clinical benefit with no disease progression within 6 months with a weekly oral dose of 150 mg [30]. Currently, MK-2206 is being tested in an ongoing phase II clinical study with concurrent treatment of anastrozole for newly diagnosed ER+/HER2− patients [30].

Although progress has been made in the development of PI3K/AKT/mTOR inhibitor-based treatment, there are still many issues that should be taken into consideration for a given patient. These factors include toxicities, level of effective inhibition, feasibility of combined therapy, phenotype of the tumor, and others [15]. Furthermore, PI3K/AKT/mTOR inhibitors are associated with a 6.7% increased propensity for high-grade hyperglycemia compared with non-PI3K/AKT/mTOR targeting agents [31]. Importantly, PI3K pathway inhibitors are also associated with several drug-related toxicities such as fatigue, nausea, diarrhea, and in rare cases, cardiac side effects [32, 33]. The mTOR inhibitors differ somewhat in their safety profile from PI3K inhibitors but also have drug-related side effects including stomatitis, rash, fatigue, diarrhea, interstitial pneumonitis, and anorexia [15, 24]. Aside from toxicities and adverse effects from PI3K/AKT/mTOR inhibitors, there are other challenges that need to be considered for their clinical use. One is the activation of a negative regulatory feedback loop triggering AKT and ERK signaling pathways by other kinases such as HER2 and HER3 that lead to limited clinically beneficial outcome [34]. Also, it still remains to be determined as to what the optimal treatment combinations are for the inhibitors of this pathway. Moreover, there is the question of whether there are other targets within the pathway yet to be identified that could be key for long-term, relapse-free survivability [28]. Answers to these questions could allow for the future design of customized therapies capable of sustained, effective treatment for endocrine therapy-refractory breast cancer patients.

2.3   IGF-1/IGF-1R Pathway

The insulin-like growth factor (IGF) signaling pathway has long been recognized to play a key role in breast cancer. The IGF signaling system consists of two ligands (IGF-1, IGF-II), two cell surface receptors (IGF-1R and IGF-IIR), and six binding proteins (IGFBP1–6) [35]. The IGF-1/IGF-1R-coupled system is the main signaling mechanism in the IGF family. IGF-1 is a single-chain 7 kDa polypeptide growth factor with a high degree of homology to insulin, and it was first identified in 1957 [36]. IGF-1R is a hetero-tetramer formed by two identical α-subunits and two β-subunits and exhibits significant homology with the insulin receptor (IR). The activation of IGF-1R by IGF-1 leads to the autophosphorylation of tyrosine residues in its cytoplasmic domain. The activated IGF-1R consequently directly phosphorylates and activates its substrates such as IRS-1/2 that in turn activate downstream signaling including PI3K/AKT/mTOR and Ras/Raf/MAPK pathways. Dysregulated IGF-1 signaling has also been involved in various diseases, particularly breast cancer with activation of IGF-1R noted in more than 50% of cases [37, 38]. Both in vitro and in vivo, as well as clinical, studies have demonstrated the significant role of the IGF-1 system in breast cancer tumorigenesis [39]. Furthermore, IGF-1, IRS-1, and IGFBP levels have all been linked to breast cancer progression, poor prognosis, and outcome. In ER+ breast cancer, the crosstalk of IGF-1R and ER has been found to contribute to tumor growth and progression [40, 41]. Importantly, recent studies have also revealed the involvement of the IGF-1 signaling pathway in breast cancer endocrine resistance [42].

Given the importance of IGF-1/IGF1R signaling in breast cancer tumorigenesis and endocrine resistance, a number of strategies have been developed to target key components of this pathway. The main strategies developed to block IGF-1R signaling in breast cancers are divided into three major categories: receptor blockade by monoclonal antibodies (mAb), small-molecule inhibitors, and, most recently, ligand sequestration/neutralizing. A number of IGF-1R mAbs, including cixutumumab, dalotuzumab, and ganitumab, have been developed to target the IGF-1R extracellular domain to inhibit the activation of its downstream signaling [37]. These receptor blockade antibodies can also induce the downregulation of insulin receptor (IR) in cells that co-express IGF-1R/IR through promoting receptor internalization and degradation. In addition, intracellular methods such as small molecular tyrosine kinase inhibitor (TKI) linsitinib, OSI-906, and BMS-754807 have been developed to target the ATP-binding site of the intracellular domain of IGF-1R to inhibit its activation [37, 43]. These IGF-1R inhibitors are not selective and can also potently inhibit insulin receptors due to their high homologies. More recently, ligand sequestration/neutralizing antibodies against IGF-1 (e.g., MEDI-573, BI836845) have also been developed to block the IGF-1R signaling by preventing its ligand-dependent receptor activation [44, 45].

In addition, the critical role of IGF-1R signaling in proliferation and survival has been confirmed in breast cancer cell cultures and tumor cell xenografts. Early clinical trials reveal promising evidence of targeting this pathway; unfortunately large randomized phase III trials have not shown clear clinical benefit of targeting IGF-1R signaling [37]. There are a number of possible explanations for these unexpected and disappointing trial results. First, although the IGF-1R mAb blocks the binding of IGF-1, the IGF-1 can still activate the downstream signaling through binding to the heterodimer formed between IGF-1R and the insulin receptor [37]. Second, IGF-IR mAb and TKI treatment also induce hyperglycemia and hyperinsulinemia due to compensatory upregulation of IGFs and insulin [37, 38]. Currently, ongoing clinical trials (e.g., I-SPY2) combine IGF-IR blockade with drugs such as metformin to help manage insulin resistance. Third, acquired resistance could be attributed to compensatory pathways (e.g., HER2, EGFR, GH) and activation of IGF-1R downstream pathways, such as PI3K/AKT/mTOR, etc., after long-term exposure to anti-IGF-1R therapeutics [37, 46]. Currently, ongoing clinical trials are testing the benefits of co-targeting IGF-1R with anti-HER2 therapies (e.g., lapatinib and trastuzumab) (NCT00684983 and NCT01479179), mTOR inhibitors (e.g., temsirolimus and ridaforolimus) (NCT00699491 and NCT01605396) [47], etc. It is worth mentioning that in addition to blocking intracellular growth signaling, mTOR inhibition might also blunt the effects of hyperinsulinemia induced by IGF-1 antibodies. Additionally IGF-1R may not be a good target candidate as its level is reduced in tamoxifen-resistant human breast cancer cells although phosphorylated IGF-1R levels are still very high in these cells [40, 48]. Moreover, optimal patient selection through appropriate markers or comprehensive molecular profiling may also be needed to maximize the clinical benefit of targeting IGF-1R [49].

Since extensive evidence supports the critical roles for IGF-1 in tumor development and endocrine resistance [40, 50, 51], another approach to target this pathway involves a IGF-1 ligand binding blockade. Currently, two fully humanized IGF-1 neutralizing monoclonal antibodies (mAbs), MEDI-573 and BI836845, are undergoing clinical trials [37]. MEDI-573 has been examined in a phase I clinical trial in patients with advanced solid tumor for safety, and now it is being tested in phase Ib/II clinical trials (NCT01446159) in combination with an aromatase inhibitor in women with ER+/HER2− metastatic breast cancer. Studies in rats have shown that BI 836845 potently reduces the serum IGF bioactivity without inducing metabolic adverse effects [45]. BI836845 is currently being tested in combination with exemestane (an aromatase inhibitor) and everolimus (an mTOR inhibitor) in a phase Ib/II clinical trial (NCT02123823) in women with ER+/HER2− advanced breast cancer. Most recently, a phase Ib clinical trial (NCT03099174) using BI 836845 in combination with CDK4/6 inhibitor abemaciclib and endocrine therapy has been completed in patients with locally advanced or metastatic hormone receptor-positive breast cancer. It will be interesting to see results from these studies. In addition, new approaches targeting IGF-1 upstream regulators to block IGF-1 production in circulation [39] and/or in tumor/stromal cells specifically may be proven as an effective future strategy.

3   Targeting ER Cofactors to Overcome Endocrine Resistance

As a transcription factor, ER recruits a number of cofactors to regulate the expression of its target genes and exert its functions. These cofactors often also serve as key crosstalk points for growth signaling pathways to control ER-mediated transcription and functions. Interestingly, some of these cofactors have been found to be amplified and overexpressed in a high percentage of human breast cancers. Overexpression of these cofactors not only promotes ER-mediated transcription but also plays key roles in the endocrine resistance of breast cancer cells. Importantly, the high expression of these cofactors correlates with poor survival of breast cancer patients who have undergone endocrine therapies. Combining with their often tissue-specific roles in vivo, these cofactors have become highly promising new therapeutic targets for breast cancer treatment. In this section, we will discuss recent development of small-molecule inhibitors of SRC family members and the use of a novel technology, namely, RNA nanotechnology, to specifically target MED1 in breast cancer to overcome endocrine resistance.

3.1   p160/SRC (Steroid Receptor Coactivator) 1/2/3

The p160/steroid receptor coactivator (SRC) family of transcriptional coactivators interacts with nuclear/steroid hormone receptors to facilitate ligand-dependent transcription [52]. The three homologous members of this coactivator family include SRC-1/ NCOA1, SRC-2/NCOA-2, and SRC-3/AIB-1, which have been shown to be amplified or overexpressed across a wide variety of human cancers, including breast cancer [53]. There are two transcriptional activation domains located in the carboxyl terminus of the SRCs, known as AD1 and AD2 [53]. CREB-binding protein (CBP) and histone acetyltransferase p300 are recruited to the chromatin through the AD1 domain of SRCs, while the second domain (AD2) interacts with histone methyltransferases coactivator-associated arginine methyltransferase 1 (CARM1) and protein arginine N-methyltransferase 1 (PRMT1) [53–56]. Although all three p160 SRCs positively regulate E2-dependent expression, they are likely to play some distinct and overlapping roles as well, depending on the cellular and biological context [57]. It was found that knockout of SRC-1 led to decreased growth and development of the mammary gland but does not affect breast tumor initiation and growth of PyMT tumors. Importantly, in this tumor model lung metastasis is significantly reduced by loss of SRC-1, likely due to the regulation of Twist1, a master regulator of metastasis. However, SRC-3 appears to have roles in both tumor growth and metastasis in a number of mammary tumor models after crossing with SRC-3 overexpression or knockout mouse models.

Both SRC-1 and SRC-3 are overexpressed in endocrine-resistant breast cancer, and treatment with tamoxifen has led to increased expression of these proteins. High expression of SRC1 has been found in approximately 19–29% of breast tumors and shown to positively correlate with HER2 expression, lymph node metastasis, poor disease-free survival, and tumor recurrence [58, 59]. SRC-3 is amplified in about 5–10% of breast cancers and is overexpressed in about 60% of breast cancer cases. Significantly, one study quantified the expression of SRC-3/AIB1 and HER-2 in clinical breast tumor samples from patients who underwent long-term clinical follow-up following either no adjuvant therapy or adjuvant tamoxifen treatment. They found that a high expression of SRC-3 in patients with no adjuvant tamoxifen therapy correlated with better disease-free survival and better overall prognoses [60]. However, in patients who received tamoxifen, high SRC-3 expression in these patients was associated with worse disease-free survival, thus correlating with endocrine therapy resistance. The co-expression of HER2 and SRC-3 together resulted in the worst prognoses and also reduced disease-free survival rates [60].

Recently, several small-molecule compounds targeting SRC family members have been identified. Gossypol was first identified based on fluorescence resonance energy transfer (FRET) screening for its ability to interfere with the binding between SRC-1 and the ERα ligand-binding domain. Further studies indicate that gossypol can inhibit both SCR-1- and SRC-3-dependent transcriptional activities [61]. Later, by fusing SRC-1 or SRC-3 to the GAL4 DNA-binding domain (DBD), GAL4-luciferase reporter activities were measured to screen for the small-molecule compound libraries. Cardiac glycoside bufalin was identified as a strong small-molecule inhibitor of both SRC-1 and SRC-3 by using the NIH-Molecular Libraries Probe Production Centers (MLPCN) chemical library. It was found that this agent was capable of not only degrading SRC-3 protein expression but also blocking cancer cell growth at nanomolar concentrations [62]. In another screen using the same strategy with an expanded library, SI-2 was identified, and functions in a similar way to bufalin to promote SRC degradations, but has significantly lower toxicity than bufalin [63]. SI-2 also functions in the nanomolar range and inhibits breast cancer growth both in vitro and in vivo in orthotopic xenograft models. Interestingly, another compound, MCB-613, was discovered in this screen and MCB-613 acts instead to promote the cellular functions of SRCs to selectively kill cancer cells through a cellular process called paraptosis [64]. With further preclinical development and clinical trials, these compounds targeting the SRC family of coactivators could become promising novel strategies for breast cancer treatment to overcome resistance.

3.2 MED1 (Mediator Subunit 1)

As discussed in the previous chapters (chapters "Estrogen Receptor-Mediated Gene Transcription and Cistrome," "Structural Studies with Coactivators for the Estrogen Receptor," and "The Estrogen-Regulated Transcriptome: Rapid, Robust, Extensive, and Transient"), in response to estrogens, the estrogen receptor (ER) needs to recruit diverse transcriptional coactivators in a sequential manner to facilitate the transcription of target genes [65, 66]. Most of these coactivators (e.g., SWI/SNF, SRCs, PRMTs) are chromatin modifiers that function to open up the chromatin structure to allow RNA polymerase II and general transcription factors (GTFs) to assemble at the transcriptional initiation site [65–67]. However, for transcriptional initiation to start, ER still needs to recruit another large transcriptional coactivator complex called Mediator [68–71]. Mediator is a multi-subunit complex, composed of approximately 25–30 subunits, that acts as a bridge between ER and RNA pol II/GTFs. Mediator Subunit 1, also known as MED1, is a key subunit of the Mediator complex that directly interacts ER through its two classical nuclear receptor interacting LxxLL motifs/NR boxes [72–75]. Further studies have confirmed a requirement of MED1 and its LxxLL motifs in ER-mediated gene transcription using both in vitro transcription assays and gene expression analyses in breast cancer cell lines. Importantly, knockdown of MED1 significantly impairs the estrogen-dependent growth of breast cancer cells [69].

Interestingly, biochemical analyses indicate that MED1 only exists in a subpopulation (less than 20%) of the Mediator complex. Further mass spectrometry analyses indicate that the MED1-containing Mediator complex is specifically enriched with RNA polymerase II and at least eight additional mediator subunits. Importantly, chromatin immunoprecipitation experiments show that the MED1-containing Mediator complex is selectively recruited to the ER-target gene promoter over those Mediator complexes lacking MED1 [69]. Consistent with that, mutation of ER-interacting LxxLL motifs of MED1 in vivo in mice only impairs the expression of selective ER-target genes in mammary epithelial cells [76]. Surprisingly, the MED1 LxxLL motif mutant knockin mice are grossly normal with only apparent defects in pubertal mammary gland development but not the development of other estrogen responsive tissues such as the uterus. Furthermore, it was found that, like ER, MED1 expression is restricted to the luminal but not basal epithelial cells and its LxxLL motifs play key roles in luminal mammary epithelial cell differentiation. Together, these studies highlight a previously unexpected tissue-, cell-, and gene-specific role of MED1 in mediating ER functions [76].

MED1 is found to be overexpressed in about 50% of human breast cancer cell lines and primary breast cancers [77, 78]. Another prominent feature of the MED1 gene is that it is located within the HER2 amplicon and co-amplifies with HER2 at almost all instances [77–79]. Recent studies have also confirmed the high association of MED1 protein expression with HER2 status using human breast cancer tissue microarray (TMA) [78]. It is well-recognized that HER2 amplification and activation is a major mechanism contributing to poor prognoses and therapy resistance of ER+ breast cancer [50, 80]. Interestingly, HER2 is able to activate MED1 by phosphorylating its key activations sites through its downstream pathways such as the MAPK pathway [78]. Importantly, this activation was found to serve as a key crosstalk point for the HER-2/neu and ERα pathways in mediating tamoxifen resistance (Fig. 1). Thus, when MED1 is activated, MED1 and phospho-MED1 are selectively recruited to ER-target gene promoters over corepressors including N-CoR and SMRT even in the presence of tamoxifen [78]. Importantly, knockdown of MED1 expression sensitizes otherwise resistant HER2-overexpressing cells to tamoxifen (TAM) treatment. In addition, a loss of MED1 or mutation of MED1 phosphorylation sites was sufficient to restore the promoter recruitment of N-CoR and SMRT to ER-target genes by tamoxifen. A later study from this group also showed that knockdown of MED1 was capable of restoring sensitivity of formerly resistant breast cancer cells to pure antiestrogen fulvestrant both in vitro and in vivo in an orthotopic xenograft mouse model [81]. Consistent with these findings, other groups have also reported a role for MED1 in endocrine resistance and a correlation of high expression of MED1 with poor response in breast cancer patients who underwent endocrine therapies [82–84].

Given the experimental and clinical evidences supporting a key role for MED1 in endocrine resistance, recent studies have further investigated the potential of MED1 as a therapeutic target to overcome endocrine resistance by using a new technology called RNA nanotechnology [85, 86]. Owing to its versatility in structure and function and propensity for bottom-up self-assembly, RNA has become an attractive biomaterial for nanoparticle drug delivery. First, these RNA nanoparticles have

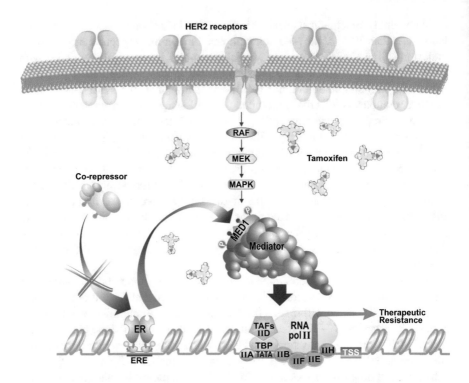

Fig. 1 MED1 is a key crosstalk point of the ER/HER2 signaling pathway in mediating tamoxifen resistance. HER2 overexpression leads to activation of the MAPK pathway and the phosphorylation of MED1. Activated p-MED1/Mediator but not corepressors is recruited to the ER-target gene promoter even in the presence of tamoxifen to allow for ER-dependent transcription and therapeutic resistance

a nanoscale size ranging from 10 to 100 nm, making them small enough for specific and targeted tissue penetration and delivery to tumor sites but also big enough not to be quickly cleared by the renal system. Second, these RNA nanostructures are also capable of incorporation of different functional moieties (e.g., imaging probes, RNA aptamers, siRNAs, and miRNAs) for simultaneous targeting, therapy, and even imaging. Importantly, these RNA nanoparticles are highly stable both in vitro and in vivo, especially with the recent development of 2′-fluoro (2′F) and other modifications to the selected RNA bases. These RNA nanoparticles exhibited impressive pharmacokinetic profiles and strong bioavailability in a number of clinical cancer and other models. Moreover, in contrast to many other small or macromolecule-based therapies, RNA nanoparticles elicit little or no immunogenicity, making them an especially promising potential therapeutic option. Due to these advantageous properties of RNA nanoparticles, RNA nanotechnology has advanced rapidly for uses in nanomedicine and bionanotechnology during the past decade.

By using RNA nanotechnology, Zhang et al. have been able to specifically target breast cancer cells to deplete MED1 and overcome tamoxifen resistance (Fig. 2) [87].

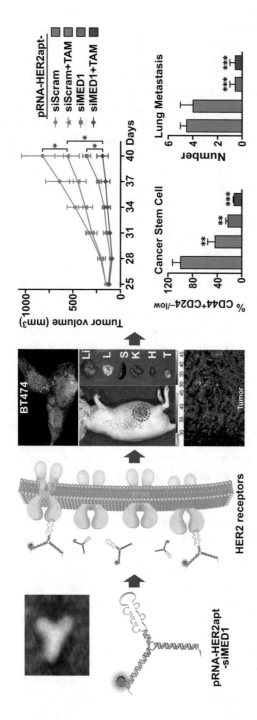

Fig. 2 Overcoming tamoxifen resistance of human breast cancer by pRNA–HER2apt–siMED1 nanoparticles. pRNA–HER2apt–siMED1 nanoparticles containing HER2 targeting aptamer and two MED1 siRNAs specifically target HER2+ breast cancer cells both in vitro and in vivo. Significantly, these RNA nanoparticles sensitized otherwise resistant BT474 tumor cells to tamoxifen treatment and greatly inhibited cancer stem cell formation and lung metastasis. Image modified with permission from [87] Copyright (2017) American Chemical Society

Using a three-way junction (3-WJ) RNA nanodelivery system, RNA nanoparticles incorporating a HER2-targeting RNA aptamer and two different MED1-targeting siRNAs have been constructed [87]. This 3-WJ RNA nanodelivery system is based on the core structure of the monomer subunits that comprise the hexameric Phi29 viral DNA packaging motor [88]. This Phi29 3-WJ motif is one of the most stable natural 3-WJ RNA motifs that exhibits extreme thermodynamic stability with high affinity and low free energy [88, 89]. It was found that 3WJ pRNA–HER2apt–siMED1 nanoparticles are also highly thermostable with a Tm value of approximately 70 °C. Additionally, these 2′F modified pRNA–HER2apt–siMED1 nanoparticles are resistant to the treatment of RNaseA, serum, and 8M urea. These RNA nanoparticles can specifically target HER2+ breast cancer cells as fluorescent microscopy and flow cytometry demonstrated a significant accumulation of pRNA–HER2apt–siMED1 nanoparticles in HER2+ BT474 breast cancer cells but not of control HER2-mutant aptamer containing nanoparticles [87]. Furthermore, it was shown that the pRNA–HER2apt–siMED1 nanoparticles selectively bound to BT474 but not HER2-negative MDA-MB-231 breast cancer cells. Importantly, systemic injection of the pRNA–HER2apt–siMED1 nanoparticles resulted in accumulation primarily in the tumor of their orthotopic xenograft tumor mouse model [87]. Subsequent analysis of multiple extracted organs and tumors further identified strong accumulation of the pRNA–HER2apt–siMED1 nanoparticles in the tumor with only residual levels in the liver and kidney and none in the heart, spleen, or lung. Importantly, the study found that mutated pRNA–HER2aptmut–siMED1 nanoparticles were capable of only accumulating on the sites of tumor blood vessels but not penetrating into tumor tissues [87].

Importantly, these pRNA–HER2apt–siMED1 nanoparticles can sensitize otherwise resistant HER2+ breast cancer cells to tamoxifen treatment both in vitro and in vivo in orthotopic xenograft mouse models [87]. It was found that the pRNA–HER2apt–siMED1 nanoparticles, but not control nanoparticles with scrambled siRNAs or a mutated HER2 aptamer, were able to reduce MED1 expression and ERα-mediated gene transcription and inhibit cell growth, migration, invasion, and stem cell formation capabilities. Moreover, co-treatment of the pRNA–HER2apt–siMED1 nanoparticles with tamoxifen further reduced cell growth, stem cell formation, and metastatic capabilities in vitro. Importantly, these RNA nanoparticles also exhibited excellent efficacy and safety when further tested in vivo by using an orthotopic xenograft mouse model. Weekly treatment with 4 mg/kg of pRNA–HER2apt–siMED1 nanoparticles significantly inhibited tumor growth, metastasis, and tumor stem cell formation better than five times weekly treatment with 0.5 mg of tamoxifen. When combined, the tumor essentially stopped growing, with tumor stem cell formation and metastasis to lung both inhibited by greater than 90%. Consistent with in vitro studies, expression of ERα target genes, such as TFF-1, c-Myc, and cyclin D1 that are involved in cell growth, metastasis, and stem cell formation, are also greatly inhibited. Importantly, the nanoparticle demonstrated a preferred biosafety profile in vivo without weight change in the mice or abnormalities in any isolated tissues, including the liver, heart, kidney, etc. [87]. Together, these findings support that pRNA–HER2apt–siMED1 nanoparticles represent a highly promising treatment modality to overcome tamoxifen resistance of breast cancer cells.

As discussed above, generation of MED1 ER-interacting LxxLL motif mutant knockin mice revealed a previously unexpected tissue-specific role for MED1 in pubertal mammary gland development [76]. Recently, Yang et al. further crossed these mice with a MMTV-HER2 mammary tumor mouse model to examine its role in mammary tumorigenesis [90]. It was found that the MED1 LxxLL motif mutant knockin mice exhibited greatly delayed tumor onset, growth, metastasis, angiogenesis, and cancer stem cell formation [90]. Interestingly, further mechanistic analyses indicated that IGF-1 is a major downstream direct target, regulated by MED1 LxxLL motifs, that contributes to these observed phenotypes [90]. Given the tissue-specific in vivo role of the MED1 LxxLL motifs, future development of innovative approaches to target these MED1 LxxLL motifs and ER/MED1 interactions could provide an alternative strategy to inhibit the IGF-1 pathway for breast cancer treatment and circumvent the toxicity seen in other systems. In addition, targeting this last "rate-limiting" step of transcription before initiation starts could also be more effective and less likely to foster resistance that often accompanies activation of upstream signaling pathways and mutations of ER itself.

4 Future Perspective/Conclusion

In addition to the discussed key growth factor signaling pathway proteins and ER cofactors, there are still many other potential targets that could be utilized for breast cancer treatment. These include all EGFR family members, the platelet-derived growth factor receptor (PDGFR)/Abl and MAPK/MEK, etc. Many inhibitors against the pathways of the EGFR family members and PDGFR have been developed and some are being evaluated in clinical trials. We will almost certainly see more combination therapies with the antiestrogens and ER degraders in double and triple therapeutic approaches. It is also clear that deregulation of epigenetic processes such as DNA methylation and histone/protein modifications (e.g., acetylation, methylation) is common in breast cancer and endocrine-resistant breast cancer. Inhibitors developed against the enzyme and effectors of these pathways (e.g., p300/CBP, CARM1, Brd4) have been developed. In addition, we now better understand that "noncoding" RNAs, such as miRNAs, lncRNAs, eRNAs, etc., can also play key roles in gene expression regulation in breast cancer. Importantly, as previously discussed, many of these noncoding RNAs (e.g., miR-21, miR-205, miR221/222) have already been shown to play important roles in mediating the endocrine resistance of breast cancer. Development of effective strategies to target these noncoding RNAs could become a new vital avenue for future therapeutic applications. Finally, immunotherapies have recently been successful in treating many different cancers with several ongoing clinical trials in breast cancer. Although breast cancer is considered particularly immunogenic, better understanding of the underlying molecular mechanisms may help the future design of new approaches to empower immunotherapies for the benefit of breast cancer treatment. In summary, Dr. Jensen's discovery of the estrogen receptor 60 years ago quickly led to breakthrough breast cancer therapies that have benefited countless patients. With our better understanding of breast cancer and the molecular mechanisms underlying its therapeutic resistance, as well as currently unprecedented rapid technology advancement, we fully expect much more to come in the next 60 years with many breakthroughs even within the next decade.

Acknowledgments We thank Zhang lab members for helpful discussion and Mr. Glenn Doerman for figure illustrations. This study was supported by NCI R01 CA197865, University of Cincinnati Cancer Center Startup, and College of Medicine Innovation Seed Grant (to X.Z.).

References

1. Ingham M, Schwartz GK (2017) Cell-cycle therapeutics come of age. J Clin Oncol 35(25):2949–2959. https://doi.org/10.1200/JCO.2016.69.0032
2. Shapiro GI (2006) Cyclin-dependent kinase pathways as targets for cancer treatment. J Clin Oncol 24(11):1770–1783. https://doi.org/10.1200/JCO.2005.03.7689
3. Mayer EL (2015) Targeting breast cancer with CDK inhibitors. Curr Oncol Rep 17(5):443. https://doi.org/10.1007/s11912-015-0443-3
4. Dean JL, Thangavel C, McClendon AK, Reed CA, Knudsen ES (2010) Therapeutic CDK4/6 inhibition in breast cancer: key mechanisms of response and failure. Oncogene 29(28):4018–4032. https://doi.org/10.1038/onc.2010.154
5. Augereau P, Patsouris A, Bourbouloux E, Gourmelon C, Abadie Lacourtoisie S, Berton Rigaud D, Soulie P, Frenel JS, Campone M (2017) Hormonoresistance in advanced breast cancer: a new revolution in endocrine therapy. Ther Adv Med Oncol 9(5):335–346. https://doi.org/10.1177/1758834017693195
6. O'Sullivan CC (2016) CDK4/6 inhibitors for the treatment of advanced hormone receptor positive breast cancer and beyond: 2016 update. Expert Opin Pharmacother 17(12):1657–1667. https://doi.org/10.1080/14656566.2016.1201072
7. Kwapisz D (2017) Cyclin-dependent kinase 4/6 inhibitors in breast cancer: palbociclib, ribociclib, and abemaciclib. Breast Cancer Res Treat 166(1):41–54. https://doi.org/10.1007/s10549-017-4385-3
8. Maurer C, Martel S, Zardavas D, Ignatiadis M (2017) New agents for endocrine resistance in breast cancer. Breast 34:1–11. https://doi.org/10.1016/j.breast.2017.04.007
9. Janni W, Alba E, Bachelot T, Diab S, Gil-Gil M, Beck TJ, Ryvo L, Lopez R, Tsai M, Esteva FJ, Aunon PZ, Kral Z, Ward P, Richards P, Pluard TJ, Sutradhar S, Miller M, Campone M (2018) First-line ribociclib plus letrozole in postmenopausal women with HR+, HER2− advanced breast cancer: tumor response and pain reduction in the phase 3 MONALEESA-2 trial. Breast Cancer Res Treat 169(3):469–479. https://doi.org/10.1007/s10549-017-4658-x
10. de Groot AF, Kuijpers CJ, Kroep JR (2017) CDK4/6 inhibition in early and metastatic breast cancer: a review. Cancer Treat Rev 60:130–138. https://doi.org/10.1016/j.ctrv.2017.09.003
11. Haricharan S, Punturi N, Singh P, Holloway KR, Anurag M, Schmelz J, Schmidt C, Lei JT, Suman V, Hunt K, Olson JA Jr, Hoog J, Li S, Huang S, Edwards DP, Kavuri SM, Bainbridge MN, Ma CX, Ellis MJ (2017) Loss of MutL disrupts CHK2-dependent cell-cycle control through CDK4/6 to promote intrinsic endocrine therapy resistance in primary breast cancer. Cancer Discov 7(10):1168–1183. https://doi.org/10.1158/2159-8290.CD-16-1179
12. Cortes J, Im SA, Holgado E, Perez-Garcia JM, Schmid P, Chavez-MacGregor M (2017) The next era of treatment for hormone receptor-positive, HER2-negative advanced breast cancer: triplet combination-based endocrine therapies. Cancer Treat Rev 61:53–60. https://doi.org/10.1016/j.ctrv.2017.09.011

13. Goel S, DeCristo MJ, Watt AC, BrinJones H, Sceneay J, Li BB, Khan N, Ubellacker JM, Xie S, Metzger-Filho O, Hoog J, Ellis MJ, Ma CX, Ramm S, Krop IE, Winer EP, Roberts TM, Kim HJ, McAllister SS, Zhao JJ (2017) CDK4/6 inhibition triggers anti-tumour immunity. Nature 548(7668):471–475. https://doi.org/10.1038/nature23465

14. Castaneda CA, Cortes-Funes H, Gomez HL, Ciruelos EM (2010) The phosphatidyl inositol 3-kinase/AKT signaling pathway in breast cancer. Cancer Metastasis Rev 29(4):751–759. https://doi.org/10.1007/s10555-010-9261-0

15. Ciruelos Gil EM (2014) Targeting the PI3K/AKT/mTOR pathway in estrogen receptor-positive breast cancer. Cancer Treat Rev 40(7):862–871. https://doi.org/10.1016/j.ctrv.2014.03.004

16. Miller TW, Balko JM, Arteaga CL (2011) Phosphatidylinositol 3-kinase and antiestrogen resistance in breast cancer. J Clin Oncol 29(33):4452–4461. https://doi.org/10.1200/JCO.2010.34.4879

17. Saal LH, Johansson P, Holm K, Gruvberger-Saal SK, She QB, Maurer M, Koujak S, Ferrando AA, Malmstrom P, Memeo L, Isola J, Bendahl PO, Rosen N, Hibshoosh H, Ringner M, Borg A, Parsons R (2007) Poor prognosis in carcinoma is associated with a gene expression signature of aberrant PTEN tumor suppressor pathway activity. Proc Natl Acad Sci U S A 104(18):7564–7569. https://doi.org/10.1073/pnas.0702507104

18. Engelman JA (2009) Targeting PI3K signalling in cancer: opportunities, challenges and limitations. Nat Rev Cancer 9(8):550–562. https://doi.org/10.1038/nrc2664

19. Campbell RA, Bhat-Nakshatri P, Patel NM, Constantinidou D, Ali S, Nakshatri H (2001) Phosphatidylinositol 3-kinase/AKT-mediated activation of estrogen receptor alpha: a new model for anti-estrogen resistance. J Biol Chem 276(13):9817–9824. https://doi.org/10.1074/jbc.M010840200

20. Creighton CJ, Fu X, Hennessy BT, Casa AJ, Zhang Y, Gonzalez-Angulo AM, Lluch A, Gray JW, Brown PH, Hilsenbeck SG, Osborne CK, Mills GB, Lee AV, Schiff R (2010) Proteomic and transcriptomic profiling reveals a link between the PI3K pathway and lower estrogen-receptor (ER) levels and activity in ER+ breast cancer. Breast Cancer Res 12(3):R40. https://doi.org/10.1186/bcr2594

21. LoPiccolo J, Blumenthal GM, Bernstein WB, Dennis PA (2008) Targeting the PI3K/Akt/mTOR pathway: effective combinations and clinical considerations. Drug Resist Updat 11(1–2):32–50. https://doi.org/10.1016/j.drup.2007.11.003

22. Ma CX, Crowder RJ, Ellis MJ (2011) Importance of PI3-kinase pathway in response/resistance to aromatase inhibitors. Steroids 76(8):750–752. https://doi.org/10.1016/j.steroids.2011.02.023

23. Baselga J, Campone M, Piccart M, Burris HA 3rd, Rugo HS, Sahmoud T, Noguchi S, Gnant M, Pritchard KI, Lebrun F, Beck JT, Ito Y, Yardley D, Deleu I, Perez A, Bachelot T, Vittori L, Xu Z, Mukhopadhyay P, Lebwohl D, Hortobagyi GN (2012) Everolimus in postmenopausal hormone-receptor-positive advanced breast cancer. N Engl J Med 366(6):520–529. https://doi.org/10.1056/NEJMoa1109653

24. Bachelot T, Bourgier C, Cropet C, Ray-Coquard I, Ferrero JM, Freyer G, Abadie-Lacourtoisie S, Eymard JC, Debled M, Spaeth D, Legouffe E, Allouache D, El Kouri C, Pujade-Lauraine E (2012) Randomized phase II trial of everolimus in combination with tamoxifen in patients with hormone receptor-positive, human epidermal growth factor receptor 2-negative metastatic breast cancer with prior exposure to aromatase inhibitors: a GINECO study. J Clin Oncol 30(22):2718–2724. https://doi.org/10.1200/JCO.2011.39.0708

25. Dienstmann R, Rodon J, Serra V, Tabernero J (2014) Picking the point of inhibition: a comparative review of PI3K/AKT/mTOR pathway inhibitors. Mol Cancer Ther 13(5):1021–1031. https://doi.org/10.1158/1535-7163.MCT-13-0639

26. Mayer IA, Abramson VG, Formisano L, Balko JM, Estrada MV, Sanders ME, Juric D, Solit D, Berger MF, Won HH, Li Y, Cantley LC, Winer E, Arteaga CL (2017) A phase Ib study of alpelisib (BYL719), a PI3Kalpha-specific inhibitor, with letrozole in ER+/HER2− metastatic breast cancer. Clin Cancer Res 23(1):26–34. https://doi.org/10.1158/1078-0432.CCR-16-0134

27. Wagner AJ, Bendell JC, Dolly S, Morgan JA, Ware JA, Fredrickson J, Mazina KE, Lauchle JO, Burris HA, Bono JSD (2011) A first-in-human phase I study to evaluate GDC-0980, an oral

PI3K/mTOR inhibitor, administered QD in patients with advanced solid tumors. J Clin Oncol 29(15_suppl):3020–3020. https://doi.org/10.1200/jco.2011.29.15_suppl.3020

28. Yap TA, Garrett MD, Walton MI, Raynaud F, de Bono JS, Workman P (2008) Targeting the PI3K-AKT-mTOR pathway: progress, pitfalls, and promises. Curr Opin Pharmacol 8(4):393–412. https://doi.org/10.1016/j.coph.2008.08.004

29. Hirai H, Sootome H, Nakatsuru Y, Miyama K, Taguchi S, Tsujioka K, Ueno Y, Hatch H, Majumder PK, Pan BS, Kotani H (2010) MK-2206, an allosteric Akt inhibitor, enhances antitumor efficacy by standard chemotherapeutic agents or molecular targeted drugs in vitro and in vivo. Mol Cancer Ther 9(7):1956–1967. https://doi.org/10.1158/1535-7163.MCT-09-1012

30. Ma CX, Sanchez C, Gao F, Crowder R, Naughton M, Pluard T, Creekmore A, Guo Z, Hoog J, Lockhart AC, Doyle A, Erlichman C, Ellis MJ (2016) A phase I study of the AKT inhibitor MK-2206 in combination with hormonal therapy in postmenopausal women with estrogen receptor-positive metastatic breast cancer. Clin Cancer Res 22(11):2650–2658. https://doi.org/10.1158/1078-0432.CCR-15-2160

31. Geuna E, Roda D, Rafii S, Jimenez B, Capelan M, Rihawi K, Montemurro F, Yap TA, Kaye SB, De Bono JS, Molife LR, Banerji U (2015) Complications of hyperglycaemia with PI3K-AKT-mTOR inhibitors in patients with advanced solid tumours on phase I clinical trials. Br J Cancer 113(11):1541–1547. https://doi.org/10.1038/bjc.2015.373

32. Hoff DDV, LoRusso P, Demetri GD, Weiss GJ, Shapiro G, Ramanathan RK, Ware JA, Raja R, Jin J, Levy GG, Mazina KE, Wagner AJ (2011) A phase I dose-escalation study to evaluate GDC-0941, a pan-PI3K inhibitor, administered QD or BID in patients with advanced or metastatic solid tumors. J Clin Oncol 29(15_suppl):3052–3052. https://doi.org/10.1200/jco.2011.29.15_suppl.3052

33. Grana B, Burris HA, Ahnert JR, Razak ARA, Jonge MJD, Eskens F, Siu LL, Ru QC, Homji NF, Demanse D, Tomaso ED, Cosaert JGCE, Quadt C, Baselga J, Bendell JC (2011) Oral PI3 kinase inhibitor BKM120 monotherapy in patients (pts) with advanced solid tumors: an update on safety and efficacy. J Clin Oncol 29(15_suppl):3043–3043. https://doi.org/10.1200/jco.2011.29.15_suppl.3043

34. Serra V, Scaltriti M, Prudkin L, Eichhorn PJ, Ibrahim YH, Chandarlapaty S, Markman B, Rodriguez O, Guzman M, Rodriguez S, Gili M, Russillo M, Parra JL, Singh S, Arribas J, Rosen N, Baselga J (2011) PI3K inhibition results in enhanced HER signaling and acquired ERK dependency in HER2-overexpressing breast cancer. Oncogene 30(22):2547–2557. https://doi.org/10.1038/onc.2010.626

35. Samani AA, Yakar S, LeRoith D, Brodt P (2007) The role of the IGF system in cancer growth and metastasis: overview and recent insights. Endocr Rev 28(1):20–47. https://doi.org/10.1210/er.2006-0001

36. Salmon WD Jr, Daughaday WH (1990) A hormonally controlled serum factor which stimulates sulfate incorporation by cartilage in vitro. 1956. J Lab Clin Med 116(3):408–419

37. Ekyalongo RC, Yee D (2017) Revisiting the IGF-1R as a breast cancer target. NPJ Precision Oncol 1. https://doi.org/10.1038/s41698-017-0017-y

38. Weroha SJ, Haluska P (2008) IGF-1 receptor inhibitors in clinical trials--early lessons. J Mammary Gland Biol Neoplasia 13(4):471–483. https://doi.org/10.1007/s10911-008-9104-6

39. Yu H, Rohan T (2000) Role of the insulin-like growth factor family in cancer development and progression. J Natl Cancer Inst 92(18):1472–1489

40. Fagan DH, Uselman RR, Sachdev D, Yee D (2012) Acquired resistance to tamoxifen is associated with loss of the type I insulin-like growth factor receptor: implications for breast cancer treatment. Cancer Res 72(13):3372–3380. https://doi.org/10.1158/0008-5472.CAN-12-0684

41. Nicholson RI, Hutcheson IR, Knowlden JM, Jones HE, Harper ME, Jordan N, Hiscox SE, Barrow D, Gee JM (2004) Nonendocrine pathways and endocrine resistance: observations with antiestrogens and signal transduction inhibitors in combination. Clin Cancer Res 10(1 Pt 2):346S–354S

42. Fox EM, Kuba MG, Miller TW, Davies BR, Arteaga CL (2013) Autocrine IGF-I/insulin receptor axis compensates for inhibition of AKT in ER-positive breast cancer cells with resistance to estrogen deprivation. Breast Cancer Res 15(4):R55. https://doi.org/10.1186/bcr3449

43. Beckwith H, Yee D (2015) Minireview: were the IGF signaling inhibitors all bad? Mol Endocrinol 29(11):1549–1557. https://doi.org/10.1210/me.2015-1157

44. Gao J, Chesebrough JW, Cartlidge SA, Ricketts SA, Incognito L, Veldman-Jones M, Blakey DC, Tabrizi M, Jallal B, Trail PA, Coats S, Bosslet K, Chang YS (2011) Dual IGF-I/II-neutralizing antibody MEDI-573 potently inhibits IGF signaling and tumor growth. Cancer Res 71(3):1029–1040. https://doi.org/10.1158/0008-5472.CAN-10-2274

45. Friedbichler K, Hofmann MH, Kroez M, Ostermann E, Lamche HR, Koessl C, Borges E, Pollak MN, Adolf G, Adam PJ (2014) Pharmacodynamic and antineoplastic activity of BI 836845, a fully human IGF ligand-neutralizing antibody, and mechanistic rationale for combination with rapamycin. Mol Cancer Ther 13(2):399–409. https://doi.org/10.1158/1535-7163. MCT-13-0598

46. Huang F, Hurlburt W, Greer A, Reeves KA, Hillerman S, Chang H, Fargnoli J, Graf Finckenstein F, Gottardis MM, Carboni JM (2010) Differential mechanisms of acquired resistance to insulin-like growth factor-i receptor antibody therapy or to a small-molecule inhibitor, BMS-754807, in a human rhabdomyosarcoma model. Cancer Res 70(18):7221–7231. https://doi.org/10.1158/0008-5472.CAN-10-0391

47. Ma CX, Suman VJ, Goetz M, Haluska P, Moynihan T, Nanda R, Olopade O, Pluard T, Guo Z, Chen HX, Erlichman C, Ellis MJ, Fleming GF (2013) A phase I trial of the IGF-1R antibody Cixutumumab in combination with temsirolimus in patients with metastatic breast cancer. Breast Cancer Res Treat 139(1):145–153. https://doi.org/10.1007/s10549-013-2528-8

48. Knowlden JM, Hutcheson IR, Barrow D, Gee JM, Nicholson RI (2005) Insulin-like growth factor-I receptor signaling in tamoxifen-resistant breast cancer: a supporting role to the epidermal growth factor receptor. Endocrinology 146(11):4609–4618. https://doi.org/10.1210/en.2005-0247

49. Johnston SR (2015) Enhancing endocrine therapy for hormone receptor-positive advanced breast cancer: cotargeting signaling pathways. J Natl Cancer Inst 107(10):djv212. https://doi.org/10.1093/jnci/djv212

50. Osborne CK, Schiff R (2011) Mechanisms of endocrine resistance in breast cancer. Annu Rev Med 62:233–247. https://doi.org/10.1146/annurev-med-070909-182917

51. Schiff R, Massarweh S, Shou J, Osborne CK (2003) Breast cancer endocrine resistance: how growth factor signaling and estrogen receptor coregulators modulate response. Clin Cancer Res 9(1 Pt 2):447S–454S

52. Anzick SL, Kononen J, Walker RL, Azorsa DO, Tanner MM, Guan XY, Sauter G, Kallioniemi OP, Trent JM, Meltzer PS (1997) AIB1, a steroid receptor coactivator amplified in breast and ovarian cancer. Science 277(5328):965–968

53. Xu J, Wu RC, O'Malley BW (2009) Normal and cancer-related functions of the p160 steroid receptor co-activator (SRC) family. Nat Rev Cancer 9(9):615–630. https://doi.org/10.1038/nrc2695

54. Anafi M, Yang YF, Barlev NA, Govindan MV, Berger SL, Butt TR, Walfish PG (2000) GCN5 and ADA adaptor proteins regulate triiodothyronine/GRIP1 and SRC-1 coactivator-dependent gene activation by the human thyroid hormone receptor. Mol Endocrinol 14(5):718–732. https://doi.org/10.1210/mend.14.5.0457

55. Brown K, Chen Y, Underhill TM, Mymryk JS, Torchia J (2003) The coactivator p/CIP/SRC-3 facilitates retinoic acid receptor signaling via recruitment of GCN5. J Biol Chem 278(41):39402–39412. https://doi.org/10.1074/jbc.M307832200

56. Chen D, Huang SM, Stallcup MR (2000) Synergistic, p160 coactivator-dependent enhancement of estrogen receptor function by CARM1 and p300. J Biol Chem 275(52):40810–40816. https://doi.org/10.1074/jbc.M005459200

57. Karmakar S, Foster EA, Smith CL (2009) Unique roles of p160 coactivators for regulation of breast cancer cell proliferation and estrogen receptor-alpha transcriptional activity. Endocrinology 150(4):1588–1596. https://doi.org/10.1210/en.2008-1001

58. Fleming FJ, Myers E, Kelly G, Crotty TB, McDermott EW, O'Higgins NJ, Hill AD, Young LS (2004) Expression of SRC-1, AIB1, and PEA3 in HER2 mediated endocrine resistant breast

cancer; a predictive role for SRC-1. J Clin Pathol 57(10):1069–1074. https://doi.org/10.1136/jcp.2004.016733

59. Redmond AM, Bane FT, Stafford AT, McIlroy M, Dillon MF, Crotty TB, Hill AD, Young LS (2009) Coassociation of estrogen receptor and p160 proteins predicts resistance to endocrine treatment; SRC-1 is an independent predictor of breast cancer recurrence. Clin Cancer Res 15(6):2098–2106. https://doi.org/10.1158/1078-0432.CCR-08-1649

60. Osborne CK, Bardou V, Hopp TA, Chamness GC, Hilsenbeck SG, Fuqua SA, Wong J, Allred DC, Clark GM, Schiff R (2003) Role of the estrogen receptor coactivator AIB1 (SRC-3) and HER-2/neu in tamoxifen resistance in breast cancer. J Natl Cancer Inst 95(5):353–361

61. Wang Y, Lonard DM, Yu Y, Chow DC, Palzkill TG, O'Malley BW (2011) Small molecule inhibition of the steroid receptor coactivators, SRC-3 and SRC-1. Mol Endocrinol 25(12):2041–2053. https://doi.org/10.1210/me.2011-1222

62. Wang Y, Lonard DM, Yu Y, Chow DC, Palzkill TG, Wang J, Qi R, Matzuk AJ, Song X, Madoux F, Hodder P, Chase P, Griffin PR, Zhou S, Liao L, Xu J, O'Malley BW (2014) Bufalin is a potent small-molecule inhibitor of the steroid receptor coactivators SRC-3 and SRC-1. Cancer Res 74(5):1506–1517. https://doi.org/10.1158/0008-5472.CAN-13-2939

63. Song X, Chen J, Zhao M, Zhang C, Yu Y, Lonard DM, Chow DC, Palzkill T, Xu J, O'Malley BW, Wang J (2016) Development of potent small-molecule inhibitors to drug the undruggable steroid receptor coactivator-3. Proc Natl Acad Sci U S A 113(18):4970–4975. https://doi.org/10.1073/pnas.1604274113

64. Wang L, Yu Y, Chow DC, Yan F, Hsu CC, Stossi F, Mancini MA, Palzkill T, Liao L, Zhou S, Xu J, Lonard DM, O'Malley BW (2015) Characterization of a steroid receptor coactivator small molecule stimulator that overstimulates cancer cells and leads to cell stress and death. Cancer Cell 28(2):240–252. https://doi.org/10.1016/j.ccell.2015.07.005

65. McKenna NJ, O'Malley BW (2002) Combinatorial control of gene expression by nuclear receptors and coregulators. Cell 108(4):465–474

66. Glass CK, Rosenfeld MG (2000) The coregulator exchange in transcriptional functions of nuclear receptors. Genes Dev 14(2):121–141

67. Roeder RG (1998) Role of general and gene-specific cofactors in the regulation of eukaryotic transcription. Cold Spring Harb Symp Quant Biol 63:201–218

68. Malik S, Roeder RG (2005) Dynamic regulation of pol II transcription by the mammalian Mediator complex. Trends Biochem Sci 30(5):256–263. https://doi.org/10.1016/j.tibs.2005.03.009

69. Zhang X, Krutchinsky A, Fukuda A, Chen W, Yamamura S, Chait BT, Roeder RG (2005) MED1/TRAP220 exists predominantly in a TRAP/Mediator subpopulation enriched in RNA polymerase II and is required for ER-mediated transcription. Mol Cell 19(1):89–100. https://doi.org/10.1016/j.molcel.2005.05.015

70. Kornberg RD (2005) Mediator and the mechanism of transcriptional activation. Trends Biochem Sci 30(5):235–239. https://doi.org/10.1016/j.tibs.2005.03.011

71. Conaway RC, Sato S, Tomomori-Sato C, Yao T, Conaway JW (2005) The mammalian Mediator complex and its role in transcriptional regulation. Trends Biochem Sci 30(5):250–255. https://doi.org/10.1016/j.tibs.2005.03.002

72. Warnmark A, Almlof T, Leers J, Gustafsson JA, Treuter E (2001) Differential recruitment of the mammalian mediator subunit TRAP220 by estrogen receptors ERalpha and ERbeta. J Biol Chem 276(26):23397–23404. https://doi.org/10.1074/jbc.M011651200

73. Plevin MJ, Mills MM, Ikura M (2005) The LxxLL motif: a multifunctional binding sequence in transcriptional regulation. Trends Biochem Sci 30(2):66–69. https://doi.org/10.1016/j.tibs.2004.12.001

74. Kang YK, Guermah M, Yuan CX, Roeder RG (2002) The TRAP/Mediator coactivator complex interacts directly with estrogen receptors alpha and beta through the TRAP220 subunit and directly enhances estrogen receptor function in vitro. Proc Natl Acad Sci U S A 99(5):2642–2647

75. Savkur RS, Burris TP (2004) The coactivator LXXLL nuclear receptor recognition motif. J Pept Res 63(3):207–212

76. Jiang P, Hu Q, Ito M, Meyer S, Waltz S, Khan S, Roeder RG, Zhang X (2010) Key roles for MED1 LxxLL motifs in pubertal mammary gland development and luminal-cell differentiation. Proc Natl Acad Sci U S A 107(15):6765–6770. https://doi.org/10.1073/pnas.1001814107
77. Zhu Y, Qi C, Jain S, Le Beau MM, Espinosa R 3rd, Atkins GB, Lazar MA, Yeldandi AV, Rao MS, Reddy JK (1999) Amplification and overexpression of peroxisome proliferator-activated receptor binding protein (PBP/PPARBP) gene in breast cancer. Proc Natl Acad Sci U S A 96(19):10848–10853
78. Cui J, Germer K, Wu T, Wang J, Luo J, Wang SC, Wang Q, Zhang X (2012) Cross-talk between HER2 and MED1 regulates tamoxifen resistance of human breast cancer cells. Cancer Res 72(21):5625–5634. https://doi.org/10.1158/0008-5472.CAN-12-1305
79. Luoh SW (2002) Amplification and expression of genes from the 17q11 approximately q12 amplicon in breast cancer cells. Cancer Genet Cytogenet 136(1):43–47
80. Bender LM, Nahta R (2008) Her2 cross talk and therapeutic resistance in breast cancer. Front Biosci 13:3906–3912
81. Zhang LCJ, Leonard M, Nephew K, Li Y, Zhang X (2013) Silencing MED1 sensitizes breast cancer cells to anti-estrogen fulvestrant therapy in vitro and in vivo. PLoS ONE 8(7):e70641. https://doi.org/10.1371/journal.pone.0070641
82. Nagalingam A, Tighiouart M, Ryden L, Joseph L, Landberg G, Saxena NK, Sharma D (2012) Med1 plays a critical role in the development of tamoxifen resistance. Carcinogenesis 33(4):918–930. https://doi.org/10.1093/carcin/bgs105
83. Ross-Innes CS, Stark R, Teschendorff AE, Holmes KA, Ali HR, Dunning MJ, Brown GD, Gojis O, Ellis IO, Green AR, Ali S, Chin SF, Palmieri C, Caldas C, Carroll JS (2012) Differential oestrogen receptor binding is associated with clinical outcome in breast cancer. Nature 481(7381):389–393. https://doi.org/10.1038/nature10730
84. Murtaza M, Dawson SJ, Tsui DW, Gale D, Forshew T, Piskorz AM, Parkinson C, Chin SF, Kingsbury Z, Wong AS, Marass F, Humphray S, Hadfield J, Bentley D, Chin TM, Brenton JD, Caldas C, Rosenfeld N (2013) Non-invasive analysis of acquired resistance to cancer therapy by sequencing of plasma DNA. Nature 497(7447):108–112. https://doi.org/10.1038/nature12065
85. Guo P (2010) The emerging field of RNA nanotechnology. Nat Nanotechnol 5(12):833–842. https://doi.org/10.1038/nnano.2010.231
86. Jasinski D, Haque F, Binzel DW, Guo P (2017) Advancement of the emerging field of RNA nanotechnology. ACS Nano 11(2):1142–1164. https://doi.org/10.1021/acsnano.6b05737
87. Zhang Y, Leonard M, Shu Y, Yang Y, Shu D, Guo P, Zhang X (2017) Overcoming tamoxifen resistance of human breast cancer by targeted gene silencing using multifunctional pRNA nanoparticles. ACS Nano 11(1):335–346. https://doi.org/10.1021/acsnano.6b05910
88. Shu D, Shu Y, Haque F, Abdelmawla S, Guo P (2011) Thermodynamically stable RNA three-way junction for constructing multifunctional nanoparticles for delivery of therapeutics. Nat Nanotechnol 6(10):658–667. https://doi.org/10.1038/nnano.2011.105
89. Zhang H, Endrizzi JA, Shu Y, Haque F, Sauter C, Shlyakhtenko LS, Lyubchenko Y, Guo P, Chi YI (2013) Crystal structure of 3WJ core revealing divalent ion-promoted thermostability and assembly of the Phi29 hexameric motor pRNA. RNA 19(9):1226–1237. https://doi.org/10.1261/rna.037077.112
90. Yang Y, Leonard M, Zhang Y, Zhao D, Mahmoud C, Khan S, Wang J, Lower EE, Zhang X (2018) HER2-driven breast tumorigenesis relies upon interactions of the estrogen receptor with coactivator MED1. Cancer Res 78(2):422–435. https://doi.org/10.1158/0008-5472.CAN-17-1533

Appendix: Photo Gallery

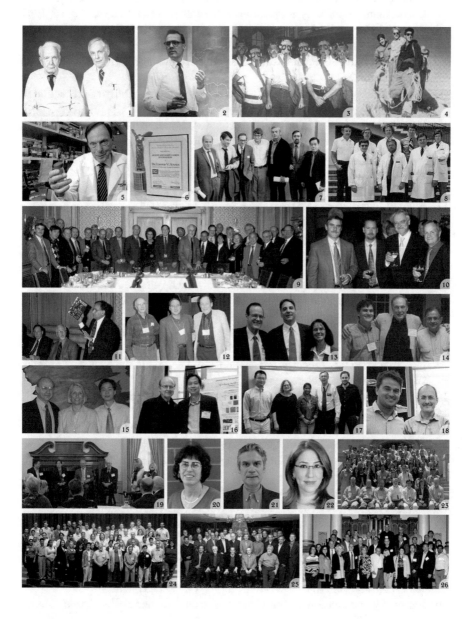

© Springer Nature Switzerland AG 2019
X. Zhang (ed.), *Estrogen Receptor and Breast Cancer*, Cancer Drug Discovery
and Development, https://doi.org/10.1007/978-3-319-99350-8

Photo Gallery Captions:

1. Charles Huggins and Elwood Jensen, circa 1975
2. Elwood Jensen at the Ben May Laboratory for Cancer Research, University of Chicago
3. Elwood Jensen (third from right) works on a National Defense Research Council project at the Department of Chemistry, University of Chicago, 1944
4. Elwood Jensen (middle) at the Summit of Mountain Matterhorn, Aug 18, 1947
5. Elwood Jensen at the University of Cincinnati College of Medicine, 2004
6. Elwood Jensen's 2004 Albert Lasker Award at Henry R. Winkler Center for the History of the Health Professions, University of Cincinnati's Donald C. Harrison Health Sciences Library
7. Bert O'Malley (third from right) and pioneers of the field of hormone action in their early days
8. William McGuire (middle, front row), C. Kent Osborne (second from left, back row), and medical oncology faculty, University of Texas Health Sciences Center at San Antonio, 1980
9. Jensen Symposium banquet at the University of Cincinnati, 2003
10. David Moore, Tom Burris, Jan-Åke Gustafsson, and Geoffrey Greene, 2003
11. Elwood Jensen, Bert O'Malley, and Sohaib Khan, 2003
12. Jack Gorski, Ken Korach, and Elwood Jensen, 2003
13. Lee Kraus (middle) with John and Benita Katzenellenbogen at Endocrine Society meeting, 2014
14. Ken Nephew, Elwood Jensen, and Sohaib Khan at the Midwest Regional Molecular Endocrinology Conference, Indiana University, 2004
15. Robert G. Roeder, Joanne Masin, and Xiaoting Zhang at Rockefeller University, 2002
16. Robert G. Roeder and Xiaoting Zhang at the Jensen Symposium on Breast Cancer 2016, University of Cincinnati
17. Drs. Xiaoyong Fu, Rachel Schiff, Jamunarani Veeraraghavan, C. Kent Osborne, and Carmine De Angelis at Baylor College of Medicine
18. Tomás Reinert and Matthew Ellis at Washington University, St. Louis, 2014
19. Drs. Jun-lin Guan, Xiaoting Zhang, Craig Jordan, and Jeff Rosen with community advocate leaders Eileen Barret and Carrie Hayden at a Jensen Symposium outreach event, Queen City Club, Cincinnati, 2016
20. Nira Ben-Jonathan at the Vontz Center for Molecular Studies, University of Cincinnati
21. Christoforos Thomas at University of Houston
22. Balkees Abderrahman at The University of Texas MD Anderson Cancer Center
23. Group photo of Midwest Regional Molecular Endocrinology Conference, Indiana University, 2004
24. Group photo of Midwest Regional Molecular Endocrinology Conference, University of Cincinnati, 2002
25. Jensen Symposium Speakers' Dinner at the Celestial, Cincinnati, 2009
26. Jensen Symposium on Breast Cancer speakers' dinner at Bell Event Centre, Cincinnati, 2016

Index

Printed in the United States
By Bookmasters